D1737693

The Biologic Basis of Dental Caries

AN ORAL BIOLOGY TEXTBOOK

Edited by

LEWIS MENAKER, D.M.D., Sc.D.

Professor, Department of Oral Biology; Senior Scientist, Institute of Dental Research
University of Alabama School of Dentistry
Birmingham, Alabama

Associate Editors

ROBERT E. MORHART, D.D.S.
Clinical Investigator, Dental Research Unit,
Veterans Administration Hospital;
Research Assistant Professor, Microbiology and Family Medicine
University of Miami School of Medicine, Miami, Florida

JUAN M. NAVIA, Ph.D.
Professor, Department of Oral Biology;
Senior Scientist, Institute of Dental Research
University of Alabama School of Dentistry, Birmingham, Alabama

With 27 Contributors

The Biologic Basis of Dental Caries

AN ORAL BIOLOGY TEXTBOOK

HARPER & ROW, PUBLISHERS

Hagerstown

Cambridge
New York
Philadelphia
San Francisco

London
Mexico City
São Paulo
Sydney

1817

1 3 5 6 4 2

Biologic Basis of Dental Caries
An Oral Biology Textbook

Copyright © 1980 by Harper & Row, Publishers, Inc. All rights reserved. No part of this book may be used or reproduced in any manner whatsoever without written permission except in the case of brief quotations embodied in critical articles and reviews. Printed in the United States of America. For information address Medical Department, Harper & Row, Publishers, Inc., 2350 Virginia Avenue, Hagerstown, Maryland 21740.

Library of Congress Cataloging in Publication Data
Main entry under title:
Biologic basis of dental caries.
    Includes index.
    1. Dental caries.   I. Menaker, Lewis
[DNLM: 1. Dental caries.   WU270.3 B615]
RK331.B56   617.6'7'07   79-26561
ISBN 0-06-141726-2

The author and publisher have exerted every effort to ensure that drug selection and dosage set forth in this text are in accord with current recommendations and practice at the time of publication. However, in view of ongoing research, changes in government regulations, and the constant flow of information relating to drug therapy and drug reactions, the reader is urged to check the package insert for each drug for any change in indications and dosage and for added warnings and precautions. This is particularly important when the recommended agent is a new and/or infrequently employed drug.

To our parents

Contents

CONTRIBUTORS ix

PREFACE xi

PART ONE. **THE HOST**

      A. Saliva and Salivary Glands 1

1. MICROANATOMY OF HUMAN SALIVARY GLANDS 3
   WALTER H. WILBORN, JOHN H. SHACKLEFORD

2. MECHANISMS OF SECRETION OF SALIVA 64
   RICHARD P. SUDDICK, FRANK J. DOWD

3. SALIVARY PROTEINS AND ORAL HEALTH 113
   ROBERT J. BOACKLE, RICHARD P. SUDDICK

4. SALIVARY WATER AND ELECTROLYTES AND ORAL HEALTH 132
   RICHARD P. SUDDICK, ROBERT J. HYDE, RALPH E. FELLER

5. NONMINERALIZED COVERINGS OF THE ENAMEL SURFACE 148
   CLYDE W. MAYHALL

      B. Tooth Composition 167

6. BIOCHEMISTRY OF TOOTH PROTEINS 168
   WILLIAM T. BUTLER, WILLIAM S. RICHARDSON, III

7. ENAMEL, APATITE AND CARIES—A CRYSTALLOGRAPHIC VIEW 191
   HOWARD M. EINSPAHR, CHARLES E. BUGG

PART TWO. **THE DISEASE**

8. ETIOLOGY, EPIDEMIOLOGY AND CLINICAL IMPLICATIONS
   OF CARIES 211
   DONALD W. LEGLER, LEWIS MENAKER

9. HISTOPATHOLOGY OF CARIES LESIONS 226
   SEYMOUR HOFFMAN

10. CLINICAL CARIOLOGY 247
    CARL A. OSTROM

PART THREE. THE AGENTS: MICROBIOLOGIC INTERACTIONS WITH ORAL TISSUE

11. COMPOSITION AND ECOLOGY OF THE ORAL FLORA 263
ROBERT MORHART, ROBERT FITZGERALD

12. ECOLOGIC DETERMINANTS OF THE ORAL MICROBIOTA 278
ROBERT MORHART, RICHARD COWMAN, ROBERT FITZGERALD

13. MICROBIAL ASPECTS OF DENTAL CARIES 297
ROBERT MORHART, ROBERT FITZGERALD

14. PLAQUE BIOCHEMISTRY 313
JUAN M. NAVIA

15. IMMUNOLOGIC ASPECTS OF DENTAL CARIES 332
ROBERT J. GENCO

PART FOUR. THE ENVIRONMENT: CARIES PREVENTION

16. NUTRITION IN DENTAL CARIES 343
MICHAEL C. ALFANO

17. NUTRITIONAL ANALYSIS AND DIETARY COUNSELING 365
MICHAEL C. ALFANO, DOMINICK P. DEPAOLA, LEWIS MENAKER

18. ANTIMICROBIAL AGENTS FOR MANAGEMENT OF CARIES 386
PAGE W. CAUFIELD, JUAN M. NAVIA

19. DYNAMICS OF BIOLOGIC MINERALIZATION APPLIED TO DENTAL CARIES 419
THEODORE KOULOURIDES

20. FLUORIDES IN DENTISTRY 445
CARL A. OSTROM

21. PIT AND FISSURE SEALANTS 461
RUSSEL N. KEMPER

22. TOOTHBRUSHES AND TOOTHBRUSHING 482
JOSEPH ALEXANDER

PART FIVE. CARIES RESEARCH

23. CARIES EXPERIMENTATION 499
LEWIS MENAKER

INDEX 515

Contributors

MICHAEL C. ALFANO, D.M.D., Ph.D.
Director, Oral Health Research Center; Associate Professor of Periodontics and Oral Medicine
Fairleigh Dickinson University School of Dentistry
Hackensack, New Jersey

JOSEPH ALEXANDER
Cooper Laboratories
Dental Division
305 Fairfield Avenue
Fairfield, New Jersey

ROBERT J. BOACKLE, Ph.D.
Assistant Professor
Department of Basic and Chemical Immunology and Microbiology
Medical University of South Carolina College of Medicine
Charleston, South Carolina

CHARLES E. BUGG, Ph.D.
Senior Scientist
Institute of Dental Research
University of Alabama School of Dentistry; Professor, Department of Biochemistry
Schools of Medicine and Dentistry
University of Alabama
Birmingham, Alabama

WILLIAM T. BUTLER, Ph.D.
Senior Scientist
Institute of Dental Research
University of Alabama School of Dentistry; Professor, Department of Biochemistry
Schools of Medicine and Dentistry
University of Alabama
Birmingham, Alabama

PAGE CAUFIELD
Assistant Professor of Dentistry
University of Alabama School of Dentistry
Birmingham, Alabama

RICHARD A. COWMAN, Ph.D.
Research Associate Professor of Microbiology
University of Miami School of Medicine; Research Microbiologist
Dental Research Unit
Veterans Administration Hospital
Miami, Florida

DOMINICK P. DEPAOLA, D.D.S., Ph.D.
Professor, Department of Pharmacology
Fairleigh Dickenson University School of Dentistry
Hackensack, New Jersey

FRANK DOWD, D.D.S., Ph.D.
Assistant Professor, Department of Oral Biology
Creighton University
Boyne School of Dental Science
Omaha, Nebraska

HOWARD M. EINSPAHR, Ph.D.
Investigator
Institute of Dental Research
University of Alabama School of Dentistry; Instructor
Department of Biochemistry
Schools of Medicine and Dentistry
University of Alabama
Birmingham, Alabama

RALPH E. FELLER, D.M.D.
Chief, Dental Service
Veterans Administration Hospital
Loma Linda, California

ROBERT J. FITZGERALD, Ph.D.
Research Microbiologist
Chief, Dental Research Unit
Veterans Administration Hospital; Professor of Oral Microbiology
Microbiology Department
University of Miami School of Medicine
Miami, Florida

ROBERT J. GENCO, D.D.S., Ph.D.
Professor and Chairman
Department of Oral Biology
School of Dentistry
State University of New York at Buffalo
Buffalo, New York

SEYMOUR HOFFMAN, D.D.S.
Professor of Pathology and Dentistry
Department of Pathology
Division of Oral Pathology
Schools of Medicine and Dentistry
University of Alabama
Birmingham, Alabama

ROBERT J. HYDE
Research Physiologist
Dental Service
Veterans Administration Hospital
Loma Linda, California

RUSSELL N. KEMPER, Ph.D.
Manager, Chemical Research
Johnson & Johnson Dental Products Company
East Windsor, New Jersey

THEODORE KOULOURIDES, D.M.D., M.S.D.
Professor, Department of Oral Biology; Senior Scientist
Institute of Dental Research
University of Alabama School of Dentistry
Birmingham, Alabama

DONALD W. LEGLER, D.D.S., Ph.D.
Professor and Chairman
Department of Oral Biology
University of Alabama School of Dentistry
Birmingham, Alabama

CLYDE W. MAYHALL, D.M.D., Ph.D.
Associate Professor, Department of Periodontics
University of Alabama School of Dentistry
Birmingham, Alabama

LEWIS MENAKER, D.M.D., Sc.D., F.R.S.H.
Professor, Department of Oral Biology; Senior Scientist
Institute of Dental Research
University of Alabama School of Dentistry
Birmingham, Alabama

ROBERT E. MORHART, D.D.S.
Clinical Investigator
Dental Research Unit
Veterans Administration Hospital; Research Assistant Professor
Microbiology and Family Medicine
University of Miami School of Medicine
Miami, Florida

JUAN M. NAVIA, Ph.D.
Professor, Department of Oral Biology; Senior Scientist
Institute of Dental Research
University of Alabama School of Dentistry
Birmingham, Alabama

CARL A. OSTROM, D.D.S., M.S.D.
Associate Professor, Department of Oral Biology
University of Alabama School of Dentistry
Birmingham, Alabama

WILLIAM S. RICHARDSON, III, Ph.D.
Assistant Professor, Department of Physical
Sciences
Auburn University at Montgomery
Montgomery, Alabama

JOHN M. SHACKLEFORD, Ph.D.
Professor and Chairman
Department of Anatomy
College of Medicine
University of South Alabama
Mobile, Alabama

RICHARD SUDDICK, D.D.S., Ph.D.
Professor and Chairman
Department of Oral Biology
School of Dentistry
Health Science Center
Louisville, Kentucky

WALTER H. WILBORN, Ph.D.
Professor of Anatomy
Department of Anatomy
College of Medicine
University of South Alabama
Mobile, Alabama

Preface

The maturation of dentistry from a craft to a healing art and science has been made possible by the changes in, and growth of, our scientific knowledge base. A progression from emphasis on removing a focus of infection by extracting a diseased tooth, to the therapeutic repair by restoration with a filling material, to the prevention of disease has been a reflection of the information available and subsequently transferred to the clinician. What is important to understand is that the driving force for the advancement of patient care has been our expanding understanding of the disease itself and the translation of this information through the educational process.

The central role of dental caries in the clinical practice of dentistry establishes without question the importance of this subject to both the student and practitioner. The present explosion in our knowledge of this subject has underscored the increased complexity of this condition as a disease process, the essentiality of a multidisciplinary approach to the understanding of this problem, and the importance of a rationale of patient care centered on the concept of preventive interception. Accepting these premises, we see the threefold goal of this text: (1) to bring the reader to a new level of appreciation of the unity of knowledge too often segregated by dental educators into clinical and basic sciences; (2) to provide the reader with current scientific evidence upon which clinical judgment must be based; and (3) to introduce the reader to the field of caries research in a manner that will provide a basis for future understanding of the burgeoning scientific literature in this field.

To accomplish these objectives this book has been designed around a framework of host, vector, and environmental factors that not only bear on the disease itself but also on those aspects that determine caries prevention. The complexity of etiology, interactions, mechanisms, and principles presented here is testimony to the advances that dentistry has made as a scientifically based profession. The need for our profession to expand knowledge continually is not optional; the responsibility to expand, understand, and apply such knowledge is mandatory. It is hoped that this book will be an aid in meeting these obligations.

Lewis Menaker
Robert E. Morhart
Juan M. Navia

PART ONE

The Host

A. Saliva and Salivary Glands

1 Microanatomy of Human Salivary Glands*

WALTER H. WILBORN

JOHN M. SHACKLEFORD

Introduction
Phylogenetic Considerations
Anatomic Classification of Glands
Structural Plan
  Terminology
Histochemical Classification
  Serous Secretions
  Mucous Secretions

Major Salivary Glands
  Parotid Gland
  Submandibular Gland
  Sublingual Gland
Minor Salivary Glands
Summary
Glossary
Suggested Readings

INTRODUCTION

Salivary glands are important glands of the digestive system that produce digestive enzymes, withdraw constituents from the plasma, and serve many other functions that directly or indirectly influence oral health in general and dental caries specifically. A knowledge of the microscopic anatomy of these glands is the keystone for understanding their function. This information also provides a basis for appreciating the multifaceted investigative work on salivary glands which includes a broad spectrum of inquiry and is reported in many scientific journals.

Because the salivary glands are convenient for extirpation, produce secretions that are easily collected, and are composed of funda-mental tissues which respond to a variety of the same stimuli as other tissues of the body, they serve as ideal models to study many areas of modern biology. They have provided much new information related to protein synthesis (See Chap. 2 and 3), ion and water transfer (See Chap. 4), epithelial-mesenchymal interactions, tissue regeneration, uptake of radioactive substances, and the pathogenesis of tumors. Ablation of salivary glands or alterations of their secretions have given insight into the initial formative stages of caries, calculus, and peridontal disease. Many biologically active substances, including nerve growth factor, parotin, serotonin, kinin, and lysozyme, have been isolated from salivary glands and are of special interest to biologists.

Salivary glands also serve as models to study the effects of hormones, diet, and the autonomic nervous system on glandular structure and function. For example, thyroxine and sex

* Supported in part by USPH Grant DE-02110 and Grant DE-02670

3

hormones alter the metabolism, histology, and histochemistry of salivary glands; liquid diets result in major ultrastructural alterations of acinar cells of the parotid gland; and the autonomic nervous system maintains the functional and structural integrity of salivary glands and plays a role in regulating the development of immature glands.

Since most previous works on salivary glands have dealt with laboratory animals, the material presented here summarizes the most significant microscopic features of normal human salivary glands. A brief account of salivary glands in other forms is also included for comparative purposes. Inclusion of the major and minor salivary glands within a single chapter benefits the student, since a report of this type has not previously been published and the information available is spread throughout many books, symposia, and journals, where it is difficult to survey.

PHYLOGENETIC CONSIDERATIONS

Salivary glands can be defined as glands that secrete into the anterior part of the digestive tract. On the basis of this broad definition, salivary glands are found in many groups of animals, invertebrates as well as vertebrates.

Among the invertebrates, salivary glands have been studied in worms, molluscs, and arthropods. The anticoagulant substances of leeches, tsetse flies, and mosquitos, the silk of certain insects, and the toxin of octopuses are examples of salivary gland secretions. In some forms, as in flatworms, the cells comprising the salivary glands are morphologically so simple that they can be distinguished from the surrounding epithelial cells only by their larger size. In contrast, salivary glands of certain insects attain marked structural and functional development and may secrete amylase, as in the case of the cockroach. The salivary glands of invertebrates and vertebrates are certainly not homologous, but in some cases, their functions of lubrication and initiation of the digestion of food are interestingly similar.

Fish, the earliest vertebrates, usually do not have salivary glands. Mucous secretions in their oral cavity are from unicellular glands constituting part of the epithelial lining of the oral cavity. One excepton is the lamprey eel, a parasite, which has large salivary glands that

open by ducts into the sucker where the juice is added to the blood and flesh ripped from the prey. Other exceptions are found in at least two species of the salt water male catfish. These fish contain deep oral crypts, also called brood pouches, where fertilized eggs are carried and kept moist by goblet cell secretions.

Beginning with amphibians, terrestrial tetrapods have characteristically large numbers of oral glands, but the number is markedly reduced in practically all aquatic tetrapods. This is no handicap because salivary glands are unnecessary for lubrication in the aqueous environment. The salivary glands of amphibians are mucous glands with ducts lined by ciliated epithelium. Although lingual glands occur in all amphibians, only anurians have internasal glands whose ducts open into the anterior part of the oral cavity. These glands in frogs secrete a sticky substance that is deposited on the tongue and assists in the capture of insects.

The oral glands of reptiles (other than the aquatic forms such as turtles and crocodiles) are more highly developed than those of amphibians. They may contain serous cells, in addition to mucous cells, and are divided into groups: 1) palatal, 2) lingual, 3) sublingual, and 4) labial. Venom glands of poisonous snakes are serous salivary glands homologous to the parotid glands of mammals. The Gila monster, the only poisonous lizard, has lingual salivary glands that produce a poison. When biting a prey, the venom travels along fanglike grooved teeth into the wound.

Salivary glands of birds are poorly developed. There are, however, aggregations of mucous cells in the lingual, sublingual, and parotid regions; smaller collections of similar cells occur in the wall of the oral cavity. The glands, as in the chicken, produce a mucous secretion that lacks digestive enzymes.

Mammals, the only animals that chew their food, possess three pairs of major salivary glands in addition to the minor salivary glands of the lips, tongue, cheeks, and palate present in other terrestrial forms. Of the major salivary glands (parotid, submandibular, and sublingual glands), only the parotid and submandibular are characteristic of all mammals. Both glands secrete *ptyalin* or *amylase*, the enzyme that hydrolyzes starches to maltose.

The position of the major salivary glands is variable with the exception of the parotid which is closely related to the external ear. In general, submandibular glands lie near the angle of the mandible in animals with flattened faces, such as man; they are in the ventral cervical region in animals with elongated faces such as rodents. Sublingual glands of man occupy a position beneath the tongue in the floor of the oral cavity. They vary in anatomic position in other forms and may be absent.

Salivary glands have not been studied in all mammals, but enough information is available to illustrate the influence of environment and feeding habits on these glands. For example, the rudimentary salivary glands of aquatic mammals, such as seals and whales, are probably related to life in water and to a lack of starch in the diet. Parotid glands are usually larger than submandibular glands in herbivorous mammals (e.g., the cow and beaver). This fact is well illustrated among bats, in whom parotid glands are larger than submandibular glands in frugivorous forms and smaller in insectivorous forms. The variation in size of salivary glands is no doubt related functionally to the needs of the organism for a particular type of secretion.

The major salivary glands of most mammals are not essential for life, but sheep die when deprived of the secretion from their parotid glands; newborn rats also die after removal of submandibular and major sublingual glands. The submandibular, parotid, and sublingual glands of man function respectively in tasting, masticating, and swallowing food. In addition to these functions, secretions of the major salivary glands keep the mouth wet and help clean the teeth. They also produce amylase which begins the digestion of starches within the oral cavity.

ANATOMIC CLASSIFICATION OF GLANDS

Salivary glands comprise an important group of glands of the digestive system. Like other glands, they are composed of specialized epithelial cells, referred to as *parenchyma*, and of connective tissue, called *stroma*. The stroma surrounds and supports the epithelial cells and serves as a passageway for nerves, blood vessels, and lymphatics. It contains collagenous fibers, fibroblasts, macrophages, plasma cells, and mast cells.

Differences in glandular morphology have given rise to various anatomic classifications of glands that must be understood to conceptualize glandular architecture. The simplest classification is based on the number of cells comprising the gland. Accordingly, glands are classified as unicellular or multicellular. The only unicellular gland in man is the goblet cell.

The terms *exocrine* and *endocrine* are used to classify glands according to the presence or absence of ducts. Salivary glands are exocrine glands because they have ducts in which the secretion is conveyed toward the oral cavity. Endocrine glands (*e.g.*, the hypophysis cerebri and the thyroid gland) lack ducts and secrete hormones directly into the blood or lymph. They are also called ductless glands or glands of internal secretion. Some glands, such as the pancreas, are both exocrine and endocrine. There is some evidence that the major salivary glands also produce hormones (e.g., parotin), but this concept remains to be firmly established before salivary glands can be classified as endocrine. Parotin is believed to stimulate growth of tissues derived from mesenchyme.

The terms *merocrine* or *eccrine*, *apocrine*, and *holocrine* are often used to classify glands according to the mode by which they liberate their secretory product. Most gland cells (e.g., parotid and pancreatic acinar cells) secrete by the merocrine method; (i.e., they discharge their secretion without any loss of cytoplasm). The process of discharging the secretion is referred to as *exocytosis*. It is the reverse of *endocytosis* or *pinocytosis*, in which a cell takes up raw materials for use within the cell, as for the synthesis of secretory products. Some gland cells, such as those of apocrine sweat glands, lose part of their apical cytoplasm during the process of discharging their secretion, and are said to secrete by the apocrine method. Electron microscopy shows that cells lining large excretory ducts also secrete by the apocrine method, and their apices have been identified in the saliva. Cells that secrete by the holocrine method are found, e.g., in sebaceous glands. Holocrine secretion requires that the cell fill itself with its own secretory product, which is liberated by the cell's breaking open and dying. Surviving cells must multiply to replace those lost if the gland is to continue its secretory activity.

Glands are also classified according to the nature of their secretion as serous, mucous, mixed, or seromucous. Serous glands contain only serous secretory cells, arranged in "grapelike" or "saclike" clusters called acini, which produce a thin, watery secretion rich in enzymes. The parotid gland and pancreas are examples of purely serous glands. Mucous glands contain only mucous secretory cells, which are usually arranged in elongated tubules, rather than as acini. The cells produce a viscid, slimy secretion. Minor salivary glands of the soft palate are examples of purely mucous glands. Mixed glands contain both serous and mucous secretory cells. Human submandibular and sublingual glands are examples of mixed glands. The consistency of the secretory product varies from thick to thin and depends on the proportion of mucous to serous cells within the gland. Seromucous glands, composed of seromucous secretory cells arranged as acini, produce a secretion intermediate between watery and viscous. Seromucous salivary glands are absent in man but

are found in certain rodents. Although other glands of the seromucous type do occur in man, as in the nasal cavity, they show considerable histophysiologic variation among individuals.

Exocrine glands can be classified according to their duct system as simple or compound. Simple glands have an unbranched duct system that connects with one or more secretory end pieces (Fig. 1-1A–D). There may be slight branching of the duct at the point of origin of the secretory end pieces (tubules or acini). Compound glands have a highly branched duct system (Fig. 1-1E–F). Secretions pass from secretory end pieces into small ducts and then into larger ducts. The site of termination of the main duct represents the point where the gland arose embryologically.

Secretory end pieces of simple or compound glands resemble tubules, alveoli, or

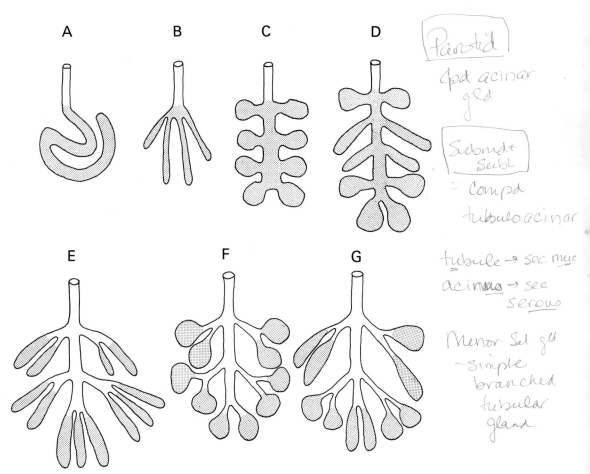

Fig. 1-1. Diagrams of various types of exocrine glands. **A–D.** Simple glands with unbranched ducts. **E–G.** Compound glands with branched ducts. **A.** Simple coiled tubular. **B.** Simple branched tubular. **C.** Simple alveolar. **D.** Simple tubuloalveolar. **E.** Compound tubular. **F.** Compound alveolar. **G.** Compound tubuloalveolar.

acini and must be named when the complete classification of a simple or compound gland is given. A *tubule* is an elongated group of secretory cells, most frequently of the mucous type, whose apices abut on a lumen and whose bases rest on a basement membrane. The lumen may be large or small. An *alveolus* is a saclike group of secretory cells, most frequently of the serous type, whose apices are arranged around a large lumen. An acinus differs from an alveolus in that the cells are arranged around a small lumen. Since an acinus and alveolus are similar, the terms are used interchangeably by many authors. When a gland has some secretory end pieces arranged as tubules and others as alveoli, it is a tubuloalveolar gland. Myoepithelial cells, as will be shown later, sometimes intervene between the basement membrane and the secretory cells. They are contractile cells characteristic of glands derived from ectoderm, as are the salivary glands.

Simple glands found in man include tubular, alveolar, and tubuloalveolar types. Simple tubular glands are illustrated by sweat glands. Since the single secretory unit is coiled, a sweat gland is a simple coiled tubular gland (Fig. 1-1A). *Minor salivary glands* are also simple tubular glands, but the duct of each gland gives rise to multiple tubules, and the glands are more precisely classified as simple branched tubular glands (Fig. 1-1B). *Sebaceous glands* are simple alveolar glands (Fig. 1-1C), while the small glands of the respiratory tract are of the simple tubuloalveolar type (Fig. 1-1D).

Compound glands, characterized by a highly branched duct system, are also of tubular, alveolar, and tubuloalveolar types. The kidney and testis are compound tubular glands (Fig. 1-1E). The mammary gland, parotid gland, and pancreas are of the compound alveolar type (Fig. 1-1F). In the strict sense the parotid gland and pancreas are compound acinar because the secretory end pieces have small lumina and are classified as acini. In contrast the mammary gland is compound alveolar because it has secretory end pieces with large lumina that fulfill the criteria of alveoli. The submandibular and sublingual glands are compound tubuloalveolar because each has ducts that connect with tubules and alveoli (Fig. 1-1G). The saclike end pieces have small lumina and are acini, as is the case with the parotid and pancreas. The submandibular and sublingual glands are, therefore, of the compound tubuloacinar type. An interesting feature of these glands is the presence of serous cells that cap the ends of some of the mucous tubules. Serous cells arranged in this fashion are called demilunes. Demilunes are also found in the tracheal glands.

STRUCTURAL PLAN

Terminology

We have seen that gland types can vary from very simple, unbranched tubules to highly complex, compound glands. The salivary glands of man are of the more complex type and are classified as *compound acinar* or *compound tubuloacinar* glands. This general classification applies to all the salivary glands, regardless of location or size.

There are three pairs of relatively large salivary glands. Because they are grossly visible and easily dissectable, they are named *major salivary glands*. Many smaller groups of salivary glands are too small to dissect easily with the unaided eye and are located within the walls of the oral cavity. These smaller glands are, therefore, named *minor salivary glands*. The term *intramural* is sometimes used to designate minor salivary glands since the term literally means "within the wall."

Major and minor salivary glands receive their individual names in accordance with their location. Thus the major salivary glands are named the *parotid*, situated near the external ear; the *submandibular*, located inferiorly with respect to the mandible; and the *sublingual*, situated in the floor of the oral cavity below the tongue. It would be wise for the student to review a gross anatomy textbook for exact positions of the major salivary glands.

Human salivary glands may be *monostomatic* (having a single duct) or *polystomatic* (having more than one duct). The parotid and submandibular glands are examples of monostomatic glands, because a single main duct carries the secretory product from these glands to the oral cavity. The sublingual gland and most minor salivary glands are polystomatic, since multiple ducts carry their secretions to the mouth. Regardless of the dispositions of main ducts of salivary glands, numerous smaller ducts unite within the substance of the gland to form the main duct(s).

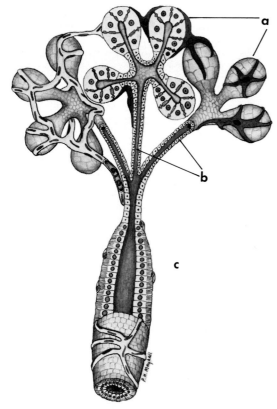

Fig. 1-2. Diagrammatic representation of serous acini and intralobular ducts showing clusters of acini (**a**) attached to three intercalated ducts (**b**) that, in turn, converge to join a striated duct (**c**). The group of acini (**right**) are unsectioned to show relationships of myoepithelial cells. The group of acini (**center**) are sectioned to show general shapes of cells; the dilated intercellular areas represent the canalicular tissue space complex. The group of acini (**left**) shows the intimate relationship of blood vascular elements.

These smaller varieties of ducts are discussed later. The remaining terms concerning the salivary glands require some knowledge of their microscopic structure.

Acini

Salivary gland acini (plural of *acinus*) are so named because they are saclike dilations bearing a resemblance to grapes. Reconstructions of a group of acini resemble a bunch of grapes (Fig. 1-2). In the past some textbooks have used the term *alveolus* (pl. *alveoli*) as synonymous with acinus. It is more common now, however, for authors to reserve the term *alveolus* for structures such as the air sacs of the lung, *viz.*, the respiratory alveoli.

The acinus is the most distal portion of the salivary gland parenchyma (with respect to the oral cavity). That is, secretion originating at the acinus must travel the entire length of the duct system before it reaches the mouth. It is the secretory unit where primary saliva originates. However, this primary saliva may be altered somewhat in its composition by action of the ducts before it reaches the oral cavity.

The acinus is composed of a single layer of epithelial cells resting on a basement membrane and surrounding an acinar lumen. The cells are somewhat pyramidal in shape, but this may vary depending on the overall shape of the acinus. Most acini are of the *serous* type and have a characteristic structure that can be related to their function. Cells composing *serous acini* exhibit two characteristic zones, i.e., a secretory zone, occupying most of the distal two-thirds of the cell, and a basal zone.

The secretory zone contains varying amounts of secretory granules that stain acidophilically, while the basal zone, which is rich in rough endoplasmic reticulum (ergastoplasm), stains basophilically. Thus the protein synthetic machinery occupies the narrow basal zone of serous acinar cells, and the product of this machinery, the secretory granules, is stored in the secretory zone (Fig. 1-3A). Sometimes the two zones are referred to simply as the acidophilic and basophilic zones.

The nucleus of a serous acinar cell tends to be spherical and located toward the cell base. It usually contains one or more nucleoli. Chromatin of the nucleus is mostly dispersed (euchromatin) but may exhibit a few small clumps (heterochromatin). Mitotic figures are rarely seen in adult salivary glands.

With the electron microscope certain features of serous acinar cells are more clearly visualized. The rough endoplasmic reticulum (RER) of the basal zone, for example, is seen to be more widely distributed than one would expect from light microscopy. Actually, the RER extends into distal areas of the secretory zone, although it is more concentrated in the basal zone (Fig. 1-3A). This arrangement is predictable since the newly synthesized proteins must eventually reach distal areas of the cell to be incorporated into the secretory granules. It is well docmented that material, synthesized on the ribosomes of the RER, passes into the RER cisternae and reaches the secretory zone *via* these channels.

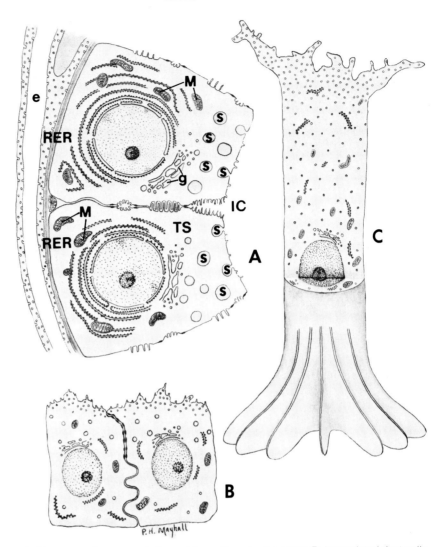

Fig. 1-3. Diagrammatic representations of **A.** sectioned acinar cells **B.** Intercalated duct cells **C,** and A striated duct cell. Symbols representing various structures are secretion granules (**S**), Golgi apparatus (**g**), rough endoplasmic reticulum (**RER**), mitochondria (**M**), intercellular canaliculus (**IC**), intercellular tissue space (**TS**), endothelium (**e**). Darkened areas on cell membranes represent desmosomes.

Eventually the new protein, destined for export from the cell, reaches the Golgi apparatus and, by means of a complex mechanism, is incorporated into the forming secretory granules. The Golgi apparatus of serous acinar cells is located just distal (apical) to the nucleus. The *Golgi apparatus* is responsible for the formation of mature secretion granules, and each of these granules is surrounded by a membrane derived from the Golgi apparatus. As the granules mature, they separate from the Golgi apparatus and move toward the luminal surface of the cell. At the point of secretory extrusion the membrane of the granules fuses with that of the cell's luminal surface. The fused area then ruptures partially, allowing the secretory material to flow into the acinar lumen (Fig. 1-3A). Remaining portions of the Golgi-derived membrane are said to repair any luminal surface discontinuity resulting from secretory granule extrusion.

Mitochondria are scattered throughout the cytoplasm of serous acinar cells, but they are more concentrated in the basal zone. Here they provide energy for peptide bond formation in the RER, whereas in more distal areas they are energy sources for other aspects of the secretory mechanism. Most of the minute details of the secretory mechanism have been worked out in pancreatic acinar cells, but these cells are structurally similar to the serous acinar cells of human salivary glands. This similarity probably extends to include at least most aspects of the secretory mechanisms.

Since space does not allow for a complete review of cell structure and function as it applies to exocrine glands, the student should reexamine basic cellular functions in relation to cellular ultrastructure. Basic to an understanding of secretory mechanisms is the ability to trace amino acids and sugars from the point of absorption from the blood stream to their incorporation into the secretory product. In the process one should be aware of the role of transfer ribonucleic acid (tRNA), messenger RNA (mRNA), ribosomes, mitochondria, and various nuclear-cytoplasmic interactions in producing secretory material.

To this point the discussion of serous acinar cells has been concerned with their internal structure. Surface morphology, (i.e., plasma membrane modification), is also an important consideration, since everything that enters or leaves the cell must pass through the plasma membrane.

At light microscopic levels the luminal surface appears to be small, and, in many instances, the plane of section excludes it from view. Actually the surface of the lumen is much larger than it first appears, since it forms tortuous extensions that pass between the acinar cells. These luminal extensions, named according to their location, are the *intercellular canaliculi* (Fig. 1-3A). One can readily visualize the extended surface area of the lumen provided by these canaliculi if the entire structure is reconstructed in three dimensions (Fig. 1-4).

A very important aspect of the luminal surface that should be recognized at the outset is the presence of tight junctions (*zonula occludens*). Tight junctions, at least indirectly, are very important to cell transport. That is, in sealing off luminal surfaces at points where adjacent cells are in contact, the tight junctions prevent substances from merely passing through intercellular spaces and reaching the lumen without impediment. In other words, if it were not for the presence of tight junctions at the luminal surface of all epithelia, an indi-

vidual would rapidly lose all substances absorbed by the bloodstream. The person would literally "ooze to death." Tight junctions appear as small densities with the electron microscope and are limited to plasma membranes of adjacent cells just deep to the luminal surface. A luminal surface that extends into intercellular canaliculi necessarily has more extensive tight junctions because they must follow contours of the canaliculi. This complication can be best visualized by again viewing a three-dimensonal reconstruction (Fig. 1-4).

Surface area of the lumen is further increased by the presence of microvilli. The *microvilli* are fingerlike extensions of the luminal plasma membrane. They are present in the intercellular canaliculi as well as in the lumen proper (Figs. 1-3A, 1-4). Microvilli of acinar cells are usually irregular in numbers and in length. They do not closely resemble the highly regular arrangement of microvilli in the small intestine, (i.e., of the striated border, or of the brush border of the kidney). Microvilli of salivary gland acini are thought to be related to secretory activity, since salivary glands of species other than man producing large volumes of saliva have a corresponding increase in numbers of acinar microvilli, (e.g., in bovine parotid glands). Thus it is probable that microvilli of salivary gland acini differ functionally as well as structurally from those of intestine and kidney.

Toward the basement membrane and deep to the luminal surface, plasma membranes of acinar cells are thrown into complex folds. At first glance in electron micrographs it is easy to confuse profiles of *acinar folds* with microvilli. Actually the folds are platelike or shelflike extensions from the acinar surface rather than the fingerlike projections of microvilli. More importantly, however, is the location of acinar folds as opposed to microvilli. Whereas microvilli are located at the luminal surface, acinar folds are characteristic of intercellular tissue spaces.

The *intercellular tissue spaces* are areas between acinar cells exhibiting varying degrees of dilation and containing *tissue fluid*. This fluid is mostly derived from the blood vessels and interstitial fluids surrounding the acini. Acinar cells are thereby bathed in tissue fluid located in the intercellular tissue spaces. The fluid contains nutrients, oxygen, and various other raw materials necessary for the proper maintenance and function of acinar cells. The fluid-filled spaces also serve as a vehicle for the removal of metabolites destined to be absorbed by the blood stream.

Intercellular tissue spaces, with their acinar folds extending into them, are difficult to visualize in sections. Therefore a three-dimensional reconstruction is provided to aid the student in conceptualizing this complex structure and its intimate relationship to the intercellular canaliculi (Fig. 1-5). In intercellular tissue spaces, the contained tissue fluid, to repeat, is prevented from entering the lumen directly by the presence of tight junctions. The intimate spatial relationship of tissue spaces and canaliculi is nevertheless important, since it allows for large surface area contact between tissue fluid and acinar cells.

At points along the interface between adjacent acinar cells, various attachment mechanisms provide a means of keeping the cells from separating. Most of this attachment is provided by desmosomes (*macula adherens*), which function as a small "spot weld", holding adjacent cells together while, at the same time, allowing for dilation of the intercellular tissue space. Just deep to the luminal surface a consistent finding is a combination tight junction (*zonula occludens*), an intermediate attachment (*zonula adherens*), and a desmosome (*macula adherens*). The three attachment devices taken together at the luminal surface make up the so-called "junctional complex" common to all epithelia of the digestive tract.

Thus far discussion of the acinus has centered on the type that predominates in the parotid and submandibular glands, the *serous acinus*. Serous acini are known to produce a watery saliva rich in salivary amylase. By contrast the mucous acini produce a viscid secretion rich in mucin. *Mucin* is a glycoprotein in which the carbohydrate moiety is formed by side chains. The carbohydrate side chains are attached to a protein core. More is said about mucin (or mucous secretions) in the next section of this chapter.

With the light microscope mucous acini are easily distinguished from the serous type. Nuclei are usually flattened toward the base of the acinar cells and darkly stained. Most of the cytoplasm is filled with droplets of mucous. Mucous acinar cells do not show the same cytoplasmic zonation as serous acinar cells. This is so because the basal zone of ergastoplasm in mucous acinar cells is restricted to a very narrow zone not visible with the light microscope. The ergastoplasm (RER) is pres-

ent, of course, and is easily visualized with the electron microscope.

The RER of mucous acinar cells appears to be reduced in amount while Golgi membranes are relatively abundant. This difference in two important organelles reflects the obvious functional differences between mucous and serous acini. The secretions of mucous-producing cells are rich in carbohydrate, as was mentioned earlier, and it is well documented that the Golgi apparatus plays an important role in the formation of this product, just as the RER is responsible for synthesis of the protein moiety. Thus, any cell producing large quantities of carbohydrate-rich mucin shows a well-developed Golgi apparatus.

In some instances the nucleus of a mucous acinar cell may appear rounded in a stained section and will have moved away from the base of the cell. This occurs with the cyclic emptying of the cell of its stored secretion. The nucleus will return to a more basal location as the cytoplasm fills with newly synthesized secretion. It is common, in any given histologic section, to see the majority of nuclei in the flattened, basal position.

With routine histologic stains such as hematoxylin and eosin the secretory product of mucous acini will be faintly stained, and, for this reason, students occasionally confuse these acini with fat cells. Close examination, however, even in hematoxylin- and eosin-stained sections, shows an enormous difference in the structure of mucous acini and adipose tissue. Mucous acini are easily identified, even to the unpracticed eye, if histochemical dyes are used to demonstrate the cell's content of mucus. Histochemical reactions and terminology associated with mucous secretions are discussed later.

Lumina of mucous acini exhibit larger diameters than those of serous acini, but, in contrast to serous acini, there are no intercellular canaliculi between mucus-secreting cells. Some acinar folds may be present, but the tissue spaces are not as well developed as those of serous acini. Again, well-developed intercellular tissue spaces and intercellular canaliculi are associated with cells producing large volumes of watery (serous) secretions.

Tubules

Many if not most of the mucous "acini" are actually tubular structures. In histologic sections, mucus-secreting cells may appear to be

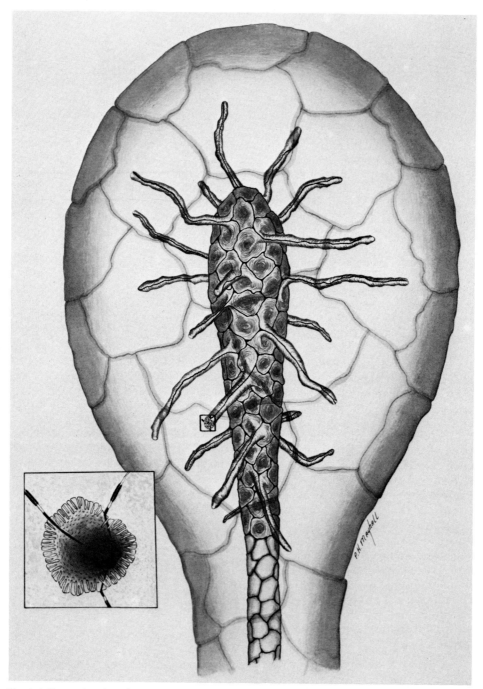

Fig. 1-4. Reconstruction of an acinar lumen from which intercellular canaliculi extend. The drawing shows bases of acinar cells in outline. The luminal aspect illustrates tight junctions (**dark lines**) and adjacent cytoplasm making up luminal and canalicular walls. Note that tight junctions of the lumen proper extend basalward onto the canaliculi. A cross section of one canaliculus (**inset**) shows three cells forming its boundary with a junctional complex at each boundary. The canaliculi are extensions of the lumen proper and, as such, must include tight junctions to prevent loss of intercellular fluids. Also note microvilli projecting into the canalicular lumen.

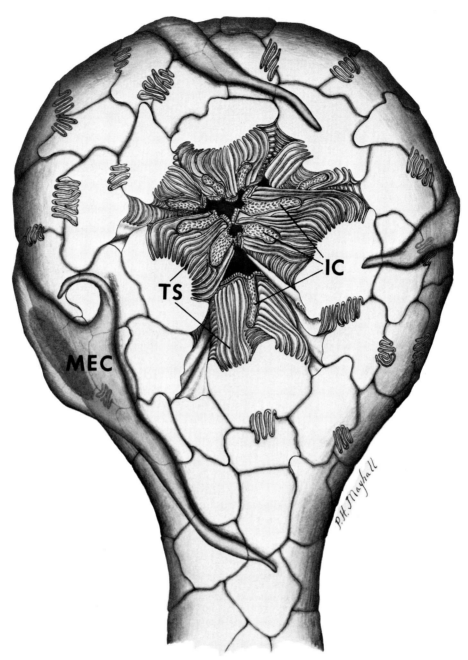

Fig. 1-5. Three-dimensional reconstruction of a serous acinus illustrating separated acinar cells. Note the intimate relationship of the intercellular canaliculi (**IC**) with the tissue spaces (**TS**). A myoepithelial cell is shown embracing the acinus (**MEC**).

grouped into acini or acinarlike secretory units. In serial sections, however, a large number of these structures are elongated to the degree that they do not resemble the true acinar shape. For practical purposes these structures continue to be called mucous acini, but the student should remember that the term may not be, in the strict sense, accurate.

Demilunes

Many of the mucous acini (or tubules) exhibit in histologic sections a crescent-shaped group of serous cells at their distal ends. These structures are named, for their histologic appearance, the *demilunes* (of Heidenhain) or *crescents* (of Gianuzzi). In three dimension they would resemble a cap of cells, but the most common reference is simply to call them demilunes.

The demilunes, as far as can be judged by their structure and histochemistry, are composed of typical serous secreting cells that are almost identical to those composing serous acini. Since they cap over the distal ends of mucous acini, the demilunes do not surround a lumen and must release their secretory product into lumina of mucous acini. Sometimes a mucous acinus, with its serous demilune, is referred to as a "mixed acinus", since both secretory cell types exist together in the same unit. Cells of serous demilunes exhibit intercellular canaliculi, intercellular tissue spaces, and the zonation of cytoplasm characteristic of serous acinar cells.

Myoepithelial Cells

Myoepithelial cells are contractile elements with long fingerlike processes extending around serous, mucous, and mixed acini (Figs. 1-2, 1-5). An oval-shaped or elongated cell body, from which the processes originate, contains the nucleus. These contractile cells lie inside the basement membrane at the basal aspect of the acinar cells. Thus, from its position and function, the name *myoepithelial cell* is derived.

The analogy of the hand squeezing an orange is commonly made for myoepithelial cell function; the hand represents the cell body and the fingers represent the processes. The orange would, of course, be analogous to the acinus. The danger in strict interpretation of the analogy lies in the obvious difference between a hand and a myoepithelial cell; (i.e., processes of the myoepithelial cells do not contain bones). The "squeezing" effect comes from contraction and shortening of the cell processes, which, in actuality, is very different from a hand squeezing an orange. Desmosomes that attach myoepithelial cells to acinar cells prevent the processes from "sliding off" when contraction occurs.

Ultrastructurally, contractile elements of the cytoplasm closely resemble those of smooth muscle cells. The myofibrils have no obvious banding as in skeletal muscle. Small nerve endings (neuroglandular junctions) may be seen in close proximity to the myoepithelial cells. Occasionally nerve endings are found between acinar cells that have no obvious relationship to the myoepithelial cells. These small endings contain "synaptic" vesicles and small mitochondria, but their function in regard to the secretory mechanism is unclear (Fig. 1-6).

Intralobular ducts

Intralobular ducts are of the two basic types, the *intercalated duct* and the *striated duct*. These ducts, in addition to other functions, carry the secretion of the acini to the periphery of the lobule where they empty into larger ducts.

The intercalated duct connects directly with the acinus. This duct is branched and has the smallest diameter of any duct associated with the salivary glands. Branches of the intercalated duct, with an acinus at the distal end of each branch, resemble a cluster of grapes with stems attached (Fig. 1-2).

There is evidence that the intercalated ducts may contribute a small amount of secretory product to the saliva. There are occasional acidophilic granules in the cell apices, and, at ultrastructural levels, a small amount of RER may be present. The Golgi apparatus is also small in comparison with that of the acinar cells. Cytoplasmic filaments are numerous and small vesicles may be present in the distal cytoplasm (Fig. 1-3B). Intercalated duct cells appear to be the most undifferentiated of all cell types present in the salivary glands. Indeed, they closely resemble the earliest form of epithelium seen in developing salivary glands from which the other elements differentiate.

The intercalated ducts terminate abruptly at the striated ducts. From this point on, the morphology of the duct system is more complex. The striated ducts (occasionally referred to as the salivary ducts) are so called because the basal aspect of the duct cells has a striated or striped appearance in stained sections viewed with the light microscope. It is well known that the striated appearance is caused by interdigitating processes between adjacent

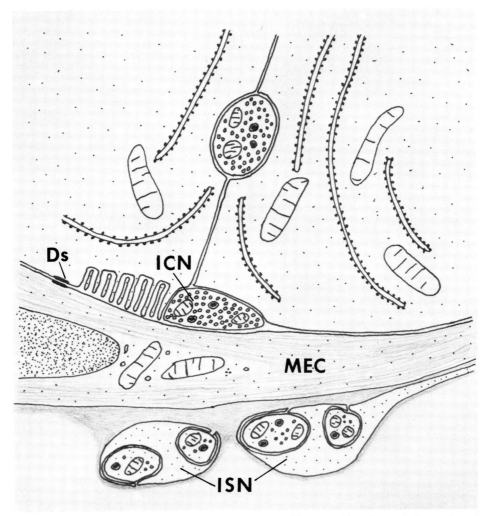

Fig. 1-6. Diagrammatic representation to show ultrastructural features at basal aspect of two adjacent acinar cells. Myoepithelial cell (**MEC**); interstitial nerve (**ISN**); intercellular nerve endings (**ICN**); and other cytoplasmic features such as RER and mitochondria. Note desmosome (**Ds**) attaching myoepithelial cell to acinar cell base.

cells. The processes of striated duct cells may be represented as finlike projections from the basal cytoplasm (Fig. 1-3C). Actually these processes are more complex than this stylized drawing, but it is helpful for understanding the principle involved in producing the striated appearance.

For the moment, if we think of the processes of striated duct cells as finlike, and the cytoplasm of each fin is examined, we find a narrow zone in the cell that is packed with large numbers of mitochondria. The mitochondria tend to be lined up in rows along the plasma membrane and thus reinforce the striated appearance. Upon sectioning of the striated ducts, the base of each cell appears to have numerous plasma membrane infoldings with rows of mitochondria lined up along the infoldings. What is actually being observed, however, are the processes of several adjacent cells in intimate contact in the form of interdigitations (Fig. 1-7).

At distal ends of striated duct cells there are scattered elements of RER and, in most instances, numerous small vesicles. At the luminal surface the cytoplasm is highly irregular and may show irregular microvilli and blebs (Figs. 1-3C, 1-7). A small Golgi apparatus and scattered mitochondria are also present distal to the nucleus.

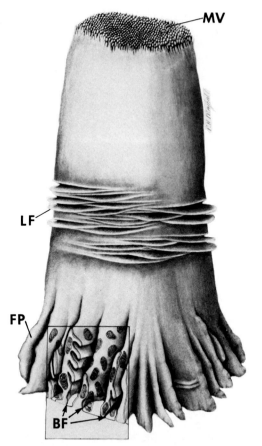

Fig. 1-7. Three-dimensional reconstruction of a striated duct cell illustrating microvilli (**MV**) at luminal surface; lateral foldings (**LF**) of cell wall at level of nucleus; and foot processes (**FP**) at cell base. The foot processes interdigitate with similar processes from adjacent cells. The **enclosed rectangular area** illustrates basal infolded appearance (**BF**). This feature results from sectioned foot processes and explains the striated picture as seen with the light microscope.

The striated ducts are believed to play an important role in regulating the final electrolyte concentration of the saliva. They usually terminate at the periphery of the gland lobule by emptying into the extralobular ducts.

Extralobular Ducts

At one time it was thought that the extralobular ducts were mere conduits and contributed very little, if any, to the final composition of saliva. Animal experiments have shown that this is not true. Indeed, the extralobular ducts not only transport the saliva from the periphery of the lobule to the oral cavity but also continue the work of ion transport which

began with the striated ducts. One may subdivide the extralobular ducts into the *interlobular ducts*, *interlobar ducts*, and the *main duct(s)*. The smallest extralobular ducts are composed of simple columnar epithelium. As these unite with one another to form larger ducts, the epithelium may become pseudostratified or stratified columnar. Just before the main duct opens into the oral cavity, the epithelium becomes stratified squamous and is continuous with that of the oral cavity.

HISTOCHEMICAL CLASSIFICATION

Serous Secretions

The serous acini are characterized by a certain morphologic appearance (Fig. 1-8) and by their carbohydrate histochemistry. The secretory product of serous acini is periodic acid Schiff (PAS) positive and alcian blue negative. This reaction (or lack of reaction) indicates that neutral polysaccharides are present and acidic polysaccharides are absent (Figs. 1-9, 1-10).

The PAS reaction tells us that, in addition to the presence of a protein (salivary amylase), there are also complex sugars located in the

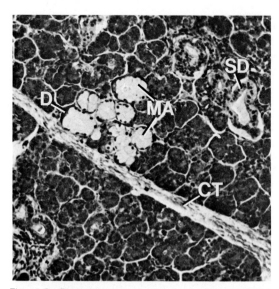

Fig. 1-8. Photomicrograph of human submandibular gland. Mucous acini (**MA**) are unstained in this preparation. Heavily stained elements are serous acini. A serous demilune (**D**), striated duct (**SD**) and a connective tissue septum (**CT**) are also shown. Orange-G, aniline blue hematoxylin stain. (× 160)

secretion granules. The exact role of these polysaccharides is unknown, but it is probable that they function in maintaining the integrity of the granule until after the stored secretion is extruded from the cell. The situation is analogous to a pharmaceutical company's making a pill with a binder. The binder is usually inert and functions simply in holding the pill together until swallowed by the patient. In the instance of digestive glands it is certainly logical that the cell producing the enzyme would possess some mechanism of protecting its cytoplasm from autodigestion. The polysaccharides demonstrated by the PAS reaction may play a role in such a mechanism.

Alcian blue is one of a number of dyes used to detect acidic polysaccharides (acid mucosubstances). These substances are present in large amounts in the mucous acini but are negligible in serous acini (Figs. 1-10, 1-13). As will be seen later on, the parotid gland is composed almost entirely of serous acini and, for this reason, is sometimes referred to as a serous gland. In spite of this classification, small amounts of acid mucosubstance may be detectable in parotid saliva, owing to the presence of an occasional mucus-secreting cell. It is well known that the main parotid duct in many species contains mucus-secreting goblet cells. The frequency of goblet cells in human parotid glands is unknown.

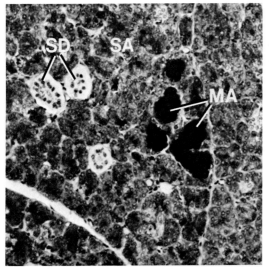

Fig. 1-9. Photomicrograph of human submandibular gland. Mucous acini (**MA**) are strongly stained by the periodic acid–Schiff reaction. Serous acini (**SA**) react moderately while striated ducts (**SD**) are unstained. Nuclei are stained with hematoxylin. PAS-hematoxylin stain. (×200)

Mucous Secretions

Mucous acini are mostly unstained in routine histologic preparations (Figs. 1-8, 1-11) but are

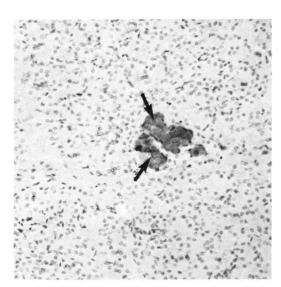

Fig. 1-10. Photomicrograph of human submandibular gland. Alcian blue (pH 2.5) selectively stains the mucous acini (**at arrows**). Nuclei are counterstained with the Feulgen reaction. Alcian blue-Feulgen stain. (×200)

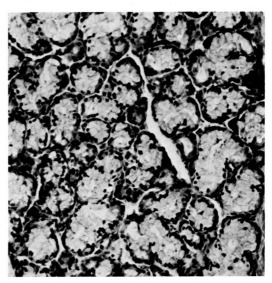

Fig. 1-11. Photomicrograph of human sublingual gland. Mucous acini predominate and are relatively unstained in this preparation. Nuclei, located at bases of acinar cells, are stained with hematoxylin. Orange-G, aniline blue and hematoxylin stain. (×200)

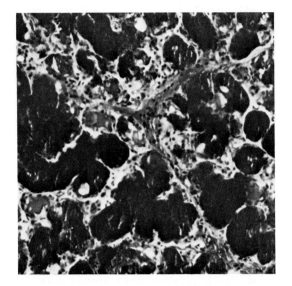

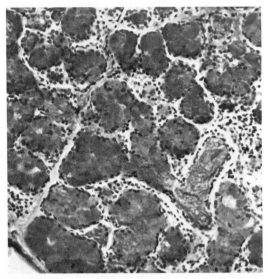

Figs. 1-12–1-13. Photomicrographs of human sublingual gland mucous acini react strongly to periodic acid–Schiff (Fig. 1-12) or alcian blue (Fig. 1-13) because of the predominance of carbohydrates. Nuclei are counterstained with hematoxylin (Fig. 1-12) or by the Feulgen reaction (Fig. 1-13). (×200)

characterized by a very strong reaction to PAS and alcian blue (Figs. 1-9, 1-10, 1-12, 1-13). Acid mucosubstances are responsible for this reaction, and it is these substances that impart viscosity to the saliva. Mucosubstances of the human salivary glands are mostly of the sialomucin variety. *Sialomucins* are composed of a protein core and carbohydrate side chains. *Sialic acid* is a terminal sugar in the side chains and plays an important role in main-

taining the viscous properties of mucin molecules.

Thus one can identify mucous acini on the basis of their histochemical reactions as well as by structural characteristics. In the case of a mixed acinus, (i.e., a mucous acinus with a serous demilune), one can compare the histochemistry of serous and mucous cells within the same secretory unit. The demilune will be moderately positive to PAS, whereas the mucous acinus will be strongly colored; alcian blue will not stain the demilune but will react strongly with the mucus-secreting cells.

MAJOR SALIVARY GLANDS

Parotid Gland

Gross Features

The *parotid* is the largest of the three large salivary glands. It weighs 20–30 g., lies beneath the skin immediately in front of the ear, and extends down over the mandible.

The gland is enclosed by fascia. The superficial layer sends deep extensions into the gland to form part of the glandular stroma and then extends upward to attach to the zygomatic arch. The deep layer thickens to form the stylomandibular ligament, which attaches to the styloid process and to the angle of the mandible. This ligament separates the parotid from the submandibular gland.

The parotid gland is shaped somewhat like an inverted pyramid with the apex directed downward toward the angle of the mandible. The anterior surface is indented by the ramus of the mandible to form lateral and medial lips. The lateral lip frequently has a more or less detached portion. The facial nerve and the transverse facial artery emerge from beneath the lateral lip.

The parotid duct is about 5 cm. long. It crosses the masseter muscle about a finger's breadth below the zygomatic arch and pierces the buccinator fat pad and buccinator muscle to open into the oral cavity opposite the crown of the second upper molar tooth. The opening is often indicated by a projection, the parotid papilla. The duct and its opening can be palpated by placing a finger inside the mouth. Injection of a radioopaque medium into the opening of the duct permits the pattern of branching of the duct to be examined radiographically. This technique is called sialography.

Several nerves are found within the gland. Most important is the facial nerve or cranial nerve (C.N.) VII, which divides to give rise to the parotid plexus (*pes anserinus*). The presence of the facial nerve within the substance of the gland makes the task of surgical excision of the parotid (e.g., for a tumor) a delicate procedure, since sufficient injury to the nerve causes paralysis of the entire ipsilateral facial musculature. Branches of the auriculotemporal nerve are also found within the gland. They convey sensory fibers (from C.N. V) and parasympathetic fibers (mainly from C.N. IX).

The gland also contains several veins and arteries. The retromandibular vein is formed within the gland by the union of two veins, the superficial temporal and maxillary. The retromandibular vein joins the posterior auricular vein near the gland apex to form the external jugular vein. The external carotid artery passes through the gland and gives rise to the posterior auricular artery before dividing into its terminal branches, the superficial temporal and maxillary arteries. The blood supply to the parotid is derived from branches of the external carotid.

The autonomic innervation of the parotid is quite complex. Like other salivary glands, it is innervated by both parasympathetic and sympathetic fibers. Preganglionic parasympathetic fibers, chiefly from C.N. IX and to some extent from C.N. VII, end in the otic ganglion. Postganglionic parasympathetic fibers pass from the otic ganglion via the auriculotemporal nerve to innervate the gland. Postganglionic sympathetic fibers to the parotid are from the superior cervical ganglion. The parotid is dependent on an intact parasympathetic and sympathetic nerve supply for its structural and functional integrity. Sectioning of the secretory fibers from one or both divisions of the autonomic nervous system results in severe glandular atrophy, diminished amylase synthesis, and loss of secretory synchrony of the acinar cells.

Light Microscopy

The parotid is a serous gland of the compound acinar (compound alveolar) type. In Table 1-1 the morphologic characteristics of the parotid and other major salivary glands are summarized. The exocrine pancreas, which bears

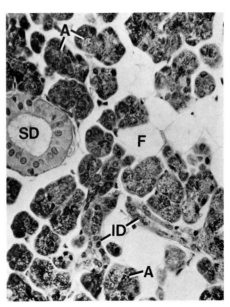

Fig. 1-14. Photomicrograph of paraffin section of parotid gland stained with H & E. Acini (**A**), intercalated ducts (**ID**), striated duct (**SD**), and fat (**F**) are shown. (× 300)

a structural and functional similarity to the salivary glands, is also included for comparative purposes.

The parenchyma and stroma of the parotid must be dealt with in describing the gland. Attention is focused first on the parenchyma and then on the stroma.

The main parenchymal components of the parotid are acini, intercalated ducts, striated ducts, and excretory ducts, which connect in the order named to convey saliva toward the oral cavity. Myoepithelial cells are parenchymal components that are sometimes neglected. They are closely associated with acini and extend into the intercalated ducts. A diagram of the parenchymal elements and the general architectural plan of the parotid is shown in Figure 1-2.

Acini are composed exclusively of serous cells that are pyramidal in shape and have round nuclei located in the basal cytoplasm. Granules are prominent in cells fixed before the onset of autolysis and subsequently stained with hematoxylin and eosin (H&E). Partially preserved granules are similar to the pale granules observed in mucous cells after H&E staining. Figure 1-14 shows acinar cells with dark granules, intercalated ducts, and a striated duct in a section stained with H&E. Fat in the stroma is characteristic of the parotid and increases with age.

The finer cytologic features of acini (and

TABLE 1-1. SUMMARY OF MORPHOLOGIC CHARACTERISTICS OF MAJOR SALIVERY GLANDS AND PANCREAS

Gland type; position; size	Parotid	Submandibular	Sublingual	Exocrine Pancreas
Gland type; position; size	Compd. acinar; around mandibular ramus; largest	Compd. tubuloacinar; beneath mandible; intermediate	Compd. tubuloacinar; floor of mouth; smallest	Compd. acinar; behind stomach; head in concavity of duodenum
Main excretory duct; interlobar ducts; inter-lobular ducts	Stenson's duct (main duct) opens op-posite 2nd upper molar; all lined by pseudostratified columnar epith.	Wharton's duct (main duct) opens on either side of frenulum of tongue; all lines by pseudo-stratified columnar epith.	Bartholin's duct (main duct) opens into or beside Wharton's duct; Rivinian ducts (minor ducts) open into oral cavity on sublingual fold; all lined by pseudost. col. epith.	Wirsung's duct (main duct) opens into 2nd part of duodenum after joining com-mon bile duct; San-torini's duct (acces-sory duct) joins main duct or empties separately into duodenum; all lined by simple columnar epithelium with oc-casional goblet cells.
Striated ducts	Single layer cuboidal to columnar cells; basal striations	Structure is same, but ducts are longer and more abundant	Structure is same, but ducts are rare	Absent
Intercalated ducts	Single layer flat to cuboidal cells; ducts are long, narrow, & branching	Structure is same, but ducts are much shorter and fewer are present	Structure is same, but ducts are rare and seldom seen	Structure is similar, but some ducts have low columnar epithelium; connect with inter-lobular ducts & end as centroacinar cells within acinus
Terminal secretory units	Serous acini	Serous acini pre-dominate; some tubules are present with demilunes	Some serous acini, but mostly mucous tubules & many demilunes	Serous acini with nonsecretory centro-acinar cells in lumina
Stroma or inter-stitial tissue	C.T. septa with much fat; lobulated	C.T. septa; lobulated	C.T. septa; lobulated	C.T. septa; lobulated

other parotid components) are better shown in 1-micron plastic sections stained with tolui-dine blue (Figs. 1-15– 1-17) than in conven-tional 6-micron paraffin sections stained with H&E. Cellular apices are close together and the lumen seldom shows. A basophilic infra-nuclear zone of ergastoplasm is present.

Raw materials are carried to the acinar base by the numerous blood vessels between the acini. These materials enter the cell and are synthesized into secretory products by the cell organelles. The products are stored as secre-tory granules until discharged from the cell. It has been determined that the granules con-tain some 30 different products in addition to amylase. Granules decrease in number after one eats. Administration of pilocarpine, a parasympathomimetic drug, also stimulates the extrusion of granules.

Myoepithelial cells, whose contractions help to expel the secretory products, can be seen near the acinar base (Figs. 1-16, 1-17). Special stains are required to show the finger-like processes of these cells at the light microscopic level. The processes, which squeeze the acinus to augment the release of secretory products, are not alkaline phosphatase positive in the human parotid as they are in the parotid of rodents.

Intercalated ducts connect with acini and join other intercalated ducts before their prox-imal ends connect with striated ducts. These ducts are longer in the parotid than they are in other major salivary glands. Segments of in-tercalated ducts nearest the acini are lined by elongated, somewhat flattened cells that often contain granules (Figs. 1-18, 1-19). Proximal segments, by contrast, are lined by cuboidal cells that usually lack secretory granules. Myoepithelial cells are more frequent in distal segments (Fig. 1-19) than in proximal seg-ments. In both segments, nuclei conform to the cell shape, and the cytoplasm is acido-philic. Although intercalated ducts have been thought to serve only as conduits for acinar secretions, the presence of granules in the

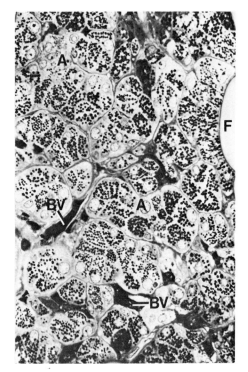

Fig. 1-15. Photomicrograph of plastic section of parotid gland stained with toluidine blue. Note acini (**A**) with granules, blood vessels (**BV**), and fat (**F**). (×480)

and have a characteristic position near the basement membrane. Of the three cell types in striated ducts, only the function of light cells in the regulation of electrolytes in saliva is well known. While functions are still being sought for dark cells and basal cells, it is possible that they are only stages in the life cycle of a light cell.

Excretory ducts course between the lobes and lobules where they are surrounded by an abundance of connective tissue (Fig. 1-22). *Striated ducts* are tributaries of interlobular excretory ducts, which, in turn, are tributaries of interlobar excretory ducts. The epithelium of excretory ducts is composed of the cell types described for striated ducts. Basal cells are, however, more numerous in excretory ducts, and because of their large number, the epithelium should be classified as pseudostratified columnar. This type of epithelium lines the main excretory duct (Stenson's duct).

Light cells of excretory ducts have basal striations, as do corresponding cells of striated

cells indicates that the cells produce one or more secretions whose nature and significance remain to be determined.

Striated ducts are shorter and less tortuous in the parotid than in the submandibular gland and are second to acini as the predominant parenchymal component (Fig. 1-20). Plastic sections of the ducts stained with toluidine blue show three types of epithelial cells, designated light cells, dark cells, and basal cells (Fig. 1-21). *Light cells*, the most numerous type, are columnar cells that extend from the basement membrane to the duct lumen. They have pale, granular cytoplasm and round to ovoid nuclei. The granular cytoplasm is produced by mitochondria, rather than secretory granules. Basal striations are present in the infranuclear region. *Dark cells* likewise reach the lumen, but in contrast to light cells, they seldom occur adjacent to each other and their cytoplasm and nuclei are intensely chromophilic. Dark cells have infranuclear processes that extend to the basement membrane. *Basal cells* resemble dark cells in staining intensity but differ in that they occur less frequently, do not extend to the lumen,

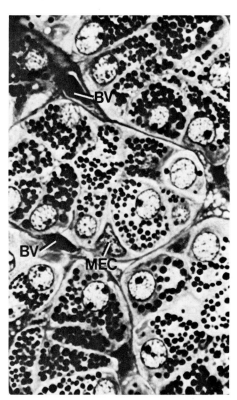

Fig. 1-16. Photomicrograph of plastic section of parotid gland stained with toluidine blue. Observe secretory granules in acini; blood vessels (**BV**); myoepithelial cell (**MEC**). (×1000)

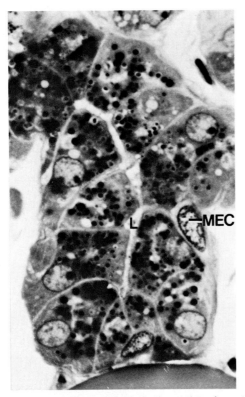

Fig. 1-17. Photomicrograph of plastic section of parotid gland stained with toluidine blue. Observe acinar lumen (**L**) and myoepithelial cell (**MEC**). In the **lower left** portion of the micrograph, note the zonation of the acinar cell cytoplasm. Secretory granules occupy most of the supranuclear zone while the infranuclear zone is rich in ergastoplasm. (×1200)

uronic acid is the chief component of the ground substance that occupies the spaces between the fibers and connective tissue cells. The ground substance, although an important stromal constituent, is not preserved in routine preparations, and only the spaces that it formerly occupied are visible. The technique of freeze drying is used to preserve the ground substance for subsequent study.

Collagenous fibers are minimal between the closely packed acini. Here the fibers are of the fine collagenous type (also called reticular or precollagenous fibers), which require special stains, such as the PAS techniques, for their demonstration. Thin layers of somewhat coarser collagenous fibers surround the striated ducts. These increase in size and number to form thick layers about excretory ducts.

Of the various types of stromal cells, fat cells are the largest (Figs. 1-14, 1-20). They are

ducts. These cells are also concerned with electrolyte regulation. Many light cells have convex apices that extend far into the lumen, where they break off according to the apocrine mode of secretion (Fig. 1-23). Light cells of striated ducts also secrete by the apocrine method but to a lesser extent. The broken apices of duct cells are components of the saliva and can be seen when saliva is examined electron microscopically.

The stroma or supporting tissue of the human parotid gland consists of loose connective tissue infiltrated with the usual cell types associated with loose connective tissue in other parts of the human body. The stroma is richly supplied with small blood vessels, which are more numerous around striated and excretory ducts (Figs. 1-21, 1-22) than around intercalated ducts or acini (Figs. 1-15, 1-16). Collagenous fibers constitute the predominant type of connective tissue fiber, and hyal-

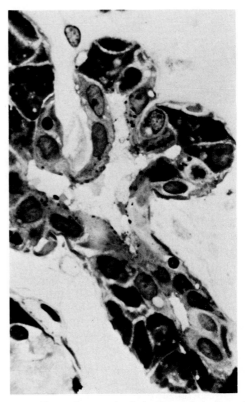

Fig. 1-18. Photomicrograph of plastic section of parotid gland stained with toluidine blue. Portions of several intercalated ducts lined by low epithelium and containing a few secretory granules are shown near their connections with acini. (×1200)

The following account of the parotid parenchyma will, therefore, serve as a basis for the study of other serous glands and their secretory mechanisms.

When examined with the electron microscope, the parotid acinar cell shows two strikingly different zones with distinctly different functions. The apical or supranuclear zone is mainly concerned with concentrating, packaging, storing, and extruding secretory products, while the basal or infranuclear zone functions mainly in protein synthesis and in the uptake of raw materials for synthesis into secretory products. The specializations of these two zones that assist in performing these functions are now discussed.

In the basal region of the parotid acinar cell, as in other cells specialized for the synthesis of protein for export, the system of RER is highly developed (Fig. 1-24), although it is somewhat less developed than in the pancreatic acinar cell. The cisternae making up this

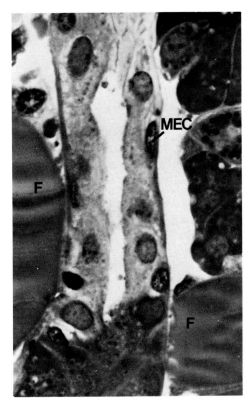

Fig. 1-19. Photomicrograph of plastic section of parotid gland stained with toluidine blue. An intercalated duct, shown in longitudinal section, connects with acinus in lower portion of micrograph. Note myoepithelial cell (**MEC**) and fat (**F**). (× 1200)

characteristic of the adult parotid but vary in number. Fibroblasts can be identified by their elongated nuclei (Fig. 1-22). They are the most numerous of the stromal cells and are responsible for the synthesis of collagen. Macrophages, second to fibroblasts in number, differentiate from monocytes, which migrate from the blood vessels. They have vacuolated cytoplasm and dark nuclei. Plasma cells, a source of salivary antibodies, are most frequently located around acini and intercalated ducts, while mast cells tend to be located in the connective tissue surrounding excretory ducts. The granules of mast cells are usually dissolved in routine preparations, making it difficult to identify the cells and to appreciate their large number in salivary glands.

Ultrastructure

The parotid gland bears many ultrastructural similarities to other serous exocrine glands.

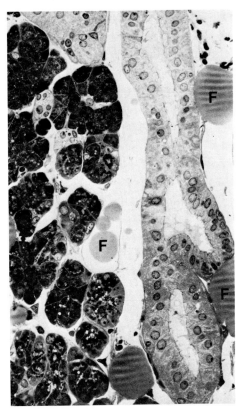

Fig. 1-20. Photomicrograph of plastic section of parotid gland stained with toluidine blue. Note the longitudinal section of striated duct (**right**), acini (**left**), and fat (**F**). (× 300)

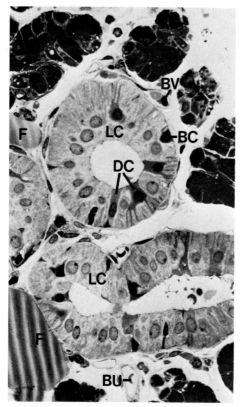

Fig. 1-21. Photomicrograph of plastic section of parotid gland stained with toluidine blue. Light cells (**LC**), dark cells (**DC**), and basal cells (**BC**) constitute three epithelial cell types of striated ducts. Blood vessels (**BV**) and fat (**F**) are present. Basal striations of light cells and infranuclear, basal processes of dark cells are shown in the cross section of striated duct near center of micrograph. (×480)

branching and anastomosing system have the form of lamellae, which in general run parallel to each other, with small particles (ribosomes) attached to their outer surfaces. The products of synthesis—in this instance mainly amylase—are sequestered in the cavities of the RER prior to transport to the Golgi apparatus for further modifications. It is the RNA of the ribosomes, including those attached to the cisternae as well as those free in the basal cytoplasm, that accounts for the basophilia of this zone in histologic sections.

The uptake of raw materials by the basal zone is facilitated by the numerous short infoldings of the basal plasma membrane and the shelflike extensions of the lateral plasma membrane. These specializations produce tissue spaces along the base and lateral margins of the acinar cell (Fig. 1-24). The spaces con-

tain nutrient-rich fluids derived from blood vessels in the vicinity. No acinar cell is more than a few microns from a capillary. The capillaries have very thin, fenestrated walls, a feature which further expedites the passage of nutrients through the vessel wall. The nutrients, once outside the capillaries, come into direct contact with the acinar base and enter the tissue spaces, where they are readily available for uptake and synthesis into secretory products (cf. Figs. 1-5, 1-24).

As noted earlier, two functions of the apical zone are concentraton and packaging of secretory products that were synthesized in the basal zone. The Golgi apparatus performs these, in addition to other functions. It is a well-developed organelle in the apical cytoplasm of parotid acinar cells. Rather than a single Golgi, as in many cells of the body, the acinar cell has multiple foci of Golgi membranes randomly distributed in the apical cytoplasm (Fig. 1-25). Each is completely functional and consists of three components:

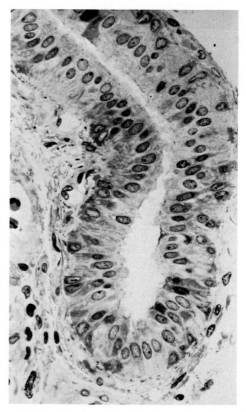

Fig. 1-22. Photomicrograph of plastic section of parotid gland excretory duct stained with toluidine blue. Collagenous fibers, cells, and small blood vessels are present in the connective tissue surrounding the duct. (×480)

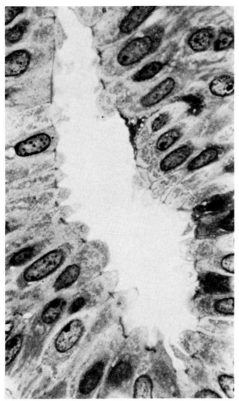

Fig. 1-23. Photomicrograph of plastic section of parotid gland excretory duct stained with toluidine blue. Note that apices of duct cells extend into the lumen. If they detach, they become a component of the saliva. (× 1200)

several saccules of smooth membranes arranged parallel to each other, small vesicles, and large condensing vacuoles. The size and extensiveness of the components fluctuate with the secretory activity of the cell, being larger in cells in the process of producing new secretory granules than in cells filled with granules.

Each Golgi component plays a vital role in the secretory process. The small vesicles, also called transfer vesicles, arise by pinching off the cisternae of RER located in the vicinity of the Golgi. They migrate toward and eventually fuse with a saccule at the forming face of the Golgi and thereby empty their contents into the lumen of the saccule. While passing through the saccule, the contents of the former vesicles are mixed, concentrated, and modified by the addition of carbohydrate. The latter is a small amount in the case of serous acinar cells of the human parotid but much larger in the case of mucous cells of the submandibular and sublingual glands. The con-

tents of several of the former vesicles, now concentrated and containing a carbohydrate moiety, leave the mature face of the Golgi as a large, membrane-bound condensing vacuole. With further maturation, a pale condensing vacuole becomes a mature, dark secretory granule.

The two zones of the acinar cell, although functionally different, work in synchrony in producing the secretory products so that there is no delay in the process. To illustrate this fact, labeled raw materials necessary for the synthesis of secretory products have been injected into the blood stream and their course has been followed from cellular uptake to the formation of condensing vacuoles and mature secretory granules. Interestingly, the whole process requires only a few minutes. Its rapidity is made possible by specific enzymes within the membranes of the RER and Golgi.

The mature secretory granules stored in the apical zone are unusual in that a small membrane-bound granule is often located within a larger granule, which is also surrounded by a membrane (Fig. 1-25). Both granules are electron dense, but the smaller granule is darker. The membrane about the small granule separates its contents from those of the larger granule, while the membrane about the larger granule prevents the mixing of its contents with that of the cytoplasm. It is certain that the large granule contains amylase, but the content of the small granule is not known. The various secretory products within the granules are biologically inactive before extrusion from the cell. This is a protective mechanism that prevents destruction of the cell by its own secretory products.

The third function of the apical region, the extrusion of secretory granules, is performed at two sites, the acinar lumen and the intercellular canaliculi (Figs. 1-26– 1-28). The process of extrusion is initiated by fusion of the membrane of the secretory granule with the plasma membrane about the lumen or intercellular canaliculus (Figs. 1-27, 1-28). The biochemical mechanisms responsible for the attraction and fusion of the two membranes have not been elucidated. Nonetheless, the fusion of the two membranes results in release of the products of the granule into the lumen of the acinus or into the lumen of the canaliculus. The latter is lined by microvilli (Fig. 1-28) and is continuous with the acinar lumen, which, in turn, continues into the lumen of an intercalated duct. The secretory products, once

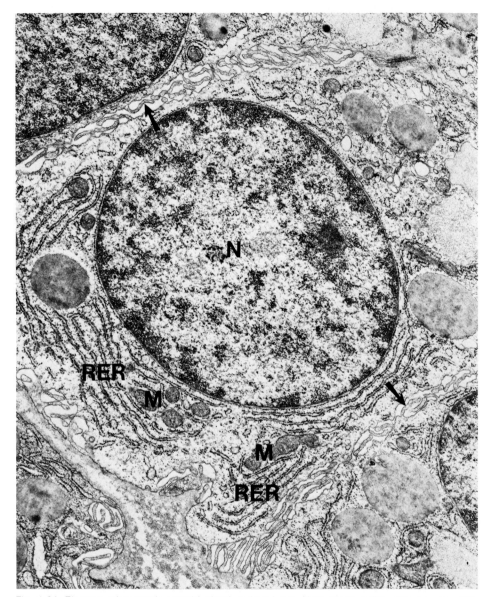

Fig. 1-24. Electron micrograph, parotid gland, acinar base. Note nucleus (**N**), mitochondria (**M**), rough endoplasmic reticulum (**RER**), and folded plasma membranes (**arrows**) at the base and lateral margins of the cell, which project into tissue spaces. (× 16,000)

extruded, lose their previously dark appearance to become pale and homogeneous.

Only a small portion of the membrane surrounding each large secretory granule is normally extruded with the secretory product. The fragments from several secretory granules tend to coalesce and can be identified as membranes within the lumen (Fig. 1-26). The membranes of secretory granules that remain in the cytoplasm, except those used to repair the cell membrane at the site of extrusion, are engulfed and digested by lysosomes (Fig. 1-26), and their constituents are returned to the cytoplasm for future synthetic activities. This process prevents the accumulation of excess membranes, which, in view of the large number of granules extruded by an acinar cell, would fill the cytoplasm if a mechanism were not available for their removal.

The small granules within the large granules are often extruded with their membranes intact (Fig. 1-28). This unusual method of ex-

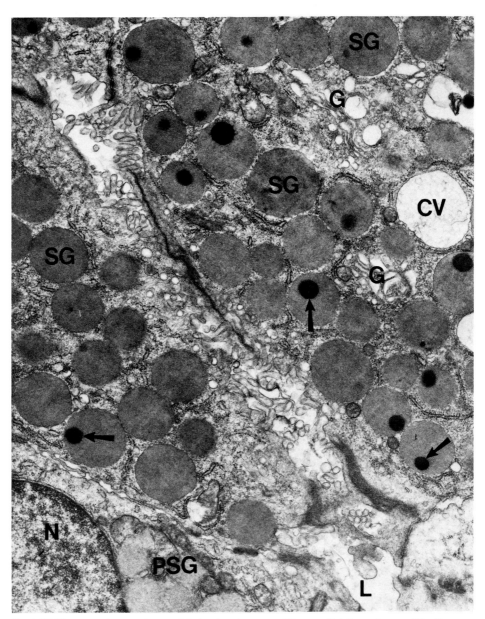

Fig. 1-25. Electron micrograph, parotid gland, acinar apex. Observe Golgi membranes (**G**) with associated vesicles, large secretory granules (**SG**), small secretory granules (**arrows**) within large secretory granules, and condensing vacuoles (**CV**). In the lower portion of the micrograph, an intercalated duct is shown connecting with the acinus. Note the nucleus (**N**), pale secretory granules (**PSG**), and the lumen (**L**) of the intercalated duct, which is continuous with the lumen of the acinus. (× 16,085)

pelling a secretory granule occurs because the small granule is extruded as part of the large granule without first fusing with the plasma membrane.

Besides the structures whose functional significance have been emphasized in the basal and apical regions of acinar cells, a variety of other organelles and inclusions are also pres-

ent. Most noteworthy are mitochondria (Fig. 1-24), which supply energy for synthetic activities; free ribosomes (Fig. 1-24), which are concerned with the synthesis of protein for intracellular use; microfilaments and microtubules (Fig. 1-27) for cell support and transport mechanisms; and intercellular attachments such as desmosomes and junctional com-

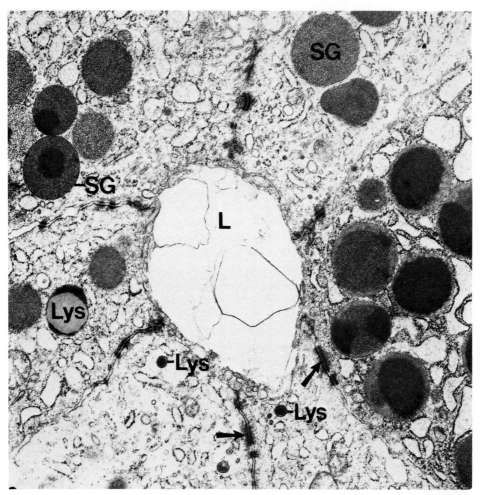

Fig. 1-26. Electron micrograph, parotid gland, showing apex and lumen of acinus. Note membranes in the lumen (**L**) and membrane-bound secretory granules (**SG**) in the cytoplasm. A few lysosomes (**Lys**) are shown. Desmosomes (**arrows**) and other components of the junctional complex separate adjacent cells. (× 19,800)

plexes (Fig. 1-25– 1-27) for maintaining acinar cells in close apposition.

Myoepithelial cells lie between the basement membrane and the bases of acinar cells (Fig. 1-29). Characterized by contractile myofilaments in their cytoplasm, these cells have a cell body in which the nucleus is located and numerous processes that extend around the periphery of the acinus. A number of thin sections have been reconstructed to show diagramatically the number and extensiveness of these processes (Figs. 1-2, 1-5), which cannot be appreciated in a single electron micrograph. Direct observations of myoepithelial contractions and the concomitant expulsion of secretion have been observed in apocrine sweat glands.

Intercalated ducts lack most of the highly specialized features of acini, which might be expected, since the main function attributed to the ducts is to convey acinar secretions to striated ducts. Electron microscopy clearly shows, however, that the duct cells contribute to the saliva a secretory product that, as reflected by the appearance of the secretory granule, is a different type of secretion than that contributed by acinar cells. The granules are most numerous in cells near the acinus-intercalated duct junction (Fig. 1-30) and gradually diminish or disappear as the striated duct is approached (Fig. 1-31). They differ from granules in acinar cells in that they are paler and, as shown by the PAS technique, are richer in carbohydrate.

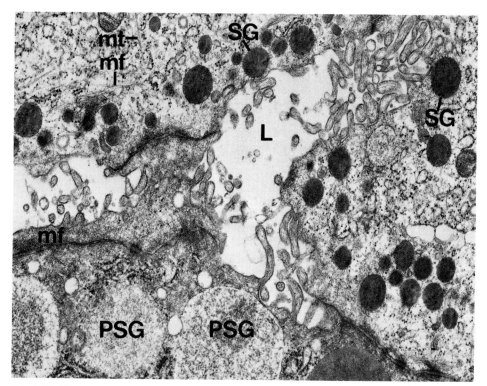

Fig. 1-27. Electron micrograph, parotid gland, showing apex of acinus at junction with intercalated duct. Note the dark secretory granules (**SG**) in the vicinity of the lumen (**L**). The pale secretory granules (**PSG**) are in an intercalated duct cell. Microtubules (**mt**) and microfilaments (**mf**) are present. (×24,750)

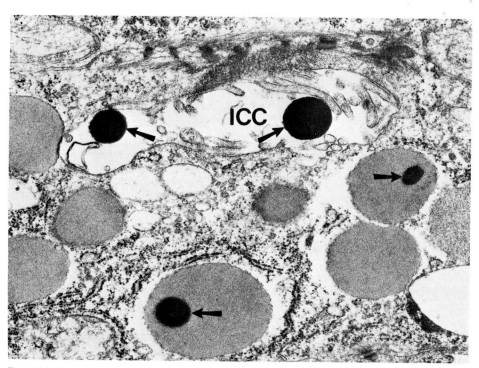

Fig. 1-28. Electron micrograph, parotid gland, showing intercellular canaliculus. Microvilli project into the lumen of the intercellular canaliculus (**ICC**). Small, dark secretory granules (**arrows**) are present in the intercellular canaliculus as well as in the large secretory granules of the acinar cell. (×25,370)

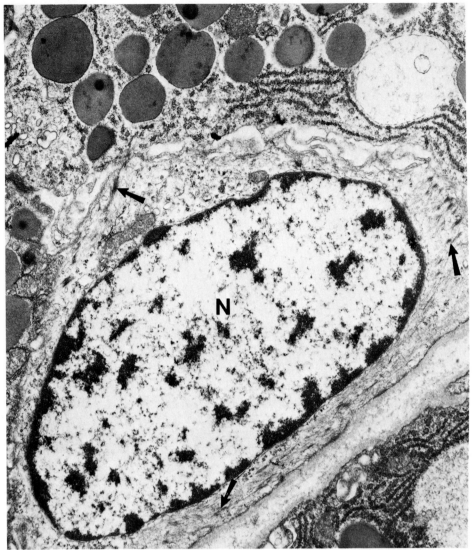

Fig. 1-29. Electron micrograph, parotid gland, showing myoepithelial cell at base of acinus. Note the nucleus (**N**) and myofilaments (**arrows**). Myofilaments are most important prominent when they occur in clumps. (× 15,000)

Although intercalated duct cells are the least specialized of the parenchymal components, they contain the same organelles previously noted in acinar cells. Intercellular canaliculi are absent, but myoepithelial cells are present to help expel the secretion (Fig. 1-31). All the cells tend to accumulate lipid, but those near intercalated-striated duct junctions, which are less active in the production of secretory granules, have a greater propensity for lipid than those closer to acini (Fig. 1-31).

Each of the three cell types of striated ducts have unique ultrastructural features that indicate their diverse functions. Light cells are characterized by a basal specialization formed by interdigitating plasma membranes associated with numerous mitochondria (Fig. 1-32). A specialization of this type increases the basal surface area and provides mitochondria for energy production. It also typifies cells of the proximal and distal tubules of the kidney, which, just as light cells of striated ducts, are concerned with ion transport. The pres-

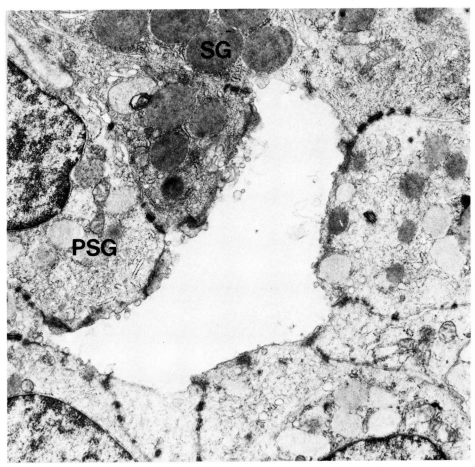

Fig. 1-30. Electron micrograph, parotid gland, showing apex of intercalated duct at junction with acinus. Dark secretory granules (**SG**) at top of micrograph belong to acinar cells while pale secretory granules (**PSG**) in lower portion of micrograph are in intercalated duct cells. (×11,800)

ence of desmosomes between the membranes indicates that interdigitating processes belong to more than one cell. Fenestrated capillaries outside the basement membrane carry products to and from the specialized basal zone (Fig. 1-33).

The apical region of light cells is also rich in mitochondria and is provided with short microvilli at the luminal surface for absorptive purposes (Fig. 1-34). Bleblike extensions project into the lumen and eventually detach to enter the saliva by the apocrine mode of secretion.

Dark cells have an abundance of mitochondria throughout their cytoplasm (Fig. 1-35), along with numerous microfilaments that account for the dark appearance of the cytoplasm (Fig. 1-36). Supranuclearly, dark cells

contain glycogen, a Golgi apparatus, and small, dense secretory granules (Fig. 1-36). The infranuclear region divides to form several processes. Each process is especially rich in mitochondria (Fig. 1-37), but lacks the infolded membranes characteristically associated with mitochondria in the basal region of light cells. Although the presence of secretory granules indicates that dark cells produce a secretory product, the chemical nature and importance of the secretion have not been determined.

Basal cells are of two types in striated ducts of human parotid glands. Type I resembles a myoepithelial cell and is similarly characterized by filaments and long cytoplasmic processes believed to be contractile (Figs. 1-37, 1-38). Type II has a greatly indented nucleus

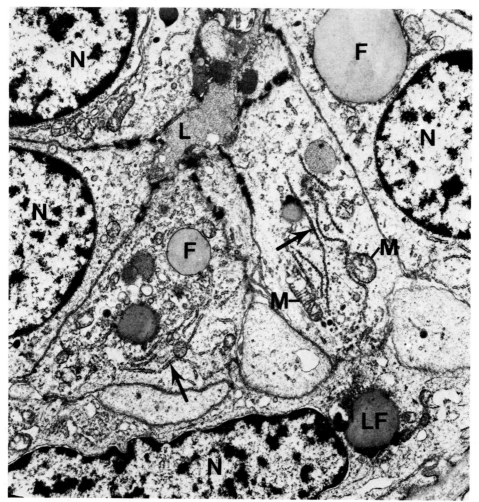

Fig. 1-31. Electron micrograph, parotid gland, depicting intercalated duct near junction with striated duct. A myoepithelial cell with an elongated nucleus (**N**) and cytoplasmic lipofuscin (**LF**) is shown near bottom of micrograph. Note the lumen (**L**) of the intercalated duct. Observe fat (**F**), mitochondria (**M**), RER (**arrows**), and nuclei of the intercalated duct. (× 11,800)

and fewer filaments than the Type I cell (Fig. 1-39). Its features indicate that it is a precursor of other cell types of the striated duct.

Excretory ducts, as noted in the section on light microscopy, have the same cell types as striated ducts; only their light cells need further comment. The supranuclear region contains more microfilaments and smooth vesicles of endoplasmic reticulum than the corresponding region in light cells of striated ducts (Fig. 1-40). On the basis of the latter feature, light cells of excretory ducts are the probable sites for degradation of steroid hormones, a process known to occur in salivary glands. The infranuclear region for electrolyte

transfer, while similar to that of light cells of striated ducts, has wider spaces between the interdigitating membranes (Fig. 1-41). Lipofuscin, representing residual products of senile lysosomes, tends to accumulate infranuclearly (Fig. 1-41) and may fluoresce when the ducts are studied with the light microscope.

The various parenchymal components of the parotid are innervated by small unmyelinated fibers from both divisions of the autonomic nervous system. The fibers permeate the gland in company with blood vessels. The terminals occur outside the basement membrane, as well as in the spaces between acinar, myoepithelial, and duct cells (Fig. 1-6). Some

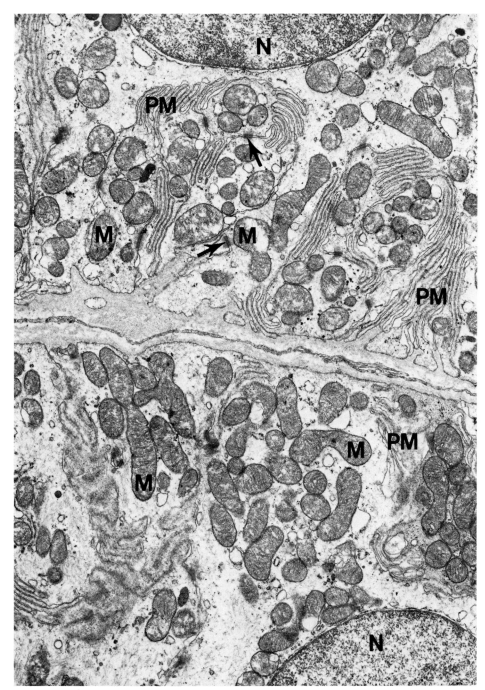

Fig. 1-32. Electron micrograph, parotid gland, showing infranuclear region of light cells and bases of two adjacent striated ducts. Note the plasma membranes (**PM**) and mitochondria (**M**), which extend the nucleus (**N**). Desmosomes (**arrows**) are present. (× 14,750)

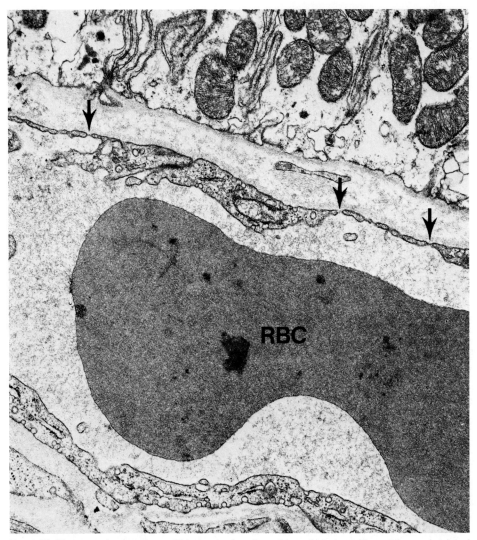

Fig. 1-33. Electron micrograph, parotid gland, of portion of fenestrated capillary at base of striated duct. A red blood cell (**RBC**) is in the capillary lumen. Fenestrations (**arrows**) are present in the capillary endothelium. (×24,750)

endings contain vesicles purely of the "clear" or cholinergic type while others contain a mixture of "clear" and "dark" adrenergic vesicles. Absence of synaptic junctions with parenchymal cells indicates that the neurotransmitters must diffuse to the parenchyma to produce their effects.

Submandibular Gland

Gross and Light Microscopic Features

The *submandibular gland* is smaller than the parotid gland and is surrounded by a well-defined capsule. It is located in the submandibular triangle with its posterior extent separated from the parotid gland by the stylomandibular ligament.

The main duct is about 5 cm. in length and exits the gland on its deep surface. It courses forward lateral to the hyoglossus and genioglossus muscles, deep to the mucous membrane of the mouth, and opens on the summit of the sublingual papilla just lateral to the frenulum of the tongue. Similar to the parotid duct, the submandibular duct is smaller in diameter at its origin and, to some extent, may serve as a reservoir for saliva. The student

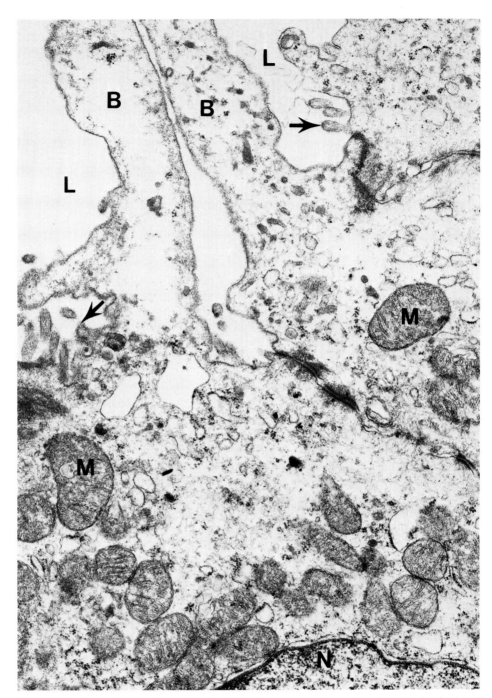

Fig. 1-34. Electron micrograph, parotid gland, showing supranuclear region of light cells of striated duct. Below the two large apical projections or blebs (**B**) that extend into the lumen (**L**), note microvilli (**arrows**), mitochondria (**M**), and the edge of a nucleus (**N**). (×24,750)

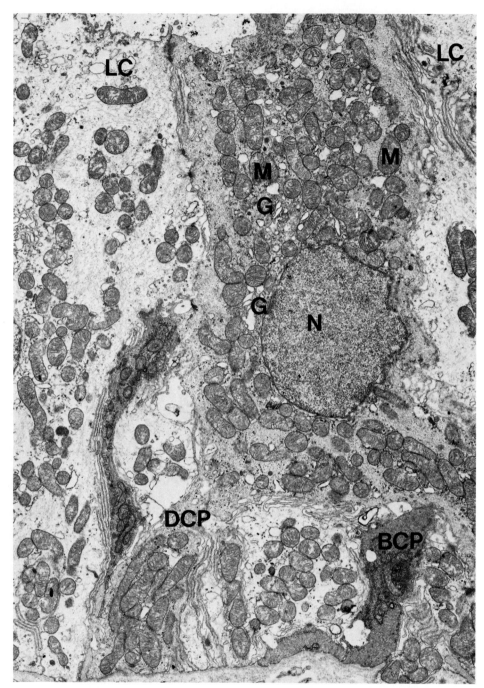

Fig. 1-35. Electron micrograph, parotid gland, showing apex and base of dark cell of striated duct. Portions of light cells (**LC**) are present on both sides of the dark cell in the center of the micrograph. Note the nucleus (**N**), Golgi membranes (**G**), and mitochondria (**M**) of the dark cell. Each infranuclear dark cell process (**DCP**) is also rich in mitochondria. A process of a Type I basal cell (**BCP**) is shown at bottom of micrograph. (×9280)

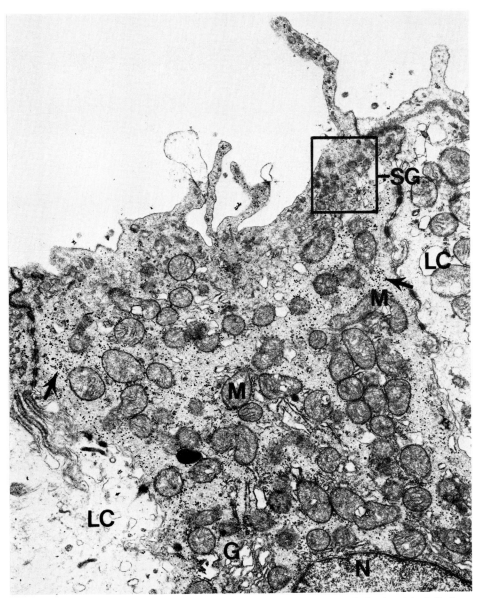

Fig. 1-36. Electron micrograph, parotid gland, illustrating apex of dark cell of striated duct. Portions of two light cells (**LC**) are also shown. In the dark cell, note Golgi membranes (**G**), edge of nucleus (**N**), mitochondria (**M**), and small secretory granules (**SG**) in enclosed area. Small, dark particles of glycogen (**arrows**) often occur in clusters. Closely packed microfilaments and glycogen account for the density of the cytoplasm. (×15,840)

should consult a gross anatomy text for detailed relationships of the gland and its duct.

The gland receives its arterial supply from the facial artery and its submental branch. Secretomotor nerves (parasympathetic) leave the brain stem with the facial nerve and run in the chorda tympani. Preganglionic fibers mostly synapse on the postganglionic cells lo-cated in the submandibular ganglion, but some pass directly into the gland to synapse on ganglion cells embedded in the gland stroma. As an interesting side note, it is common for postganglionic cells to migrate into the substance of submandibular glands of many species. By contrast this phenomenon is not known to occur in the parotid gland.

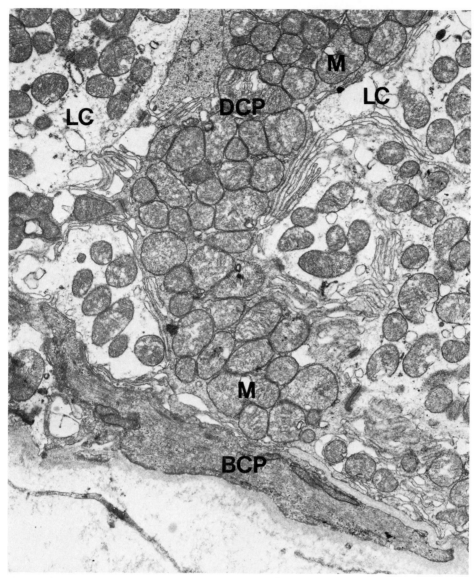

Fig. 1-37. Electron micrograph, parotid gland, showing basal process of dark cell of striated duct. Light cells (**LC**) are adjacent to the dark cell process (**DCP**), is almost filled with mitochondria (**M**). A process of a Type I basal cell (**BCP**) is also shown. (× 16,300)

Connective tissue septa pass into the gland from the capsule and divide it into lobes and lobules. The extralobular ducts run in the septa and are, to some extent, enveloped by the connective tissue. Plasma cells, lymphocytes, mast cells, fibroblasts, and macrophages are present in interstitial areas between the gland cells or are enmeshed in the connective tissue between lobes and lobules.

Parenchymal elements of submandibular glands show a predominance of serous acini (Fig. 1-8–1-10). Fewer mucous acini are present, and these are commonly capped with serous demilunes. The striated ducts are longest in the submandibular gland and comprise most of the intralobular portion of the duct system. Intercalated ducts are present but are shorter than those of the parotid gland.

Ultrastructure

Serous acini of the submandibular gland contain secretory granules that closely resemble

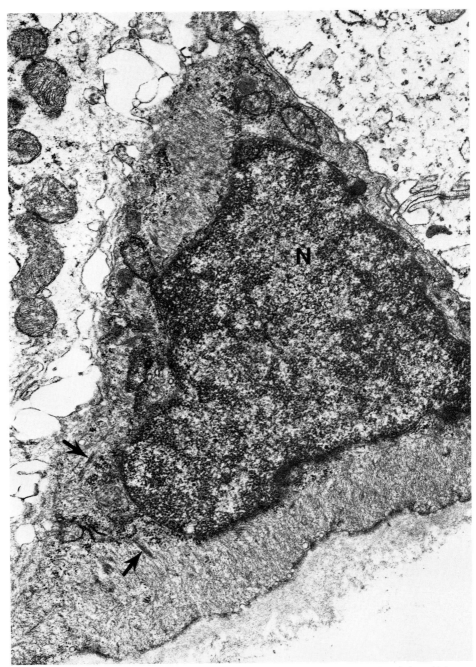

Fig. 1-38. Electron micrograph, parotid gland, showing Type I basal cell of striated duct. Note nucleus (**N**) and dense cytoplasmic filaments, which are especially prominent where they are clumped together (**arrows**). (×24,750)

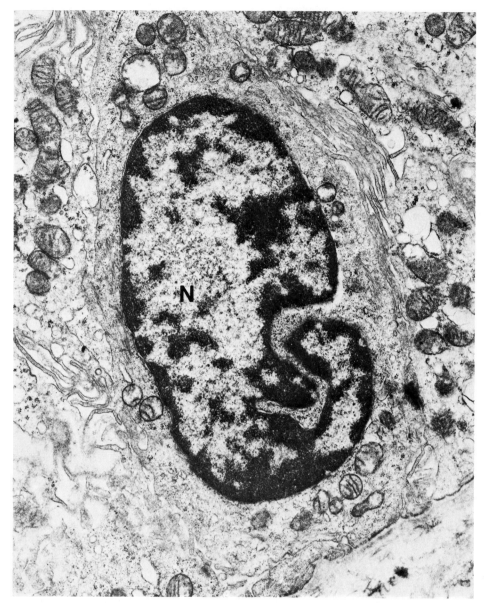

Fig. 1-39. Electron micrograph, parotid gland, depicting Type II basal cell of striated duct. Note the indented nucleus (**N**). (×18,750)

those of the parotid gland (Fig. 1-28). The granules consist of a spherical shaped structure containing a smaller, electron-dense component. A third component of intermediate density is reported to occur at the periphery of the granule. In regard to the organelles of serous acinar cells, the description given for the parotid gland exemplifies the structure of serous cells in submandibular glands.

Mucous acini of human submandibular glands have not been extensively investigated at ultrastructural levels. The reports that do mention them indicate features common to submandibular mucous acini of many species. Large electron lucent secretory granules originate from an extensive system of Golgi membranes. Intercellular canaliculi and tissue spaces are poorly developed or totally absent. The RER and nucleus tend to be compressed toward the base of the cell, especially in cells filled with stored secretion. The secretory

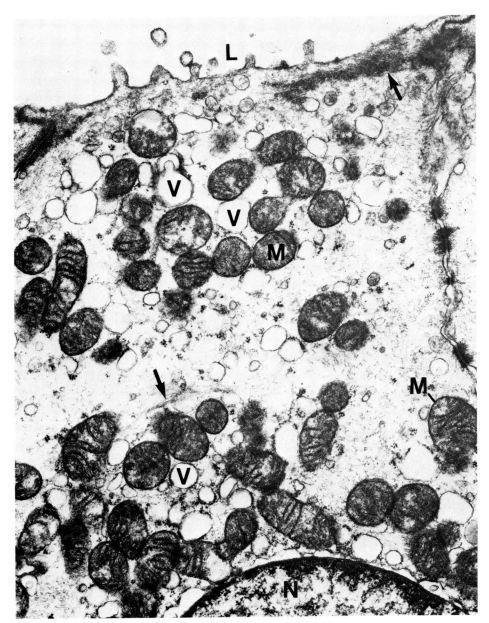

Fig. 1-40. Electron micrograph, parotid gland, showing apex of light cell of excretory duct. Short microvilli project into the lumen (**L**). Many mitochondria (**M**) are located above the nucleus (**N**). Vesicles (**V**) and microfilaments (**arrows**) are present. (×24,750)

granules exhibit varying degrees of coalescence, whereas remaining areas between the granules contain foci of Golgi membranes and RER (Fig. 1-42). Higher magnifications of the secretory granules often show linear densities that have been interpreted as protein cores of mucin molecules.

Ultrastructural features of intercalated ducts (Figs. 1-30, 1-31) and striated ducts (Figs. 1-32–1-39) of the human parotid and submandibular glands are essentially identical.

The so-called dark cell is common to striated ducts of all mammalian species, including the striated ducts of man. Dark cells of submandibular glands have been more extensively investigated than those of parotid glands, and some special mention of them here is appropriate. It was once thought that

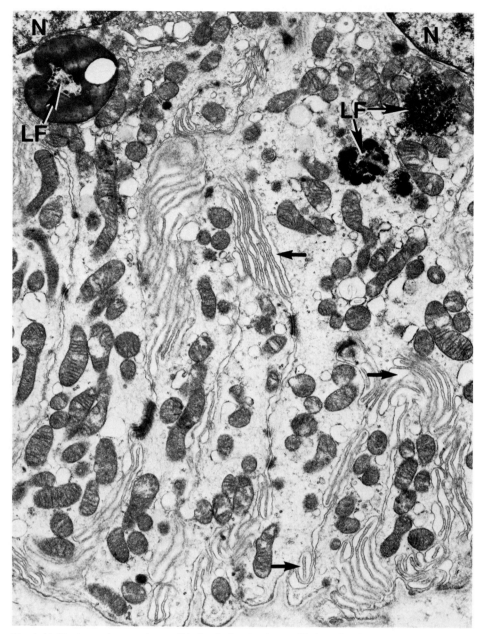

Fig. 1-41. Electron micrograph, parotid gland, showing base of light cells of excretory duct. Note the prominent spaces (**arrows**) between the membranes. Lipofuscin (**LF**) lies below each nucleus (**N**). (× 14,750)

dark cells could represent the remains of degenerating light cells and no special significance was attached to them. With electron microscopic examination, however, it became apparent that dark cells possessed a highly specialized morphology totally distinct from that of light cells (Figs. 1-35– 1-37). In several species specialized microvilli are present and, for this reason, are easily identified as a distinct cell type (Fig. 1-43). Dark cells are not limited to striated ducts but extend into the main excretory duct, where they can be identified with the scanning electron microscope (Fig. 1-44).

The phenomenon of bleb formation, so characteristic of cells that secrete by the apo-

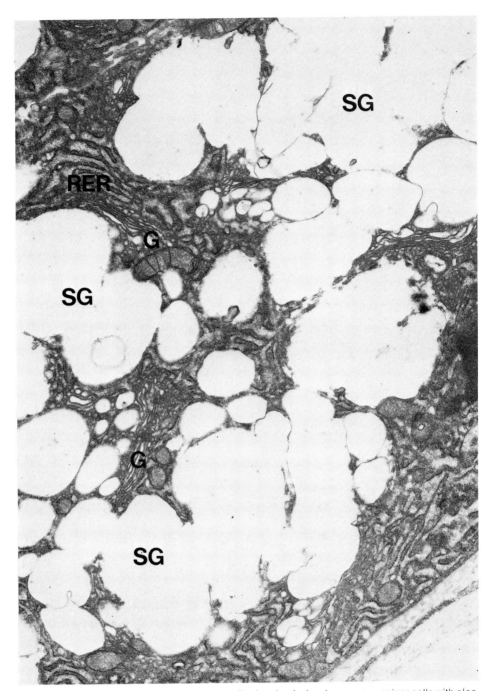

Fig. 1-42. Electron micrograph, bovine submandicular gland, showing mucous acinar cells with electron lucent secret granules (**SG**). Note that many granules have coalesced to form larger aggregates of stored secretion. Rough endoplasmic reticulum (**RER**) and Golgi membranes occupy areas between the secretory granules. (×14,000)

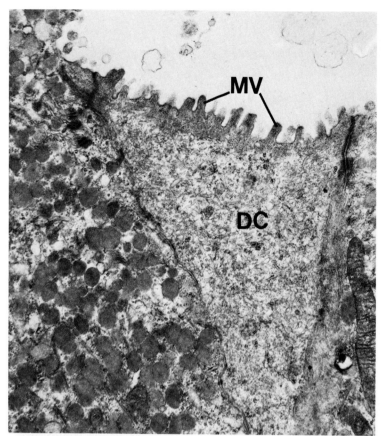

Fig. 1-43. Electron micrograph, cat submandibular gland, illustrating dark cell (**DC**) of a striated duct with prominent microvilli (**MV**). (×15,000)

crine method, is also a common feature of striated ducts and excretory ducts. At one time blebs were thought by some investigators to be artifacts. Now it has been established that blebs represent a special method of secretion in which saclike accumulations of cytoplasm are released from the cell. Intact blebs have been identified in human saliva obtained from the parotid duct. Scanning electron microscopy is capable of demonstrating varying degrees of bleb formation in the main excretory duct of submandibular glands (Fig. 1-45). In the process of formation the bleb first shows a broad base at its point of attachment to the cell. This base becomes progressively narrowed until the bleb assumes a spherical shape. At this point the bleb pinches off from the underlying cytoplasm and thus prevents discontinuities in the apical cell membrane.

Sublingual Gland

Gross and Light Microscopic Features

The sublingual glands are the smallest of the major salivary glands. Laterally the gland lies in the sublingual fossa on the inner surface of the mandible, while the medial surface is in contact with the genioglossus and hyoglossus muscles. The upper border of the gland lies immediately below the mucous membrane of the sublingual fold.

The sublingual gland is actually a composite of a number of smaller glands. This, in part, explains the polystomatic nature of the gland with its multiple duct openings. A larger portion of the gland complex has a main duct (of Bartholin) that opens into the oral cavity near the duct of the submandibular gland.

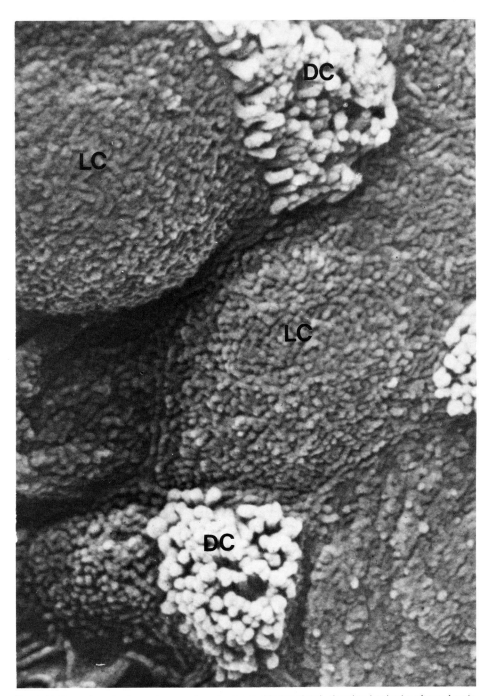

Fig. 1-44. Scanning electron micrograph, rat submandibular gland, showing luminal surface of main excretory duct. The contrast between dark cell microvilli (**DC**) and those of light cells (**LC**) is striking. (× 12,000)

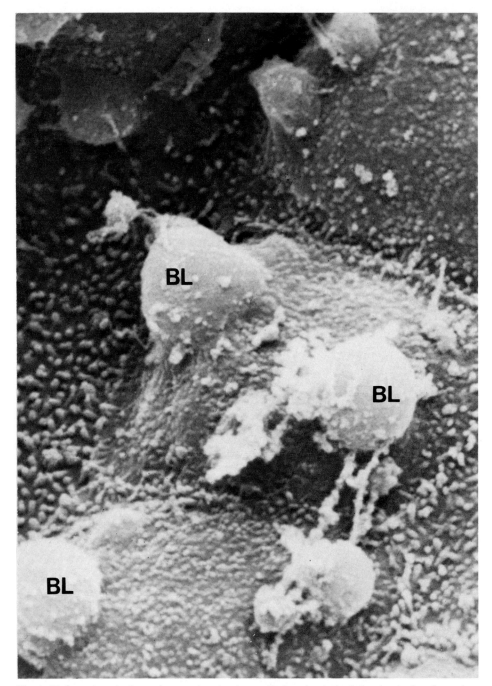

Fig. 1-45. Scanning electron micrograph, rat submandibular gland, depicting luminal surface of an excretory duct. Note blebs (**BL**) in various stages of formation. The spherical blebs are about to be released from the underlying cytoplasm. (×10,000)

Ducts of the smaller components (8–20 in number) mostly open independently along the sublingual fold.

The gland capsule is ill defined or absent, but pronounced connective tissue septa separate the gland into lobes and lobules. Interstitial elements are otherwise similar to those present in parotid and submandibular glands.

Parenchymal elements show a predominance of mucous acini, some of which are capped with serous demilunes, but serous acini are rare (Figs. 1-11–1-13). Striated and intercalated ducts are also rare or, in some instances, absent from the gland.

Blood supply is received from branches of the sublingual and submental arteries. Postganglionic parasympathetic fibers pass to the gland from the submandibular ganglion.

Ultrastructure

Of all the major salivary glands, the sublingual gland of man has been investigated the least. Secretory granules of the serous demilunes are not as electron dense as those of submandibular and parotid glands. An inner component may form a single mass or be fragmented into several smaller foci.

Most of the sublingual gland parenchyma consists of mucous acini with ultrastructural characteristics similar to those of many species, i.e., electron lucent secretion granules that tend to coalesce, a well-developed Golgi apparatus, RER, and nuclei that occupy a relatively narrow zone toward the cell base (Fig. 1-46). Myoepithelial cells are present and enclosed by the basement membrane of mucous acini just as with serous acini of submandibular and parotid glands.

MINOR SALIVARY GLANDS

Distribution, Function, and Structure

In addition to the major salivary glands, there are numerous intraoral glands, referred to as *minor salivary glands*, that empty their secretions into the oral cavity. Minor glands are found in all parts of the oral mucosa with the exception of the gingiva and anterior portion of the hard palate. Named according to their location, the minor glands include 1) labial, 2) buccal, 3) minor sublingual, 4) glossopalatine, 5) lingual, and 6) palatine glands. Whereas the major glands secrete only in response to mechanical, thermal, chemical, and certain psychic or olfactory stimuli, the minor glands secrete continuously. Therefore, they constantly moisten and lubricate the oral mucosa.

Copious amounts of mucins are secreted by the minor glands, but little information is available concerning other constituents of the secretion. Amylase, the main secretory product of the major glands, is absent or barely detectable in secretions of the minor glands. On the other hand, high concentrations of blood group antigens and virus hemagglutination activity have been found in secretions of minor glands.

From 8–10 per cent of the total saliva (resting or stimulated) is contributed by the minor glands. Although this volume in terms of total saliva is relatively small, secretions from the minor glands are in intimate contact with the enamel surfaces of the teeth. When flow from the major glands is reduced, as during sleep, the dental plaque, gingiva, and enamel surfaces of the teeth are in contact mainly with the secretions of the minor glands. The secretions are, therefore, believed to play a role in the physiology of these structures and in the formation of the acquired pellicle (See Chap. 5).

Minor glands are simple branched tubuloalveolar glands and, with the exception of the lingual glands of von Ebner, are classified as mucous glands. It was previously thought that some of the minor glands were mixed glands, but electron microscopy has not confirmed the presence of serous cells. Since one group of minor glands continues into the next group and all groups are similar microscopically, it is appropriate to consider the general features of the various glands and to give the details of only one group. The palatal glands will be considered in greatest detail because of their importance as the most frequent site of tumors, both benign and malignant, and because of their tendency to atrophy with the wearing of dentures.

The parenchyma of all the minor glands consists of tubules, alveoli, intercalated ducts, striated ducts, and excretory ducts. The stroma is similar to that of major glands.

Mucous cells of the tubules and alveoli are columnar in shape and vary in appearance according to their functional activity. Cells that have emptied their secretion are narrower than others, and their nuclei, though at the cell base and transversely oval, are not as flat

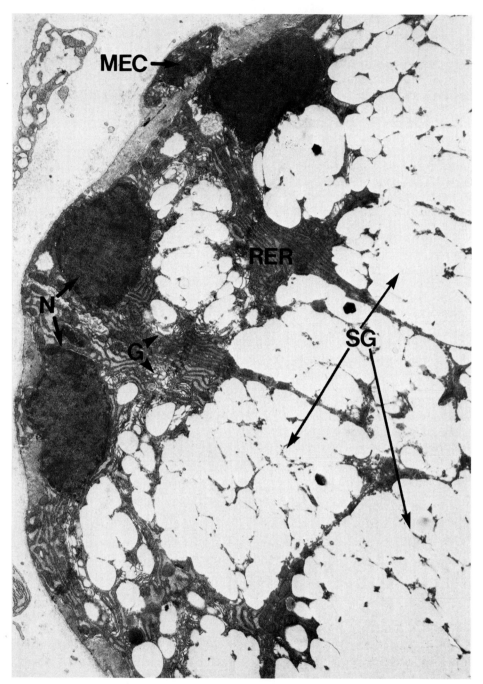

Fig. 1-46. Electron micrograph, rat sublingual gland, showing mucous cells almost filled with electron lucent secretory granules (**SG**). Rough endoplasmic reticulum (**RER**), Golgi membranes (**G**) and acinar nuclei (**N**) are visible in basal cytoplasm. The nucleus of a myoepithelial cell (**MEC**) is shown. (×5625)

as in cells full of secretion. A single tubule may contain cells in widely different phases of secretory activity. Ultrastructural features of the secretory cells of the palatine glands are noted later.

Secretory end pieces connect with intercalated ducts whose cells have the potential to develop into mucus-producing cells. The remaining segments of the duct system, *i.e.*, striated and excretory ducts, have microscopic features comparable to those present in major salivary glands.

Labial Glands

Labial glands are small, nonencapsulated clusters of mucous glands embedded in the submucosa of the upper and lower lips (Figs. 1-47, 1-48). Secretory cells are entirely of the mucous type and show various stages of secretory activity. In the early synthetic phase of their secretory cycle they resemble serous cells histologically. Consequently, labial glands were erroneously classified as mixed glands until electron micrographs showed that true serous cells were absent. Intercalated ducts are short, and only one large excretory

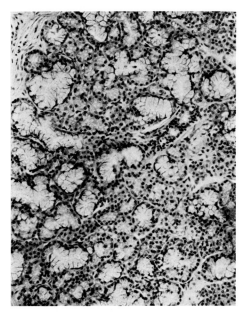

Fig. 1-48. Photomicrograph of paraffin section of labial glands stained with H&E. Mucous cells filled with secretory product are paler and larger than those with little or no secretory material. (× 120)

duct from each lobule opens onto the inner surface of the lip.

Buccal Glands

Buccal glands are continuous with the labial glands. They are embedded in the mucous membrane of the cheek external to the buccinator muscle. Buccal glands near the opening of the parotid duct drain into the third molar region and are sometimes called molar glands. Since intercalated ducts are exceptionally short in buccal glands, the secretory end pieces may empty directly into striated ducts.

Minor Sublingual Glands

Minor sublingual glands are mucous glands that lie near the major sublingual gland but are quite distinct from it. They consist of 5–15 tubuloalveolar glands of variable size whose ducts open along a fold of mucous membrane, the *plica sublingualis*.

Glossopalatine Glands

The *glossopalatine* (isthmian or faucial) *glands* are continuous with the posterior por-

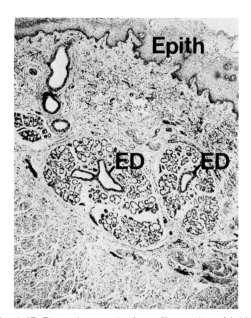

Fig. 1-47. Photomicrograph of paraffin section of labial glands stained with H&E. Lobules of glands are shown in the connective tissue beneath the moist stratified squamous epithelium (**Epith**). A large excretory duct (**ED**) associated with each lobule conveys the secretion to the surface. (× 30)

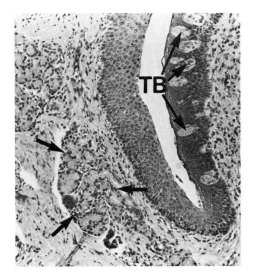

Fig. 1-49. Photomicrograph of paraffin section stained with H&E showing serous glands of von Ebner (**arrows)** at base of circumvallate papilla. Numerous taste buds (**TB**) are in wall of papilla. (×120)

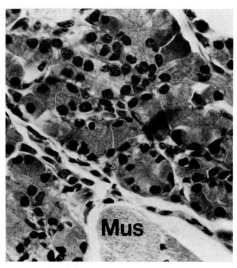

Fig. 1-50. Photomicrograph of paraffin section stained with H&E depicting serous glands of von Ebner. Skeletal muscle (**Mus**) of tongue is near bottom of micrograph. (×480)

tions of the minor sublingual glands. They ascend in the mucosa of the glossopalatine fold and may be confined to the anterior faucial pillar, or extend into the soft palate to become continuous with the palatine glands proper. They may also be present in the retromolar area of the mandible.

Lingual Glands

Lingual glands are found on the dorsum of the tongue in association with the circumvallate papillae (the glands of von Ebner) and in the body, root, and tip of tongue. Glands in the tip of tongue are located on each side of the frenulum and are referred to as the anterior lingual glands (glands of Nuhn or Blandin). Approximately five excretory ducts extend from the secretory portions of these glands to open on the *plicae fimbriate* of the undersurface of the tongue. The openings are small and difficult to distinguish in the living subject. Glands of the body and root of the tongue occur in clusters surrounded by connective tissue and skeletal muscle (Figs. 1-49, 1-50). They are more numerous in the root than in the body of the tongue.

The serous glands of von Ebner are confined to the region of the circumvallate papillae (Figs. 1-51, 1-52). They produce a watery secretion that washes away debris from the furrows of the circumvallate papillae. The

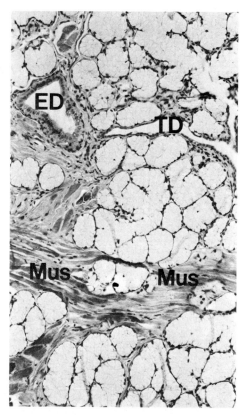

Fig. 1-51. Photomicrograph of paraffin section of lingual glands stained with H&E. Secretory units of mucous glands are very pale and lie between the skeletal muscle fibers (**Mus**) of tongue. Note intercalated duct (**ID**) and excretory duct (**ED**). (×120)

secretory cells are serous and similar to serous cells of the major salivary glands.

Palatine Glands

The *palatine glands* can be divided into glands of the hard palate and glands of the soft palate and uvula. Each gland group is composed of separate lobules, which number about 250 in the hard palate, 100 in the soft palate, and 12 in the uvula.

Histologic sections show that mucous secretory cells comprise most of the parenchyma (Fig. 1-53). Nuclei of mucous cells are located at the cell base. The supranuclear cytoplasm is filled with pale or slightly chromophilic granules when sections are stained with conventional stains such as H&E or toluidine blue (Fig. 1-54). The contents of the granules are rich in carbohydrates, sialomucins, and sulfomucins (Figs. 1-55, 1-56). Granules are

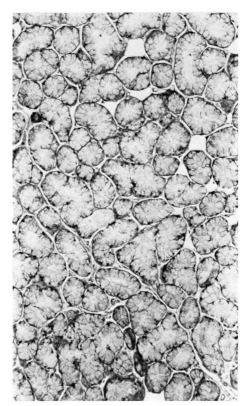

Fig. 1-53. Photomicrograph of paraffin section of palatine glands stained with H&E showing tubuloalveoli of mucous secretory cells. (×120)

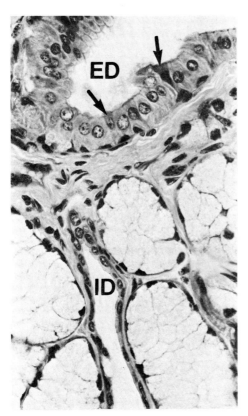

Fig. 1-52. Photomicrograph of paraffin section of lingual glands stained with H&E. An intercalated duct (**ID**) lies between the pale-staining, mucous secretory tubules. Observe the large excretory duct (**ED**) with light cells and dark cells (**arrows**). (×480)

discharged by apocrine and holocrine methods of secretion. Apocrine secretion has already been described, and features of holocrine secretion are discussed below.

Intercalated ducts of variable length and morphology occur singly and in clusters (Figs. 1-57, 1-58). Although the cells are typically flattened, they can develop into mucous cells. When this occurs, a mucous tubule elongates at the expense of the intercalated duct and may connect directly with the intralobular duct.

Striated and excretory ducts resemble corresponding ducts in major salivary glands. The epithelium of excretory ducts changes from pseudostratified columnar or stratified columnar to stratified squamous as the ducts pierce the palatal epithelium to open into the oral cavity (Fig. 1-59).

The stroma of the palatine glands is rich in fat, nerves, and blood vessels (Fig. 1-60). Connective tissue fibers, mainly of the collagenous type intermingled with the elastic

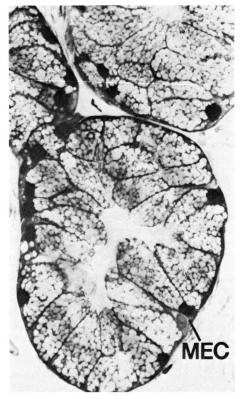

Fig. 1-54. Photomicrograph of plastic section of mucous secretory cells of palatine glands stained with toluidine blue. Granules fill cytoplasm above dark nuclei. A myoepithelial cell (**MEC**) is shown. (× 750)

variety, form septa that divide the glands into lobules.

The ultrastructure of mucous cells of the palatine glands is complicated by the fact that cells are in various stages of the secretory cycle. On the basis of cytologic features, four stages can be identified: presecretory, secretory, mature, and resting. The secretory cycle is, however, a continuous process during which each stage merges with the next, making it impossible in most cases to recognize the end of one stage and the beginning of the next.

In the early stage of the cycle—the presecretory stage—mucous cells are characterized by a few randomly distributed Golgi membranes and several lamallae of RER with flattened cisternae. Synthetic activity is absent or minimal. The presence of only a few cells with characteristics solely of this stage suggests that the presecretory stage is brief.

As the secretory cycle continues, there is

hypertrophy of the Golgi membranes, and the once flattened cisternae of RER become distended with flocculent material (Figs. 1-61, 1-62). Many vacuoles and vesicles of varying densities are associated with the Golgi membranes (Fig. 1-63). These changes in organelles usher in the first half of the secretory stage, which is characterized by the production of numerous secretory granules.

During the second half of the secretory stage the supranuclear cytoplasm becomes packed with secretory granules that tend to coalesce. There is a concomitant decrease in cisternal size and extensiveness of the Golgi membranes. Most granules are electron lucent, but a few are filled with fibrils (Figs. 1-64, 1-65).

In the mature stage of the secretory cycle, cell apices are filled with secretory granules and bulge into the lumen (Fig. 1-66). Nuclei are displaced basally and are often flattened or irregularly shaped. Only a few Golgi membranes and segments of RER are present among the secretory granules.

Discharge of secretory granules is accomplished by three methods: rupture of the api-

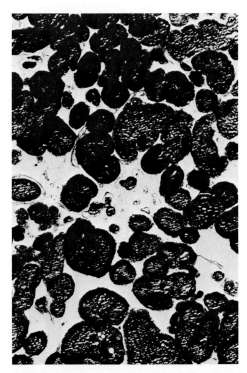

Fig. 1-55. Photomicrograph of paraffin section of palatine glands stained with PAS. Mucous cells are intensely PAS-positive. (× 120)

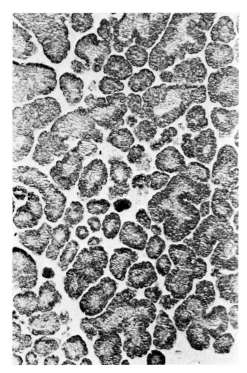

Fig. 1-56. Photomicrograph of paraffin section of palatine glands stained with alcian blue, pH 0.5. Mucous cells are stained, and this indicates the presence of sulfomucins. More intense staining occurs at pH 2.6, and this suggests that sialomucins are major constituents of the secretory product. (×120)

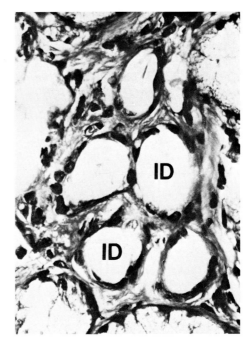

Fig. 1-58. Photomicrograph of paraffin section of palatine glands stained with H&E showing a group of intercalated ducts (**ID**). (×480)

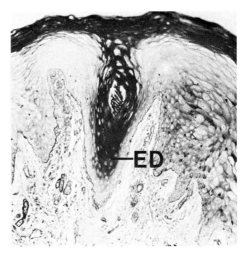

Fig. 1-59. Photomicrograph of paraffin section stained with PAS showing an excretory duct (**ED**) in the stratified squamous epithelium of the palate. (×120)

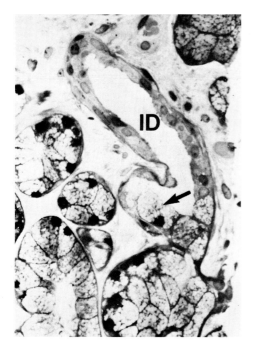

Fig. 1-57. Photomicrograph of plastic section of palatine glands stained with toluidine blue. Some cells lining the intercalated duct (**ID**) are mucous cells (**arrows**). (×480)

cal plasma membrane with release of the contents of the granules into the lumen (Fig. 1-67), apocrine secretion (Fig. 1-66), and holocrine secretion (Fig. 1-68). In the latter method the cell dies and enters the lumen as part of the secretory product. When this

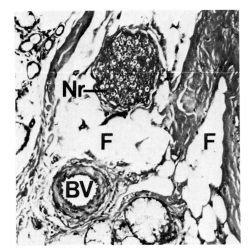

Fig. 1-60. Photomicrograph of paraffin section stained with H&E showing fat (**F**), nerve (**Nr**), artery (**BV**), and connective tissue fibers in palatal stroma. (×120)

occurs, the lumen is separated from the extracellular space only by a myoepithelial cell, or in the absence of a myoepithelial cell, only by the basal lamina (Fig. 1-69). Cells that discharge their products by either of the first two methods enter a brief quiescent or resting stage before beginning a new secretory cycle. Cells lost by holocrine secretion are replaced by mitosis of neighboring cells.

Ducts of palatine glands are similar ultrastructurally to corresponding ducts of major salivary glands. The stroma also closely approximates that of the major glands.

SUMMARY

Understanding the structure of the salivary glands is basic to a knowledge of their importance in the functioning organism. There is more variation of salivary gland structure among different species than in most other organs, and these variations generally reflect special dietary and environmental dependences of the organism.

The salivary glands of man comprise three pairs of major glands and numerous minor glands. Taken totally, the saliva from these glands provides the oral environment with a lubricating mucus and the enzyme amylase. The parotid and submandibular glands provide most of the salivary amylase, whereas most of the mucous secretions derive from the

sublingual gland. The parotid gland contains serous acini only, and the submandibular gland is composed predominantly of serous acini, whereas the sublingual gland contains a predominance of mucous acini.

The duct system is important in regulating the final composition of the saliva, particularly in relation to its ionic concentration. The striated ducts are especially implicated in contributing to the final composition of the saliva, but the larger ducts, up to and including the main ducts, are also important in this activity. Striated ducts are longest in the submandibular gland but are also well developed in the parotid gland. Striated ducts are very short and rarely present in human sublingual glands.

Other substances produced by the various parenchymal elements are numerous and are more properly studied in Chapters 2, 3 and 4. Note, however, that certain components of the saliva are not produced by either the acini or the duct system. Immunoglobulins appearing in the saliva, for example, are made in plasma cells located in the glandular interstices. The striated ducts, however, play an important role in transporting immunoglobulins into the saliva.

Ultrastructure of the salivary glands reveals a complex array of biosynthetic machinery and the morphologic expression of a sophisticated transport mechanism. A high level of protein synthesis for export is reflected in the well-developed rough endoplasmic reticulum (RER) of serous acinar cells. Protein synthesis for export also occurs in mucous acinar cells, but in this instance the protein becomes a fraction of a large molecule of mucin in which the major moiety is composed of carbohydrate. The elevated carbohydrate synthesis of mucus-secreting cells is reflected in this cell's extensive system of Golgi membranes.

The striated duct's elegant system of "basal infoldings", and large numbers of associated mitochondria, are structural expressions of the work involved in active transport. Any cell showing a comparatively large surface area, in combination with increased numbers of mitochondria, may be suspected of transporting substances against a concentration and/or pressure gradient. Striated ducts and kidney tubules, although located in organs with obvious functional differences, are similar in structure because both are involved in the same type of work.

Thus the structural-functional relationships,

(Text continued on p. 60)

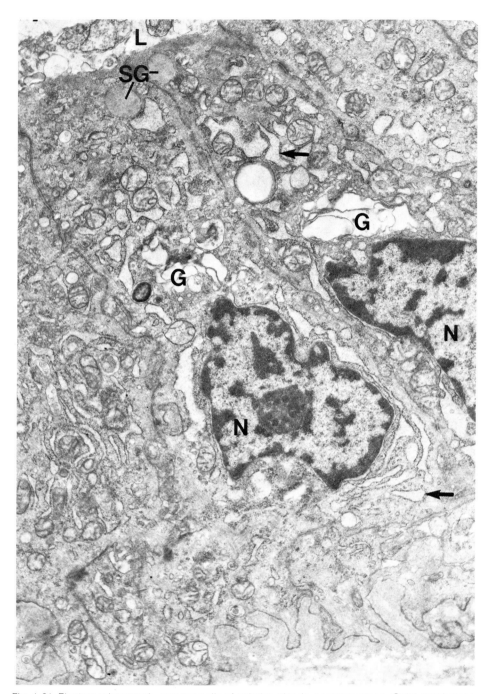

Fig. 1-61. Electron micrograph, mucous cells of palatine glands, secretory stage. Golgi membranes (**G**) are above each nucleus (**N**), cisternae (**arrows**) of the RER are dilated, and secretory granules (**SG**) are sparse. Some debris is in lumen (**L**). (× 14,705)

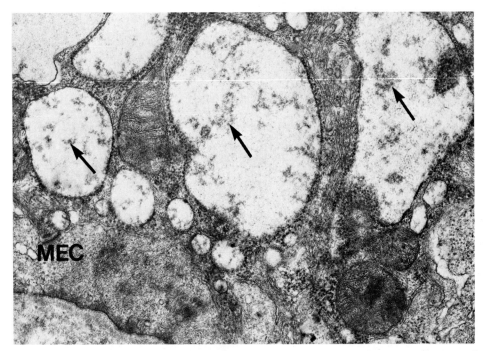

Fig. 1-62. Electron micrograph, base of mucous cell of palatine glands, secretory stage. Cisternae of RER are distended with flocculent material (**arrows**). The process of a myoepithelial cell (**MEC**) occupies the lower left portion of the micrograph. (×31,250)

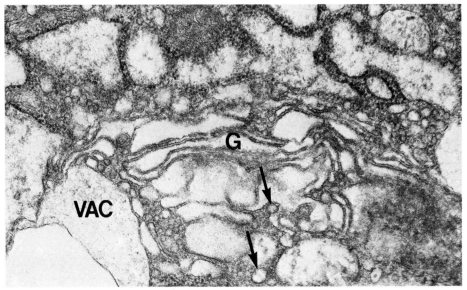

Fig. 1-63. Electron micrograph illustrating focus of Golgi membranes (**G**) in mucous cell of palatine glands. Vesicles (**arrows**) and vacuoles (**VAC**) of secretory material are associated with the membranes. (×31,250)

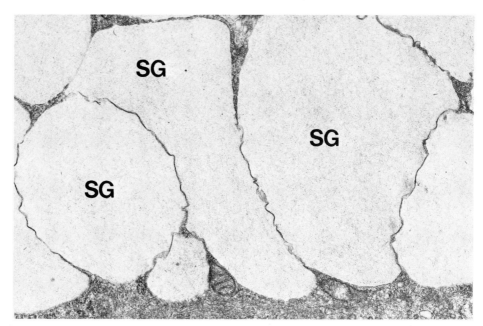

Fig. 1-64. Electron micrograph showing large pale secretory granules (**SG**) in mucous cells of palatine glands during secretory stage. (×24,750)

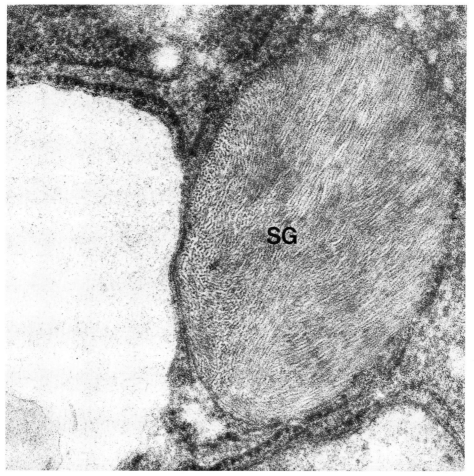

Fig. 1-65. Electron micrograph, mucous cell of palatine glands, secretory stage, showing a secretory granule (**SG**) filled with fibrils. To the left of the fibrillar granule is a pale or electron lucent granule. (×76,250)

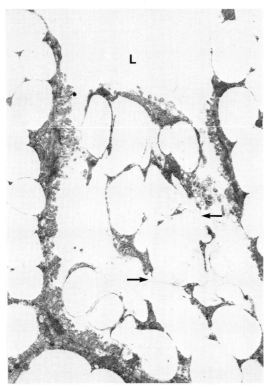

Fig. 1-66. Electron micrograph, apices of mucous cells, palatine glands, mature stage. Cells at margins of micrograph extend further into lumen (**L**) than cells in center of micrograph. Apex of central cell appears to be breaking off by the apocrine method (**arrows**). (× 14,750)

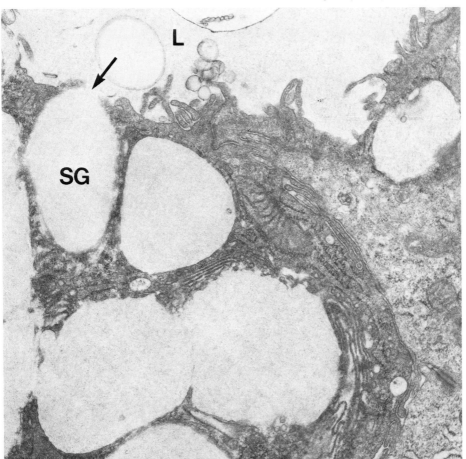

Fig. 1-67. Electron micrograph, mucous cells, palatine glands. Note ruptured plasma membrane (**arrow**) and its relationship to the secretory granule (**SG**) whose contents are entering the lumen (**L**). (× 24,750)

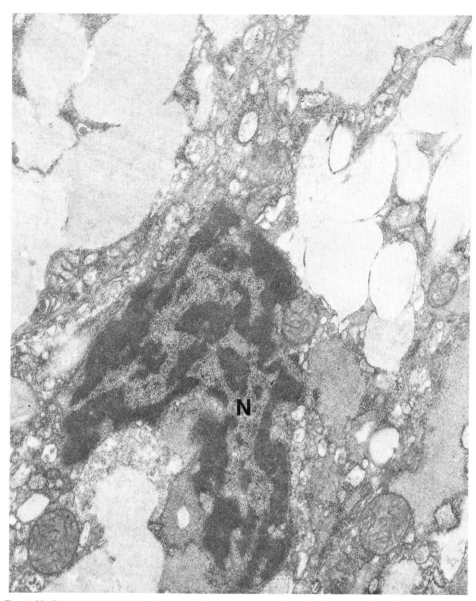

Fig. 1-68. Electron micrograph, mucous cell, palatine glands, holocrine secretion. The pyknotic nucleus (**N**), indistinct organelles, and vesiculated cytoplasm with areas of lysis indicate impending cell death. (×24,750)

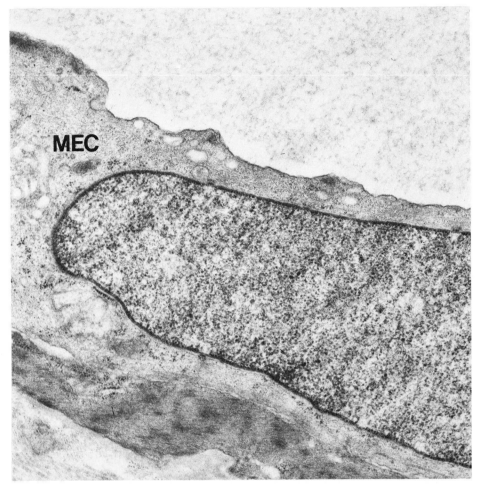

Fig. 1-69. Electron micrograph, myoepithelial cell, palatine glands. The pale area with flocculent material above the myoepithelial cell (**MEC**) was previously occupied by a mucous cell that was lost by holocrine secretion. (×24,750)

as revealed in studies of the salivary glands, form a basis for understanding mechanisms of other organs of the body. Indeed, the salivary glands are not only important organs to the clinical practitioner but also are excellent models for experimentation.

GLOSSARY

Acid mucosubstance. A term referring to epithelial mucins with an acidic component located on carbohydrate side chains. Sialomucins and sulfomucins are grouped under this general heading.

Acidophilic. Acid loving. Refers to cells and tissues that react with acidic stains such as eosin.

Acinar folds. Platelike cytoplasmic projections or lamellae located on acinar cells. The folds may interdigitate across an intercellular tissue space between adjacent acinar cells.

Acinus. (pl. acini). A grapelike cluster of cells surrounding a lumen. Used in connection with secretory cells of salivary glands. See text for special significance of this term.

Active transport. Transport of water, electrolytes and other substances against a concentration or pressure gradient.

Adrenergic. Secreting epinephrine or substances with similar activity, such as sympathomimetic substances.

Alcian blue. A stain used to demonstrate the presence of acid mucosubstances and other acid polysaccharides.

Alkaline phosphatase. An enzyme, active in an alkaline medium, that hydrolyzes monophosphoric esters, with liberation of inorganic phosphate.

Alveolus. A saclike cluster of cells grouped around a lumen. See text for specific use of this term.

Amylase. An enzyme that catalyzes the hydrolysis of starch into smaller molecules.

Apical. Refers to the distal end of a cell; that is, away from the cell base. Commonly used in connection with pyramidal shaped cells, such as serous acinar cells.

Apocrine. Refers to a type of secretion in which a portion of the apical cytoplasm is cast off along with the secretory product.

Autolysis. Cellular disintegration by action of autogenous enzymes.

Basal. Toward the basement membrane of an epithelial cell. Opposite of distal or apical.

Basal cell. A cuboidal- or pyramidal-shaped cell located among taller columnar cells of an epithelium. The basal cell rests on a basement membrane but its apex does not reach the luminal surface.

Basal infolding. The sectioned appearance of striated duct cells, reflecting the complex interdigitation of cytoplasmic lamellae between adjacent epithelial cells.

Basal striations. Striated or striped appearance of basal infoldings and associated mitochondria as seen with the light microscope.

Basal zone. A specific reference to the basal area of acinar cells in which ergastoplasm (RER) predominates.

Basement membrane. A membrane rich in carbohydrate, tropo-collagen, and reticular fibers located at the base of epithelial cells.

Basophilic. Base loving. Refers to the affinity of a cell or tissue to basic stains.

Bleb. Specifically refers to apical protrusions of cytoplasm. Usually associated with cells that secrete by the apocrine method.

Cholinergic. Refers to acetylcholine activity or drugs with similar activity (parasympathomimetic).

Chromophilic. Color loving. Refers to heavily stained portions of a cell.

Cisternae. A closed space serving as a reservoir; for example, the cisternae of RER which contain peptides and proteins synthesized on the ribosomes.

Condensing vacuole. A saccule of the Golgi apparatus in which newly formed secretory product is being concentrated.

Cytoplasmic filaments. A threadlike organelle of the cytoplasm, composed of fibrous protein and measuring about 50 angstroms in diameter.

DNA. Deoxyribonucleic acid.

Dark cell. Specifically refers to electron dense cells (also stain darkly with basic dyes) found in striated ducts and excretory ducts of salivary glands.

Demilune. Half-moon appearance of collections of serous cells which cap distal ends of mucous acini.

Desmosome. A cell attachment device (macula adherens) limited to a small focal area.

Distal. Portion of cell adjacent to the lumen (apical). Also used in reference to segment of a gland; that is, the acinus is distal to the duct system (cf. proximal).

Eccrine. Refers to eccrine sweat glands. Secretion by the merocrine method in contrast to the apocrine sweat glands.

Electrolyte. A substance that dissociates into ions when fused or in solution.

Eosin. A rose-colored, acid stain.

Endocrine. Refers to the endocrine method of secretion of ductless glands. A gland of internal secretion.

Endocytosis. Uptake by a cell of particles too large to diffuse through its wall. Includes phagocytosis and pinocytosis.

Ergastoplasm. Rough endoplasmic reticulum or (usually) its light microscopic appearance.

Exocrine. Secretion by means of a duct system as in an exocrine gland (cf. endocrine).

Exocytosis. The discharge of particles from a cell. The opposite of endocytosis.

Extralobular duct. Refers to exocrine gland ducts not located within the gland lobule. Includes interlobular and interlobar ducts.

Fenestrated. Pierced by small openings, such as fenestrated capillaries.

Fibroblast. A connective tissue cell that makes collagen and certain components of ground substance.

Frugivorous. Eating or subsisting on fruit.

Ganglion. A collection of nerve cell bodies located outside the central nervous system.

Goblet cell. A unicellular gland found in large numbers in the epithelia of the digestive and respiratory tracts. Secretes a lubricating mucous in tubular organs or ducts.

Golgi apparatus. A system of membranes, vesicles, and vacuoles in which secretory product is formed. Located adjacent to the nucleus (sometimes perinuclear) of all cells.

Golgi membranes. Individual membranes, or stacks of membranes, belonging to the Golgi apparatus.

Ground substance. Substance filling in spaces between cells and fibers of the connective tissues. Contains variable amounts of water, polysaccharide, nutrients, and other organic and inorganic components.

Hematoxylin. Used as a basic stain following exposure of the tissue to a mordant.

Herbivorous. Eating or subsisting on a vegetable diet.

Histochemistry. Specifically refers to chemical reactions in cells and tissues involving or yielding colored compounds that can be assessed with the light microscope.

Holocrine. A method of secretion in which the entire cell, along with its stored substances, disintegrates to form the secretion.

Hyaluronic acid. An acidic polysaccharide found in ground substance.

Inclusion. A lifeless or temporary constituent of the cell, such as secretory granules, fat droplets (cf. organelle), etc.

Infranuclear. Basal to the nucleus.

Insectivorous. Eating or subsisting on insects.

Intercalated duct. A small diameter duct interposed between acinus and striated duct in the submandibular and parotid glands.

Intercellular canaliculus. A basalward extension of the lumen between adjacent acinar cells.

Intercellular tissue space. A "space" filled with tissue fluid located between acinar cells, across which acinar folds interdigitate. In salivary glands it closely approximates intercellular canaliculi but is not confluent with them.

Interlobar duct. Specifically, a duct located between lobes of salivary glands.

Intermediate junction. A member of the junctional complex. A zonula adherens.

Interstitial. Located between parts, usually in the stroma between parenchymal elements.

Intralobular duct. A duct within the lobule, such as intercalated and striated ducts.

Intramural. Within a wall. Specifically used in reference to minor salivary glands.

Ion. An atom or group of atoms having a positive charge (cation) or negative charge (anion).

Junctional complex. A group of attachment devices that includes a desmosome (macula adherens), an intermediate junction (zonula adherens), and a tight junction (zonula adherens).

Lamella. A leaf or platelike projection.

Light cell. Specifically refers to lightly stained cells in salivary gland ducts (cf. dark cells).

Lipofuscin. A lipid body of the cytoplasm containing dissolved pigment. Sometimes referred to as "wear and tear" pigment. A residual body found in older cells.

Lumen. A cavity or channel lined by an epithelium.

Luminal surface. The epithelial cell surface adjacent to a lumen.

Lysosome. An organelle surrounded by a single membrane and containing acid hydrolases.

Macula adherens. A type of attachment device between cells; a desmosome.

Main duct. The largest duct of an exocrine gland into which the smaller ducts empty. Main ducts of salivary glands carry secretions to the oral cavity.

Merocrine. A type of secretion in which the secretory cell remains intact; no cytoplasm is lost with the secretory product.

Microfilament. Specifically, a threadlike, fibrous protein of the cytoplasm.

Microtubule. A cylindrical, hollow-appearing structure of the cytoplasm measuring *ca.* 200 angstroms in diameter and of indefinite length.

Microvilli. Small fingerlike processes projecting from free surfaces of a cell.

Minor salivary glands. Small groups of salivary glands embedded in the wall of the oral cavity.

Mitochondrion. An organelle surrounded by a double membrane with cristae projecting into its matrix from the inner member of the double membrane. Most of the energy needs of the cell are provided by the mitochondria.

Mixed gland. Specifically, a gland containing mucous and serous acini.

Monostomatic. A term applied to a salivary gland with one main duct (cf. polystomatic).

mRNA. Messenger RNA. A species of RNA conveying genetic information to ribosomes.

Mucin. A glycoprotein. Specifically, a product of secretory epithelia composed of a protein core and carbohydrate side chains.

Mucosubstance. A general term including sialomucins and sulfomucins.

Mucus. The noun form (adj. mucous) referring to the viscous properties of secretions containing mucin.

Mucous acinus. An acinus (or tubule) whose principal secretory product is mucin.

Myoepithelial cell. A contractile cell located between the basement membrane and the bases of secretory cells of ectodermal origin.

Nerve ending. The terminal portion of a neuron containing synaptic vesicles and located in close association with another cell.

Neutral polysaccharide. A polysaccharide with a neutral charge. The molecule is periodic acid Schiff positive and alcian blue negative.

Organelle. A living part of the cell necessary for normal function (e.g., mitochondria, Golgi apparatus).

Parenchyma. The functional part of an organ as opposed to its supportive elements.

Parotin. A factor extractable from parotid glands reported to possess hormonal properties.

Periodic acid Schiff. Specifically, a histochemical stain demonstrating the presence of 1–2 glycols (cf. alcian blue).

Pinocytosis. Cell drinking. The means of taking liquids into a cell by vesicle formation.

Plasma membrane. The unit membrane surrounding a cell.

Plastic section. A section of tissue embedded in a plastic medium and cut thinner (usually one micron or less) than is possible with paraffin embedding.

Polystomatic. Having more than one main duct.

Postganglionic. Second order autonomic neurons whose cell bodies lie in a ganglion.

Preganglionic. First order autonomic neurons whose cell bodies lie in the central nervous system.

Protein core. Specifically, the protein component of a mucin molecule.

Proximal. Close to, or toward, the embryologic origin of a gland. Thus the acinus of a gland is the most distal segment, whereas the main duct is most proximal.

Pseudostratified. Specifically, an epithelium having the appearance of a many layered structure. It is not truely stratified because all cells rest on the basement membrane.

Ptyalin. An older term denoting salivary amylase.

RER. Rough endoplasmic reticulum (ergastoplasm).

RNA. Ribonucleic acid.

Reticular fiber. A type of collagen fiber associated with higher levels of polysaccharide which is argyrophilic. It is present in basement membranes, certain lymph organs and, to a lesser extent, in most connective tissues.

Ribosome. Ribonucleoprotein particles concerned with protein synthesis.

Rough endoplasmic reticulum. A system of membranes studded with ribosomes and enclosing cisternae.

Secretion. A product of a gland derived from its secretory epithelium.

Secretion granule. A discrete, saccular inclusion containing secretory product.

Secretomotor. A term describing the activity of autonomic nerves supplying glands.

Secretory zone. The distal or supranuclear area of an acinar cell.

Septum. A dividing wall or a partition.

Seromucous. A cell or acinus producing a combination of serous and mucous secretions.

Serous acinus. An acinus producing a watery, nonviscous secretion.

Sialic acid. Also neurominic acid. A nine carbon amino acid sugar.

Sialography. Radiographic demonstration of salivary gland ducts.

Sialomucin. A mucin in which some of the carbohydrate side chains contain a molecule of sialic acid.

Smooth endoplasmic reticulum. A system of cytoplasmic membranes without attached ribosomes.

Striated duct. A portion of the intralobular duct system of salivary glands. They are highly developed in the submandibular glands.

Stroma. The supportive elements of an organ (cf. parenchyma).

Supranuclear. Distal or apical to the nucleus.

Synaptic vesicles. Vesicular structures (300–500 angstroms in diameter) located in nerve endings. They are involved in neurotransmission.

Tight junction. A zonula occludens. The most distal member of the junctional complex.

Tissue fluid. Fluid derived from blood and lymph, containing dissolved nutrients and cellular metabolites.

Tissue space. A potential space containing tissue fluid. An intercellular space.

Toluidine blue. A basic dye.

Transfer vesicle. A vesicle thought to transfer materials from the RER cisternae to the Golgi apparatus.

tRNA. Transfer RNA. A type of RNA involved in transporting amino acids to sites of peptide formation on the ribosomes.

Tubule. An elongated structure containing a lumen and lined with an epithelium.

Ultrastructure. Those structures that can only be resolved with the electron microscope.

Zonula adherens. An intermediate junction. A member of the junctional complex.

Zonula occludens. A tight junction. A member of the junctional complex.

SUGGESTED READINGS

Babkin BP: Secretory mechanisms of the Digestive Glands. Paul B. Hoeber, Inc., New York, 1950.

Burgen ASV, Emmelin, NG: Physiology of the Salivary Glands. Edward Arnold, Ltd., London, 1961.

Riva A, Motta G, Riva-Testa F: Ultrastructural diversity in secretory granules of human major salivary glands. Am J Anat 139: 293–298, 1974.

Shackleford JM, Wilborn WH: Structural and histochemical diversity in mammalian salivary glands. Ala J Med Sci 5: 180–203, 1968.

Tandler B: Ultrastructure of the human submaxillary gland. I. Architecture and histological relationships of the secretory cells. Am J Anat 111: 287–307, 1962.

Tandler B: Ultrastructure of the human submaxillary gland. III. Myoepithelium. Z Zellforsch 68: 852–863, 1965.

Tandler B, Erlandson RA: Ultrastructure of the human submaxillary gland. IV. Serous granules. Am J Anat 135: 419–434, 1972.

Tandler B, Denning CR, Mandel ID, Kutscher AH: Ultrastructure of human labial salivary glands. I. Acinar secretory cells. J Morph 127: 383–408, 1969.

Wilborn WH, Schneyer CA: Ultrastructural changes of rat parotid glands induced by a diet of liquid Metrecal. Z Zellforsch 103: 1–11, 1970.

Wilborn WH, Schneyer CA: Effects of postganglionic sympathectomy on the ultrastructure of the rat parotid gland. Z Zellforsch 130: 471–480, 1972.

2 Mechanisms of Secretion of Saliva

RICHARD P. SUDDICK

FRANK J. DOWD

Introduction: An Initial Perspective on Secretion
History of Investigations of Salivary Secretion
Physiological Secretion: Oral Reflexes and Nerve Pathways
Energetics of Secretion
Gland Structure and Innervation
Vascular Elements
Innervation
Sympathetic Effects on Vasculature
Sympathetic Effects on Myoepithelial Cells
Autonomic Effects on Acinar and Ductal Cells
Protein Secretion
Background
The Secretory Cycle
Simple Proteins and Glycoproteins
Structure of Secretory Granules
Timing of Granule Formation
The Terminal Secretory Event: Exocytosis
Role of β-Adrenergic Stimulation in Protein Secretion
Cyclic AMP: Intracellular Mediator in the Secretory Process
Protein Kinase
Role of Transmethylation in Exocytosis
Possible Sequential Enzymatic Events in Exocytosis
Terminating or Controlling the Secretory Cycle

Function of Calcium in the Secretory Process
Summary of Events Leading to Protein Secretion
Fluid and Electrolyte Secretion
Saliva: A Hypotonic Fluid
The Energetics of Fluid Secretion
Micropuncture Studies
A Recent Hypothesis of Fluid Secretion: Vascular Events
Fluid Transfer Channels
Hypotonic Saliva: Result of a Transepithelial Countercurrent Mechanism
Experimental Evidence Relative to Hypothesis of Fluid Secretion
Source of Experimental High Secretory Pressures
Evidence of Hemodynamic Changes in the Glands
Evidence for Fluid Transfer Channels
Evidence for Cellular Site of Water and Electrolyte Secretion
Other Observations Related to the Hypothesis
Evidence for Direct Generation of Hypotonic Fluid Through Gap Junctions
Summary
Resting Secretion
Eating Reflex Secretion
Glossary
Suggested Readings

INTRODUCTION: AN INITIAL PERSPECTIVE ON SECRETION

The secretion of saliva may be viewed in two ways. One is that salivation is a specific homeokinetic response of specialized organs (salivary glands) which enable terrestrial animals to chew and swallow food. The salivary glands accomplish this by producing a relatively large and continuing supply of dilute electrolyte fluid (on the order of 1 to 3 ml./min. of whole saliva in the human adult), which contains glycoproteins or mucins whenever food enters the mouth. This rather "slippery" fluid facilitates the chewing and swallowing of food by its lubricating qualities and, in humans, salivation also facilitates the ability to speak. Young rats deprived of the three major pairs of salivary glands by extirpation or duct ligation gain weight much more slowly than their littermate, sham-operated brethren and drink much more water during periods of eating, perhaps in an attempt to compensate for the loss of the natural lubricant, saliva.

Salivary glands also secrete when the oral receptors are not being overtly stimulated by eating or other activities. This state is known as "resting secretion" and the flow rates from the glands in the human may be 50 to 100 times less than the oral reflex-elicited secretion stimulated by chewing food. The receptors that elicit resting secretion in human beings lie at least in part outside the oral cavity. It has been found that the normal, steady rate of resting secretory flow from the parotid glands, which is characteristic for each individual, will decline and virtually cease when the individual is blindfolded or placed in a completely darkened room. Apparently photic stimulation of retinal receptors provides at least a necessary background reflex stimulus for human parotid gland resting secretion. Thus while we are awake and alert, our salivary glands are secreting at a more or less continuous slow rate of flow. This resting flow plays a major role in maintaining the health of the oral and pharyngeal mucosal epithelia, as well as the preservation of an optimal environment for maintenance of the teeth. The specific constituents of this fluid and the mechanisms involved in these vital functions of saliva are subjects of Chapters 3 and 4. In the context being discussed, however, we may view resting secretion as the second and per-

haps the more important of the homeokinetic responses of the salivary glands in maintaining homeostasis in intact animals, including the human being. While the eating reflex response of the glands is undeniably a burst of dramatic activity and energy, resting secretion procedes continuously while we are awake and provides the necessary fluid environment to maintain optimum health of the oral mucosa and teeth. The importance of this function cannot be overstated. Individuals who have suffered the loss of salivary glands or secretion through radical surgery or radiation therapy usually become jeopardized secondarily by deterioration of the mucous membranes of the mouth and throat, and/or carious destruction of teeth, leading at times to severe life threatening infections.

History of Investigations of Salivary Secretion

Until the past few years, the major investigative interests in the salivary gland field have been the mechanisms of fluid and electrolyte secretion, and the mechanisms of protein secretion. The great interest in fluid and electrolyte secretion is documented by the excellent reviews of this subject which have appeared in the Handbook of Physiology and other scientific journals (See Suggested Readings). Perhaps a major reason for the devoted attention to this subject over the years lies in the fact that saliva from the major salivary glands of nearly all species which have been examined is markedly hypotonic to other bodily fluids. Investigators have considered it a great challenge to unravel the mechanisms by which the glands are able to elaborate such a fluid.

The interest in protein and glycoprotein secretory mechanisms also has a long history. Over the past few years there seems to have been greater interest and work in this area, while published investigations of fluid and electrolyte secretion have declined in frequency. However, the greatest share of published investigative interest in the salivary gland field in recent years has been in the make-up and functions of the fluid itself, particularly in the molecular identification of specific proteins and glycoproteins and how they function in oral homeostasis. This is the subject of Chapter 3 of this book.

Physiological Secretion: Oral Reflexes and Nerve Pathways

It is important to note that physiological secretion is the result of autonomic reflexes with receptors located primarily in the oral cavity. There is good evidence that stimulation of mechanoreceptors and chemoreceptors located in the oral cavity, pharynx, nasopharynx, and nose will elicit salivary secretion. Some of the mechanoreceptors involved in secretion are touch and pressure receptors located widely throughout the mucous membranes in the mouth, but concentrated largely in the tongue and palate. The chemoreceptors involved are taste buds in the tongue and palate primarily, and the olfactory sense organ in the nose. Other mechanoreceptors that elicit secretion when stimulated are proprioceptors in the jaw muscles and sensory endings around the roots of the teeth. Mechanical (or electrical) stimulation of pulpal nerve endings will also elicit secretion. Thus, the sensory modalities and surface areas involved in the physiological stimulation of salivary secretion are, respectively, diverse and large.

The efferent pathways regulating physiological secretion involve both divisions of the autonomic nervous system: sympathetic and parasympathetic. This is an important concept. In the rest of this chapter the reader will encounter discussions of many experiments in which one or the other of the respective receptors of these autonomic nerves have been stimulated by drugs (α- or β- adrenergic (sympathomimetic) or cholinergic (parasympathomimetic)) or by electrical stimulation of the appropriate efferent nerves. However, in the real life (physiologic) situation, the animal, whether rat, cat, or human, in chewing food stimulates sensory receptors which cause vollies of impulses to be sent to the salivary glands via both parasympathetic and sympathetic nerves. This undoubtedly results in a wide array of efferent nerve receptors being activated in cells of the salivary glands; cholinergic, and α- and β-adrenergic receptors located on secretory cells, myoepithelial cells, and vascular smooth muscle cells. It is also likely that a complex modulation of these receptor responses occurs within the glands during prolonged reflex activity, mediated by the release of ions or other cellular products from the secretory cells. The overall result is a more or less steady flow of hypotonic electrolyte fluid containing predominately sodium, potassium, chloride and bicarbonate ions and an array of proteins and glycoproteins, the functions of which we are only beginning to understand. The point to be made here, however, is that our current state of understanding of the mechanisms of salivary secretion have come about by studies in which investigators have examined and analyzed the secretory effects of stimulation of specific autonomic efferent receptors on salivary gland cells either by use of the appropriate autonomic drugs or by stimulation of the appropriate efferent nerves. We are now beginning to be able to piece together, often times by inference, the overall events which occur in the salivary glands during normal reflex secretion.

Energetics of Secretion

The means by which the major salivary glands are able to produce on demand abundant and seemingly unlimited quantities of saliva has intrigued physiologists for well over 100 years. During the middle years of the nineteenth century the great French scientist, Claude Bernard, conducted numerous investigations of the salivary glands and salivary secretion. Bernard is generally considered to be the father of modern physiology. He was the first to investigate the relationship of salivary gland blood flow to secretion. As many investigators have done since, Bernard observed the venous blood outflow from the gland when the nerves to the gland were electrically stimulated. Bernard's observations are much more descriptive than the style of scientific writing permits today. He remarked that the venous outflow became so vigorous that it reflected the arterial pulse, and that the venous blood from the gland during this interval became more reddish in hue such as to resemble the arterial blood.

Experiments conducted by another famous physiologist, Carl Von Ludwig, during these same years were more penetrating in concept and enduring in effect. In 1850, Ludwig presented to the Natural History Society of Zurich the results of these experiments and they were published in the same year. Over the years since, the promulgation and interpretation of these startlingly simple experiments by successive generations of physiologists have resulted in the establishment of a dogma about the mechanisms underlying the secretion of saliva that have persisted unchallenged until very recently.

Ludwig connected a cannula from the excretory duct of the dog submandibular gland to a mercury manometer and monitored systemic arterial pressure from the femoral artery by the same means. When he stimulated the chorda tympani nerve to the gland, the gland secreted a volume of fluid sufficient to raise the column of mercury to a pressure which was somewhat above the recorded arterial pressure. From this Ludwig deduced that the energy for secretion was derived from the gland itself and not from the vascular pressure generated by the heart. He believed, in other words, that secretion was *not* analogous to the ultrafiltration of plasma by the glomerulus of the kidney. This conclusion was remarkably prescient and discerning considering that it predated virtually all knowledge of cell biochemistry by more than one half-century and specific knowledge of active transport processes and exocrine gland exocytosis by about 100 years. Unfortunately Ludwig's conclusion appears to have been in error in at least the totality of his generalizations. As indicated, however, the error now lies more in the manner in which physiologists have continued to reiterate Ludwig's conclusions with little or no additional critical experimentation.

Philosophers have long recognized a natural tendency of man to try to create order by applying simple principles and unified concepts to explain complex phenomena. We have introduced here one of the more prominent and interesting examples of this tendency in the field of physiology, (i.e. the promulgation of the basic concept of secretion which Ludwig initiated), that has subsequently developed into a widely accepted but seldom explicitly stated dogma. This dogma is that salivary secretion *in toto* is a product of the metabolic activity of the secretory cells, these cells providing *all* of the energy for secretion of the proteins, electrolytes and water of the secretory fluid. As will be discussed fully later in this chapter, there is now reason to believe that this concept may be erroneous. While there is no doubt that the energy for protein secretion comes from the metabolic processes of the acinar cells, recent evidence indicates that the major source of energy for fluid and electrolyte secretion may, indeed, reside in the hydrostatic pressure differential across the secretory epithelium which originates in the vasculature of the gland. Thus, to present an overall viewpoint of both the energetics involved and the composition of the fluid itself, secretion may be considered as a two compartment model. Particulate secretion is one of these compartments, and the energy for secretion of particulates (i.e. proteins and glycoproteins, and perhaps certain ions) is derived from metabolic processes occurring within the secretory cells. Fluid and electrolyte secretion constitutes the other compartment. The energy for fluid and electrolyte secretion is derived from energy generated by the pumping of the heart. To coin terms for this distinction, we might say that the energy for protein secretion is *endocellular* in origin, while that for fluid and electrolyte secretion is *exocellular* in origin. This would reserve for traditional usage the terms *intracellular* and *extracellular* to apply to description of volumes and chemical compositions of these two respective fluid compartments.

To gain an initial perspective on the processes of secretion associated with the anatomical and histological structures discussed in the following pages, it may be useful to picture the secretory parenchyma as a number of functional units composed of sheets of epithelial cells tightly bound to each other and rolled into a blind-ended tube. A very large number of these tubes make up a major salivary gland. The contents of each tube in any part of the gland are always separated from the interstitial fluid and plasma within the gland by this continuous layer of cells. The processes of secretion involve two principal activities. One is the biosynthesis of protein and glycoproteins within the cells of the tubes and the export of these products into the lumen. This undoubtedly occurs predominantly in the acinar cells at the closed end of the blind tube. The other process involves the transfer of water and electrolytes across the continuous sheet of cells into the lumen of the tube. This probably occurs to some degree concurrently with protein secretion in the acini. However, we suggest that the primary site for fluid and electrolyte secretion is in the secretory tubules (i.e. striated ducts, and granular ducts, perhaps also in other intralobular ducts distal to the striated ducts). The main point here is that these are two completely distinct homeokinetic mechanisms occurring simultaneously which together constitute the secretory process. Energy which drives the first of these mechanisms is endocellular in origin, while the driving energy for the second is exocellular.

GLAND STRUCTURE AND INNERVATION

Before attempting to understand secretory mechanisms readers should have a basic understanding of the structure of salivary glands and their innervation. The following descriptions represent only the bare rudiments of these complex subjects. Furthermore, we describe these structures in a general way, but the reader should realize there are variations from gland to gland and from species to species. For a more detailed presentation see Chapter 1.

When discussing secretion there are three basic structures to consider, the *acinus* (pl., acini), the *intercalated ducts* and the *secretory tubules* or *ducts*. In addition, there are other intraglandular ductal elements which are thought to serve mainly as conduits to the excretory ducts.

The **acinus** is a ball of cells which, when cut in section, shows large pyramidal cells arranged in a circle around a minute lumen (Fig. 2-1). The narrow portion of the cell facing the lumen is the *apex*. The membrane bordering the lumen is the *apical membrane*. The opposite pole of the cell facing the interstitial fluid is known as the *basal portion*. The outer cell membrane is known as the *basal membrane*. The lateral membranes of adjacent cells lie close to each other and near the basal pole of the cell they are tightly joined by structures known as *desmosomes* (also referred to junctional complexes, subcategorized as tight junctions and gap junctions). During secretory activity the lateral membranes become less closely apposed to each other giving the appearance of channels or canaliculi. We will refer to these channels as *canaliculi* when they are continuous with the lumen. From the lumen they appear to course between the cells, but only as far as the tight junctions at the base. Thus, it appears that substances may enter the lumen of the acinus by being extruded from the cells at the apical membrane; by coursing through the cells passing through both basal and apical membranes; by moving between the cells through the tight junctions and canaliculi; and, finally, by moving through the lateral membrane into

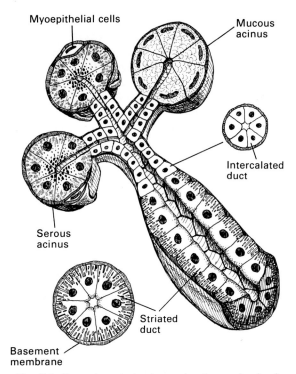

Fig. 2-1. Parenchymal structures of salivary glands. A composite drawing showing the types of parenchymal elements and cells found in salivary glands. Structures shown here are those which would be found at the most distal (i.e., "distal" from the excretory duct at the entrance or hilus of the gland) parts of the secretory parenchymal tree, and all can be considered to be "secretory structures" in that they contribute in some respect to the secretory product of the gland. The cluster of three acini in the figure shows two serous acini and one mucous acinus emptying, via the short intercalated duct segment, into a striated duct. In actual sections, coalescence of several acini into a common duct is rarely observed, and it is improbable that serous and mucous acini ever empty into a common duct. Not shown are larger downstream ductal structures, the intra- and interlobular collecting ducts, all of which empty into a central excretory duct. Walls of these larger ducts become successively thicker eventually composed of several flattened epithelial cell layers. For a detailed review of the histology of salivary glands see Chapter 1.

the canaliculi and then into the lumen. Several of these events or processes must occur during physiological secretion.

The intercalated ducts are composed of small cuboidal cells with few remarkable or highly characteristic cytological features. They are connected to the secretory tubules which in turn join the intralobular collecting ducts. The latter collect fluid from other secretory tubules within the lobule before joining an interlobular duct or ducts which in turn, at the hilus, empties into the extraglandular excretory duct. The latter carries the secretions from the gland to the oral cavity.

In humans the major salivary glands develop as invaginations of the oral epithelium beginning about the sixth week *in vitro*. The simple epithelial infolding gradually deepens and branches in a tree like manner. In some species (e.g., rat) the glands of a newborn lack acini; the acinar elements develop during the first few weeks after birth from tree-like buds from the terminal ends of the intercalated ducts. Thus, the intercalated ducts from several acini join at one secretory tubule.

The secretory tubules are composed of tall columnar epithelial cells (20 to 30μ from luminal border to base) with distinctive cytological features. Several different types of cells occur in the secretory tubules, and these tubules have been subcategorized according to the appearance of the two main types of cells. One has a characteristic striated appearance in the basal portion, probably due to a heavy concentration of mitochondria visible when viewed with the light microscope. These make up the striated ducts. The other is known as the granular duct cell because of the appearance of numerous granules predominantly in the apical half of the cell. The secretory ducts of the parotid glands of man and many other species appear to be composed entirely of striated ducts, whereas the secretory ducts of the submandibular glands of many mammals including man contain both granular and striated cells, both arranged as distinctive segments. The granular duct segment in these circumstances lies closest to the acini.

These different ductal cells also possess apical, basal, and lateral borders and membranes. Thus, as was pointed out above, any substance which enters or leaves the ductal structures must either pass through the cells or between the cells via the tight junctions for secretion into the lumina of the acini.

Vascular Elements

The blood vessels in the salivary glands run parallel to the ductal-acinar tree of the secretory parenchyma. Branching of intraglandular arteries and veins occurs as the excretory ducts are followed from the hilus. In the rat submandibular gland each ductal branch off the intraglandular excretory duct(s) is accompanied by one artery and two veins. Similarly,

each secretory tubule is supplied by one artery and two veins, all running parallel to the tubule. In the striated duct region, numerous capillaries cross the tubule transversely, forming an actual gridwork around the duct. This ductal network becomes more sparse as more distal tubular regions are reached. The intercalated ducts and acini appear to be served by a common capillary bed consisting of long terminal capillary loops which vary in their proximity to the different structures. Blood returns from this bed and the separate striated duct capillary bed via the two veins mentioned above. The point at which these veins originate has not been ascertained.

Other vascular structures of interest have been observed in rat and guinea pig submandibular glands. Both of these species appear to have a central system of arteriovenous anastomoses in anatomical studies, but physiological studies have failed to substantiate this. In the guinea pig and rabbit valves have been observed in the veins which drain the separate lobes of gland. These structures have very significant implications regarding secretory mechanisms, but there have been very few studies of salivary gland vasculature, and virtually none from a comparative viewpoint.

Innervation

Nerve endings or terminals can be observed on cells throughout the glands on both parenchymal cells and blood vessels. The main branches of the intraglandular nerve fibers follow the course of the vessels, breaking up into terminal plexuses in the connective tissue adjacent to the terminal portions of the parenchyma. Nerve bundles, consisting of unmyelinated axons embedded within Schwann cell cytoplasm, are distributed to the smooth muscle of the arterioles, to the acinar cells, to myoepithelial cells, and possibly to the intercalated and striated duct cells.

The secretory cells receive their innervation by one of two patterns, *intraepithelial* and *subepithelial*. In the intraepithelial type, the axons split off from the nerve bundle and penetrate the basal lamina that lies adjacent to or between the secretory cells. The site of innervation (neuroeffector site) is considered to be at varicosities of the axon which contain small vesicles and mitochondria. A single axon may have several varicosities along its length making contact with one secretory cell or with two or more cells. The vesicles are believed to contain the chemical neurotransmitters norepinephrine and acetylcholine and presumably release them by an exocytosis-like process. The membranes of the axon and secretory cell are separated by a space of only 100 to 200 Å, but no specializations of the secretory cell membranes have been detected at these sites.

In the subepithelial type of innervation, instead of penetrating the basal lamina, the axons remain associated with the nerve bundle in the connective tissue. Where the nerve bundles approach the secretory cells, some axonal varicosities lose their covering of Schwann cell cytoplasm. Presumably these bared varicosities are the sites of transmitter release from the vesicles. These neuroeffector sites of the axons are separated from the secretory cells by 1000 to 2000 Å, and the transmitters must diffuse across this space, which includes the nerve bundle and the basal lamina of the secretory cells. It is also conceivable that neurotransmitters released above the basal lamina may affect vascular networks that lie in this same tissue space or compartment.

Both divisions of the autonomic nervous system participate in the innervation of the secretory cells. In some glands both sympathetic (adrenergic) and parasympathetic (cholinergic) terminals have been observed in proximity to the acinar cells. These terminals are distinguished by special fixation and cytochemical techniques. The adrenergic terminals are further distinguished on the basis of the underlying receptors, (i.e., some being α—receptors and others β—receptors). From the pharmacologic viewpoint, these receptors can be explained in the most simple terms as follows. The α—receptor can be conceived of as the receptor most responsive to epinephrine or norepinephrine and less sensitive to isoproterenol. It is blocked by phenoxybenzamine, phentolamine (Regitine) and other classical α—blocking agents. Beta—receptors, by contrast, are most responsive to isoproterenol and least responsive to norepinephrine. They are blocked by propranolol, pronethalol and other blocking agents. The parasympathetic nerves affect target cells in both acini and ducts, and receptors on these cells mediate cholinergic (more precisely muscarinic) effects on fluid and electrolyte secretion. On the other hand sympathetic (adrenergic) nerve

endings tend to be concentrated more in the vicinity of acinar cells compared to ductal regions. Protein secretion is due primarily to acinar cell function. The predominant effect of secretory sympathetic activity is on protein secretion, and sympathetic nerve activity (in animal studies in which the sympathetic nerves can be isolated) is characterized by a secretory product of high protein concentration. However, the effects of sympathetic activity are numerous and include many distinct actions which probably have an influence on secretion.

Sympathetic Effects on Vasculature

Sympathetic innervation is evident in the vasculature of the glands. The adrenergic receptors are characteristically α in type. Thus sympathetic stimulation of salivary glands is characterized by a reduction in blood flow through the gland due to vasoconstriction as is characteristic of many other vascular beds. The relative effect of sympathetic-induced generalized vasoconstriction on secretion is not known with certainty, but such an effect may be secondary to other sympathetic influences as explained below.

Recent research indicates that some β-adrenergic receptors may also be present in salivary gland vasculature. In the rat submandibular gland increased blood flow, presumably by vasodilation, occurs when α-adrenergic blocking agents are administered prior to sympathetic stimulation. This vasodilation is abolished by a β-adrenergic antagonist. Despite this interesting phenomenon however, β-receptor mediated vasodilatation is an unknown entity as far as its effect on secretion is concerned. (The effects of the parasympathetic nerves on the vasculature is considered later in this chapter.)

Sympathetic Effects on Myoepithelial Cells

Sympathetic nerves also affect myoepithelial cell function. These cells are closely associated with acinar cells. The adrenergic receptors on myoepithelial cells are α in type and stimulation of the sympathetic nerve leads to contraction of these smooth muscle cells. The effect of this process may actually be measured *in vivo*, by measuring glandular ductal pressure increases upon nerve stimulation. This effect can be seen using nerve stimulation techniques (i.e., a single shock or impulse) which do not elicit secretion. In these cases the pressure increases in salivary ducts are attributed to actual squeezing of the ends of ducts by the myoepithelial cells rather than to an increase in volume due to secretion.

Autonomic Effects on Acinar and Ductal Cells

Alpha- and β-receptors, as well as cholinergic receptors, are present on acinar cell membranes. Beta-receptor stimulation is largely responsible for protein secretion from acinar cell secretory granules. Alpha—receptor stimulation on the other hand, leads to a much different response with far less protein secretion, at least in the majority of experiments conducted to date. Cholinergic (muscarinic) receptor activation leads to considerable fluid and electrolyte secretion but only modest protein secretion. These differences in autonomic control over secretion are discussed in this section and in the following pages.

Some secretory effects of stimulation of cholinergic receptors and α-receptor stimulation have distinct similarities and it is likely that they are mediated in part by a common biochemical pathway which is distinct from that mediating β-adrenergic effects. However, certainly not all effects of α-adrenergic stimulation and cholinergic stimulation on salivary glands are the same. In fact, copious secretion is elicited by cholinergic (muscarinic) stimulation, whereas far less fluid secretion occurs with α-adrenergic stimulation. Furthermore, some investigators have shown the α- and β-receptor stimulation have a cooperative effect in promoting protein secretion in at least some salivary glands. The most obvious distinguishing characteristic between β-receptor stimulation on the one hand, and either α-adrenergic or cholinergic receptor stimulation on the other, is the nature of the secretory product and the biochemical pathways leading to the observed effect.

The overall physiologic effect of this complex array of nerve influences on salivary glands is one in which sympathetic nerve stimulation modifies rather than reverses the effects of parasympathetic nerve stimulation. In effect, sympathetic nerve stimulation, largely through β-receptor activation, leads to enhanced protein secretion and, therefore, modifies the secretory product of parasympathetic stimulation. The predominant tone of the salivary gland is parasympathetic. Intuitively, this is of functional value since maximum parasympathetic effects are characterized by large volumes of secretion, whereas, maximum sympathetic effects are not. In addition, without parasympathetic effects, sympathetic stimulation (especially β) would conceivably lead to clogging of the salivary ducts due to a high protein and low water content. Although sympathetic nerve stimulation also leads to α-receptor stimulation in salivary glands, the β-receptor appears more sensitive than the α-receptor. As a result, at low levels of adrenergic stimulation, β-effects are probably predominant. In summary, salivary glands have a dual autonomic innervation with variable sympathetic secretory effects due to the presence of both α- and β-adrenergic receptors.

Physiologic studies indicate that acinar cells respond to both sympathetic and parasympathetic stimulation; each response is associated with specific and different changes in the acinar membrane potentials. The innervation of duct cells is not as clear. Intraepithelial terminals in ducts have been observed only rarely, but histochemical studies suggest that cholinergic and adrenergic nerves are found in the connective tissue around the ducts. Physiologic studies of changes in membrane potentials and ion exchanges indicate that the ductal system is responsive to autonomic stimulation or administration of autonomic drugs. A few investigators have suggested that the copious secretion seen with parasympathetic nerve stimulation is due largely to activation of cholinergic receptors in this ductal region of salivary glands.

Motor control of secretion resides in the salivary center in the medulla. This center contains two distinct nuclei, the superior and inferior salivary nuclei. Afferent impulses to the salivary center may arise from normal stimuli associated with eating. Both chemoreceptor and mechanoreceptors are involved; chemoreceptors in olfaction and taste, and mechanoreceptors, which sense pressure and movement of the jaw during chewing. Pain and irritation of the oral tissues and pharynx will also stimulate secretion.

In summary, the processes of secretion involve two principal activities both of which are under strict neural control. One is the biosynthesis of protein and glycoproteins within the cells of the gland and the export of these products into the lumen. The other involves the transfer of water and electrolytes across the continuous sheet of epithelial cells into the lumen. These are two completely distinct biologic processes and they may in fact occur at different sites along the parenchymal tube. Under physiologic conditions, both processes occur simultaneously. This is also true during certain experimental conditions, such as electrical stimulation and pilocarpine stimulation. Stimulation of most mammalian salivary glands electrically via either the sympathetic nerves, on the one hand, or the parasympathetic nerves on the other, produces distinctly different salivary secretory effects. Sympathetic stimulation produces a thick viscous fluid, but very little of it. Stimulation of the parasympathetic nerves on the other hand produces a profuse flow of a watery electrolyte containing secretion, and this flow continues as long as the parasympathetic nerves continue to be stimulated. It is interesting to note that the salivary glands, in contrast to the pancreas, have not often been used as a model for demonstration of the distinctly different nature of these two secretory processes. In the pancreas the gastrointestinal hormones, Pancreozymin-CCK and Secretin, can be used to demonstrate this fact. Pancreozymin-CCK stimulates a low-volume secretion with high protein (enzyme) content while Secretin causes a profuse watery secretion high in bicarbonate content but low in enzyme content. In the salivary glands electrical stimulation of the sympathetic nerves or the parasympathetic nerves, respectively, produces salivary secretory effects which are somwhat analogous to these different hormonal effects. Parasympathetic nerve stimulation, however, often elicits substantial protein secretion along with the copious flow it produces.

The cellular and glandular phenomena which are associated or involved with these two secretory processes will be discussed and explained on the following pages with the mechanisms which underlie protein secretion being covered first, followed by a discussion of the mechanisms involved in fluid and electrolyte secretion.

PROTEIN SECRETION

Background

Much of the knowledge of exocrine gland protein secretion comes as a result of work on the synthesis and secretion of proteins in the pancreas. A good deal of this information was derived by following the incorporation of radioactive-labeled amino acids into protein microscopically, the subsequent cellular transport of these macromolecules, their condensation into secretory granules, and the eventual emptying of these granules into the lumen (exocytosis). Salivary glands, particularly the parotid, bear many similarities to the exocrine pancreas, and much of what is known about pancreatic protein secretion also applies to salivary gland secretion. The present discussion results from a synthesis of our general knowledge of exocrine glands applied specifically to salivary glands.

It is important to keep in mind that there are significant structural and biochemical differences between mucous type and serous type salivary glands. Most of the information on protein secretory mechanisms is derived from serous glands. Despite this precaution the basic elements of the protein secretory mechanisms in both types of glands have many similarities. Many of the basic concepts therefore, apply to mucous glands as well as serous glands. This appears to be particularly true for one of the most important and readily observable activities occurring during protein secretion, an activity best described as secretory granule formation or "packaging" of proteins and glycoproteins.

A major task of salivary glands is to organize proteins into forms which will enable their ready secretion on demand. Serous type glands do this by packaging them into membrane-bound secretory or zymogen granules. These are spherical sacks about 1.0 μm in diameter which contain a high concentration of protein (see Fig. 2-2). Mucous type glands contain mucin droplets which also act as secretory organelles. Secretion takes place by a process of extrusion of the granule contents. Important events precede the packaging of

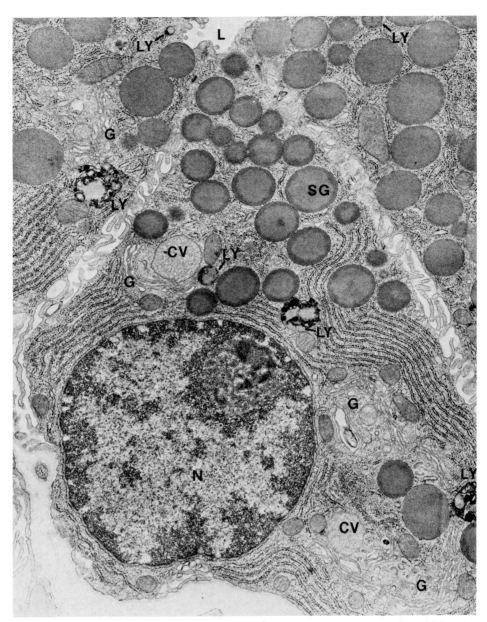

Fig. 2-2. Portions of three parotid acinar cells from an *ad libitum* fed rat. The acinar lumen (L) is at the top of the figure. Six lysosomes (LY) can be recognized in this figure. The Golgi apparatus (G) is extensive in these cells, and usually one or more condensing vacuoles (CV) are present. Parallel arrays of endoplasmic reticulum are prominent in the basal portion of the cell, while shorter segments course irregularly between the secretory granules in the apical regions. The secretory granules (SG), although exhibiting some slight variation, are homogeneously electron-dense. × 14,000. (Reprinted with permission from: Hand, AR "The effects of acute starvation on parotid acinar cells. Ultrastructural and cytochemical observations on *ad libitum* fed and starved rats." (Am. J Anato 135: 71, 1972)

proteins into granules. Some of these events are basic to protein synthesis as a general process in all cells, while other events appear to be specialized phenomena peculiar to protein secretory cells, (i.e., cells which synthesize and organize specific proteins and glycoproteins for export). With respect to those proteins which are synthesized for export, all of these events, basic and specialized, must be considered together as a series of cell functions required to secrete proteins. We will refer to these collective events henceforth as the (protein) secretory cycle. The culmination of the secretory cycle is the extrusion of the contents of the secretory granules from the cell, a process termed **exocytosis**. In effect, exocytosis *is* protein or glycoprotein secretion.

The Secretory Cycle

The basic processes by which messenger RNA is synthesized using DNA as template, and by which the protein synthetic machinery is regulated at the ribosomes, take place in much the same manner whether the protein is destined for secretion or not. Some differences in location of synthesis may exist. After this, however, the fate of the secretory proteins is unique and complex. The transport and packaging of secretory proteins involves a number of intracellular membrane structures resulting in the movement of the secretory protein from one site to another. The transport of protein progresses from the basal or contraluminal portion of the cell near the nucleus to the apical or luminal portion near the extrusion site or lumen.

Protein synthesis takes place on ribosomes which are attached to membranes arranged in sheets concentrated largely in the basal half of the acinar cell. This entire structure is called the rough endoplasmic reticulum (RER). The RER membrane sheets have enclosed spaces between them called cisternae. Following synthesis, secretory protein is segregated from non-secretory protein by being sequestered in the cisternal space. Entry into this space is made possible by *signal peptides* which enable the protein destined for secretion to penetrate the membrane of the endoplasmic reticulum. These peptides act then as segregators of secretory protein. Lysosomal proteins may also enter the same pathway. Proteins then migrate within the cisternal space to terminal areas within that space. These terminal areas are called transitional elements.

At this point the membranes of the transitional elements begin to bud off from the rest of the RER and become totally enclosed vesicles. This process at some point requires metabolic energy. Next, a complex association of proteins takes place in which the products of budding from RER appear to become part of the Golgi complex. Membranes in the Golgi

combine to form a third distinct structure called the condensing vacuole which is distinct in that it is similar in size but less dense than the final product, the secretory granule. Secretory protein is handled during this entire process so as to be included within the confines of these limiting membranes within the cell, in order: the RER, the transitional elements, the Golgi, the condensing vacuole and the secretory granule. Metabolic energy may be required for conversion of Golgi elements to condensing vacuoles, but evidence to support this theory is lacking.

If protein synthesis is blocked with drugs, proteins including secretory proteins, will not continue to be formed. However, all of the described processes of secretory granule formation, and protein secretion itself, continue uninhibited until protein is depleted. This illustrates that the packaging and secretion of proteins are separate processes from protein synthesis. As one would expect, the rate of protein synthesis is governed largely by the requirement for new protein, (i.e., by the rate of protein secretion). This ensures an adequate supply of protein for the demands of secretion.

Simple Proteins and Glycoproteins

Proteins secreted by exocrine glands, including salivary glands, represent various kinds. They can be arbitrarily divided into two types, simple proteins and conjugated proteins. *Simple proteins* are proteins with no chemical components other than amino acids. *Conjugated proteins* are proteins which contain components other than amino acids. One class of such proteins that is an important constituent of salivary gland secretions, particularly those from mucous glands, is glycoprotein. The molecular structure of glycoproteins is a protein core with side chains comprised of carbohydrate moieties branching off the protein core. During synthesis of these molecules, the protein core is constructed first followed by addition of single carbohydrate components to form carbohydrate side chains of various lengths.

The manner in which glycoproteins are synthesized in salivary gland cells has been the subject of recent research. The protein cores are synthesized in the RER in much the same manner as simple secretable proteins. In many cases the initial carbohydrate components are also attached to these cores in the RER. However, the major carbohydrate synthetic process takes place at a location outside the RER. Using radioactive-labeled monosaccharides which are utilized in the synthesis of glycoproteins, it has been shown that many of these sugar components are chemically attached to the glycoprotein molecule in the region of the Golgi. This is further indicated by the fact that enzymes responsible for catalyzing the conjugation of monosaccharides to protein to form glycoproteins have been identified in the Golgi region.

Other chemical additions can also occur after synthesis in the RER is completed. It has been shown, for instance, that addition of sulfate to various secretory products also takes place in the Golgi region. Thus, significant synthetic activity responsible for production of secretory material continues even into the Golgi region.

Structure of Secretory Granules

Conversion from condensing vacuoles to mature secretory granules involves a noticeable increase in density of the structures as seen in the electron microscope. This is due in part to an aggregation of protein. Presumably condensing vacuoles also continue to acquire protein once they are formed. This would account for the higher density of the secretory granules compared to condensing vacuoles of similar size. Golgi may continually contribute secretory protein to pre-existing condensing vacuoles resulting in an increase in the amount of protein present in the vacuole. Microscopically the membrane border of the condensing vacuole is rough whereas that of the mature secretory granule is smooth. This is consistent with the relative amount of protein present in each structure. Thus, tight aggregation of protein permits compression of the limiting membrane, giving the secretory granule a smooth spherical appearance.

Secretory granules can actually be isolated intact from salivary gland tissue. Parotid glands have been extensively used in these procedures. The granules are usually about 1.0 μm in diameter possessing a complete limiting membrane about 80 to 100 Å thick. The limiting membranes look very similar to plasma membranes with their three-layered structure. Over 95 per cent of the total protein of secretory granules is exportable (secretory

protein) whereas the remainder is membrane-associated. Alpha amylase is the secretory protein of highest occurrence in most parotid gland tissue and it is commonly used as an indicator both of secretory granule contents and secretory product. An electron microscopic picture of an unstimulated rat parotid acinar cell is given in Figure 2-2.

Timing of Granule Formation

By using radioactive amino acids it has been shown that in the exocrine pancreas the radioactive label follows an ordered temporal sequence from synthesis into protein at the RER to maturation of secretory granules. Under experimental conditions the label reaches a peak in the Golgi at about seven minutes after addition of a labeled amino acid, and is present in mature secretory granules by 80 minutes. The formation and packaging of secretory product, therefore, is able to take place within that time period. This aspect has not been as extensively researched in salivary glands, but the time frame for secretory granule formation is, in all probability, similar.

The Terminal Secretory Event: Exocytosis

Secretion of protein is ultimately realized when secretory granule contents are discharged into the lumen of salivary gland ducts. This process is termed exocytosis and is by no means unique to salivary glands. The key event is the fusion of two membranes, secretory granule membranes and plasma membranes. This fusion is followed by a conversion of the double membrane into one common membrane separating lumen from granule content, and then fission of the common membrane structure resulting in the expulsion of granule content into the lumen. This process is characterized as a "fusion-fission" event and necessitates the close approximation of secretory granules with the apical portion of the plasma membrane. Figure 2-3 shows a scheme of important events in protein secretion.

Intracellular structures are located in an ordered arrangement with the basal to apical progression generally being in the same order as the progression of the "packaging" events, (i.e., RER → Golgi → condensing vacuole →

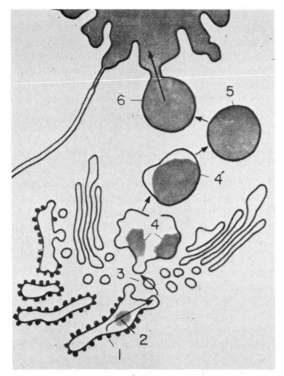

Fig. 2-3. Schematic representation of the pancreatic acinar cell. The postulated sequence of events from synthesis to discharge of secretory proteins is indicated by the numbers and arrows. (1) Synthesis on the bound ribosomes of the rough endoplasmic reticulum and discharge into the cisternal space. (2) Intermediary aggregation as "intracisternal granules" which is observed only under particular conditions of starvation and refeeding. (3) Transport via small smooth surfaced "Golgi vesicles" which bud from the transitional elements of the rough endoplasmic reticulum. (4) Accumulation within condensing vacuoles. (4) Condensation within condensing vacuoles. (5) Storage as mature zymogen granules. (6) Discharge to the acinar lumen. (Tartakoff, AM, Greene, LJ, Jamieson, JD, and Palade, GE: Parallelism in the processing of pancreatic proteins. In Ceccarelli, B, Clementi, F, and Meldoles, J: Advances in cytopharmacology. vol 2. p 180, New York, Raven Press, 1974)

secretory granule → apical plasma membrane). As expected the secretion of older secretory granules precedes that of newer ones. As secretion takes place granule membrane becomes one with plasma membrane and the acinar or tubular lumen enlarges at the expense of cell volume. The "oldest" secretory granules, which are located closest to the apical plasma membrane, are the first to interact with the apical plasma membrane and their contents are the first to be secreted.

After secretion of a large amount of protein, (e.g. after isoproterenol administration)

the lumen of the salivary gland acinar unit is much larger than in the resting state, and often shows several circular profiles due to incorporation of secretory granule membranes. The extent of enlargement of the lumen or invagination into the acinar cells is directly proportional to the strength and duration of the secretory stimulus. Acinar cells appear to be essentially depleted of secretory granules after only a few (e.g. 30) minutes of maximal stimulation.

Microscopically, communication between and fusion of adjoining secretory granules is not often seen in serous glands of most species. However, this probably occurs with greater frequency in mucous droplets of mucous glands than in secretory granules of serous type glands. Thus the interaction appears to be specific in that secretory granule membranes interact to the greatest extent with apical plasma membrane sites and to a lesser extent, or not at all, with other granule membranes or plasma membranes on the internal lateral aspects of the acinar cells.

The definitive molecular trigger for the fusion event is not known, but recent research indicates that specific sites on either plasma membranes of granule membranes (or both) become available when the gland is stimulated to secrete. Some investigators have shown, for example, that secretion by certain secretory cells is accompanied or preceded by a clumping or aggregation of membrane-bound proteins away from sites of fusion in both plasma membranes and secretory granule membranes. It has been postulated that this exposes lipid elements of both plasma membranes and secretory granule membranes so that they are attracted to each other and fuse.

Another area of recent speculation is the role of microtubules and microfilaments in secretion. There is indirect evidence that either or both of these structures may function in exocytosis. Microfilaments are composed of contractile proteins, principally actomyosin, which are positioned near plasma membranes and appear to act as a network for controlling cell shape or for supporting specialized contractile activities of the cell. Microtubules are somewhat larger in diameter than microfilaments and appear to form a cytoskeleton. Disruption of the microfilaments by drugs reduces parotid gland protein secretion under certain conditions. It has been proposed that microtubules act as the framework through which secretory granules travel during protein secretion, while microfilaments aid in a contractile process associated with secretion.

These speculations are consistent with previously discussed membrane changes during secretion, because microtubules or microfilaments could induce the process of membrane fusion by promoting close proximity between plasma membranes and membranes of secretory granules. This area has been the subject of recent speculation. However, further evidence is needed before microtubules or microfilaments can be considered as full participants in secretion.

Under certain circumstances, exocrine glands can secrete protein in the absence of sizable numbers of secretory granules. In these cases protein secretion appears to continue even after degranulation. Thus it has been proposed that protein secretion is possible without the mediation of secretory granules. Furthermore, it is possible that secretion, even in the presence of secretory granules, takes place by extrusion or movement of protein from granule to cytoplasm and then to the lumen of the duct. This, of course, would reduce the importance in the secretory process of direct membrane interaction between secretory granules and plasma membranes. It is conceivable that intervening microtubules and/or microfilaments could also play a role in such an indirect route of secretion. While it remains to be proven that fusion of plasma membranes and secretory granules account for a major part of protein secretion, microscopic evidence is overwhelming that the process of exocytosis, involving membrane fusion, plays a dominant role in protein secretion when secretory granules are present. A minor alternate pathway may operate in the absence of secretory granules and/or concurrently, in parallel with exocytosis.

Secretion is followed by a conservation of at least part of the secretory granule membrane for use in synthesis of new membranes. Secretory granule membranes appear to be constructed from both recently synthesized and older components. It is not known to what extent this conservation of membrane material involves digestion of old membranes but in all likelihood membrane components are preserved by pinching off vesicular portions of the enlarged acinar lumen, and fragments from these vesicles are again utilized for gran-

ule production at the level of the Golgi complex. Microscopic evidence is consistent with this theory in that small vesicles located near the lateral aspects of the apical plasma membrane are observed during the post secretory or recovery phase. Lysosomes may play a role in digesting membrane material for resynthesis (see Fig. 2-2). Conservation of all membrane proteins does not seem to occur to the same extent, however, and therefore reutilization of membrane material appears to be somewhat of a selective process.

Role of β-Adrenergic Stimulation in Protein Secretion

It has been mentioned that the effect of β-adrenergic stimulation on the parotid acinar cell is distinctly different from that of α-adrenergic stimulation. Beta-adrenergic stimulation is associated with heightened protein secretion, far surpassing that seen with α-adrenergic stimulation. Alpha-adrenergic stimulation is associated with its own set of acinar cell responses. In addition to these differences, the internal cell machinery for producing the appropriate responses is quite different when comparing α- and β-adrenergic stimulation. The previous discussion on the dynamics of protein secretion relates very closely and characteristically to the β-adrenergic response in parotid acinar cells.

It can be seen in Figure 2-4 that certain cellular changes, such as vacuole formation, occur with stimulation of the α-receptors but are not apparent with β-receptor stimulation. Rapid release of intracellular potassium also occurs with α-receptor stimulation in the parotid gland but this effect is likewise not observed with β-adrenergic stimulation. These facts further emphasize the uniqueness of β-adrenergic effects relative to α-adrenergic effects in the parotid gland.

One key biochemical response characteristic of β-adrenergic stimulation is a discernible increase in intracellular cyclic AMP (cAMP). Alpha-adrenergic stimulation, or for that matter cholinergic stimulation, is *not* accompanied by such changes in cAMP. Receptor specificity can also be demonstrated by the fact that β-adrenergic receptor blockage by β-adrenergic antagonists (e.g., propranolol) abolishes the effects of the β-receptor agonist on both secretion and cAMP synthesis. The

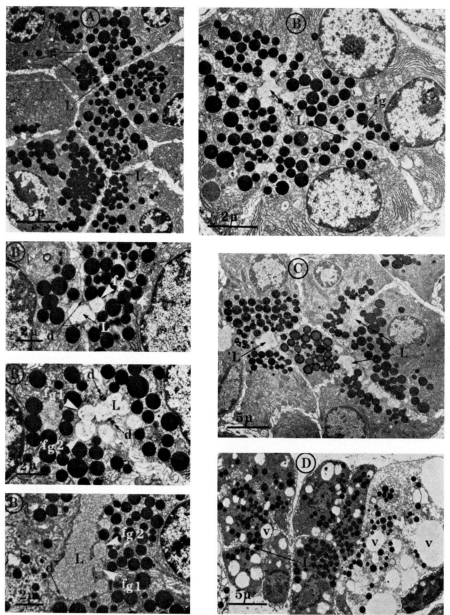

Fig. 2-4. Ultrastructural changes in rat parotid slices caused by isoproterenol butyryl cAMP and phenylephrine. **A.** control slices have been incubated for 10 minutes in absence of hormone. Groups of cells situated around a common lumen (L) are seen. The lumen appears empty and small, about the size of a secretory granule (g). **B.** B_1, B_2, B_3, slices have been incubated for 10 minutes in presence of 20 μM isoproterenol. **B,** the lumen (L) is filled with secretory material and is already quite enlarged as compared to A. The lumen appears to have grown through fusion with the secretory granules (fg). B_1, B_2, B_3, detail of lumens fused with secretory granules. fg1 and fg2 are secretory granules fused in sequence to the lumen. The desmosomes (d) delineate the cell borders which form the common lumen. **C.** slices have been incubated for 20 minutes with 1 mM butyryl cAMP. The structural changes resemble those obtained with isoproterenol. Enlarged lumens filled with secretory material are seen. **D.** slices have been incubated for 10 minutes in presence of 20 μM phenylephrine. In contrast to isoproterenol and butyryl CAMP, phenylephrine causes appearance of numerous vacuoles (V) which distort the shape and structure of the cells. The *right side* of the micrograph shows extensive vacuolization which appears to have destroyed the major cellular structures. A few constricted lumens can be observed (Batzri, S, Selinger, Z, Schramm, M et al.: Potassium release mediated by the epinephrine α-receptor in rat parotid slices. Properties and relations to enzyme secretion. (J Biol. Chem. 248: 365, 1973)

increase in intracellular cAMP seen with β-adrenergic stimulation is in turn associated with protein secretion. In fact, secretion of protein from the parotid acinar cell can be elicited by cAMP itself. (Experimentally, more lipid soluble derivatives like dibutyryl cyclic AMP are used because they can more easily penetrate into the cell than cAMP, and they are not as readily metabolized as cAMP.) Microscopic evidence for the effects of isoproterenol, cAMP, and phenylephrine (an α-adrenergic agonist) on rat parotid acini is shown in Figure 2-4.

Cyclic AMP: Intracellular Mediator in the Secretory Process

There is now abundant evidence that cyclic AMP plays a key and broad role in cell function. In addition to carbohydrate and lipid metabolism where its role has been established, cyclic AMP may mediate specific events which relate to a variety of cell functions including secretion by salivary glands. Most of the evidence relating protein secretion and cAMP is derived from the parotid gland and to a lesser extent from serous submandibular glands. Conclusions regarding cAMP may or may not apply in the same manner to mucous submandibular secretory units or to sublingual glands. Since the parotid glands from various species are often quite similar, the role played by cAMP in the parotid gland may be generally applied. Future evidence may support a common mechanism of cAMP-mediated secretion for virtually all salivary glands.

The use of salivary gland slice systems, (i.e., an experimental procedure in which salivary glands are sliced into small fragments and incubated under various experimental protocols) and a more recently developed technique using dissociated acinar cells or cell clumps has led to a good deal of the information available concerning salivary gland secretion and the role of cAMP. In such tissue slice and cell systems stimulation of parotid gland β-receptors by the appropriate drug, hormone or neurotransmitter leads to stimulation of the activity of adenylate cyclase, the enzyme responsible for catalyzing the synthesis of cAMP from ATP (Fig. 2-5). This response is dose related, (i.e., increasing the concentration of the agonist leads to a greater rate of synthesis of cAMP).

Adenylate cyclase is localized in plasma membranes and is susceptible to influences by β-adrenergic receptor neurotransmitters or agonists. (β–receptors also reside in the plasma membrane.) The exact nature of the connection between adenylate cyclase and the β-receptor is unknown although they appear to be distinct sites within the membrane. The β-receptor is influenced by agents external to the cell while adenylate cyclase faces the internal aspect of the cell where ATP is available and where cAMP is discharged. This arrangement allows substances external to the cell to alter intracellular cAMP levels (see Fig. 2-5).

Since cAMP mediates the action of a number of hormones and other substances it is often termed the "second messenger". In the body a message is sent via the release and distribution of the appropriate hormone or

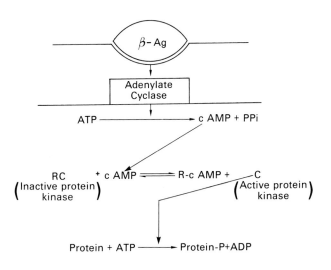

Fig. 2-5. Sequence of events from β-receptor occupation to protein phosphorylation. Beta receptor agonists (β-Ag) stimulate adenylate cyclase activity in the plasma membrane. Adenylate cyclase catalyzes the formation of cyclic AMP (cAMP) and pyrophosphate (PPi) from ATP. Cyclic AMP in turn stimulates the enzyme protein kinase. Protein kinase is composed of two types of subunits: regulatory subunits (R) and catalytic subunits (C). The enzyme is inactive in the associated form (RC). By combining with the regulatory subunits, cyclic AMP dissociates the two types of subunits of the enzyme and permits the catalytic subunits to express themselves. Active protein kinase (the catalytic subunit) then catalyzes the phosphorylation of protein (Protein-P) leading to an appropriate response.

neurotransmitter (first messenger) whose message is translated to yield an increase in intracellular cAMP (second messenger) concentration. The same effect takes place when β-receptors are stimulated in acinar cell membranes of the parotid gland. The message of the agonist is translated to a rise in cAMP, with cAMP in this case acting as the mediator of protein secretion. The concentration of cAMP directly parallels the rate of protein secretion. Furthermore, the increase in cAMP appears temporally to precede or coincide with the protein secretory response. Bypassing the receptor is possible *in vitro* by the use of cAMP (dibutyryl cAMP). Administration of dibutyryl cAMP is accompanied by a prompt protein secretion not blocked by β-receptor antagonists. Dibutyryl cAMP stimulated protein secretion is not increased beyond maximal β-receptor stimulated levels (i.e., by β-receptor agonists) even when no antagonist is present. Collectively this is good evidence for a common pathway for protein secretion elicited by both cAMP and β-adrenergic agonists and supports the theory that cAMP is the second messenger for parotid gland protein secretion.

Protein Kinase

The most obvious influence of cAMP on salivary gland protein secretion is on the final event, exocytosis. While the exact mechanism is speculative, it is known that virtually all of the effects of cAMP in mammalian tissues are mediated via its action on the enzyme cAMP-dependent protein kinase, referred to here as simply protein kinase. Protein kinase is available to interact with cAMP since it appears to be present both in the soluble cell fraction (cytoplasm) and in membrane structures. This enzyme is markedly stimulated in the presence of cAMP (see Fig. 2-5). Protein kinase is responsible for mediating the effect of cAMP on carbohydrate and lipid metabolism in cells and quite likely on a whole host of other cellular functions. One area of recent research interest has been the interaction of protein kinase with membranes and the possible control of some membrane functions by protein kinase. This includes protein secretion by salivary glands.

The reaction catalyzed by protein kinase is the phosphorylation of a protein using ATP as phosphate donor (Fig. 2-6). Several proteins have been shown to act as substrates for pro-

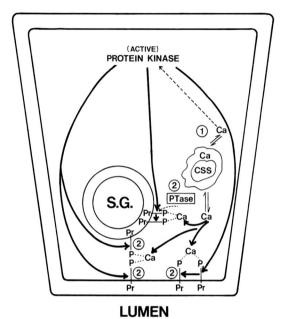

LUMEN

Fig. 2-6. Possible sequence of events leading to protein secretion by the parotid acinar cell after activation of protein kinase. Arrows refer to the stimulation or inhibition of reactions. Activated protein kinase catalyzes the phosphorylation of specific proteins at membrane sites. Intracellular calcium dynamics may be changed by protein kinase activity at some intracellular calcium storage site allowing redistribution of calcium to areas critical for secretion. Phosphoproteins aggregate as a result of calcium mediation (possibly as ionic bridges) permitting fusion of the membranes and exocytosis. The numbers in circles represent two possible control points in the process (i.e., places where secretion can be inhibited or modified). ① Calcium may also play a physiological role as a negative feedback modifier of secretion, inhibiting protein kinase, thus making a discrete secretory stimulus self-limiting. ② Phosphatases may catalyze the hydrolysis of phosphoesters resulting in removal of phosphate groups from membrane proteins. Many other possible control points exist but are not pictured. Abbreviations: CSS, calcium storage site(s); –P, state of phosphorylation; Pr, protein; PTase, phosphatase; SG, secretory granule; ⟶, stimulatory for protein secretion; ⟶, inhibitory for protein secretion; ⇌, reversible calcium interaction with calcium storage sites. (Calcium release from these sites is shown to be both stimulatory and inhibitory for secretion.)

tein kinase including some located in plasma membranes and in membranes of secretory granules. Although identification of these substrates alone does not prove physiologic significance, there remains a strong possibility that protein kinase plays an integral role in secretion. The fact that ATP seems to be required for protein secretion is consistent with this proposed role of protein kinase.

Just exactly how phosphorylation of membrane components could lead to membrane fusion, fission, and secretion is only a matter of speculation at the present time. Phospholipids in the membranes may play a role in the secretory process, but protein kinase does not appear to influence phospholipid phosphorylation. Since protein kinase directly interacts only with *protein* substrates, proteins must be considered instrumental in any effect protein kinase may have on secretion. Phosphorylation catalyzed by protein kinase, for instance, may lead to aggregation of proteins within and/or between membranes (see Fig. 2-6). This would be consistent with previous indications of membrane protein aggregation during the secretory process and an increase in attraction of the membranes involved. Phosphorylation would therefore be the trigger for membrane fusion due to interactions of specific membrane proteins.

Protein kinase may also catalyze the phosphorylation of a protein component(s) of the microtubule or microfilament network. By so doing, and there is some evidence for this, the phosphorylation mechanism could stimulate a change in the state of aggregation of the microfilaments or microtubules. This in turn could promote the migration of secretory granules to the plasma membrane secretory sites.

Role of Transmethylation in Exocytosis

Another enzymatic reaction which appears to play an important role in exocytosis is one that transfers a methyl group from S-adenosyl-L-methionine to the carboxyl side chains of proteins. The enzyme involved in this reaction was first discovered in the pituitary gland and reported as a methanol-forming enzyme. Subsequent studies have shown that the methanol-forming enzyme is actually a protein carboxyl-methylase (PCM; S-adenosyl-L-methionine: protein carboxyl-O-methyltransferase, EC.2.1.1.24). The transmethylation reaction results in the neutralization of negative charges on the protein substrates. Protein-methyl esters are unstable at physiological pH and temperature and undergo rapid hydrolysis to yield methanol.

The enzyme, PCM, is widely distributed in the body. *In vivo* and *in vitro* studies have suggested a role for PCM in exocytotic secretion in the adrenal medulla, pituitary gland,

and parotid gland. Recent studies on the parotid gland of rats have centered on the effects of β-adrenergic stimulation on PCM activity, amylase secretion, and the cellular distribution of PCM and methyl acceptor protein (MAP) substrates. The results show a rapid and reversible increase in both PCM activity and MAP capacity following stimulation of the parotid gland by isoproterenol. Injection of this β-adrenergic agonist causes a rapid secretion of amylase, a significant increase in PCM activity, and a significant increase in the methyl acceptor capacity of the parotid proteins (MAP capacity).

The molecular weight of the methyl acceptor proteins appears to be less than 25,000, but subcellular localization of MAP's in the parotid has not yet been determined. In the adrenal medulla, however, the largest MAP capacity has been localized in the chromaffin granules, whose contents are also secreted by exocytosis. In the parotid, the time course of the increase in PCM activity and MAP capacity associated with isoproterenol administration matches the time course of amylase secretion, suggesting a relationship to the process of exocytosis.

The inner surface of cell membranes and the outer surface of secretory granules are both negatively charged which creates an electrostatic barrier to contact. This would inhibit fusion of the granule-limiting membrane and the inner surface of the plasma membrane. There is evidence that the negative charge on granules is due to carboxyl groups of proteins. Methylation of these groups would reduce the electrostatic barrier and favor fusion of the granule and plasma membranes. The same phenomenon may explain the distinct separation between secretory granules that is nearly always evident in micrographs of serous secretory cells. By the same token, it also raises questions about the observed differences between serous granules in serous cells and the mucous droplets observed in mucin secretory cells. The latter are usually observed in a crowded or compacted condition with limiting membranes apparently touching and often indistinct.

Possible Sequential Enzymatic Events in Exocytosis

These findings concerning the protein carboxyl-methylase enzyme and methyl acceptor proteins in parotid glands raise a question concerning a possible relationship of trans-methylation to the protein kinase-mediated phosphorylation mechanisms discussed in detail above. It is conceivable that both of these enzyme-mediated reactions are necessary to bring about exocytosis. The reactions may occur concurrently or sequentially. A plausible explanation can be presented for sequential reactions. Elimination or reduction of the electrostatic barrier between granules and plasma membrane would be a logical first step permitting approximation of the membranes. This process would then be followed by the kinase-mediated phosphorylation reaction which may signal the fusion and fission events resulting in release of granule contents into the lumen. However, an equally plausible picture can be presented for concurrent reactions, with the protein kinase mediated phosphorylation reactions being primarily *intramembranous*. This would "clear" certain membrane lipid areas of protein and permit fusion of the granule and plasma membrane lipid layers. Apposition of these membranes would occur as a result of reduction of the electrostatic barrier by the concurrent CPM-mediated transmethylation reaction.

Terminating or Controlling the Secretory Cycle

Physiologic requirements dictate that not only must there be control over the initiation of the secretory cycle but also continuing control of the events after initiation. This includes in particular the ability to terminate the process. Relative to cAMP and protein kinase, there are several potential control points that may regulate the protein secretory process. Termination of the secretory process may take place by way of the phosphodiesterase enzymes, which break down cyclic nucleotides, (e.g., cAMP). Secondly, a specific protein which inhibits protein kinase has been isolated from some tissue and such a protein, although apparently not in high concentrations in the parotid gland, may also control protein kinase activity in salivary glands. Still another possibility is that phosphatases could account for a reduction in the secretory rate by removing phosphate from specific proteins and thus reversing the process catalyzed by protein kinase. Finally, more subtle mechanisms may

retard or halt the secretory process such as inhibition of adenylate cyclase activity; compartmentalization of critical secretory stimulating agents; a reduction in ATP; and changes in intracellular electrolytes. It has been suggested in fact that loss of intracellular potassium and/or loss of intracellular cyclic AMP due to vacuolization (both α-adrenergic effects) may account for the rapid retardation of protein secretion seen when α- and β-receptors are stimulated simultaneously. Conceptually any of these mechanisms could prevent complete elimination of secretory protein from the cell except under conditions of maximal β-adrenergic stimulation. It must be remembered, however, that while there are ample possibilities for control of the secretory process once initiated, it is impossible at the present to be more precise as to their relative importance in salivary gland function.

Mention should be made of another cyclic nucleotide which is normally present in mammalian tissue, cyclic GMP. Its role in protein secretion appears doubtful but has been implicated in mediating some of the effects resulting from cholinergic and α-adrenergic stimulation of salivary glands. These effects may include the low level of protein secreted when those receptors are stimulated. Suffice it to say that cyclic GMP may mediate some secretory events by mechanisms that bear resemblence to cyclic AMP's action. Compared to cyclic AMP however, much less is known about its function in cell processes.

Function of Calcium in the Secretory Process

Not only is calcium present in the secretions, but it probably plays a significant role in the structure and content of the secretory granules. It is also an important modifier or regulator of both protein secretion and fluid and electrolyte secretion. Aggregation of protein within secretory granules appears to be due in part to the presence of calcium. Calcium may play a key role in establishing complexes of proteins required for filling condensing vacuoles and maturation of secretory granules. It is widely known that salivary glands contain high levels of calcium especially within secretory granules. A large component of calcium is secreted in parallel with protein and some is tightly bound to protein.

It has been shown that extracellular calcium (at millimolar levels) is required for certain cholinergic (muscarinic) and α-adrenergic parotid gland effects and has a major influence on fluid and electrolyte secretion. Cyclic AMP, on the other hand, appears to have its major influence in mediating β-adrenergic effects on protein secretion. Calcium and cAMP to this extent regulate separate functions and do so relatively independently. Another important difference between calcium and cAMP is that for many cholinergic and α-adrenergic effects at least some calcium must enter the cell when the cell is appropriately stimulated, whereas cyclic AMP is synthesized totally within the cell.

Salivary gland acinar cells (at least in the parotid gland) can effectively secrete protein for some time without *extracellular* calcium; this β-adrenergic effect, therefore, does not require the presence of extracellular calcium. This does not rule out the need for *intracellular* calcium for protein secretion, (e.g., from calcium stores in mitochondria, endoplasmic reticulum, or other locations). In fact, intracellular calcium, as opposed to extracellular calcium, appears to influence protein secretion in the parotid gland.

Several possible intracellular calcium effects exist. Calcium could be required for the membrane fusion or fission process by acting at some membrane site predisposed to calcium influences by the action of protein kinase. Such interaction could involve a redistribution of membrane protein, perhaps with calcium acting as an ionic bridge between phosphorylated proteins. On the other hand, in much the same way calcium could regulate the degree of aggregation of microtubules and/or microfilaments. When one considers that protein kinase has profound influences on calcium distribution in many tissues, it would not be surprising to discover that the presence of calcium at key regulatory sites is required for exocytosis.

Calcium may also act as a *regulator* of protein secretion by inhibiting the process at certain discrete steps. Thus calcium could both stimulate and inhibit secretion depending on its intracellular location or concentration. Negative feedback loops are well known in a variety of biological systems. Calcium could act in such a capacity in protein secretion (i.e., calcium may not only act as an ionic bridge for exciting exocytosis but may also act

as a feedback inhibitor on the action of protein kinase). The consequences of this reaction imply that secretion of protein would have built in limitations via intracellular regulatory mechanisms. Therefore, duration of effective β-adrenergic stimulation of protein secretion may be limited by a negative feedback loop involving increased intracellular calcium concentrations. These possible control points are summarized in Figure 2-6.

Summary of Events Leading to Protein Secretion

Autonomic innervation controls salivary gland secretion. Cholinergic and α-adrenergic agonists mainly, but not entirely, control fluid and electrolyte secretion, whereas β-adrenergic agonists control mainly protein secretion. The secretory product reflects the relative degree of influence by each receptor type. Although protein synthesis is required for formation of secretory granules it is not required for the act of protein secretion as such. The protein synthetic mechanism resides in the ribosomes located in the rough endoplasmic reticulum (RER). Deposition of synthesized protein into the cisternae of the RER follows protein synthesis. From this point secretory product can be followed microscopically from terminal buds of the cisternae to condensing vacuoles via the Golgi complex. This procedure ensures packaging of secretory proteins and transport of these proteins to the apical or luminal aspect of the acinar cell. Maturation to the secretory granule from condensing vacuole takes place by concentration and aggregation of protein. Large concentrations of calcium are also stored in the granule and may aid in the aggregation process.

The secretory event itself consists of a process by which apical plasma membranes fuse with secretory granule membranes. This event is influenced by cAMP which mediates the action of β-adrenergic agonists on protein secretion in all likelihood by stimulating the enzymatic activity of protein kinase. A redistribution or aggregation of membrane protein may occur and may be mediated by a phosphorylation mechanism involving membrane proteins. Conceivably the aggregation could be either intramembraneous or intermembraneous (between granule membrane and cell membrane). Another enzyme-mediated reaction which seems to be involved is the methylation of membrane carboxyl groups catalyzed by protein-carboxyl methylase (CPM). The action of this enzyme could result in the neutralization of negative charges on the limiting membranes of the secretory granules and perhaps also on the plasma membrane which could eliminate or reduce an electrostatic barrier to fusion of granules and apical membrane. There is yet, however, no evidence indicating a concerted relationship between CPM and cAMP dependent protein kinase in salivary gland protein secretion.

The physical movement of the granules toward the apical cell membrane may involve microtubules and microfilaments. Microtubules may play a role in acting as channels for secretory granule movement, whereas microfilaments, by a contractile process, may physically move the granules to secretory sites. Another possible source of energy for granule migration, however, is simply the bulk flow of fluid through the acinar cell. (The means by which this may occur is explained in the following section of this chapter.)

Small amounts of intracellular calcium may be required for the protein secretory process acting for example as an ionic bridge between membrane phosphoproteins. Calcium may also be required for microtubule or microfilament function. The membrane fusion process is followed by a fission of the common membrane formed from the secretory granule membrane and plasma membrane. Extrusion of the content of the granule into the duct lumen follows.

Portions of the expanded plasma membrane are pinched off to preserve some components of the membrane for synthesis of new secretory granule membranes. Thus some components in the secretory process are reutilized for multiple secretory cycles.

Several possibilities exist for limiting and controlling the protein secretory process. These controlling factors could influence the action or net effect of protein kinase activity at membrane sites. Figure 2-6 shows several biochemical steps where reversal or inhibition of protein secretion may occur. In addition, a postulated negative feedback loop involving calcium is also plausible.

Finally, the acinar cell may possess alternate methods of secreting proteins. These processes may be operative in the absence of secretory granules or may utilize secretory granules as storage organelles only. Their contribution is probably minor under most physiologic conditions.

FLUID AND ELECTROLYTE SECRETION

Fluid and electrolyte secretion may be defined as the controlled transfer of water and electrolytes across the secretory epithelium into the lumen. Since a single gland will secrete much more than its own volume during an observed period of secretion, the source of the fluid of secretion is the blood supply to the gland. In addition, an electrically stimulated salivary gland will gain in volume, weight, and water content during an observed period of secretion. Such gains are brought about by fluid filtration from the glandular capillaries. While the blood supply is the source of fluid, this fluid is modified in its electrolyte content as it undergoes transfer across the secretory epithelium, and/or as it passes along the lumen of the tubules and ducts of the gland. Both of these processes probably operate to modify the electrolyte levels. Ultimately, energy-requiring transport mechanisms must be invoked to explain the electrolyte composition of the secretory fluid during normal physiologic secretion. In certain pathologic states, however, the electrolyte composition of the salivary glands becomes essentially plasma-like, suggesting a true ultrafiltration-like process unmodified by cellular transport phenomena.

Saliva: A Hypotonic Fluid

The great interest in saliva as a physiologic fluid arises in part from the fact that it is hypotonic with respect to the other fluids in the body, (i.e., plasma, interstitial fluid, lymph, aqueous humor, cerebrospinal fluid and the cytoplasmic fluid in cells in general). It has been of consuming interest to investigators to try to unravel the mechanisms by which these glands are able to elaborate a fluid that is hypo-osmotic to other body fluids. In human parotid saliva, for example, osmolarity rarely exceeds 120 mOsm per kilogram during the highest levels of physiologic secretion. Levels much lower than this predominate at lower levels of secretion, reaching values as low as 60 mOsm per kilogram. In comparison, the osmolarity of blood plasma is approximately 290 mOsm per kilogram. The major question is how salivary glands are able to elaborate a fluid across the tubular epithelial sheet and maintain it against this osmotic gradient.

The Energetics of Fluid Secretion

Major differences exist among modern salivary exocrinologists in their views of the energetics of fluid and electrolyte transfer across the secretory epithelium. Most investigators have continued to treat secretion of protein, electrolytes and water, (i.e., secretion *in toto*) as a cellular energy requiring continuum. These investigators continue to operate and interpret experiments within the framework of the dogma of secretion (cited earlier in the chapter) developed over the decades following the classical experiment of Ludwig. In modern terms they hold that fluid and electrolyte secretion is the result of active, metabolic energy-requiring mechanisms within the fluid secreting cell. Most would suggest that these energy requiring mechanisms involve the active transport of one or more of the major electrolytes (Na^+, K^+, Cl^- and HCO_3^-), that in turn provides an osmotic driving force for the transfer of water across the secretory epithelium. The osmotic pressure of saliva secreted from virtually any gland at virtually any rate of flow can be accounted for on the basis of the sum of the concentrations of Na^+, K^+, Cl^- and HCO_3^- (see Chap. 4). Thus, if active transport processes are responsible for an osmotic gradient which drives secretion, it would be reasonable to assume that it must be one or another or some combination of these four ions that is transported and responsible for fluid secretion.

The advent of the modern view of salivary fluid and electrolyte secretion occurred in the early and mid 1950's with the publication of studies on Na^+, K^+, Cl^- and HCO_3^- secretion in human parotid saliva. In these studies the secretory responses were produced by the parasympathomimetic drug methacholine. It was proposed that the final salivary electrolyte composition during normal secretion was the result of a two stage secretory mechanism. In the first stage it was suggested that a "primary secretion" was elaborated by the acini with a constant electrolyte composition irrespective of the degree of gland stimulation. In the second stage salivary electrolyte composition was

altered during passage of the primary secretion along the gland duct system by a process of sodium reabsorption, the reabsorption process having a transport capacity uninfluenced by gland stimulation. Together this two-stage mechanism would produce the hypotonic secretion. Evidence from the micropuncture studies conducted much later has been interpreted by many investigators to verify this concept. Further it has continued to be assumed by many that the energy to drive the primary secretion stems from the active transport of one or more of the four major osmolytes.

A few investigators have adopted a much different explanation for the energetics of fluid transfer. This explanation was first proposed in the form of a hypothesis to explain the results of a series of experiments on rats during which the influence of systemic and glandular vascular pressures on secretory pressures were measured while vascular pressures were manipulated. *The results of these experiments depart from current concepts of secretion by suggesting that the energy for fluid and electrolyte secretion is derived from a hydrostatic pressure differential across the secretory epithelium, extending from the vascular capillaries surrounding the epithelium to the lumen* (see A Recent Hypothesis, below).

Micropuncture Studies

The micropuncture techniques were first developed for studies of the contents of kidney tubules. They were adapted for use in salivary and sweat glands in the mid 1960's. The acini, intercalated ducts, and granular tubules occupy the most superficial layers of each glandular lobule, whereas striated ducts lie deep within the gland substance. According to experienced investigators, a micropuncture pipette can penetrate only to a depth of about 300μ below the gland surface before tip localization becomes impossible; thus it is not usually possible to micropuncture striated ducts. The excretory ducts lie almost wholly outside the glandular lobules so they can be seen quite readily. Since they are ensheathed in connective tissue, they are difficult to study by micropuncture but can easily be cannulated with fine bore polyethylene tubing which can then be passed for some distance along their length.

When a micropuncture pipette is inserted

into a salivary gland the tip can be localized if necessary by the injection of a small droplet of the colored oil. Using this technique, whenever the pipette has been found to lie not in a duct but in the interstitium, it has always proven impossible to aspirate a sample of fluid. This indicates that micropuncture samples are not of interstitial origin. It is also improbable that samples are composed of cell fluid since their volume (10^{-1}nl) is 100 to 1000 times greater than that of a single cell. Further, the samples have little protein in them, and their electrolyte composition also speaks against their having an intracellular origin.

If it is accepted that the micropuncture samples come from the lumen of the duct system, it is argued by the investigators that almost all samples must have come from acini or intercalated ducts (or granular ducts in the special case of the rat submandibular gland), since they feel that puncture of striated ducts is rarely possible. They argue further that a sample of volume 10^{-1}nl must come not from a single acinus or intercalated duct but from a number of intercalated ducts draining together (diameter of the intercalated ducts is 4-6μ) based upon the volume involved and the usual sample collection time (2-5 min).

The composition of the primary secretion studied by micropuncture in the rat submandibular, parotid, and sublingual glands, cat submandibular and sublingual glands, the rabbit pancreas, human sweat glands, the exorbital lacrimal glands, and thyroid acini of the rat are remarkably similar, having sodium concentrations of about 120 to 180 mEq/liter and potassium concentrations of about 5 to 18 mEq/liter. Of those glands in which the osmolality of primary fluid has been measured by freezing point determination, three (sweat glands, thyroid acini and immature rat submandibular glands) have primary secretions that are apparently hypertonic, while the primary secretion in the remaining two (rat submandibular and parotid glands) is isotonic. From their sodium, potassium, and chloride concentrations it may be inferred that the primary secretions of the rat sublingual and lacrimal glands are also isotonic.

The effect of artificial stimulation on the composition of the primary secretion has been studied in the rat submandibular (pilocarpine, carbachol and isoproterenol), the rat sublingual (carbachol), the rat parotid (pilocarpine), the cat submandibular, the cat sublingual (carbachol and isoproterenol), and the rabbit pancreas (pancreozymin and secretin). Pilocarpine, carbachol and isoproterenol have no significant effect on the sodium and chloride concentrations of the primary secretion of any salivary gland so far studied. In the rat submandibular the primary fluid potassium concentration after both carbachol and isoproterenol stimulation falls from values significantly greater than those in plasma to plasma-like values. In the cat submandibular this fall did not occur.

The general interpretation of the results of micropuncture experiments is that the acinus elaborates a primary secretory fluid that is isosmotic to plasma and isotonic in its major electrolyte content. This appears to be true regardless of the rate at which the primary secretion is elaborated. In contrast, the secretory fluid collected at the orifice of mammalian parotid and submandibular glands is markedly hypo-osmotic, and its electrolyte profile is much different from that collected by the micropuncture techniques at the intercalated ducts. Since the fluid collected from the latter sites is isosmotic to plasma, *the main interpretation of the micropuncture experiments is that the glands elaborate a primary isosmotic fluid in the acinus that is modified by subsequent resorptive processes as this fluid passes out through the striated ducts and the intraglandular excretory ducts.* It is further assumed that the tubular structures are relatively impermeable to water and that the resorptive processes are capable of extracting ions in excess of water molecules, thus rendering the fluid hypotonic. The ions that appear to be resorbed and cause the saliva to become hypotonic are sodium and chloride. In certain glands this type of evidence suggests that potassium is secreted by the tubules in at least a partial exchange for the resorption of sodium so that the potassium concentration, which is essentially plasma-like at the acinus (around 4 to 5 mEq/L), becomes more concentrated in the tubular structures, perhaps reaching values of 10 to 20 mEq/L. If all of the prior assumptions upon which these interpretations are based are accepted, then the micropuncture two-stage theory on secretion and electrolytes is perfectly reasonable. However, without any direct evidence it seems unwise to accept the major primary assumption that the acinus is the primary site for secretion of all the fluid entering the parenchymal tubules of the salivary glands during the complete range of physiologic-stimulated secretion.

A Recent Hypothesis of Fluid Secretion

The vascular pressure oriented experimental approach yields an hypothesis that includes both vascular and cellular events which are mediated primarily by the parasympathetic (cholinergic) nerves. These events enable the gland to develop high pressures in blood capillaries surrounding tubules which are secreting, and permit this pressure energy to be converted into the kinetic energy of fluid transfer across the tubular epithelium. Thus, the hypothesis is concerned primarily with the eating reflex secretion, or that secretion which under experimental conditions is induced by electrical stimulation of the parasympathetic nerves to the glands.

Vascular Events

The vascular events are accomplished by cholinergic-mediated changes in the glandular blood vessels resulting in an immediate and dramatic increase in glandular blood flow. The blood flow increase is accomplished by dilatation of the main arterial supply to the gland and opening of the very dense capillary networks which surround the ducts (Fig. 2-7). This blood flow and pressure increase within the gland, is closely followed by a blockage of blood flow in the capillary beds surrounding some of the secretory tubules. During active secretion such blood flow blockage seems to occur intermittently and selectively in the different lobules. This causes an increase in the pressure differential across these particular secretory tubules while allowing blood flow to proceed in other lobules. (In the latter there is a pressure drop and a simultaneous cessation of fluid and electrolyte secretion.) Altogether these vascular changes result in a greatly increased net flow of blood and an increased arterial pressure head in the gland. The overall effect is an increased pressure-flow shunt to the salivary glands at the expense, at least initially, of other extraglandular tissues in the head (Fig. 2-7).

The selective blood flow blockage phenomenon may or may not be the result of valves

known to exist in the lobular veins. It is well known that veins and venules contain contractile smooth muscle. The release of the neurotransmitter may cause a contraction in key segments or junctions which have the effect of blocking blood flow. It is also possible that neurotransmitter release into the blood causes, directly or indirectly, transitory changes in the surface charge or structure of the red blood cells and vascular endothelial cells increasing cell to cell adherence which would block flow. Of course a combination of these factors, (i.e., venule contraction, closure of valves, and red cell surface changes) could cause the stop-flow and red blood cell packing phenomenon. Whichever is the mechanism, the result is identical to what would be expected if there occurred a sudden actuation and closure of the venous valves that have been found in the lobular veins. Thus, the phenomenon may be as simple as it is represented in Figure 2-7.

The second nerve-mediated glandular event occurs simultaneously with the vascular changes but at the secretory cell level. The cholinergic neurotransmitter causes an increase in permeability of the striated duct epithelium (and perhaps other ducts as well) to water and electrolytes, and this increase in permeability permits the transfer of water and small solutes across this fluid secretory epithelium.

Fluid Transfer Channels

Although the observed vascular changes represent a thermodynamic engine capable of driving fluid and electrolyte secretion, it still remains unclear as to exactly how and by what pathway water and the principal ionic solutes cross the secretory epithelium. Since an electrolyte fluid is the principal volumetric product of the gland, and the immediate supply of secreted water and electrolytes is from the blood, then pathways or channels must exist for transfer of the fluid from the blood capillaries to and across the secretory epithelium. Fluid transfer may occur predominantly *through* the epithelial cells proper or *between* the cells (through the lateral channels and gap junctions). We shall refer to the former pathway as *transcellular transfer*, while the latter represents *paracellular transfer* (see Fig. 2-8).

There is limited information which bears upon the size of these fluid transfer channels

A. Unstimulated or "resting" gland

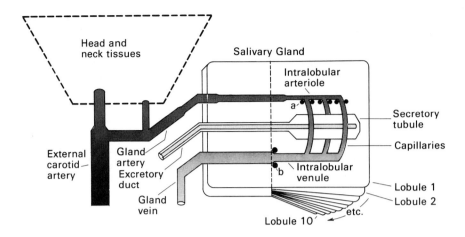

B. Eating Reflex Stimulated Gland

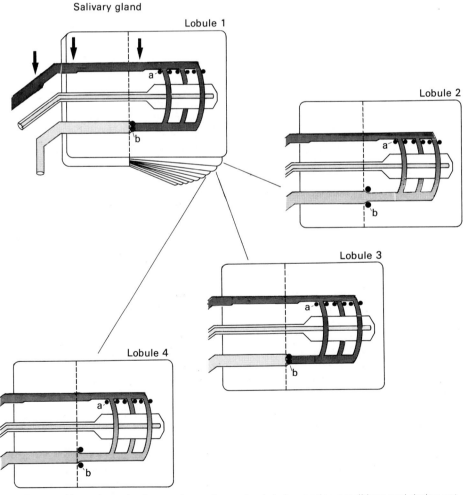

Fig. 2-7. Proposed hemodynamic changes in a salivary gland during resting conditions and during eating reflex stimulated secretion. This schema has been modified from a model presented by Suddick to explain gland hemodynamics during nerve-stimulated secretion. (*continued on facing page*)

based on evidence of possible molecular sieving. If data were available concerning the salivary clearance of noncharged molecules representing an array of different molecular diameters, the molecular sieving equation that has been used to characterize the glomerular capillaries of intact animals and man, could be used to characterize channels in the salivary glands. Some relevant inferences in this regard can be derived from the studies of salivary urea in human dialysis patients. In these studies parotid saliva and plasma urea nitrogen concentrations were compared in patients with renal failure and in normal subjects. With widely differing plasma urea levels, a near perfect correlation (r = 0.97) was found with salivary urea. Salivary clearance of urea remained constant at these widely varying plasma concentrations (clearance of urea =

$$\frac{\text{Salivary Urea Concentration}}{\text{Plasma Urea Concentration}} \times \text{salivary flow}$$

rate. The saliva to plasma concentration ratio in the stimulated saliva averaged 0.66, and the highest saliva to plasma correlation coefficients were at the highest stimulated flow rates. In unstimulated (resting) saliva the reverse was true. The saliva to plasma ratio of urea was 1.3 and saliva to plasma correlation coefficients were not as high. These results support the concept that resting secretion and

stimulated secretion are the result of different processes. Secondly, they support the concept that urea, during stimulated secretion, may be moving in bulk flow with water through channels or pores which are partially restrictive to urea as compared to water. These conclusions rest on the fact that the saliva to urea concentration ratio was lower at the highest rates of flow and yet was more predictive of the plasma concentration. This indicates that the plasma to saliva pathway is consistently more direct at the highest flow rates and that urea passage by bulk flow in aqueous channels becomes more predominant as flow rate increases. These conclusions and findings are in conflict with the notion offered by other investigators who say that urea enters the ducts solely by simple diffusion during active secretion, with all secreted water entering the system at the acinar level.

The resting urea saliva to plasma ratio of 1.3 is equally interesting since urea is not known to be actively transported by the salivary glands or other tissues. The higher urea concentration in the unstimulated saliva can be explained by the resting secretion concept presented in this chapter. During resting secretion urea would be expected to diffuse into the acinar lumen at the same concentration found in plasma. Then, as sodium and water are reabsorbed in the striated ducts, urea passage outward through aqueous channels

Fig. 2-7 (*continued*) **A.** The gland is shown in the resting or "unstimulated" state, while in **B** the gland is shown after the onset of reflex elicited (predominantly parasympathetic nerve) stimulation.

Parenchymal structures identified in **A** are: a central excretory duct shown coursing into the gland where it divides into intralobular collecting ducts serving specific secretory tubules. The tubule shown lies within secretory lobule 1. (To simplify the drawing, the secretory tubule is shown as the terminal secretory structure of the parenchymal tree; the acinus and its vascular bed are not shown). Ten secretory lobules are represented beyond the branching meridian, each as a separate slice, or leaflet.

Upon reflex stimulation of the gland, a marked increase in glandular blood flow occurs within 2 to 5 seconds. The vascular events following such stimulation are shown in B. This massive increase in capillary flow could be brought about by opening of precapillary sphincters ("valves" a.) combined with arterial dilation (arrows). This will cause increased glandular blood flow and development of a pressure-flow shunt to the salivary glands at the expense of blood pressure-flow energy to other head and neck tissues. As stimulation is continued, the glandular blood flow increase is followed, after a delay of 3 to 10 seconds, by secretory fluid flow from the excretory duct. It is suggested that the energy for this fluid flow is derived from the hydrostatic pressure differential between the capillaries and lumina of the secretory tubules (see Fig. 2-8). High capillary pressures will be generated by blockage of blood flow occurring on the venous side of these capillary beds ("valves" in lobules 1 and 3). The capillary pressures will approach the pressures in the artery serving the gland causing a rapid transfer of plasma into the tissue spaces surrounding the secretory tubules.

Thus three sequential events occur in *each lobule* as follows: 1) massive capillary dilatation and greatly increased overall blood flow; 2) venous blockage causing a sudden and marked rise in capillary pressure coupled with the onset of fluid secretion in the secretory tubules; 3) "release" or cessation of venous blockage with rapid reestablishment of blood flow, and a concomitant drop in capillary pressures and fluid secretion. This sequence *will repeat and continue to repeat in each lobule*, though in different phase relationships, as long as parasympathetic nerve stimulation continues to be elicited by physiologic reflexes.

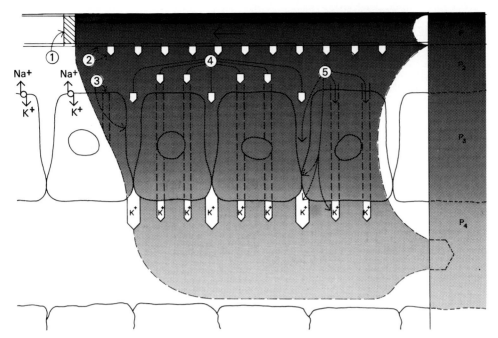

Fig. 2-8. Schematic of the fluid secretory mechanisms during eating reflex stimulated secretion. A blood capillary is shown at the top lying in close approximation to the secretory tubule. The tubular fluid secreting cells are shown in section with their basolateral borders facing the capillary and opposite luminal borders facing the tubular lumen. Four potential spaces are shown: the capillary lumen (P_1); the interstitial fluid compartment surrounding the tubular cells (P_2); the intracellular compartment (P_3); and the lumenal space (P_4).

Five events are depicted, not as distinct physiologically defined entities, but as a means of explaining the processes which are believed to occur after stimulation of the glands. The first event ① is a combination of vascular mechanisms that result initially in greatly increased capillary flow and intraglandular arterial pressure, followed quickly by a venous blockage downstream of the particular capillary depicted here (a "valve" or obstruction to flow is shown at ① for simplicity). This results in a sudden marked increase in transmural capillary pressure (the hydrostatic pressure in P_1 minus that in P_2) and a rapid movement of plasma-like fluid (event ②) out of the capillary. The pressure differentials P_2-P_3 and P_3-P_4 also increase and an equilibrium state is quickly reached with a relatively constant net rate of fluid transfer from capillary to tubular lumen and a continuous hydrostatic pressure gradient throughout the four compartments. Effects of the neurotransmitter on the secretory cell membrane result in a general increase in membrane permeability (event ③), resulting in a large increase in K^+ efflux. The combined vascular and cell membrane effects causes movement of fluid into the lateral channels (event ④) and across the epithelium, passing through the gap junctions (event ⑤). As the plasma-like fluid passes through the lateral channels sodium diffuses into the cells down its concentration gradient and potassium diffuses out of the cells into the channels. This results in transformation of the plasma-like fluid as it passes through the epithelium, with sodium being extracted and potassium becoming elevated. Altogether these processes amount to secretion of a hypotonic fluid at the site of fluid transfer during eating reflex stimulation.

The figure depicts a Na^+, K^+ ATPase transport system in the basolateral membrane, transporting sodium out and potassium into the cells. This maintains low intracellular $[Na^+]$ and a concentration gradient for passive sodium extraction along the lateral channels (and also from the luminal fluid column).

would be hindered by the same steric considerations as was the case for its transfer into the ducts during stimulated secretion. Thus the fact that the resting saliva urea to plasma ratio (1.3) is the reciprocal of the reflex stimulated ratio (0.66) may not be coincidental, but may accurately reflect the stearic hindrance to this molecule in passage through aqueous channels in the duct cells. This im-

plies that urea and water reabsorption in the striated ducts occurs via channels which have the same diameter as those through which these molecules pass in the opposite direction during secretion. It is suggested that the direction of the net force which drives water transfer in the ducts changes 180° when going from resting secretion to eating reflex secretion. At low capillary pressures during resting secretion the active transport of sodium at the basolateral membrane causes net sodium movement from lumen toward the capillaries and a net osmotic driving force for a small degree of water reabsorption. In the eating reflex stimulated secretion, activation of vascular mechanisms produces a hydrostatic pressure differential which pushes water through the epithelium toward the lumen. This "secreted" water carries large amounts of Na^+ of extracellular origin and large amounts of K^+ of cellular origin (this will be explained further below).

Calculated from its diffusion coefficient water presents a molecular radius of 1.0Å. By the same methods the molecular radius of urea can be calculated to be 1.6Å. The molecular diameter of inulin, which does not enter saliva to any significant extent, is about 14.8Å. Steric hindrance simply means that a molecule whose diameter is a significant fraction of the pore diameter is far more likely to strike the edge of the pore and be deflected than to enter. The greater the diameter of the molecule relative to the pore, the less frequently it will strike sufficiently head on to enter. Thus we might propose by inference that the fluid transfer channels in the salivary secretory epithelium during stimulated secretion are probably less than 15Å in diameter, and in all likelihood, greater than 5Å in diameter. The channels present a complete barrier to inulin transfer, but inhibit urea transfer only slightly compared to water. We are presenting the viewpoint then that the salivary secretion of water is by bulk filtration, a mechanism essentially analogous to glomerular filtration in the kidney. Unlike the glomerular filtrate, however, the salivary fluid is transformed in its electrolyte content during its transit through the secretory cells.

It must be conceded that the physical presence of aqueous pores through the secretory cell membranes and the presence of fluid transfer channels through the complete glandular secretory epithelium are tenuous concepts. Glomerular capillaries, for example, seem to have aqueous pores because of their molecular sieving characteristics. However, some researchers have maintained that the glomerular capillary membranes are hydrated gels, and that glomerular fluid is formed by a process of diffusion, not by bulk filtration. According to this view, the entire glomerular capillary surface is involved in the production of glomerular fluid; pores as such, do not

exist. Water and small molecules have essentially the same diffusivities in this gel. An increase in hydrostatic pressure increases the electrochemical potential of water and solutes and so increases their ability to diffuse in the membrane, with larger molecules having progressively smaller ability as particle size increases.

The application of these concepts to the salivary glands is much more complex because molecules must traverse not only the capillary membrane and basement membrane, but also the epithelial cell layer. However, the fluid transfer channel concept is useful if certain reservations are kept in mind. The channels may not have the postulated uniform dimensions (5 to 15Å) which the limited data suggests. Indeed, the channels may not be stable anatomic structures at all. There may well be several filtering membranes involved, including those of the capillaries, the basement membrane, and the epithelium itself, either via the junctional complexes or possibly, the basolateral and apical membranes of the secretory cells. Water and dissolved molecules may migrate along devious aqueous channels that have no permanence in the membranes or between the membranes (in the gap junctions). Such channels might be continually collapsing and reforming.

If transepithelial fluid transfer occurs at least partly through the cells (transcellular), water and dissolved solutes, once into the aqueous medium of the secretory cell, probably move in bulk flow along channels of least resistance. A major source of intracellular resistance to fluid movement must be considered to be intracellular organelles composed of the same type of lipid-protein unit membranes by which the cells are bounded. Thus, water and dissolved solutes may move rather freely through the secretory cells alongside and around such organelles which make up the structural framework of these cells. If such membranes (for example, those of the basal invaginations of the striated duct cells) become activated simultaneously with respect to active transport activities (such as Na^+ and K^+ transport), it is conceivable that membrane-limited invaginations, organelles, and vesicles could serve as Na^+ extraction and storage sites, thus altering the electrolyte content of the fluid as it moves alongside these intracellular membranes.

In the *resting secretion* it is proposed that the reabsorption of water is *through* the cells (transcellular) from striated duct lumen toward the blood capillary with urea being concentrated in the duct. In the *eating reflex secretion*, capillary pressures become markedly elevated and fluid movement is from blood capillary to striated duct lumen; *this represents fluid and electrolyte secretion*. In this case, it is proposed that water and electrolytes traverse the epithelium *via the lateral channels and gap junctions* (paracellular). Thus, *secretion is paracellular, reabsorption is transcellular* according to this hypothesis. In both instances the net direction or vector of active sodium transport is from lumen to capillary. In the eating reflex secretion, however, the net total flow of sodium is from capillary to lumen. In the case of the resting secretion, active sodium transport provides the driving force for water reabsorption with the resultant urea concentration in the ducts.

The question of whether the water and solutes of secretion are driven through the various membranes and cells by gradients of electrochemical potential (diffusion) created by the hydrostatic pressure differential, or whether the pressure differential itself drives the fluid by bulk filtration, is in a sense, academic. The main point is that the source of energy for fluid transfer is the hydrostatic pressure differential between the blood capillaries and secretory tubular lumen.

From one viewpoint the fluid transfer channels might be considered, *de facto*, potassium channels during eating reflex secretion. It is well known that activation of cholinergic receptors on secretory cells causes an increase in their potassium permeability and conductance, both at the basal and apical cell membranes. This increased potassium leakage causes hyperpolarization of the cell membrane, the so called secretory potential of the acinar cells. Although it is not known with certainty that striated duct cells respond to cholinergic stimuli in the same manner, it is reasonable to expect that volleys of parasympathetic impulses will also increase the membrane permeability of these tubular cells. Perhaps the increase in potassium permeability is an integral part of fluid transfer across the epithelial cell barrier. The leakage of K^+ into the lateral channels, for example, may in some way permit the transepithelial pressure differential to be manifested in transcellular fluid flow, carrying potassium ions back through the basolateral channel membrane and then out through pores in the apical membrane.

The favored viewpoint, however, is that the augmented leakage of K^+ into the lateral channels, combined with the vascular induced pressure gradient, may force much of the potassium and virtually all secreted water into the lumen via the gap junctions. Under this concept the gap junctions of the striated duct cells represent the fluid transfer channels, and these channels would seem to require an optimum K^+ concentration to maintain their fluid transfer capabilities. Ultimately, whether fluid transfer is paracellular via the gap junction, or transcellular, it is very tempting to consider that it occurs via potassium channels. If paracellular, the potassium channels are within the gap junctions; if transcellular, the potassium channels may be located either in the basolateral membrane or in the apical membrane. As mentioned, we favor the view that fluid is transferred via the gap junctions, and that transcellular transfer occurs only under extreme experimental conditions in laboratory animals such as intense and prolonged electrical stimulation, or strong pilocarpine-induced stimulation, or in humans, under certain pathologic salivary gland disease states. When this does occur, it probably damages the fluid secretory epithelium.

Hypotonic Saliva: Result of a Transepithelial Countercurrent Mechanism

Another question which logically arises during assimilation of this new view of fluid and electrolyte secretion is just how these concepts explain the ability of the salivary glands to produce a hypotonic fluid with sodium levels much below those of blood plasma and the interstitial fluids. We have explained that the secreted fluid is transformed in its electrolyte content as it passes through the secretory epithelium. The potassium channel concept explains the elevation of potassium from plasma levels of 4 to 5 mEq/L to secretory fluid levels of around 15 to 20 mEq/L. In addition, passage of the secretory fluid through the lateral channels also permits an explanation of how sodium can be extracted as fluid moves through the epithelium. This concept explains how salivary glands are able to elaborate a hypotonic fluid as a "primary" secretion, (i.e., how the secretory epithelium is able to produce directly, at the cellular site of fluid transfer, a hypotonic, low sodium fluid).

This is a totally different concept from the current broadly promulgated notion that the salivary glands produce a hypotonic fluid by virtue of a two stage mechanism which involves ductal sodium reabsorption from an acinar derived primary secretion.

It is suggested that sodium is passively transported (or absorbed) through the plasma membrane which lines the lateral channels. This occurs as fluid moves along these channels toward the gap junctions. Concomitantly sodium pumping throughout the basolateral membrane is enhanced, and the active transport of sodium out of the cell maintains a steep concentration gradient across the lateral channel plasma membrane which favors sodium entry into the cell. Sodium pumping may be enhanced as a result of the increase in sodium concentration in the cell which occurs as sodium diffuses into the cell. Another possibility is that the cholinergic transmitter may in some way directly stimulate sodium pumping.

Regardless of the mechanism for enhanced basolateral sodium transport, it would represent part of a circular and fruitless exercise were it not for the striking cytologic characteristics of the fully differentiated striated duct epithelium (see Chap. 1). The multitude of deep invaginations of the basolateral membrane provide a sodium sink, or temporary storage site, for each cell that enables the sodium gradient to be maintained along the lateral channels. A certain amount of sodium must be transported out of the cell across the basal membrane in sites other than the basal membrane invaginations, and will thus be at least potentially recyclable back into the lateral channels. However, the huge expansion of the surface area of the basolateral membrane that the basal invaginations represent also involves a very large expansion of sodium pump sites, the direction of pumping activity being *into* the basal membrane invaginations (though still outward with respect to the cell interior). This permits at least a temporary sequestering of sodium in and around these invaginations. As the sodium concentration within the invaginations builds up, sodium will move passively in increasingly larger amounts back into the cell. Eventually, an equilibrium will be reached where the diffusional sodium flux back into the cell matches the active transport flux outward, and that part of the striated duct cell where the basal invaginations are concentrated will be a zone

of relatively high sodium concentration. This will be true both outside and inside of the cell-limiting plasma membranes of the basal invaginations. This means that sodium will tend to become more concentrated in the basal half of the cell, and within this half the highest sodium levels could be expected in the central core of the cell, away from the lateral channels. This permits sodium to diffuse into the cell from the lateral channels during secretion. In effect, the remarkable cytologic differentiation of these cells permits a *transepithelial countercurrent multiplier effect* to operate during the transfer of fluid across the epithelium.

Biologically, such a mechanism is simple and exceedingly economical. Conceptually, however, it may be difficult to master and perhaps should be explained further.

As the high sodium, low potassium fluid filters out of the tubular capillaries and moves into the lateral channels, sodium moves passively into the tubular cell, and potassium moves from the cell passively into the lateral channel (see Fig. 2-8). As sodium is passively absorbed into the cell from the moving fluid column in the lateral channel, it will tend to become concentrated and sequestered in the central core of the basal half of the cell by virtue of active transport of sodium into the basal invaginations. This amounts to generation of a high sodium, hypertonic fluid in the central core of the cell, that tends to move and become more concentrated near the basal pole of the cell. Simultaneously a low sodium hypotonic fluid is generated and moves in columns around the periphery of the cell in the opposite direction toward the tubular lumen. This is a true countercurrent multiplier effect. It produces a *hypertonic* fluid that eventually moves toward the blood capillaries, and in the process simultaneously creates a *hypotonic* fluid that moves into the ductal lumen. The whole process is made possible by virtue of the hydrostatic pressure gradient from blood capillaries to ductal lumen which drives the secretory fluid transfer. In this sense, the mechanism is analogous to the countercurrent multiplier effect in the nephron of the kidney, which is made possible by the fact that the fluid column in the loop of Henle is driven by the vascular pressure head in the glomerulus. The difference between these countercurrent mechanisms is in scale; the salivary gland countercurrent multiplier is a micromechanism compared to the kidney mechanism.

The former is operating at the cellular level while the latter operates at organ level. The former represents an exquisite cellular mechanism for the singular generation of the hypotonic fluid which bathes the oral mucosa, while the latter, is capable of a vast range of regulatory responses in terms of the osmolarity of the excreted fluid (urine ranges from very hypertonic to very hypotonic depending on hormonal and cardiovascular status at a given time). To function, both mechanisms hold in common the requirement of the thermodynamic engine represented by the vascular pressure.

Experimental Evidence Relative to Hypothesis of Fluid Secretion

The evidence has become more and more convincing concerning the main hypothesis that the energy for water and electrolyte secretion is derived from the hydrostatic pressure differential between the capillaries and secretory tubules. Investigators have studied blood flow relationships to fluid secretion in the rat submandibular gland. In examination of the rate and duration of secretory flow following arterial occlusion and venous occlusion they found that secretory flow declines in parallel to venous outflow and stops completely at the same time that venous outflow ceases, both within 2 to 3 minutes following ligation of the submandibular artery. Thus, a vascular pressure head and glandular blood flow are immediately coupled and essential to the secretion of fluid. The fact that venous occlusion does not halt secretory flow provided additional support for the contention that an arterial pressure head is required for normal secretion, and that secretion is blood pressure dependent but does not require continuous blood flow through the gland. These studies established that there is an *immediate* dynamic pressure-flow relationship between the various fluid compartments involved in secretion, (i.e., vascular fluid→interstitial fluid→cellular fluid→secretory fluid).

In further studies of rat submandibular glands it was found that the secretory pressure head from the submandibular gland (i.e., that developed by the gland during secretion as a gradually rising vertical column of fluid) is always near to or just below the vascular pressure head through the gland, (as measured by a parallel column of fluid connected to the isolated venous outflow from the gland). This is true under a variety of experimental conditions which causes major changes in the systemic blood pressure of the experimental rats. Parallel decreases and increases in systemic blood pressure, the glandular venous pressure head, and the secretory fluid pressure head are found when the animals are bled, causing a decline in the systemic arterial pressure (monitored via the glandular venous pressure head) and a simultaneous decline in the secretory pressure. When the animals are subsequently transfused with solutions of mannitol and saline both arterial and secretory pressures rise. In other experiments, drugs which block active transport processes, including ouabain, ethacrynic acid, and dinitrophenol, affect the secretory pressures head only to the extent that they also affect (decrease) the glandular venous pressure head. (Some of these drugs do however, inhibit the reabsorption of the secretory fluid by the gland under these "pressurized" conditions.) It was concluded that fluid and electrolyte secretion in the rat is an ultrafiltration-like process driven by the vascular hydrostatic pressure in the gland.

Recently, similar experiments have been performed using the dog as the experimental model. While the results are sufficiently similar to those described for the rat, there are some major differences in the development of the secretory pressure heads in the dog (vs. the rat) submandibular gland which lead to a better understanding of the overall energetics of salivary secretion. The dog gland is capable of producing an immediate and prolonged increase in secretory pressure that carries well above (e.g., 10 to 20 torr) the systemic arterial pressure (monitored via the contralateral carotid artery). However, when this experimental "stage one" secretion is exhausted (the usual duration of this response is about 15 minutes), fluid and electrolyte secretion will continue for a very long period (e.g., 2 hrs.), apparently as long as the parasympathetic nerves continue to be stimulated electrically. The secretory pressure head measured continuously during this experimental second stage of secretion behaves in a similar way as that of the rat gland; it remains near to or just below the systemic arterial pressure and declines and ascends in a parallel response to bleeding- and transfusion-induced changes in the systemic arterial pressure. Serial samples of saliva were measured for protein and electrolytes during these studies. Protein concentrations peak during stage one secretion and fall to very low constant values during stage two secretion.

In a parallel study of the histology of the dog submandibular glands subjected to prolonged periods of electrical stimulation, extensive degranulation and vacuolization of the predominent mucous acini was noted. All of these studies indicate differences in secretory pressure behaviors of the dog versus the rat submandibular glands is an expression of the fact that these are two entirely different types of salivary glands. The dog submandibular gland is composed predominently of mucous acini with few serous acini and striated ducts, while the rat gland is predominantly serous in acinar composition and contains a comparatively larger proportion of striated ducts. It is suggested that secretory pressures which are higher initially than arterial pressures in the dog are produced by virtue of extensive secretion of the mucopolysaccharides in addition to the protein and glycoprotein secretory mechanisms described earlier in this chapter.

In addition these studies support the concept that a two compartment model can explain the overall energetics of secretion (Fig. 2-9). The first compartment is coincident with protein secretion and predominates during stage one secretion. It is thus responsible for the ability of the glands to maintain secretory pressures higher than arterial pressures for limited periods. Its energy source is derived from the acinar secretory cells, (i.e., the processes associated with exocytosis). We might say, in fact, that exocytosis is not only driven by but it essentially defines what we call the first energy compartment. This first energy compartment is thus endocellular in origin. The second energy compartment is coincident with fluid and electrolyte secretion. Experimentally, it predominates during stage two secretion and its energy source is derived from the vascular pressures. Thus, the second energy compartment is exocellular in origin.

During normal eating reflex secretion when there is no artificial resistance to secretory flow, both compartments are active concurrently during the reflex initiated volleys of efferent impulses to the secretory cells. However, even during normal reflex elicited secretion it is possible to exhaust the first compartment. Under conditions of prolonged reflex stimulation of human parotid secretion,

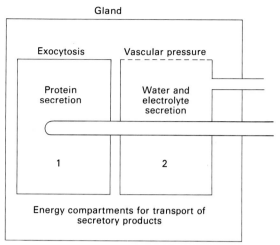

Fig. 2-9. Energetics of salivary secretion. Two distinct energy sources are involved in the mechanisms of salivary secretion. As shown, one of these drives protein secretion (energy compartment 1) and is derived from metabolic energy within the secretory cells. As described in the text, distinct metabolic mechanisms are involved not only in secretory protein synthesis, but are also associated with chemical transformations which result in extrusion of these proteins from the cells (exocytosis). Compartment one thus can be said to be endocellular.

The second energy source is the vascular pressure within glandular blood vessels (energy compartment 2) which drives fluid and electrolyte secretion. This energy source is dependent on a continual dynamic link to extraglandular blood pressure and fluid supply due to pumping of the heart. From the perspective of the secretory cells of the gland, the second energy compartment is thus exocellular.

protein concentrations peak during the first hour and then markedly decline to very low and constant concentrations during the third hour. Throughout the three-hour period, however, flow rate remains constant and the key electrolytes, Na^+, K^+, and Cl^-, also remain constant and remain at the same level found in the initial samples. Altogether these studies support the notion that the second energy compartment is derived from vascular pressures, and is an inexhaustable compartment as far as secretory mechanims are concerned. Thus, stage one and stage two secretions in the dog experiments are experimental entities, not distinguishable as such during normal secretion except under extreme conditions as explained above. Under prolonged reflex stimulation of 2 to 3 hours, the first compartment (i.e., protein secretion) becomes depleted, permitting, in a sense, detection of the second energy compartment (i.e., which drives fluid and electrolyte secretion).

Source of Experimental High Secretory Pressures

Events associated with exocytosis which might be expected to cause elevations in secretory pressure are contraction of contractile proteins (e.g., the microfilaments of the microtubular system); the fusion-fission event involving the interactions of secretory granule membranes with the apical cell membranes; the dispersion of secretory granule contents into the acinar lumen; and physicochemical changes in the granular "condensed" secretory products that could enhance osmotic water transfer across the epithelium once they enter the lumen.

Once the stores of glycoproteins become depleted, fluid and electrolyte secretion remains the dominant physiologic activity of the dog gland, and the secretory pressure head closely follows changes in systemic or glandular arterial pressure. In serous glands, fluid and electrolyte secretion is the dominant activity from the very beginning of electrical or eating reflex stimulated secretion (in so far as total secretory output is considered). It is interesting to note, however, that even in the rat submandibular gland experimental conditions may be arranged such that the secretory pressure exceeds systemic arterial pressure during initial brief periods of electrical stimulation. When the main excretory duct is cannulated and connected to a "Y" connector (one limb of which is open and the other is connected to a pressure transducer), and the parasympathetic nerves to the gland are stimulated electrically, secretory flow commences through the open end of the cannula beyond the Y connector. When this cannula is suddenly clamped, secretory pressure measured by the transducer open to the gland quickly rises and sometimes exceeds systemic arterial pressure for short periods. It is proposed that this phenomenon in the rat submandibular gland is also caused by the protein and glycoprotein secretory mechanisms described earlier, and further, that myoepithelial cell contraction may be associated with these high pressures. The myoepithelial cells which are closely associated with the serous acini may be stimulated to contract in unison during such electrical stimulation. It is thought that this contributes to the elevation of the secretory pressure to values above arterial pressure under these particular experimental conditions. These conditions differ from those previously utilized for both rat and dog secretory pressure studies since the gland is not able *to secrete significant quantities of fluid and electrolytes* after the secretory cannula beyond the Y connector is clamped. From that instant, there is essentially a closed, fluid-filled column compartment extending from the face of the secretory cells to the face or diaphragm of the pressure transducer. This is in contrast with studies of secretory pressures conducted in the rat and in the dog in which the salivary glands secrete abundant quantities of fluid, producing a steady increase in the secretory pressure head as a consequence of fluid accumulation. The latter may be described as an open system and the former as a closed system; the open system provides a more realistic means of assessing the energetics of fluid secretion.

As noted, forces other than fluid transfer or protein secretion can cause elevation of pressures in the secretory fluid column in the closed system. One such force is contraction of the myoepithelial cells which surround the acini. Another such force is contraction of the acinar units, the individual acinar cells undergoing a coordinated contraction via the microfilament system. There is evidence for such contraction in microcinematographic studies of isolated acinar units. In these films the movements of the isolated acini appear to represent coordinated contractions of the complete acinar units.

Evidence for Hemodynamic Changes in the Glands

As discussed earlier, the eating reflex results in two cholinergic—mediated effects in the glands, one causing hemodynamic changes (Fig. 2-7), the other causing secretory cell membrane responses (Fig. 2-8). The vascular effects described in Figure 2-7 are hypothesized to occur during normal reflex stimulation of the glands, such as that elicited by chewing a morsel of food. The vascular effects which are seen upon electrical stimulation of the parasympathetic nerve in the dog or rat submandibular glands are somewhat different, but the overall principles and effects are the same in the active fluid secreting lobules. Stimulation of the parasympathetic nerves to the gland causes a marked increase in glandular blood flow (as monitored by venous outflow, for example) within 2 to 5 seconds. This event is probably due to a massive increase in capillary blood flow as a result of a synchronized simultaneous opening of all "precapillary sphincters" or valves, particularly in the ductal capillary networks, and an overall dilatation of the gland artery and intraglandular arterioles (Fig. 2-7). This creates a pressure-flow shunt to the salivary gland at the expense of other head and neck tissues. Furthermore, either electrical or reflex stimulation causes closure of venous valves in the lobular venous plexus leading from the striated ducts. When the pressure-flow energy increase to the glands is combined with closure of the venous valves downstream of the secretory tubular capillaries, flow in the capillaries slows and stops and the glands quickly develop high pressures in these capillary beds. The high capillary pressures cause a rapid transfer of fluid into the glandular interstitium surrounding the tubular cells. Recent histologic studies of the dog submandibular gland present clear evidence that the striated duct tubular capillaries become engorged and distended with red blood cells in the electrically stimulated glands. This is not seen in unstimulated control glands. Eating reflex stimulated human parotid secretion demonstrates much more variance in flow from minute to minute than glands of experimental animals which are stimulated artificially either via electrical stimulation of the parasympathetic nerves or by parasympathomimetic drugs. Thus, fluid secretion in artificially stimulated glands may represent the product of relatively greater numbers of "synchronized" secretory lobules. The tubular capillaries of these artificially stimulated glands may be locked into a continuous state of blockage and stopped-flow throughout the period of stimulation, induced either by electrical stimulation of the parasympathetic nerves or by parasympathomimetic drug induced stimulation (such as methacholine or pilocarpine). This would account for secretory flow rates being much greater per unit of gland weight, and for relatively constant secretory flow rates under these experimental conditions.

A recent study of the effects of salicylates on secretion of the dog parotid gland produced intriguing results that may be related to the hemodynamic changes in the glands during stimulated secretion. It was found that intravenous administration of acetysalicylate or sodium salicylate (25–125 mg/kg) in the dog during pilocarpine stimulated parotid secretion causes a doubling of flow rate with concomitant increases in Na^+ and Cl^- levels, and a decrease in K^+ concentration. Possibly salicylates act via their known effects on prostaglandin synthetase and cause changes in intraglandular prostaglandin levels that in turn result in an accentuated hemodynamic response to the pilocarpine, increased capillary pressures, and greater fluid transfer. However, it seems more likely that the effect of salicylates is linked to an effect on potassium permeability of the secretory cells. Irrespective of the mechanism of the salicylate effect on flow rate, these results suggest that the salicylates may provide a highly useful tool to study the mechanisms of fluid and electrolyte secretion.

Evidence for Fluid Transfer Channels

There is no direct evidence concerning the existence of fluid transfer channels in salivary glands. Inferentially, it must be presumed that there are pathways for water and electrolyte transfer across the secretory epithelium. There is a considerable amount of information about channels in epithelial cell membranes and junctions, particularly of gallbladder, small intestine, choroid plexus, and renal proximal tubule. In general, epithelia contain at least two well characterized transepithelial channels: the sodium channel in the apical cell membrane of "tight" epithelia, and the gap junctional (paracellular) channel of "leaky" epithelia. Epithelia have been classified as "tight" or "leaky" according to their transepithelial electrical resistance and, inferentially, according to whether there is a significant pathway for paracellular transepithelial ion transfer. The electrical resistance of "leaky" epithelia containing the paracellular (junctional) channel is very low (generally about one hundred Ω-cm²) compared to "tight" epithelia (generally several thousand Ω-cm²). In the "leaky" epithelia the resistance of the gap junctions is so low compared to the epithelium as a whole that the junctional resistance dominates the transepithelial resistance measurement.

The resistance of the paracellular channel may depend partly on structures visible in the electron microscope and partly on fixed charges on the walls of the channel. Electron micrographs suggest that the gap junction channel is not a straight tube but is partly occluded by one or more strands. Epithelia with very low junctional resistance are reported to have only one strand, while those with high junctional resistance may have up to seven strands. In isolated epithelia preparations the addition of osmotically active solutes, or passage of electric currents that cause solute accumulation in the junctions, produce visible junctional dilatation in electron micrographs and correlated increases in junctional conductance. Thus, there is a morphologic basis to differences in junctional resistance in these "leaky" epithelia.

There is strong suggestive evidence that fixed charges in the walls of the gap junctions determine whether the channel is preferentially cation or anion selective. In the gallbladder, graphs of partial ionic conductance against pH suggest control of cation conductance by acidic wall groups (e.g., $-COO^- \rightleftarrows COOH$) with a $pKa \sim 4.5$, and control of anion conductance by basic groups (e.g., $NH_3^+ \rightleftarrows NH_2$) with a pKa below 3. At neutral pH the ion permeability channel in the gap junctions of gallbladder, small intestine, choroid plexus, and renal proximal tubule are preferentially cation-selective.

The molecular dimensions of the permeability barrier in the gallbladder junctional channel has been assessed by measuring the permeabilities of nitrogenous cations of various sizes. Permeability decreases rapidly with increasing molecular radius, and quantitative analysis has indicated an effective pore diameter of around 10Å for rabbit gallbladder and around 16Å for bullfrog gallbladder. This does not mean that the entire junctional channel is as narrow, only the portions that represent the chief barrier to the cations.

When corrected for sieving effects in these narrow channels, an extremely interesting pattern is evident for the permeabilities of the various nitrogenous cations. Permeability increases with the number of protons that the cation has available for formation of hydrogen bonds with proton acceptors such as oxygens. It appears that the molecular group in the channel wall behaves as if it consists of four oxygens that form strong hydrogen bonds. It may seem paradoxical that strongly hydrogen bonding cations have a high permeability in such channels. However, binding increases the concentration of the cations in the channel, and the increase in concentration in the channel more than offsets the decrease in mobility due to binding. Thus increases in concentration of cations in the junctional chan-

nel increases the permeability of the channel to these ions.

Virtually all tight epithelia that carry out active Na^+ reabsorption contain a channel that admits Na^+ in their apical cell membrane. This channel is blocked by the pyrazine diuretic amiloride. In the kidney, amiloride's diuretic action arises because it blocks the Na^+ channel in the distal nephron, thus blocking Na^+ reabsorption and the ability of the distal nephron to extract an equivalent amount of water. To date, the Na^+ channel has been described in urinary bladders and colons of a variety of species; skins of frogs and toads; renal distal tubule and collecting duct; sweat duct; and salivary duct. The function of this channel is to control Na^+ entrance from the luminal solution into the cell where it is then actively transported out the other end of the cell across the basolateral membrane by the usual $Na^+ - K^+$ ATPase pump. The hormone aldosterone increases both basolateral Na^+ pumping and apical Na^+ permeability. The mechanism of action of this hormone might involve activation or production of apical Na^+ channels, leading to increased Na^+ entry and thus increased basolateral pumping. It is also possible that aldosterone may somehow increase the rate of Na^+ pumping, causing an increase in apical Na^+ conductance.

The question of how water and nonelectrolytes may permeate the junctional channel of the Na^+ channel remains a major unsolved question in physiology. In salivary glands there is virtually no information even with regard to the ion channels themselves. An interesting morphologic observation has been made however, of the permeation of the marker protein horseradish peroxidase into the salivary gland tubules. It has been demonstrated with electronmicroscopy in the dog submandibular gland that horseradish peroxidase fills the lateral channels of striated ducts and *enters the lumina* when it is injected into the arterial supply during artificial stimulation. This is supportive of the contention that the striated duct is a leaky epithelium, and may indicate that water and electrolytes cross this epithelium by passing through the lateral channels and gap junctions during eating reflex stimulated secretion. However, water transfer through the epithelial cells proper (i.e., transcellular) cannot be excluded on the basis of this evidence.

Similarly, there is no direct evidence related to the suggestion that the fluid transfer channels are "K^+ channels" with water permeability maintained by a minimum concentration of K^+. The work of several investigators, however, indicates that both acetylcholine and epinephrine cause an increase in cell membrane conductance to potassium in salivary gland acinar cells. A nearly universal finding is that K^+ concentrations in both the secretory fluid and in the venous effluent from salivary glands rapidly rises immediately following nerve stimulation. Another well known phenomenon of interest is that K^+ concentration in reflex stimulated human parotid secretions and in nerve stimulated secretions from experimental animals is several times higher than plasma concentrations, and furthermore does not normally change in concentration when stimulation intensity is increased and flow rates rise. In the *in vitro* studies of leaky epithelia, the increase in concentration of permeant cations (up to a limit) in the junctional channel leading to increased cation permeability also might be considered supportive of the concept that the fluid transfer channel is a potassium channel, and that a minimum potassium concentration in the channel is tied to fluid permeation.

The presence of optimal potassium concentrations entrained in the fluid columns moving through these junctions may provide a constant electrostatic effect related to maintaining conformation of the channel. The previously discussed effects of salicylates on secretion may prove to be a major piece of evidence to unravel this aspect of secretory dynamics. Salicylates are known to cause the leakage of potassium from mammalian red cells, neurones, and yeast cells. The salivary experiments indicate that they cause a large increase in pilocarpine stimulated flow, and a corresponding increase in the rate of potassium secretion. This increased potassium output is maintained for relatively long periods in these experiments. Since the potassium levels of the saliva is much higher than the plasma levels, the increased output can be only from secretory cell stores. All of this supports a linkage between optimum potassium permeability and efflux, and transepithelial fluid transfer. If the secreted fluid moves via the paracellular route, the linkage of potassium to fluid transfer truly supports the idea of potassium channels in the gap junctions.

Another cation of critical importance, of course, is calcium. Extracellular calcium is required to maintain fluid and electrolyte secretion. This may be tied to an effect of this divalent cation on conformational changes in structural proteins associated with the gap junctions which *establishes* the fluid transfer channels, while potassium may help maintain the channels through electrostatic effects.

The alternative to paracellular transfer is fluid movement directly through the cells (transcellular). If this is the case, then the secretory cell membrane, rather than the junctional channel, will limit the rate of fluid transfer. In all probability *either* the basolateral *or* the apical plasma membrane will be rate-limiting with respect to the volume transferred per unit area with time, and thus regulate fluid secretion. If the apical unit membrane is a rate-limiting barrier, the collapse of the tubular lumina may occassionly occur and be observed in histologic and cytologic studies of salivary glands fixed during active secretion. We are not aware of published observations of this nature, but there have been reports and published electromicrographs of cytoplasmic "blebs" (small irregular bulges of the apical membrane and cytoplasm into the lumen). These apical bulges are reported to occur *only* in striated ducts. If the basolateral membrane is the rate-limiting barrier, a collapse of the secretory cell during very active secretion may be expected to occur. We are not aware of observations of this nature either. *Indeed, if fluid transfer is largely transcellular and not paracellular, the fluid secretory process would appear to pose serious problems in the cellular economy for management of cell volume and osmolarity.* It is indeed far less troublesome to conceptualize fluid transfer occurring via the paracellular route.

Evidence for Cellular Site of Water and Electrolyte Secretion

There is no direct evidence concerning the site of water and electrolyte secretion, (i.e., does it occur predominantly in the acini, the striated ducts, or in the intralobular collecting ducts for salivary glands?). It is interesting to find that most investigators have assumed that the acini are the sites where most or all of the fluid of secretion is transferred. Although the evidence to support the fact that these cells are primarily responsible for protein secretion is irrefutable, there is no direct evidence to support the assumption that they are responsible for most of the fluid secretion. This assumption probably arose simply because the acinus is the anatomical end point of the branching tubular secretory structure. In order to obtain direct evidence that most fluid is transferred in the acinar units, one would have to be able to demonstrate quantitatively the amount of fluid transferred in a single acinus per unit time, and to multiply this by the number of active acinar units in a gland. This value would have to equal approximately the amount of fluid secreted. The only types of experiments using techniques that permit sampling of fluid within the glandular tubular structures are the micropuncture experiments described earlier. However, it is not yet possible to determine how much fluid is transferred in a single acinus, nor in the clumps of acini draining toward the pipettes. Thus, it is simply not possible to state with certainty that most of the fluid secretion enters the tubular structure in the acini of the gland.

Inferential evidence indicates that tubular structures of the gland are capable of elaborating significant amounts of fluid and electrolytes. It has been suggested that these secretory tubular structures (the striated ducts and perhaps the intralobular collecting ducts) are able to elaborate most of the fluid and electrolytes of secretion during eating reflex stimulation or during artificial cholinergic stimulation. This evidence is based largely on the histologic and cytologic appearance of the cells in the different elements of the gland. In contrast to acinar cells which appear to be specialized for protein secretion, there are cells in other tissues that appear to be specialized for transfer of fluids. These are epithelial sheets of cells which line organs such as the proximal kidney tubule, stomach, small intestine, large intestine, gallbladder, and choroid plexus. *Cytologically, these epithelia resemble salivary gland tubular cells, not acinar cells.*

Perhaps the most appropriate organ to compare to the salivary glands is the kidney, because of similarities in the cytologic features of the component cells. The striated duct cells of the salivary glands are very similar in appearance to the proximal tubular cells of the kidney. As a generalization, epithelial cells of organs that appear to be involved in water and electrolyte transfer functions seem to present a characteristic appearance involving most of the cytological features of the striated duct cells, as described in this chapter.

Another feature of the striated ducts which connotes a secretory function is their intense vascularity. These tubules have a dense capillary network that lies very close to the base of the cells. The acinar units, in contrast, have a relatively sparse blood supply as judged by the numbers and proximity of blood capillaries. Since fluid secretion shows an immediate dynamic relationship to glandular blood pressures and flow, it is difficult not to consider that the striated ducts are involved in fluid secretion. It must be conceded, however, that there is little or no direct evidence concerning this matter. Studies on the timed appearance of radioactively labelled substances in artificially stimulated dog saliva after arterial injection provides perhaps the most direct physiologic evidence. From these studies a "map" was proposed for the entry sites of a variety of substances. Of all of these substances, water and urea were shown to enter the tubules in the proximal ducts. Thus, this could be considered supportive evidence that striated ducts are the site of water transfer (i.e., fluid secretion), though this was not the author's conclusion.

Other Observations Related to the Hypothesis

The neural activation of the fluid secretory cells produces both direct and indirect effects. First it causes changes in the cell membranes (e.g., an increase in K^+ permeability). *This indirectly results in major changes in the extracellular ionic composition* that *surrounds the cells.* This latter response may play a key role in the integration of the intermittent blood flow characteristics in the secretory lobules as shown in Figure 2-7. For example, a rapid transient increase in extracellular $[Ca^{++}]$ and $[K^+]$ occurs, followed by a prolonged steady increase in extracellular $[Na^+]$. These ions (and others, as well as other metabolic products) will enter the capillaries, and can be expected to influence the tone of vascular smooth muscle. These changes in the local environment of the vascular smooth muscle may influence both the onset and the cessation of the intermittent blood flow blockage phenomenon in locallized vascular beds.

Large sodium and potassium ion shifts might be expected to stimulate the $Na^+ - K^+$ ATPase pump in the basolateral membranes. The possibility exists, therefore, that the potassium link to water secretion is one which is associated with the $Na^+ - K^+$ pump, and that the movement of water molecules into the cells is associated with active K^+ transport into the cells. The hydrostatic pressure gradient would prevent the outward movement of water molecules associated with outward transport of Na^+. Fluid and electrolyte secretion would be transcellular in this case. However, whether the potassium link to water transfer is strictly passive (maintenance of fluid transfer channels), or associated with active potassium transport, the energy for water transfer must be considered to be the hydrostatic pressure gradient.

There is some evidence that water reabsorption is linked to the $Na^+ - K^+$ pump. In studies of rates of secretory fluid reabsorption caused by an elevation of secretory pressures, it was found that ouabain and dinitrophenol cause a slowing of reabsorption, but do not slow the rate of secretion or interfere with the ability of the glands to develop maximal secretory pressures. This is consistent with the concepts previously developed in this chapter stating that the direction of fluid movement across the striated ducts is dependent on the direction of the hydrostatic or osmotic pressure gradient. It also supports the concept that reabsorption is linked to active Na^+ transport in the basolateral membrane (toward the capillaries), while secretion is linked to passive K^+ leakage outward through the basolateral membranes, with fluid then moving toward the lumen via the junctional channel. Since reabsorption of fluid appears to be tied to Na^+ reabsorption, this suggests that fluid reabsorption occurs predominantly through the cells proper (transcellular route). Thus, while the hydrostatic pressure differential generated by the cholinergic effects on the vasculature is the driving force for fluid transfer during the parasympathetic (eating) reflex secretion, fluid reabsorption is not a normal phenomenon during such activity. It suggests that fluid reabsorption normally occurs only during resting secretion in the relative absence of overt parasympathetic reflex activity. It also suggests that such fluid reabsorption occurs at the same glandular site (i.e., striated ducts) that fluid secretion occurs during parasympathetic reflex activity.

Evidence for Direct Generation of Hypotonic Fluid Through Gap Junctions

When the micropuncture studies are interpreted differently they can also be considered as direct evidence that the lobular ducts produce a hypotonic fluid. An alternative explanation can be presented for the fact that the acinar secretion obtained by micropuncture during pilocarpine-stimulated secretion has a composition that is isosmotic to plasma with plasma-like sodium and potassium concentrations, but that fluid existing from the lobular ducts is very hyposmotic to plasma with very low sodium concentrations. As discussed previously, the interpretation of these findings by the micropuncture investigators was that the acini elaborates all of the secreted fluid and, that it is transformed into a hypotonic secretion in the lobular ducts by ductal sodium reabsorption. An alternate interpretation is that pilocarpine stimulation "turns on" the striated duct fluid secretory mechanism, producing large quantities of low sodium hypotonic secretion *directly* by the transepithelial countercurrent mechanism outlined earlier. This low sodium, elevated potassium hypotonic fluid dilutes the primary acinar fluid and produces the lobular fluid that can be sampled by investigators with cannulaes in the interlobular excretory ducts. At this point, no one can say that this interpreation of the micropuncture studies is not as valid as that offered by the micropuncture investigators.

Evidence that the transepithelial fluid transfer occurs via the gap junction in the ducts is inferential. It comes largely from studies of other epithelial tissues involved in fluid and electrolyte transfer which have cytologic similarities to the striated ducts. In toad bladder, induction of hypertonicities of the mucosal fluid by the addition of NaCl, KCl, mannitol, urea, sucrose, or raffinose reduces the electrical resistance across the epithelium and causes development of swelling in the apical gap junctions. Subsequent removal of solutes completely reverses both phenomena. These changes are not due to or connected with active sodium transport as shown by comparable effects in the presence or absence of sodium pump inhibition by ouabain, and during replacement of sodium by choline. The simplest interpretation of such data is that the apical tight junctions are permeable to water and small solutes. Addition of solute to the mucosal medium leads to diffusion of water into the junction and subsequent transfer of water from the lateral channels that deforms the junctional channel, and thus reduces the electrical resistance (or resistance to ionic conductance across the epithelium). The presence of a luminal-serosal concentration gradient appears to be crucial for "bubble" formation in the gap junction. In cross section the central compartments appear dilated while contact is maintained at the top and bottom. When horseradish peroxidase is added to the luminal (mucosal) side it penetrates into the bubble. When barium is added to the mucosal side and sulfate to the serosal, dense precipitates form in the lateral channels and widened junctions. All of these findings can be seen in the toad bladder, an epithelium that has been classified as "very tight" because of its very high electrical resistance (1000–2000 Ω cm²) and the presence of 5–11 strands in the junction. In contrast, the proximal convoluted tubule of the dog and rat has a transepithelial resistance of less than 10 Ω cm² and 1–2 junctional strands. On the "leaky-tight" scale these gap junctions have been classified as "very leaky." Again, the mammalian renal proximal tubule provides the most apt comparison to striated ducts.

Freeze-fracture studies have been carried out on the faces of the "fractured" zonulae occludens (gap junctions) of a variety of "tight" and "leaky" epithelia. The zonula occludens of the proximal convoluted tubule of the mouse is found to be extremely shallow in the apical-basal direction, consisting in most places of only one junctional strand. In contrast, the "very tight" frog urinary bladder exhibits zonulae occludens that are relatively deep in the apical-basal direction consisting of five or more interconnected junctional strands interposed between the luminal surface and lateral channel. When physiologic data on transepithelial resistance is compared to such morphological data, epithelia with the highest junctional resistance correlate with those having the highest number of junctional strands, while those with the lowest resistance have the fewest stands. Epithelia of intermediate permeabilities exhibit junctions with intermediate or variable morphology. Epithelia which have been studied with respect to such comparisons include toad urinary bladder, mouse stomach, jejunum and distal tubule, rabbit gallbladder, and *Necturus* kidney and gallbladder.

Unfortunately no information is available with respect to transepithelial resistance compared to junctional morphology in the salivary glands. While there have been a number of interesting studies of the main excretory ducts, it would be very useful to have information of this nature about the different parenchymal sites in the glands, the acini, intercalated ducts, striated ducts, and intralobular collecting or excretory ducts. Furthermore, it seems unlikely that information about transepithe-

lial resistance will be forthcoming very soon because an accurate measurement across each segment will require some type of isolation of that segment. It is difficult to project how such experiments could be conducted in the salivary gland acini and secretory tubules. Only the excretory ducts lend themselves readily to such measurements, and several researchers have conducted such experiments on the main (extraglandular) excretory duct of the submandibular gland. Their findings have led them to suggest that the epithelium of this duct should be classified paradoxically, as "leaky" with tight junctions. They suggest, in other words, that the low electrical resistance is due to leaky cell membranes, but that the junctions between cells should be classified as "tight". If the intraglandular ducts possess these same properties, perhaps secretory fluid transfer is transcellular instead of paracellular as discussed earlier. However, at this point salivary gland physiologists must continue to rely upon interpretations of other types of experiments and morphologic studies (such as the studies of horseradish peroxidase distribution mentioned previously) to assess the potential parenchymal site and the transepithelial pathway of fluid secretion.

SUMMARY

The mechanisms which underlie the secretion of saliva from the major salivary glands may be considered in several sets of twos. They have been discussed above as protein secretion vs. fluid and electrolyte secretion; resting secretion vs. eating reflex stimulated secretion; endocellular energy vs. exocellular energy; and adrenergic agonist, or sympathetic nerve stimulated secretion vs. cholinergic agonist, or parasympathetic nerve stimulated secretion. This summary attempts to pull all of these concepts, structures, and mechanisms together into an overall perspective of salivary secretion considered separately as resting secretion and eating reflex secretion. The different cellular mechanisms involved in protein secretion and fluid and electrolyte secretion are summarized as they pertain to each of these two homeokinetic responses of the glands. The reader should bear in mind that this overall viewpoint of salivary secretory mechanisms as two entirely different types of glandular mechanisms is a new concept, and that many of the details of these two mechanisms are conjectural, particulary as they apply to human salivary secretion.

Resting Secretion

Under physiologic conditions, the resting secretion prevails during most of our waking hours. It seems to be stimulated by activation of retinal receptors by light. The efferent limb of this light reflex may reach the acinar secretory cells predominantly via sympathetic nerves (although there is little convincing evidence concerning the efferent pathway(s) involved in resting secretion). The secretion that results is acinar in origin, contains a relatively high protein and glycoprotein content, flows at an unsteady very low rate, and is extremely hypotonic (e.g., 60–80 mOsm/kg in parotid secretion vs. about 290 mOsm/kg for other body fluids). (See Fig. 4-1). The energy for resting secretion is endocellular in origin, as it is derived from the acinar cell metabolic and kinetic processes associated with exocytosis. The low level protein secretory activity from acinar cells generates fluid transfer from osmotic forces, probably via sodium transport into the intercellular canaliculi. In this respect, fluid generation during resting secretion can be considered to result from a "standing osmotic gradient" generated by active sodium transport into the intercellular canaliculi. This fluid is comparable to the "primary secretion" referred to by those who favor the two-stage hypothesis (primary acinar secretion-ductal sodium reabsorption theory). The acinar fluid thus is isotonic with respect to cellular and extracellular fluids. The acinar basolateral *and* apical membranes contain the usual ouabain inhibited $Na^+ - K^+$ ATPase pump. The apical pump maintains Na^+ and K^+ concentrations in the acinar fluid that are very close to Na^+ and K^+ concentrations in the extracellular fluid and plasma. The acinar fluid moves past the intercalated ducts into the secretory tubules or striated ducts by virtue of its continuous generation, with flow aided by occasional contractions of the myoepithelial cells. As the primary secretion traverses the striated ducts, sodium is reabsorbed and potassium is secreted, thereby transforming the electrolyte content of the fluid. More sodium is reabsorbed from the striated duct fluid as the result of excess Na^+ extraction and slow discontinuous movement of the secretory fluid column within the lumen, thereby creating the hypotonic fluid of the resting secretion (Fig. 2-10).

In this resting state, the dense capillary network around the striated ducts is not "working". That is, these capillaries exhibit low flows and low pressures. This represents the "off" position of the exocellular energy switch. In other words, the striated duct capillaries represent a potential energy machine, and they are switched into a working status by the eating reflexes. Without this potential energy to oppose outward movement of water, some of the water of the primary secretion is lost (reabsorbed) during transit through the striated ducts.

The $Na^+ - K^+$ ATPase pumps of the striated ducts are located along the basolateral membranes. Outward sodium transport into the interstitial fluid creates a steep sodium gradient at the apical membrane causing Na^+ to diffuse into the cells from the lumen. Potassium transport into the cells at the basolateral membrane maintains high intracellular K^+, and outward diffusion into the lumina of the striated ducts raises the potassium content of the primary secretion to levels much higher than plasma K^+ concentrations. Thus, the mechanisms involved in the secretion of the resting fluid are essentially identical to the two-stage hypothesis favored by micropuncture investigators.

While the homeokinetic response of the resting secretion plays a major functional role in the homeostatic maintenance of oral tissues, another probable function is to prepare the gland for the much heavier work involved during the secretory activity associated with the eating reflex. Thus, the reflexes which are involved in resting secretion are partly trophic in nature. The low level release of the adrenergic transmitter stimulates acinar cell protein synthesis machinery to produce more proteins and glycoproteins than are released during the low level resting secretion. These products are stored in the secretory granules and are available for large scale release during eating reflex stimulated secretion.

Eating Reflex Secretion

In humans, the mechanisms involved in eating reflex secretion usually become initially activated when food enters the mouth. Contrary to usual descriptions in physiology text-

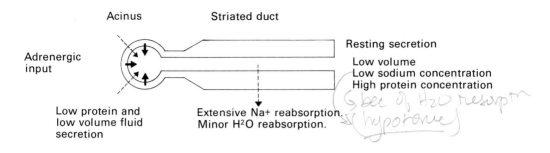

Adrenergic input

Acinus

Striated duct

Resting secretion

Low volume
Low sodium concentration
High protein concentration

sec of H₂O resorp
(hypotonic)

Low protein and
low volume fluid
secretion

Extensive Na⁺ reabsorption.
Minor H²O reabsorption.

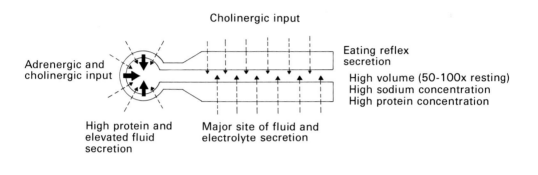

Cholinergic input

Adrenergic and
cholinergic input

Eating reflex
secretion

High volume (50-100x resting)
High sodium concentration
High protein concentration

High protein and
elevated fluid
secretion

Major site of fluid and
electrolyte secretion

➡ Low level protein secretion

➡ High level protein secretion (~100x resting levels)

--➤ Net direction of fluid and electrolyte transfer across epithelium;
relative volumes suggested by numbers of arrows

Fig. 2-10. Proposed general mechanisms of resting vs. reflex stimulated secretion. In resting secretion (top) all products, protein, water and electrolytes are elaborated by the acinus. Sodium is reabsorbed by the striated ducts (and by collecting ducts, not shown) which renders the fluid hypotonic to other body fluids. Some potassium is secreted by the ducts in exchange for sodium. More sodium is reabsorbed than potassium is excreted however, and a small amount of water is also reabsorbed with the sodium during passage through the ducts. This water reabsorption concentrates some substances which enter with the primary acinar secretion. The resting secretion is characterized by a very low flow rate, a high protein and glycoprotein content, high potassium concentrations (e.g., 20-30 mEq/l), a very low sodium concentration (e.g., 2-15 mEq/l); and it is very hypo-osmotic to other body fluids. The primary stimulus for the predominant low level efferent adrenergic input to the acinar cells is light reception on retinal receptors.

During eating (bottom) many receptors are stimulated in and around the mouth, including taste receptors, pressure receptors, and proprioceptors. This results in a profound glandular response with efferent signals carried over both cholinergic and adrenergic efferent nerves. These nerve impulses cause a very large increase (50−100 ×) in protein and glycoprotein secretion and a correspondingly large increase in fluid and electrolyte secretion. The former is due to a great increase in the rate of exocytosis in the acini, while the latter is due largely to transductal transfer of water and electrolytes. A vascular shunt mechanism which causes high capillary pressures in the ductal capillary network, provides the energy for water and electrolyte transfer across the epithelium. An increased amount of water and electrolytes also enters the parenchymal tree at the acinar level together with the increased protein secretion. The final product resembles the resting secretion in its protein content, but contains much more sodium (e.g., 30-60 mEq/l), much more biocarbonate, more chloride and less potassium. The latter ion however, always remains above serum levels (e.g., 10-20mEq/l).

books, the sight or smell of food has little or no effect on secretory flow rates in humans. Sensory receptors which activate this reflex are taste receptors in the tongue and palate, and mechanoreceptors in the teeth and jaw muscles that are stimulated by mastication. The efferent limbs of the reflex arcs involve both sympathetic and parasympathetic nerves. However, the parasympathetic division plays a predominant role in the eating reflex response of the glands (Fig. 2-10).

Events within the salivary glands themselves are varied and profound. The increase in fluid flow from a single gland is $10\times$ to $100\times$ greater than the resting flow. Protein concentrations rise over resting levels and can be maintained at relatively high concentrations for about one hour. In experimental studies where the eating reflex secretion from the human parotid gland has been prolonged for up to three hours, protein concentrations peak during the first hour and decline markedly to very low levels by the end of the third hour. Fluid and electrolyte output, however, remains steady at the same high levels throughout the three hour period.

Responses within the gland include activation of vascular smooth muscle cells, myoepthelial cells, acinar cells, striated duct cells, and possibly lobular and excretory duct cells. Neurotransmitter effects on the vascular smooth muscle produces profound vasodilation of arterial vessels and filling of the dense ductal capillary network. Activation of valves in the lobular veins results in immediate development of high pressures in the capillary network surrounding the striated ducts and lobular ducts, and perhaps also in the long capillary loops which serve the acini.

Several neurotransmitter-mediated responses of the parenchymal cells are involved. They include profound effects on the acinar cells that result in protein secretion. One of these effects is an enzyme-catalyzed transmethylation reaction resulting in methylation of membrane carboxyl groups. This neutralizes surface negative charge on secretory granules and apical membrane eliminating (or reducing) an electrostatic barrier to approximation of secretory granules and apical membrane.

A second (but perhaps concurrent) set of enzyme-mediated responses of the acinar cell to β-adrenergic stimulation of cyclic AMP and active protein kinase formation produces kinase-catalyzed phosphorylation of proteins within the plasma membranes of the secretory granules and within the plasma membranes of the cells themselves, the release of calcium ions from storage sites within the cells, and complexing of phosphate groups between the phosphorylated proteins of the secretory granules and the apical plasma membranes by cal-

cium. This then results in fusion and fission of the respective membranes. All of these reactions result in emptying the contents of the secretory granules into the acinar lumen, a process known as exocytosis. Since the rate of protein secretion is increased enormously over the resting level, the rate of migration of granules toward the apical membrane increases accordingly. Such migration may be brought about by contraction of microfilaments or by the movement of fluid through the cell from the basal membrane toward the apical membrane. Fluid movement may be generated by the vascular pressure differential, by contractions of the myoepithelial cells, or by osmotic forces created by the initial release of granule contents into the acinar lumen. Another element involved in the rapid exocytosis during eating reflex secretion is movement of the apical membrane toward the granules. This occurs as degranulation proceeds with fusion of the membranes of those granules nearest to the apical membrane. Under experimental conditions a noticeable enlargement of the acinar lumen occurs because of this phenomenon. Microcinematography of *in vitro* intact acinar units during exocytosis has revealed that the acinar cells themselves appear to contract in unison during exocytosis in the absence of myoepithelial cells. The force for this process is probably generated by the microfilaments. The effect undoubtedly aids the process of exocytosis and it may also be expected to expel a certain amount of fluid from the cells.

The other major neurotransmitter-mediated effect on the parenchymal cells during eating reflex secretion is on the striated duct cells (Fig. 2-9). This is mediated by cholinergic nerves and causes increases in the permeabilities of these cells to K^+ and Na^+ and perhaps also to water and other small solutes. This membrane effect appears to be connected in some way to water and electrolyte secretion. It has been proposed that the increase in potassium conductance is connected to the establishment of fluid transfer channels in the gap junctions with a minimum of K^+ required in the fluid column to maintain flow-through capability. In this sense these channels might also be considered to be potassium channels. The increased K^+ conductance of ductal cells results in an immediate elevation of K^+ concentration in the lateral channels forcing the fluid in these channels through

106 THE HOST

the gap junctions by the vascular hydrostatic pressure gradient. The cholinergic-mediated membrane effects on the striated duct cells *permits* the pressure differential to be manifested in fluid flow through the junctional channel. The energy for fluid transfer during eating reflex secretion is thus exocellular in origin.

Sodium is extracted as the plasma-like fluid passes into and through the lateral channels of the striated ducts. The moving fluid columns in the lateral channels pass alongside large sheets of plasma membranes lining these channels. The plasma-like sodium concentrations in the channels are presented with a steep concentration gradient, allowing these ions to be passively absorbed into the striated duct cells. This concentration gradient is maintained by an enhanced active transport of sodium into the basal membrane invaginations of these cells. Altogether, the process amounts to a transepithelial countercurrent multiplier effect for sodium, with the sodium ion becoming more and more concentrated (up to a limit) in the central core of the basal half of the striated ducts cells. This concentrating effect permits development of a hypotonic low sodium fluid within the lateral channel as this fluid moves toward the tubular lumen. This mechanism explains the ability of the salivary glands to generate a hypotonic fluid directly, (i.e., at the cellular site of fluid transfer). This direct mechanism occurs during the eating reflex stimulated secretion. It

may play little or no role during resting secretion.

In summary, the eating reflex secretion involves relatively frenetic activity of the acinar units with extensive exocytosis and contractions of the myoepithelial cells. This propels the protein and glycoprotein laden fluid past the intercalated ducts into the ductal secretory tubules. In these tubules, water and electrolytes are secreted. They stream into the lumen through the gap junctions driven by the vascular pressure in the dense periductal capillary network. Here the secreted fluid dilutes the acinar product, and then carries it out of the gland. Sodium is extracted from the plasma-like fluid as it passes between the cells of the striated duct epithelium by virtue of a transepithelial countercurrent multiplier effect. Potassium becomes elevated due to the outflow of cellular K^+ into the fluid as it passes through the lateral channels. (Sodium may continue to be lowered and potassium elevated by basal membrane $Na^+ - K^+$ pumps after the fluid enters the tubular system and continues downstream past the larger collecting and excretory ducts.) By these mechanisms the major salivary glands are able to increase their hypotonic fluid and protein output up to 100X the steady resting output without damage to the integrity of the secretory cells. Furthermore, high levels of hypotonic fluid output may be maintained physiologically for extended periods of time without damaging the glands.

GLOSSARY

Acinus (pl. acini). The functional unit for protein or mucin secretion, composed of pyramidally shaped cells arranged in a spherical ball with the predominant characteristic of secretory granules in the apical half of the cell. The acinus usually contains 8 to 12 cells, with a sparse blood supply as judged by adjacent capillaries.

Adenylate cyclase. (adenyl cyclase). A plasma-membrane-bound enzyme that catalyzes the conversion of ATP to cyclic AMP and pyrophosphate. It acts as an important factor for controlling intracellular cyclic AMP concentrations.

Agonist. A pharmacologic term referring to a substance such as a drug, neurotransmitter, or hormone that is capable of binding to a given class of receptors and activating a response.

α-Adrenergic. A term referring to a class of receptors located in some effector organs of the sympathetic

(adrenergic) nervous system, – to drugs, neurotransmitters, hormones, or other substances that act on those receptors, – and to the effects they produce. Typical systemic α-adrenergic effects include vasoconstriction and contraction of the radial muscle in the eye.

α-Amylase. A salivary enzyme that catalyzes the breakdown of polysaccharides to maltose, maltotriose, and α-dextrin. It is the most abundant of salivary enzymes.

Antagonist. A pharmacologic term referring to a substance such as a drug, hormone, or neurotransmitter that is capable of preventing the action of an agonist. Alpha and β-adrenergic antagonists bind to α- and β-adrenergic receptors, respectively, and thereby prevent the action of the appropriate agonist.

Apical (or luminal). A term referring to that side of the salivary gland cell that is closest to the duct lumen.

ATP (Adenosine triphosphate). An adenine nucleotide that supplies energy to numerous biochemical reactions and acts as a phosphate donor in many phosphorylation reactions.

Basal (or contraluminal). A term referring to that side of the salivary gland cell that is opposite that of the duct lumen and next to the interstitial space.

β-Adrenergic. A term referring to a class of receptors located in some effector organs of the sympathetic (adrenergic) nervous system—to drugs, neurotransmitters, hormones, or other substances that act on those receptors—and to the effects that they produce. Typical β-adrenergic effects include vasodilation in certain blood vessels and increase in rate and force of contraction of the heart.

Cholinergic. A term referring to receptors susceptible to occupation by acetylcholine, to effects resulting from acetylcholine, and to substances that have acetylcholinelike activity. Since the neurotransmitter at parasympathetic neuroeffector sites is acetylcholine, cholinergic is often used in reference to parasympathetic. In this case, however, its meaning is restricted to those situations more precisely termed muscarinic, a class of acetylcholine receptor sites. (See muscarinic for further amplification.)

Cisternae. The spaces enclosed by layers of intracellular membranes such as *rough endoplasmic reticulum* (RER). See rough endoplasmic reticulum.

Condensing vacuole. The vesicular structure whose maturation results in the secretory granule.

Contraluminal. See basal.

Cyclic AMP (adenosine 3′,5′-monophosphoric acid). An adenine nucleotide that activates protein kinase and regulates several cellular functions.

Cyclic GMP (guanosine 3′,5′-monophosphoric acid). A guanine nucleotide that is similar in structure to cyclic AMP. It is thought to regulate some cellular functions and may play a complementary role to that of cyclic AMP.

Cytoskeleton. An internal structural framework of the cell made up of membranelike material.

Degranulation. The state of secretory cells depleted of secretory granules. (See exocytosis.)

DNA (deoxyribonucleic acid). The principle chemical component of genetic material.

Endocellular energy. A term that reflects the origin of the energy for a particular secretory process; also referred to as the first energy compartment. Used to denote that the energy for protein, glycoprotein, and mucin secretion is derived solely from the metabolic energy produced in and by the protein secretory cells. These cells are usually found only in the acinus, the granular ducts, or in mucinous end secretory tubules.

End secretory tubule. The mucin-secreting cells of mucous glands or mixed glands; these cells are often arranged in blind-ended tubules instead of acini, which have a sparse blood supply compared to adjacent secretory tubules.

Epinephrine (adrenaline). A naturally occurring hormone released by the adrenal gland that has both α- and β-adrenergic activity.

Exocellular energy. A term that reflects the origin of the energy for a particular secretory process; also referred to as the second energy compartment. Used to denote that the energy for water and electrolyte secretion during eating reflex stimulation is derived from a hydrostatic pressure differential across the glandular epithelium; the origin of this pressure differential is the blood pressure in the gland capillaries.

Exocrine gland. A gland that secretes its product onto a body surface or into a lumen or cavity of an organ as opposed to into a blood vessel or lymph vessel.

Exocytosis. The process by which a cell secretes substances contained within a granular or vesicular structure so that the contents of the granule are released within the lumen or cavity as a result of unification of granule membrane and plasma membrane.

Fission. The process of fracturing; in this case the breaking of the fused membranes from secretory granules and plasma membranes allowing secretory material to exit from the secreting cell.

Fluid transfer channel. A term to describe the transepithelial pathway that water and electrolytes take when passing from the interstitial fluid compartment of the salivary glands to the tubular lumen of the secretory parenchyma.

Flux. A term that describes a quantitative movement or transfer specific to an ion or other substance across a cell membrane, usually measured by radioactive isotopes: efflux–outward flux or transfer, influx–flux into the cell.

Fusion. The process of joining or uniting; in this case the uniting of two membrane structures into a common membrane.

Gap junction. The membranous and fibrillar structures and fluid-filled spaces associated with the minute area where adjacent membranes of separate cells meet and are joined. By physiologic and anatomic evidence there are definite fluid-filled channels through these junctions. A type of desmosone found in "leaky epithelia" characterized by only one or two junctional strands and low transepithelial resistance.

Golgi complex. An intracellular complex of smooth-surfaced membranes evident in secretory cells and usually arranged in a layered pattern. It is thought to play a dominant role in formation of condensing vacuoles.

Granular ducts. Secretory tubules found in the submandibular gland between the striated ducts and intercalated ducts. Cells are columnar with secretory granules found in apical half of cell; intermediate blood supply judged by adjacent capillaries.

Homeostasis. This is the regulation of the internal degrees of freedom of a complex autonomous system, independent of variations or fluctuations in the external milieu. The implication is that such regulation persists for a long time, the lifetime of a system.

Homeokinesis. This is the achievement of homeostasis by

means of a dynamic regulation scheme whereby the mean states of the internal variables are attained by the physical action of thermodynamic engines.

Homeokinetic response. A specific component of a given dynamic regulation scheme; in the context used herein, related to maintaining homeostasis of the oral cavity.

Intercalated ducts. Short ducts connecting acini to secretory tubules; sparse blood supply.

Interlobular ducts. Ducts within the gland capsule but outside of secretory lobules. They generally lie in the center of gland mass with a very large lumen, multilayered epithelial walls, and a very great blood supply.

Intralobular ducts. Within a secretory lobule, the intralobular collecting ducts lie between the secretory tubules and interlobular ducts; they have more than one cell layer in their epithelial walls, and a very great blood supply.

Isoproterenol. An adrenergic drug that has almost total β-adrenergic activity.

Leaky epithelia. Epithelia between compartments characterized by low transepithelial electrical resistance and by junctional complexes (desmosomes) of only one or two strands.

Luminal. See apical.

Lysosome. An intracellular vesicular structure that contains digestive enzymes and that is important in digestion of cell components and foreign substances.

Membrane conductance. The electrical current (in ohms cm^2) across a membrane. It is the reciprocal of the resistance and can be determined if the potential difference, net flux, and area of the membrane are known.

Membrane potential difference (P.D.). A term referring to the electrical potential difference (P.D.) across a biological membrane; that is, the electrical charge inside a cell relative to the outside.

Membrane resistance. The electrical resistance (in ohms cm^2) across a membrane; can be measured directly by transmembrane electrodes.

Messenger RNA. That portion of ribonucleic acid (RNA) that transmits the genetic message from DNA to the ribosomes for protein synthesis.

Metabolic energy. Energy required to conduct certain cellular and biochemical processes. Energy is usually supplied in the form of ATP, which is in turn largely the product of mitochondrial metabolic processes.

Micropuncture experiments. The technique of withdrawing minute fluid samples (nanoliter quantities) from tiny biological tubules by micropipettes maneuvered by micromanipulators.

Mitochondrion. An intracellular structure composed of a double membrane and internal cristae that supplies the framework and machinery for oxidative phosphorylation and for the formation of ATP as well as for other important processes.

Muscarinic. A term referring to receptors susceptible to occupation by the alkaloid muscarine, to the effects of such receptor activation, or to drugs that have effects similar to that of muscarine. Muscarinic sites usually refer, as they do in this chapter, to neuroeffector receptors affected by acetylcholine released from parasympathetic nerve endings. They are not restricted to these areas, however.

Myoepithelial cell. A smooth muscle cell in close proximity to the acinar unit of exocrine glands. It is thought to play a role in squeezing the acinar cells possibly aiding secretion.

Negative feedback. A biologic process in which a product of a biochemical reaction sequence or physiologic event reduces the rate of the reaction sequence or event. By such feedback, biologic processes can be controlled within certain limits.

Neurotransmitter. A chemical substance released in the central nervous system, in ganglia, and by nerve endings at neuroeffector sites and neuromuscular junctions. This substance is responsible for transmission of a signal from nerve to muscle or effector, or across a synapse.

Nucleotide. A chemical of biologic origin composed of one mole of an organic base, either a pyrimidine or purine, one mole of a sugar, either ribose or deoxyribose, and at least one mole of phosphate joined together in specific linkages.

Paracellular. Referring to "between the cells" or passage through lateral channels and gap junctions in context of water and ion transfers.

Parasympathetic. One of the two divisions of the autonomic nervous system. (See cholinergic and muscarinic.)

Phenylephrine. An α-adrenergic agonist.

Phosphatase. An enzyme that catalyzes the hydrolysis of a phosphoester bond.

Phosphodiesterase. An enzyme that catalyzes the hydrolysis of the 3′ phosphoester bond of the phosphodiesters cyclic AMP or cyclic GMP.

Phospholipids. Phosphoesters of diglycerides such as phosphotidylcholine and phosphatidylethanolamine or phosphoesters of sphingosine.

Phosphorylation. The process by which a chemical substance is covalently bound to phosphate.

Potassium channel. A term for a theoretical channel in salivary gland epithelia that is linked to fluid transfer in a permissive manner (i.e., passage of water and small solutes through the epithelium requires a minimum concentration of K^+ in the permeating fluid). It is proposed that this permeation occurs in channels maintained by minimum concentrations of K^+. Are also referred to as the fluid transfer channels.

Propranolol. A β-adrenergic blocking agent.

Protein kinase. The enzyme activated by cyclic AMP that catalyzes the phosphorylation of various protein substrates. The enzyme is important in carbohydrate and lipid metabolism and possibly in secretion.

Protein synthesis. The biochemical process by which proteins are manufactured from amino acids.

Radioactive-labelled. A term referring to the state of any compound to which has been attached a radioactive atom or which is composed of a radioactive atom. These compounds are very useful experimentally, because their radioactivity makes it easy to monitor their location and fate.

Receptor. A molecule or group of molecules often present in plasma membranes of cells to which drugs, hormones, neurotransmitters, and other substances specifically bind with high affinity.

Recovery phase. The time period following protein secretion in which the acinar cells are regranulated with secretory granules.

Ribosome. A spherical intracellular structure attached to endoplasmic reticulum giving it a "rough" appearance; hence the term *rough endoplasmic reticulum* (RER). The ribosome is the location of protein synthesis.

Rough endoplasmic reticulum (RER). A series of intracellular membranes to which are attached ribosomes. These membranes enclose spaces called cisternae into which secretory proteins are released subsequent to synthesis.

Secretory granule. The spherical membrane-bound intracellular structure that contains secretory product.

Secretory potential. A hyperpolarizing change in the membrane potential of a secretory cell that occurs on nerve- or neurotransmitter-induced stimulation of the glands. It is due to elevated potassium leakage out of the cell.

Sodium channel. A channel in the plasma membrane(s) of epithelia that is permeable only to sodium ions and that becomes selectively activated (i.e., the membrane becomes measurably more permeable to sodium) by certain events or conditions, such as an increase in sodium concentration in the channels. Sodium permeation through these channels is blocked by amiloride and enhanced by aldosterone.

Stage one secretion. Under the experimental condition of electrical stimulation of chorda tympani, that secretion that exists during the first 10 to 20 minutes, contains a high protein, glycoprotein, and mucin content, and is capable of sustaining secretory pressures that exceed arterial pressures. The energy source for this secretion is both endocellular and exocellular but the exocellular source is masked; it thus exposes and defines the first energy compartment (i.e., endocellular energy).

Stage two secretion. Under the experimental conditions of electrical stimulation of chorda tympani, that secretion that will continue indefinitely following the first stage. It contains declining and then constant low protein levels and is characterized by the inability to cause secretory pressures to rise above arterial pressures – and by parallel changes in secretory pressures, and systemic arterial pressures (increases and decreases) induced by arterial bleeding and blood transfusions. It thus exposes and defines the second energy compartment (exocellular energy).

Striated ducts. Secretory tubules containing remarkable basal specialization including deep infoldings of the basal membrane and large numbers of mitochondria aligned in parallel to these infoldings. It has a great blood supply judged by the numerous capillaries adjacent to its basal membranes.

Sympathetic. One of the two divisions of the autonomic nervous system. The term *adrenergic* is often used in reference to sympathetic. Norepinephrine (noradrenalin) is the neurotransmitter at most sympathetic neuroeffector sites. (See α- and β-adrenergic).

Tight epithelia. Epithelia that divide or separate two compartments characterized by low transepithelial electrical resistance and by junctional complexes (desmosomes) of four or more strands.

Tight junctions. Similar to "gap junction" but characterized by four or more junctional strands. A type of desmosome found in "tight epithelia" characterized by high transepithelial resistance.

Transcellular. Referring to "through the cell" in the context of water and ion transfers (as opposed to paracellular transit).

Transepithelial. Referring to "across the epithelium;" used both for defining water and ion transfer and for descriptions of ionic gradients and pressure gradients.

Transitional element. The terminal area of the rough endoplasmic reticulum from which smooth membranes appear to bud and out of which small vesicles are formed.

Zymogen granule. See secretory granule.

SUGGESTED READINGS

Albano J, Bholla KD, Heap PF, Lemon MJC: Stimulus secretion coupling: role of cyclic AMP, cyclic GMP and calcium in mediating enzyme (kallikrein) secretion in the submandibular gland. J Physiol (Lond) 258: 631–658, 1976

Allison AC, Davies P: Interactions of membranes, microfilaments and microtubules in endocytosis and exocytosis. In Ceccarelli B, Glementi F, Meldolesi J (eds): Advances in Cytopharmacology, Vol 2, Cytopharmacology of Secretion. New York, Raven Press, 1974, pp 237–248

Augustus J, Bijman J, van Os CH: Electrical resistance of rabbit submaxillary main duct: a tight epithelium with leaky cell membranes. J Membr Biol 43: 203–226, 1978

Augustus J, Bijman J, van Os CH, Slegers JFG.: High conductance in an epithelial membrane not due to extracellular shunting. Nature 268: 657–658, 1977

Axelrod J, Daly J: Pituitary gland enzymic formation of methanol from s-adenosyl-methionine. Science 150: 892–893, 1965

Batzri S, Selinger Z: Enzyme secretion mediated by the epinephrine β-receptor in rat parotid slices. J Biol Chem 248: 356–360, 1973

Bogart BI: Secretory dynamics of the rat submandibular gland. An ultrastructural and cytochemical study of the isoproterenol-induced secretory cycle. J Ultrastruct Res 52: 139–155, 1975

Bundgaard M, Moller M, Poulsen JH: Localization of sodium pump sites in cat salivary glands. J Physiol (Lond) 273: 339–353, 1977

Burgen ASV: Secretory processes in salivary glands. In Handbook of Physiology, Section 6, Alimentary Canal, Vol II. Washington DC, American Physiological Society, 1967, pp 561–579

Burgan ASV, Seeman P: The role of the salivary duct system in the formation of the saliva. Can J Biochem Physiol 36: 119–143, 1958

Butcher FR: The role of calcium and cyclic nucleotides in α-amylase release from slices of rat parotid: studies with the divalent cation ionophone A–23187. Metabolism 24: 409–418, 1975

Butcher FR, McBride PA, Rudich L: Cholinergic regulation of cyclic nucleotide levels, amylase release, and K⁺ efflux from rat parotid glands. Molec Cell Endocrinol 5: 243–254, 1976

Chiu HI, Franks DJ, Rowe R, Malamud D: Cyclic A, P metabolism is mouse parotid glands. Properties of adenylate cyclase, protein kinase and phosphodiesterase. Biochim Biophys Acta 541: 29–40, 1976

Claude P, Goodenough DA: Fracture faces of Zonulae Occludentes from "tight" and "leaky" epithelia. J Cell Biol 58: 390–400, 1973

De Camilli P, Peluchetti D, Meldolesi J: Dynamic changes of the luminal plasmalemma in stimulated parotid acinar cells: a freeze-fractured study. J Cell Biol 70: 59–74, 1976

Diamond JM: Channels in epithelial cell membranes and junctions. Fed Proc 37: 2639–2644, 1978

Diamond JM, Bossert WH: Standing gradient osmotic flow. A mechanism for coupling of water and solute transport in epithelia. J Gen Physiol 50: 2061–2083, 1967

Di Bona DR, Civan MM: Pathways for movement of ions and water across toad urinary bladder. I. Anatomic site of transepithelial shunt pathway. J Membr Biol 12: 101–128, 1973

Ellison SA: The identification of salivary components. In Kleinberg I, Ellison SA, Mandel ID (eds): Proceedings Saliva and Dental Caries (abstr). Microbiology [Suppl] New York, Information Retrieval, 1979, pp 13–29

Emmelin A, Gjorstrup P: The physiology of the salivary myoepithelial cells. In Thorn NA, Petersen OH (eds): Secretory Mechanisms of Exocrine Glands. New York, Academic Press, 1974, pp 29–41

Emmelin N, Gjorstrup P: Secretory responses to sympathetic stimulation of the cat's salivary glands in the state of resting secretion. Q J Exp Physiol 60: 325–332, 1975

Fraser PH, Smaje LH: The organization of the salivary gland microcirculation. J Physiol (Lond) 272: 121–136, 1977

Fritz ME, Grampp W: The action of dibutyryl adenosine-3′: 5′-cyclic monophosphoric acid and theophylline on the isolated cat parotid gland. Acta Physiol Scand 93: 352–363, 1975

Gagnon C, Bardin CW, Strittmatter W, Axelrod J: Protein carboxylmethylation in the parotid gland and in the male reproductive system. In Usdin E, Borchardt R, Creveling C (eds): Transmethylation. Amsterdam, Elsevier, 1979 (in press)

Garrett JR, Parsons PA: Movement of horseradish peroxidase in submandibular glands of rabbits after arterial infection. J Physiol (Lond) 237: 3–4, 1973

Garrett JR, Thulin A: Changes in parotid acinar cells accompanying salivary secretion in rats on sympathetic or parasympathetic nerve stimulation. Cell Tissue Res 159: 179–193, 1975

Grand RJ, Gross PR: Independent stimulation of secretion and protein synthesis in the rat parotid gland. The influence of epinephrine and dibutyryl cyclic adenosine 3′, 5′-monophosphate. J Biol Chem 244: 5608–5615, 1969

Hammer MG, Sheridon JD: Electrical coupling and dye transfer between acinar cells in rat salivary glands. J Physiol (Lond) 275: 495–505, 1978

Hand AR: Secretory granules, membranes and lysosomes. In Han SS, Screebny L, Suddick R (eds): Symposium on the Mechanism of Exocrine Secretion. Ann Arbor, University of Michigan Press, 1973, pp 129–151

Hyde R, Feller R, Suddick R: Influence of salicylates on dog parotid saliva (abstr). Intern Assoc Dent Res, Special Issue A, 58: 289, 1979

Jamieson JD, Palade GE: Synthesis, intracellular transport, and discharge of secretory proteins in stimulated pancreatic exocrine cells. J Cell Biol 50: 135–158, 1971

Johnson DA, Sreebny LM: Effect of increased mastication on the secretory processes of the rat parotid gland. Arch Oral Biol 18: 1555–1558, 1973

Kanamori T, Harakawa T, Nagatsu T: Characterization of protein kinases from bovine parotid glands. The effect of tolbutamide and its derivative on these partially purified enzymes. Biochim Biophys Acta 429: 147–162, 1976

Langley LL, Brown RS: Relationship of salivary flow and pressure in dog submaxillary and parotid glands. Am J Physiol 201: 285–286, 1961

Lawson D, Raff MC, Comperts B, Fewtrell C, Gilula NB: Molecular events during membrane fusion, a study of exocytosis in rat peritoneal most cells. J Cell Biol 70: 59–74, 1976

Levintan H, Barker JL: Effect of non-narcotic analgesics on membrane permeability of molluscan neurones. Nature 239: 55–57, 1972.

Leslie BA, Putney JW, Sherman JM: α-Adrenergic, β-adrenergic and cholinergic mechanisms for amylase secretion by rat parotid gland in vitro. J Physiol (Lond) 260: 351–370, 1976

Lillie JH, Han SS: Secretory protein synthesis in the stimulated rat parotid gland. Temporal dissociation of the maximal response from secretion. J Cell Biol 59: 708–721, 1973

Ludwig C, Becker E, Rahn C: Nerve Versuche iiber die Beihilfe der Nerven zur Speichelobsonderung. Z Rat Med 1: 255–277, 1851

Lundberg A: Electrophysiology of salivary glands. Physiol Rev 38: 21–40, 1958

Mangos JA, Braun G, Hamann KF: Micropuncture study of sodium and potassium excretion in the rat parotid saliva. Pflugers Arch 291: 99–106, 1966

Mangos JA, Braun-Schubert G: Micropuncture study of the rat parotid gland. In Rossi E, Stroll E (eds): Modern Problems in Pediatrics, Vol 10, Basel, Karger S, 1967, pp 107–117

Mangos JA, McSherry NR, Barber T: Dispersed rat parotid acinar cells. III. Characterization of cholinergic receptors. Am J Physiol 229: 566–569, 1975

Mangos JA, McSherry NR, Barber T, Arvanitakis SN, Wagner V: Dispersed rat parotid acinar cells. II. Characterization of adrenergic receptors. Am J Physiol 229: 560–565, 1975

Martin CJ, Fromter E, Gevler B, Knauf H, Young JA: Electrolyte transport in the excurrent duct system of the submaxillary gland II. In Emmelin N, Zotterman Y (eds): Oral Physiology. Oxford, Pergamon Press, 1972, pp 115–125

Martinez JR: Water and electrolyte secretion by submaxillary gland. In Botelho SY, Brooks FP, Shelley WB (eds): Exocrine Glands. Philadelphia, University of Pennsylvania Press, 1969, pp 20–30

Martinez JR, Holzgreve H, Frick A: Micropuncture study of submaxillary glands of adult rats. Pflugers Arch 290: 124–133, 1966

Peterson OH: The dependence of the transmembrane salivary secretory potential on the external potassium and sodium concentration. J Physiol 210: 205–215, 1970

Peterson OH: Formation of saliva and potassium transport in the perfused cat submandibular gland. J Physiol 216: 129–142, 1971

Peterson OH, Poulsen JG: Secretory Transmembrane potentials and electrolyte transients in salivary glands. In Botelho SY, Brooks FP, Shelley WB (eds): Exocrine Glands. Philadelphia, University of Pennsylvania Press, 1969, pp 3–20

Putney JW, Jr. VanDewalle CM, Leslie BA: Receptor control of calcium influx in parotid acinar cells. Mol Pharm 14: 1046–1053, 1978

Robinovitch MR, Keller PJ, Iversen J, Kauffman DL: Demonstration of a class of proteins loosely associated with secretory granule membranes. Biochim Biophys Acta 382: 260–264, 1975

Rothman SS: Enzyme secretion in the absence of zymogen granules. Am J Physiol 228: 1828–1834, 1975

Rubin RP: Calcium and the Secretory Process. New York, Plenum Press, 1974, pp 101–150

Schneyer LH: Secretion of potassium. In Han SS, Sreebny L, Suddick RP (eds): Symposium on the Mechanism of Exocrine Secretion. Ann Arbor, University of Michigan Press, 1973, pp 18–32

Schneyer LH, Emmelin N: Salivary secretion. In Jacobson ED, Shanbour LL (eds): Gastrointestinal Physiology. London, Butterworth, 1973, pp 183–226

Schneyer LH, Young JA, Schneyer CH: Salivary secretion of electrolytes. Physiol Rev 52: 720–777, 1972

Schramm M, Selinger Z: The function of α- and β-adrenergic receptors and a cholingergic receptor in the secretory cell of rat parotid gland. In Ceccarelli B, Clementi F, Meldolesi J (eds): Advances in Cytopharmacology, Vol 2, Cytopharmacology of Secretion. New York, Raven Press, 1974, pp 29–32

Schramm M, Selinger Z: The functions of cyclic AMP and calcium as alternative second messengers in parotid gland and pancreas. J Cyclic Necleotide Res 1: 181–192, 1976

Schwartz A, Moore CA: Highly active Na$^+$, K$^+$-ATPase in rat submaxillary gland bearing on salivary secretion. Am J Physiol 214: 1163–1167, 1968

Shannon IL, Feller RP, Eknoyan G, Suddick RP: Human parotid saliva urea in renal failure and during dialysis. Arch Oral Biol 22: 83–86, 1977

Shannon IL, Feller, RP, Suddick RP: Light deprivation and parotid flow in the human. J Dent Res 51: 1642–1645, 1972

Shannon IL, Suddick RP: Effects of light and darkness on human parotid saliva flow rate and chemical composition. Arch Oral Biol 18: 601–608, 1973

Shannon IL, Suddick RP, Chauncey HH: Effect of atropine-induced flow rate depression on the composition of unstimulated human parotid fluid. Arch Oral Biol 14: 761–770, 1969

Shannon IL, Suddick RP, Dowd FJ: Saliva: composition and secretion. In Myers HM (ed): Monographs in Oral Science, Vol 2. Basel, S Karger, 1974

Shannon IL, Suddick RP, Edmonds EJ: Effect of rate of gland function on parotid saliva fluoride concentration in the human. Caries Res 7: 1–10, 1973

Sharoni Y, Eimerl S, Schramm M: Secretion of old versus new exportable protein in rat parotid slices: control of neurotransmitters. J Cell Biol 71: 107–122, 1976

Simson JAV, Spicer SS, Hall BJ: Morphology and cytochemistry of rat salivary acinar secretory granules and their alteration by isoproterenol. Z Zellforsch 101: 175–191, 1969

Soodak H, Iberall A: Homeokinetics: a physical science of complex systems. Science 201: 579–582, 1978

Spanner R: Der abkurzungskreislauf der Glandala submaxillaris. Z Anat Entw Gesh 107: 124–153, 1937

Speirs RL, Herring J, Cooper WD, Hardy CC, Hind CRK: The influence of sympathetic activity and isopronaline on the secretion of amylase from the human parotid gland. Arch Oral Biol 19: 747–752, 1974

Sreebny LM, Johnson DA, Robinovitch MR: Functional regulation of protein synthesis in the rat parotid gland. J Biol Chem 246: 3879–3884, 1971

Suddick RP: Does transepithelial hydrostatic pressure provide energy for fluid secretion? In Han SS, Sreebny LM, Suddick RP (eds): Symposium on the Mechanism of Exocrine Secretion. Ann Arbor, University of Michigan Press, 1973, pp 44–60

Suddick RP, Calhoon TB, Giammara BL: Dog submandibular secretory pressures compared to systemic arterial pressures (abstr). Intern Assoc Dent Res, Special Issue A, 58: 289, 1979

Suddick RP, Dowd FJ: The microvascular architecture of the rat submaxillary gland: possible relationship to secretory mechanisms. Arch Oral Biol 14: 567–576, 1969

Suddick RP, Dowd FJ, Shannon IL: Effects of arterial and venous occlusion on submaxillary gland secretion in rats. Arch Oral Biol 16: 509–516, 1971

Tamarin A, Pickering R, Johnson D, Robinovitch M: Correlative studies of biochemical and kinematic aspects of acinar secretion in dissociated rat parotid glands. In Han SS, Sreebny L, Suddick RP (eds): Symposium on the Mechanisms of Exocrine Secretion. Ann Arbor, University of Michigan Press, 1973, pp 1–9

Tamarin A, Sreebny LM: The rat submaxillary salivary gland. A correlative study of light and electronmicroscopy. J Morphol 117: 295–352, 1965

Tandler B, Poulsen JH: Fusion of the envelope of mucous droplets with the luminal plasma membrane in acinar cells of the cat submandibular gland. J Cell Biol 68: 775–781, 1976

Thaysen JH, Thorn NA, Schwartz IL: Excretion of sodium, potassium, chloride, and carbon dioxide in human parotid saliva. Am J Physiol 178: 155–159, 1954

Thulin A: Influence of autonomic nerves and drugs on myoepithelial cells in parotid gland of cat. Acta Physiol Scand 93: 477–482, 1975

Thulin A: Blood flow changes in the submaxillary gland of the rat on parasympathetic and sympathetic nerve stimulation. Acta Physiol Scand 97: 104–109, 1976

Voute CL, Ussing HH: Quantitative relation between hydrostatic pressure gradient, extracellular volume and active sodium transport in the epithelium of frog skin. Exp Cell Res 62: 375–383, 1970

Wade JB, Revel JP, DiScula VA: Effect of osmotic gradients on intercellular junctions of the toad bladder. Am J Physiol 224: 407–415, 1973

Wallach D, Kirshner N, Schramm M: Non-parallel transport of membrane protein and content proteins during assembly of the secretory granule in rat parotid gland. Biochim Biophys Acta 375: 87–105, 1975

Wallach D, Schramm M: Calcium and the exportable protein in rat parotid gland. Parallel subcellular distribution and concomitant secretion. Eur J Biochem 21: 433–437, 1971

Watson EL, Williams JA, Siegel IA: Calcium mediation of cholinergic-stimulated amylase release from mouse parotid gland. Am J Physiol 236: C-233-C-237, 1979

Wieth JO: Paradoxical temperature dependence of sodium and potassium fluxes in human red cells. J Physiol 207: 563–580, 1970

Wojcik JD, Grand RJ, Kimberg DV: Amylase secretion by rabbit parotid gland. Role of cyclic AMP and cyclic GMP. Biochim Biophys Acta 411: 250–262, 1975

Yoshida H, Mike N, Ishida H, Yamamoto I: Release of amylase from zymogen granules by ATP and a low concentration of Ca^{2+}. Biochim Biophys Acta 158: 489–490, 1968

Young JA: Electrolyte transport by salivary epithelia. Proc Aust Physiol Pharmacol Soc 2: 101–121, 1973

Young JA, Fromter E, Schogel E, Hamann KF: A microperfusion investigation of sodium resorption and potassium secretion by the main excretory duct of the rat submaxillary gland. Pflugers Arch 295: 157–172, 1967

3 Salivary Proteins and Oral Health

ROBERT J. BOACKLE

RICHARD P. SUDDICK

Introduction
General Classification of Salivary Proteins
  Biochemical and Immunological Aspects
  Glandular Saliva and Whole Saliva
    Digestion of Salivary Proteins
    Mucins and Salivary Precipitates
Biochemical Considerations and Biologic Significance
  Salivary Proteins Rich in Proline
  Acidic Proline-Rich Salivary Proteins (phosphoproteins)
    Detergent-Like Properties
    Charge-Charge Interactions
    Remineralization
    Model for Surface Ion Stabilization
  Salivary Proteins Rich in Aromatic Components
  Quantitative Analysis of Salivary Proteins
  Salivary Agglutinins
    Interaction of Saliva with Bacterial Polysaccharides

What is the Nature of the "Specific" Agglutinins?
Selected Salivary Enzymes
  Amylase
  Lactoperoxidase
  Lysozyme
  Lipolytic Activity (Lipases)
Nonenzymatic Antimicrobial Salivary Proteins
  Lactoferrin
  Salivary Immunoglobulins
  Protease Inhibitors in Mucosal Secretion
  Modified Salivary Proteins
Salivary Proteins and Mucosal Defense Mechanisms: New Concepts
Conclusion
Glossary
Suggested Readings

INTRODUCTION

While the previous chapter was devoted to an explanation of the mechanisms by which saliva is secreted, the following two chapters of this textbook will specifically investigate the roles played by the constituents of saliva in affecting oral health. In this first chapter the proteins in saliva will be discussed in an effort to learn their identity, uncover their functions, and investigate their involvement in maintaining the balance between health and disease in the oral cavity.

113

GENERAL CLASSIFICATION OF SALIVARY PROTEINS

Biochemical and Immunological Aspects

One of the most important functions of the salivary secretions is to continually provide the constituents of the protein coats for the teeth and for oral mucosa. In this regard, salivary secretions may be involved in processes such as lubrication of mucosa, remineralization of decayed tooth surfaces, reduction of microbial attachment to the teeth, neutralization of microbes and their products, and maintenance of taste acuity by interacting with the taste buds.

In addition to studying salivary proteins from a functional viewpoint, it is advantageous to classify them on the basis of their relative concentrations and physical properties. Using a system in which a salivary secretion is applied to a porous gel and then put under the influence of an electric current, salivary proteins can be separated from each other. The more negative proteins migrate toward the positive electrode (the anode) and the positive proteins toward the cathode. This system will also separate proteins based on their relative size if the proper gel is used. Thus, the negatively charged smaller salivary proteins will migrate rapidly through the pores of the gel while larger molecules sustain more resistance in their migration and thus move slowly. Using an alkaline acrylamide gel with defined pore sizes, the proteins of an individual parotid secretion give a distinct pattern. It should be noted that although the overall composition is generally similar for different individuals, significant genetic differences exist. Any inherited changes in size and/or charge within a population of proteins will result in a different relative migration of those proteins in the gel.

Most of the negative protein bands which are located closest to the positive electrode (Fig. 3-1) are generally referred to as the low molecular weight acidic proline-rich phosphoproteins. They comprise about twenty per cent of the total proteins in parotid and submandibular secretions. The isotypes of the amylase enzymes, another predominant group of salivary bands of higher molecular weight (60,000), are located nearer the opposite (negative) electrode (Fig. 3-1). Each band of pro-

tein, although slightly different from the others in charge because of differences in carbohydrate moieties or deaminations, has amylase activity. The electrophoretic pattern provided by the proline-rich phosphoproteins and by the amylase isozymes on these gels is an inherited characteristic. A third group of salivary proteins which can be identified using this type of electrophoretic technique are the two classes of secretory IgA. Since secretory IgA is a large molecule (400,000 molecular weight) with only a slightly negative charge at the pH used in the electrophoresis (8.6), it is located at the very top of the gel (Fig. 3-1). Secretory IgA is the predominant immunoglobulin in salivary secretions and its levels increase in the presence of active, soft tissue penetrating mucosal infections.

Although many similarities exist between the major and minor salivary gland secretions, each secretion has certain distinctive protein constituents. For example, the high molecular weight viscous mucoproteins and mucoprotein-like substances are localized to submandibular, sublingual, and minor salivary secretions; they are not found in parotid saliva. These mucoproteins (also called mucins), although very negatively charged, are so large that they cannot begin to penetrate acrylamide gels such as those shown in Figure 3-1. Special gels containing a mixture of agarose and acrylamide have been used in order to generate very large pores into which these molecules can migrate. Unlike most of the other salivary molecules, mucins contain 70 per cent carbohydrate. Therefore, a carbohydrate stain is used to visualize these components after electrophoresis. The viscous mucoproteins are responsible for the lubricating properties of saliva and have several other functions.

Those salivary proteins with an overall positive charge at the pH used in the electrophoresis procedure do *not* enter the gel (toward the positive electrode). These positively charged (basic) salivary proteins include the basic histidine-rich proteins, the basic proteins and glycoproteins rich in proline, and salivary lysozyme.

Included in the first group is the histidine-rich salivary protein gustin, a zinc protein in salivary secretions which is believed to interact with taste buds to stimulate their growth and to activate the proper sensation of taste. Perhaps it is the unusually high content of tightly bound zinc that provides the overall positive character to this otherwise aspartic

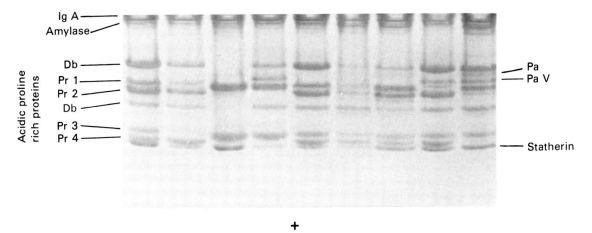

Fig. 3-1. Alkaline acrylamide gel electrophoresis of 9 parotid saliva samples from different individuals. Note that individuals inherit different salivary proteins.

and glutamic acid—rich protein. Lactoperoxidase and lysozyme are salivary enzymes which may be important in mediating a controlled defense against oral microbes. It is interesting that these enzymes have a high affinity for the hydrated calcium phosphate mineral in teeth (hydroxyapatite) and maintain their activity after binding. In addition to these proteins, salivary secretions contain substantial amounts of albumin, which tends to stabilize the conformation of the salivary proteins at the air-liquid interfaces on the surfaces of the oral cavity.

Glandular Saliva and Whole Saliva

Glandular saliva or glandular secretions are terms used to describe the various salivary secretions as they enter the oral cavity. Once in the oral cavity, these secretions are instantly contaminated with a large variety of microorganisms, microbial enzymes, sloughed epithelial cells, degenerating polymorphonuclear leukocytes, and serous crevicular fluid. This complex mixture is referred to as the **whole saliva** (see Contents of Whole Saliva).

Digestion of Salivary Proteins

Digestive enzymes, primarily from microbes but also from degenerating host cells, begin to catabolize salivary proteins, with the relative exception of albumin, which appears for the most part to be resistant to the various bacterial proteases. Perhaps this resistance explains the relatively large amount of albumin

(derived from saliva and from serous crevicular fluid) that remains unaltered in the bacterial dental plaque. Most of the other salivary proteins are not as fortunate, and many are rapidly degraded into small peptides and carbohydrate moieties. When whole saliva is expectorated into a test tube and incubated for 10 minutes to 1 hour at 37°C, little intact salivary protein remains with the exception of albumin. Of course, new salivary secretions continually enter the oral cavity providing a constant source of new proteins.

Each individual has a delicate balance in his oral cavity between the level of functionally intact salivary proteins and the level of bacterial digestive enzymes which destroy those host salivary proteins.

Mucins and Salivary Precipitates

Upon collecting whole saliva it is readily noticed that a salivary precipitate instantly forms. It is believed that this precipitate consists of partially digested salivary proteins, including salivary glycoproteins and the large molecular weight molecules of the mucins. Mucins have a protein core onto which carbohydrate groups attach via O-glycosidic ester linkages to the hydroxyl groups of serine and threonine. In the glands mucins are synthesized in a multiple step process during which the peptide core is first transported to the endoplasmic reticulum. (See Chapter 2). At this site glycosyltransferases assemble the oligosaccharide chains of varying length. Many of the side chains terminate in sialic acid, and in general the mucins are sulfated. These two types of groups give the mucins their charge and their binding tendency for microorganisms and for hydroxyapatite surfaces. The oligosaccharide side chains are structurally variable; some carry blood group activity whereas others do not.

One of the main reasons for the mucin precipitation is the action of bacterial glycosidases, such as the bacterial neuraminidases, which cleave sialic acid residues from the external surface of the molecule. Loss of mutually repulsive negative charges allows rapid folding and aggregation with other denatured salivary mucins. The large complexes then precipitate from solution. The cloudy appearance of the whole saliva is also a function of the oral bacteria, the sloughed, sometimes fragmented epithelial cells (which are coated with bacteria), and the degenerating polymorphonuclear leukocytes. It is of interest that this salivary precipitate, like the dental plaque, is one of the most potentially inflammatory substances which contacts host tissues. For example, the salivary sediment is a potent activator of the complement system. It is postulated that bacterial desialation of host proteins such as mucins generates an effective activator of the alternative complement pathway (present in serum and crevicular exudates). It is obvious that many of the experiments performed with whole saliva should have profoundly different results from those performed with the pure secretions. Indeed, the pure secretions, collected just as they enter the oral cavity are anti-inflammatory with regard to classical complement pathway activation.

BIOCHEMICAL CONSIDERATIONS AND BIOLOGIC SIGNIFICANCE

Salivary Proteins Rich in Proline

Many of the salivary proteins are rich in proline. This amino acid provides a structual rigidity within the molecules. Other host molecules with relatively high proportions of proline (e.g., collagen) serve a structural or supportive role rather than an enzymatic function. This same reasoning applies to the proline-rich proteins in saliva as these proteins have no known enzymatic function yet serve important structural roles. In general, the proline-rich proteins include what are termed the acidic proline-rich proteins (phosphoproteins), the acidic glycoproteins, the basic proline-rich proteins, the basic glycoproteins, and the salivary mucins. Two of their most important structural roles are to form the coat protein layer for mucosal surfaces, and to form the acquired pellicle on the surfaces of the teeth (see Chap. 5). These chemical interactions result in response to regions on a part(s) of these molecules which are highly charged. Such salivary proteins rapidly bind to clean tooth surfaces via ionic charge-charge interactions. The binding is with the charged hydroxyapatite mineral in the enamel. These salivary constituents form a psuedomembrane that fits tightly around the tooth like a glove. Since the charged groups on hydroxyapatite (due to calcium and phosphate ions) are in a fixed arrangement, the charged proline-rich proteins should have a structural rigidity. Therefore one might expect a certain protein pattern to form in the dental pellicle.

Acidic Proline-Rich Salivary Proteins (Phosphoproteins)

About ten years ago it was realized that phosphate ions competitively inhibited the attachment of a group of acidic salivary proteins to hydroxyapatite. Later it was determined that these proteins have little or no carbohydrate but do possess relatively large amounts of proline, serine phosphates, and glutamic acid. Thus they have been termed by some scientists as the acidic proline-rich proteins (phosphoproteins) (Fig. 3-1 and Table 3-1). At present proteins in this group are named upper and lower double bands (Db); protein acidic Pa (also called X) and its Pa variant; and acidic proline-rich proteins (Pr1, Pr2, Pr3, and Pr4). In addition, a small tyrosine-rich protein (statherin), which is an acidic phosphoprotein containing substantial amounts of proline, has some binding properties in common with this group.

The salivary proline-rich phosphoproteins are some of the most important constituents of the acquired dental pellicle present at the tooth-saliva interface. The high affinity of these proteins for the hydrated calcium phosphate mineral in tooth surfaces (hydroxyapatite) explains the very rapid rate of dental pellicle formation. The highly acidic proline-rich

TABLE 3-1. SELECTED PROTEINS IN SALIVARY SECRETIONS

	Principal Amino Acids	Carbohydrate %	Approximate Molecular Weight (daltons)
Acidic Proline-Rich Phosphoproteins			
Pr1	Glutamic acid	—	12,000
	Proline		
	Glycine		
Pr2	Same as above	—	12,000
Pr3	Same as above	—	6,000
Pr4	Same as above	—	6,000
Pa protein (X)	Proline		
	Glutamic acid		
	Glycine	(5%?)	50,000–150,000
Taste Protein			
Gustin-	Aspartic acid	—	37,000
	Glutaminic acid		
	Leucine		
	(Histidine)		
Histidine-Rich Proteins			
HRAP	Histidine	—	4,500
	Aspartic acid		
	Arginine		
HRPI (basic)	Histidine		
	Asparagine, tyrosine, arginine	—	5,800
Tyrosine-Rich Phosphoproteins			
Statherin	Glutamic acid		
	Proline		
	Tyrosine	—	5,200
Viscous Mucoproteins			
Mucins	Proline		
	Serine		
	Threonine	(70%)	$>5 \times 10^5$
Basic Proline-Rich Glycoprotein			
Basic glycoprotein	Proline		
	Glycine		
	Glutamic acid	(40%)	35,000

salivary proteins and statherin interact with the hydroxyapatite via their negatively charged carboxylic and phosphate groups which are located primarily on one end of the protein; the other end of the protein lacks this charge density and is relatively nonpolar (hydrophobic).

Detergent-Like Properties

Molecules which have a hydrophilic and a hydrophobic region are referred to as **detergents.** There is speculation that these acidic proline-rich molecules are very mild oral detergents which coat tooth surfaces as well as oral microbiota, and act to retard dental plaque formation. Coinciding with possible detergent-like effects, these proteins may play a role in dissolution of microbial membranes, as well as a role in emulsification of fatty food stuffs. *In vivo*, the biological half-life of these molecules is a function of the concentration of bacterial protease enzymes that readily digest these proteins, as bacteria probably use them as part of their nutrient source.

Charge-Charge Interactions

As will become apparent, charge-charge interactions are of extreme importance in the oral cavity due to the very low NaCl concentrations in saliva. The relative salt concentration in saliva (0.035 to 0.075 M) is about ¼ to ½ that in serum (approximately 0.15 M). High concentrations of salt theoretically interfere with many of the charge-charge interactions that occur in the oral cavity by inserting themselves between the charged species.

The biologic consequences of ion-ion interactions become significant in attempting to understand the role of salivary proteins in the formation of dental pellicle and dental plaque. It is hypothesized that after proper brushing with a detergent-containing toothpaste, most of the salivary proteins are stripped from the tooth surface and concomitantly some of the mucosal surfaces are also cleaned of a mucin-protein layer. At this time taste acuity is changed, perhaps because of the temporary removal of the taste protein, gustin, from some of the taste buds. In addition, the hydroxyapatite on the tooth surface is exposed to a rinsed oral cavity with fewer bacteria. This allows the rapid formation of a new dental pellicle relatively free of organisms. Within a few minutes a new coat of salivary proteins exists on all of the oral structures. Some of these proteins bind directly, while others, such as the acidic phosphoproteins and mucins, may bind via calcium ion bridges. Most of the oral streptococci have a cell wall that contains negatively charged groups due to the presence of lipoteichoic acid and peptidoglycan. In general these negatively charged bacteria (such as streptococci) are probably coated with many of the same proteins that form the dental pellicle. The intact salivary protein coat on the microbes partially nullifies or coats their charges and prevents direct bacterial attachment (via ion-ion interactions) to the salivary coated tooth surface. Recall, however, that salivary organisms produce substantial amounts of proteases which rapidly digest those host salivary proteins. It is speculated that when the oral concentration of microbes reaches the point where the microbes are able to remove (destroy) the protein coats on both themselves and the tooth as rapidly as those coats form, that bacterial attachment to the tooth is enhanced. Subsequently the adapted bacteria begin proliferating on the tooth surface, and dental plaque develops to the point where it becomes visible to the naked eye. Most, if not all, of the oral microbiota are potent producers of proteases. *Streptococcus sanguis* is believed to be one of the most potent microorganisms. It is interesting that this organism is one of the first to colonize the pellicle—coated tooth surface after brushing. These, however, are not the only mechanisms involved in the initial colonization of the tooth surface nor in the macroscopic development of dental plaque (see Chaps. 11 and 12).

Organisms such as the streptococci also secrete negatively charged extracellular polysaccharides that stick on to their surface. Certain strains of *Streptococcus sanguis* (OPA-1) and of *Streptococcus mutans* (K1-R) produce extracellular polysaccharides (i.e., dextrans) which can actually cause aggregation of small hydroxyapatite particles. It is speculated that these surface-bound, negatively charged polymers, if not previously coated and neutralized with intact salivary proteins, adhere strongly to charged hydrated surfaces on the hydroxyapatite mineral of the tooth (see Chap. 7).

Again, the prior addition of native salivary proteins to a suspension of oral microbes and to the tooth surface lowers the number of microbes able to adhere via ionic interactions. Thus, *intact* salivary constituents may be mitigating plaque formation. However, after bacterial degradation (digestion) of the proline-rich salivary proteins, for example, these salivary constituents may exert entirely different effects. It is possible that they may simply provide a carbohydrate and/or a nitrogen source for the organisms. Recent studies suggest, in fact, that individuals who inherit the double band (Db) acidic proline-rich proteins may have a more rapid rate of plaque formation than those who do not inherit these bands. This hypothesis is based on the increased nutrient source which the Db proteins provide and the effects of their partially digested charged fragments, which may continue to adhere to the organisms, add to their charge, and promote rather than inhibit bacterial adherence to other charged surfaces. It should be asserted that most of the postulated mechanisms for the role of saliva in plaque formation are working hypotheses.

Remineralization

Some of the acidic, proline-rich salivary phosphoproteins may also be involved in another biologically important phenomenon, regulation of the remineralization of decayed tooth surfaces (see Chap 19). These salivary proteins, having an affinity for calcium ions in saliva and for hydroxyapatite, may be actively involved in the process of transport and deposition of calcium ions in the hydroxyapatite lattice on the tooth surface. The precise mechanism(s) which regulates the rate of deposition of salivary calcium and phosphate ions is unknown, but may be directly or indirectly related to physical conditions such as pH. A role for salivary acid phosphatases that may conceivably cleave the phosphate groups from the acidic phosphoproteins has not been provided to date.

Another related function associated with the acidic proline-rich phosphoproteins is the stabilization of the supersaturated calcium and phosphate ions in salivary secretions whose formation into various insoluble lattice structures is thermodynamically favored. Perhaps the same types of mechanisms responsible for binding to hydroxyapatite and regulating its specific proper reformation on tooth surfaces are also operative in stabilization of supersaturated calcium and phosphate ions in salivary secretions. It is postulated that the relatively small charge density that exists within any small nucleus of calcium phosphate ions is insufficient to cause their release from surrounding proteins, whereas a reaction on an exposed hydroxyapatite surface with its large multiple ionic binding sites causes release of the phosphoprotein-bound calcium ions into the enamel matrix. Salivary phosphate ions would then join in forming a new hydroxyapatite surface. It is believed that most of the salivary acidic phosphoproteins are involved in these processes. Perhaps one which has received the reputation of being most potent in regulating remineralization processes and in supersaturated calcium ion stabilization in statherine (Table 3-1, Fig. 3-1).

Again, the salivary proteins in the absence of a hydroxyapatite surface may inhibit spontaneous precipitation by preventing crystal nuclei formation. Obviously, then, these proteins serve an important physiologic role in allowing the secretion of supersaturated calcium and phosphate ions from the glandular tissue. Statherin, like the other low molecular weight acidic-rich phosphoproteins, contains both a negatively charged (polar) region and a relatively nonpolar, more hydrophobic region. However, its distinguishing characteristic is its relatively large content of aromatic tyrosine residues. Preliminary studies indicate that in order to completely remove statherin from enamel either acid, detergent, or a chelator of calcium is required.

Model for Surface Ion Stabilization

Since saliva is supersaturated with respect to calcium phosphate, the thermodynamic pressure at neutral pH is for little or no net dissolution of the enamel matrix. However, a significant local decrease in pH shifts the equilibrium on that surface so that hydroxyapatite becomes more soluble or, by definition, the fluid phase calcium phosphate ions in that region no longer exist in a supersaturated state. A role for surface ion stabilization under such conditions may be provided by the salivary secretions. It is postulated that salivary calcium ions initially bound to certain salivary pellicle phosphoproteins and glycoproteins are attracted to an exposed hydroxyapatite surface of the tooth, and become part of the surface. Concomitantly, calcium ions leave the enamel surface at a very slow rate at basic pH and at a faster rate under acidic conditions (where hydroxyapatite is more soluble). In a sense the salivary proteins not only participate in the acid-induced remineralization of decalcified (decayed) tooth surfaces, but also protect the mineral from dissolution thermodynamically by stabilizing and supplying a relatively high fluid phase calcium (and phosphate) concentration. Although at present absolutely no evidence has been reported for any salivary enzyme in this process, it seems likely that salivary phosphatases activated by low pH may be involved in cleaving the (hydroxyapatite bound) phosphates from the salivary phosphoproteins. This would supply a locally high concentration of phosphates.

Some clues to understanding dental calculus formation can be found if one assumes that when bacterial enzymatic digestion of the various sites on salivary molecules responsible for stabilizing the supersaturated calcium phosphate ions occurs, so too does spontaneous calcium phosphate precipitation. Furthermore, the precipitate need not be the exact type of hydrated calcium phosphate lattice (hydroxyapatite) found in teeth since organized ionic structures as found on a tooth surface template do not exist on the plaque. Thus the bacterial dental plaque becomes calcified with various calcium phosphate minerals in a relatively disorderly fashion and does *not* give rise to a smooth surface.

Salivary Proteins Rich in Aromatic Components

Recall that the generalization concerning salivary proteins rich in proline is that they primarily serve structural or interfacial roles (i.e., surface binding). However, when proteins contain large quantities of aromatic amino acids such as histidine or tyrosine, one must assume that additional "specialized" functions are possessed. A good example of this is the tyrosine-rich acidic phosphoprotein, statherin. In addition to coating the tooth surface, statherin is involved in stabilizing the supersaturated salivary calcium and phosphate ions, and in participating in the remineralization process through an unknown mechanism. Specific reactions with mucosal cell surfaces are yet to be studied.

Another specialized function of a salivary

protein is seen in the histidine-rich protein gustin, which not only adheres to the mucosal cells but also carries zinc, and is believed to be involved in promoting the proper growth and function of the taste buds.

In general, the histidine-rich proteins are small (5,000 to 6,000 molecular weight), lack carbohydrate, and in their native state (i.e., with metals) are either neutral or slightly basic. Their small size indicates that these proteins probably have no enzymatic function. Perhaps, like gustin, the other histidine-rich proteins are also involved in carrying metals to surfaces in the oral cavity. The years ahead should provide interesting information on the precise functions of the different histidine-rich salivary proteins.

Lactoferrin is another slightly basic salivary protein with aromatic components (i.e., porphyrins). Lactoferrin is secreted as a potent iron-binding protein which acts to deplete free forms of this metal on mucosal surfaces. If microorganisms do not obtain iron needed for their metabolism, their growth is retarded.

The large size of lactoferrin (molecular weight approximately 80,000) indicates that this salivary molecule may have several different reactions in the oral cavity. One recent report suggests that lactoferrin has a site which binds to salivary antibodies. Thus lactoferrin can be specifically directed to the surface of the antibody-coated microbe.

In addition to lactoferrin, at least one other salivary protein has aromatic porphyrin rings and also binds iron. This is lactoperoxidase, which in the presence of hydrogen peroxide is a potent antimicrobial enzyme (see below). As a general rule the peroxidase enzymes, like lactoperoxidase, utilize their iron as an electron carrier in the biological oxidation of microbial components.

Quantitative Analysis of Salivary Protein

The reported concentration of total salivary protein (2 to 5 mg./ml.) varies according to salivary flow rate, genetic differences (protein phenotypes), and the particular quantitative analytical method used. It should be realized that many of the analytical methods used for the determination of protein concentration rely to some extent on the percentage of aromatic amino acids within the tested proteins. For example, quantitative assays that employ color reagents such as the Lowry method give results directly related to the phenylalanine, tyrosine, and tryptophan content of the salivary proteins. Similarly, direct measurement of the optical density at wave lengths around 275 to 280 nanometers also measures only the aromatic-containing salivary proteins. From the previous sections on aromatic rich proteins and proline-rich proteins it is obvious that only about one half of the salivary proteins contain substantial amounts of aromatic residues. The direct absorbance method can be improved by simultaneous measurement of optical density at several wavelengths including those in the 206 to 220 nanometer region where the proline-rich proteins effectively absorb light.

The accurate measurement of the total protein concentration in whole saliva is more difficult than for pure salivary secretions. The spontaneously-formed insoluble salivary sediment in whole saliva contains a significant amount of denatured and absorbed salivary proteins. In fact, recent experiments have clearly demonstrated that a more accurate method for the measurement of certain individual proteins in salivary secretions, for example, lysozyme and immunoglobulins A, G and M can be best accomplished if the whole saliva is first acidified. This procedure elutes most of these proteins from the sediment, since they are bound via ionic interactions, and enables a more accurate quantitative determination to be made.

Quantitative measurements of individual proteins can be made enzymatically if the protein has enzymatic activity. Often the method of choice is immunochemical if a specific antisera (animal serum containing antibody to the particular salivary molecule) is available. Several antigen-antibody precipitin tests can be used for the determination. One of the most recent and successful of these tests is the nephelometric method which is a measurement of turbidity accomplished by measuring the light scattering by the antigen-antibody complexes when a laser beam is passed through the saliva-antiserum mixtures.

Salivary Agglutinins

When salivary secretions such as parotid saliva or submandibular saliva, and particularly whole saliva, are added to suspension of microbes (that are initially isolated from the oral cavity), a specific spontaneous aggregation often occurs. The bacterial aggregates become so large that they sediment to the bottom of the test tube, sometimes within a few minutes. The aggregation phenomenon can usually be inhibited by the concomitant addition of normal human serum to the mixture. Serum enzymes, such as those of the complement system which bind to the bacteria, may interfere with usual salivary protein binding.

Salivary proteins bind to microorganisms via many different types of reactions. The calcium binding acidic phosphoproteins with a detergent-like (polar-nonpolar) character tend to neutralize the negative charge on the microbes by interacting with (via their polar regions and calcium ion intermediates) the negative charges on the cell wall.

Salivary glycoproteins such as the mucins may in fact have multiple or polyvalent reactions with several bacteria, causing a low level of agglutination. In that event, the presence of trace amounts of any specific salivary agglutinin for a particular organism (i.e., specific antibody) would cause a dramatic enhancement of aggregation. It is not unreasonable then, that the minor salivary glands secrete mucin-like salivary glycoproteins which, like mucin, agglutinate various microorganisms. Similar to the submandibular mucins, some of these high molecular weight mucoproteins have blood group activity and may agglutinate a variety of different types of microorganisms via both charge-charge interactions and specific carbohydrate receptors. Since mucosal epithelial cells also have blood group and similar carbohydrate sequences on their surface, the salivary glycoproteins may provide a limited competitive inhibition for these binding sites on the bacteria. It should be pointed out, however, that *in vivo* sloughed, degenerating oral epithelial cells are literally covered with microorganisms. This indicates that binding sites are exposed on the surfaces of these cells.

Interaction of Saliva with Bacterial Polysaccharides

As has been stated, extracellular polysaccharide polyanions (i.e., dextrans) have a very high affinity for untreated hydroxyapatite, probably for Ca^{++} sites. However, after treatment of hydroxyapatite with salivary secretions the binding of dextran is much weaker. It is postulated that Ca^{++} bridges interpose between the negatively charged polar regions of the *intact* acidic salivary proteins and mucoproteins and the negatively charged bacteria. These coating phenomena tend to interfere with bacterial adherence to the tooth surfaces.

What is the Nature of the "Specific" Agglutinins?

First, because an agglutinin by definition must interact with at least two bacteria simultaneously in order to cause aggregation, one would expect an agglutinin to be a molecule of relatively high molecular weight. Second, because of the supposed specificity of the agglutinins (that is, one individual's saliva will agglutinate certain types of organisms while another's saliva preferentially agglutinates different types), the responsible agglutinins must have different forms or binding sites.

Some scientists believe that salivary antibodies play no critical role in certain agglutination reactions because they have not detected immunoglobulins in any of their "purified" agglutinin preparations. However, their detection techniques may not have been sensitive enough to detect the trace amounts of antibody required to agglutinate saliva-coated organisms. In other words, agglutination, or clumping of organisms by saliva, is a complex reaction. It is likely that a variety of salivary proteins, (i.e., the mucins), salivary glycoproteins, and the charge neutralizing salivary phosphoproteins bind to the bacterial surface. Each additional large molecular weight protein, glycoprotein, or mucinous protein which binds to the bacteria generates an additional potential for agglutination if not a background agglutination in itself. In the presence of even trace amounts of a specific agglutinating substance like salivary antibodies, bacterial clumping should readily occur. Since many of the reactions of the negative salivary mucoproteins and phosphoproteins with negative bacteria are mediated by positive calcium ion bridges, it is anticipated that most of the aggregating phenomena can be reversed in the presence of Ca^{++} chelators.

In addition to salivary antibodies, it is possible that some salivary glycoproteins with blood group activity have broad spectrum interactions with certain types of microorganisms. The nature of these types of interactions may be similar to reactions that occur between bacteria and the molecules on the membrane surface of mucosal epithelial cells.

In this regard it is noteworthy that these epithelial cell receptors also have a carbohydrate character. Identifying the precise reactive nature of specific non-immunoglobulin agglutinins has proved to be a difficult task because of the ever present possibility of contamination with minute amounts of salivary antibody which would tend to confuse the interpretations.

Selected Salivary Enzymes

Amylase

By far the most concentrated and most active enzymes in parotid and submandibular saliva are the amylases. Salivary amylase is alpha-amylase, which catalyzes the hydrolysis of alpha-1, 4-glucosidic bonds of starch, but not of maltose, in a random fashion. Recall that these enzymes have polymorphic forms. It is believed that in the cells of the salivary glands, amylase is first produced as a protein core and then sequentially glycosylated. The isozymes are produced perhaps as a consequence of genetically distinct glycosylation, post-transcriptional and post-secretory modifications involving the carbohydrate, or sequential deamidations. In any event, the isozymes of amylase differ from one another as determined by isoelectric focusing, which separates the molecules only on the basis of charge (isoelectric point). In Figure 3-2 these proteins were focused electrophoretically and then incubated with a warm starch solution that penetrated the gel. Subsequently each enzyme band digested an area of starch which could then be identified by exposure to an iodine solution. Unlike the proline-rich proteins, amylase does not have a strong affinity for the tooth surface. The purpose of this enzyme

seems to be strictly to catalyze the breakdown of starch. Often the contact time between salivary amylase and foodstuffs is only brief. However, this enzyme is in very high concentration in saliva, making it probable that at least a portion of the starch is partially digested while in the oral cavity.

It is of interest that dogs, cats, and horses do not have amylase in their salivary secretions, and that some of these same species have less dental caries than man. Perhaps providing simpler carbohydrates (sugars) to microorganisms enhances their cariogenic potential. However, many other differences exist between animal and human saliva, particularly the presence or absence of protease inhibitors (see below), as well as other oral characteristics that may explain the differences in caries susceptibility.

Lactoperoxidase

Human peroxidase activity is relatively localized to the secretions coating mucosal surfaces (lactoperoxidase) and to the lysosomes of phagocytic cells (myeloperoxidase). These peroxidase enzymes participate in killing microorganisms by catalyzing the hydrogen peroxide—mediated oxidation of a variety of substances in or on the microbes. Utilizing thiocyanate ions in saliva or halide ions in the phagocyte system, peroxidases and peroxide generate highly reactive chemical compounds that bind and inactivate several intracellular microbial enzyme systems, as well as microbial surface components. The precise details of microbial killing are as yet unknown. However, oxidation of almost any vital component, from those on the membrane to those in the genetic material of the foreign organism, results in neutralization.

Since lactoperoxidase has a high affinity for

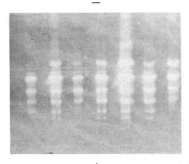

PH 9.5

PH 3.5

+

Fig. 3-2. Isoelectric focusing of amylase on acrylamide gel (pH 3.5 to 9.5). The amylase enzymes move on the gel until they are no longer charged (at their respective isoelectric points).

the enamel surface and maintains its activity after binding, it may be an important defense mechanism limiting early microbial colonization of tooth surfaces. Lactoperoxidase contains porphyrin rings and iron similar to the heme group in hemoglobin. At present there have been no reports that this 80,000 molecular weight glycoprotein has any receptor sites for immunoglobulin as found for lactoferrin.

Lysozyme

The sources of human lysozymes are the glands supplying the mucosal secretions and the host phagocytic cells. These are the same sources as those for human peroxidases. Lysozyme is a small highly positive enzyme that catalyzes the degradation of the negatively charged peptidoglycan matrix of microbial cell walls. In general, bacterial peptidoglycan is a large, insoluble, repeating disaccharide of N-acetylmuramic acid - $\beta1$, 4 N-acetylglucosamine. The β-1, 4 bond is hydrolyzed by lysozyme and after partial digestion the peptidoglycan becomes soluble. It should be pointed out that, depending on the microorganism, its particular type of peptidoglycan may be highly inflammatory. Native purified peptidoglycan causes direct activation of a biologically potent series of enzymes called complement which is present in serum and in gingival crevicular exudates. Furthermore, peptidoglycan is interwoven with the other major bacterial cell wall component, the lipoteichoic acid lattice. Together these subtances have a high affinity not only for mucosal cells but also for the hydroxyapatite in the tooth surface. It is of interest that in individuals with periodontal disease this cell wall material likely adheres to most of the host's surfaces in the periodontal pocket. Complete digestion of the peptidoglycan by lysozyme removes its complement activating inflammatory properties. Most of the lysozyme in the gingival cervicular fluid arrives there via phagocytes.

There is strong evidence that lysozyme, which is highly positively charged, binds to hydroxyapatite and maintains its activity after binding. Also because of its positive charge, lysozyme tends to have strong ionic interactions with bacterial cell walls and with the large negative mucoproteins (mucins) in saliva. It is reasonable then, that the addition of acid ions would competitively interfere with many of the above charge-charge interactions and free the lysozyme both from the hydrox-

yapatite surface and from any mucin complexes. In areas of large plaque deposits, a low local pH may interfere with optimal lysozyme binding and function.

Lipolytic Activity (Lipases)

Secretions from the serous Ebner glands (which are located beneath the circumvallate papillae on the dorsum of the tongue) enter the oral cavity via ducts at the base of the papillae. It has been postulated that a function of these secretions is to wash out taste buds located on the walls of the papillae. A recent study has clearly demonstrated that these secretions contain a potent lipase that hydrolyzes long chain triglycerides to free fatty acids and partial glycerides. Similar lipolytic activity present in esophageal and gastric aspirates in man is stable at acidic pH.

Nonenzymatic Antimicrobial Salivary Proteins

Lactoferrin

Lactoferrin is an iron binding basic protein found in saliva and other mucosal secretions with a molecular weight near 80,000. It is normally secreted in an unsaturated state with respect to iron. Thus, when in the oral cavity, this salivary protein tends to bind and limit the amount of free iron. Since iron is essential for microbial growth, this salivary protein is an active host defense mechanism. The question is, how are the organisms in the oral cavity able to sequester their needed iron in the presence of this protein? It is believed that some types of microorganisms produce their own iron chelating (binding) substances, however, no precise data are available on oral flora in this regard. Another possible source may be the free iron many foods have which could briefly provide a source of the metal on the mucosal surfaces or in trapped areas between the teeth. Crevicular exudates may also be an important source of iron, since lysed host cells and cellular debris, including erythrocytes, enter the oral cavity and contact the bacterial dental plaque.

Salivary Immunoglobulins

Secretory IgA is the predominant immunoglobulin in mucosal secretions with concentrations for stimulated parotid saliva and whole saliva averaging about 6 mg% (or about 3% of the total protein concentration in secretions). Salivary IgG and IgM concentrations are about 10 times less than the IgA concentration.

Secretory IgA is an effective agglutinin because each molecule possesses four antigen binding sites (see Chap. 15). Under normal conditions, the biologic functions of immunoglobulins in saliva are somewhat different from immunoglobulin functions in serum.

In the serum, antibodies of the IgG and IgM class activate and react with a variety of systems in the blood (i.e., classical complement pathway) after binding to antigens. Antibody and complement-coated foreign cells then bind to phagocytes and lymphocytes which have antibody and/or complement receptors. In normal healthy individuals (without significant amounts of crevicular exudates or injured mucosa), the blood enzyme systems are either not present in saliva or are not functional. Therefore, the salivary antibodies must serve other mucosal functions in the oral cavity of healthy individuals.

Protease Inhibitors in Mucosal Secretions

Host inhibition of microbial enzymes that have digestive activity (proteases and glycosidases) can theoretically protect both the mucosal surfaces and the function of other salivary proteins. Such enzyme inhibitors can include specific salivary antibodies to bacterial digestive enzymes and many other types of salivary molecules which act nonspecifically as competitive substrates.

Although several potent broad spectrum protease inhibitors have been studied in dog submandibular saliva, little has been reported on such factors in human salivary secretions. Likewise, specific inhibitors of important bacterial glycosidases such as neuraminidases have received little attention. Perhaps in the years ahead researchers will investigate human secretions of the major and minor salivary glands as a possible source of these inhibitors.

Regulation of bacterial digestive enzymes may be an important determinant in minimizing dental caries and gingivitis. Consider the delicate balance between the protective role of salivary proteins, glycoproteins, and mucoproteins that coat the teeth and oral mucosal membranes and the bacterial digestive enzymes which destroy those substances. If these destructive enzymes are inhibited, local mucosal tissue receives less insult. In addition, bacterial attachment to the tooth might be minimized because the coat salivary proteins would have a longer half-life.

Modified Salivary Proteins

There is evidence which suggests that bacterial glycosidases (neuraminidases), as well as proteases, after interacting with salivary mucoproteins and proteins, yield modified (partially digested) molecules with an extremely high inflammatory potential. Part of this potential may not be expressed until contact is made with the complement enzymes in serum or serous exudates (i.e., gingival crevicular fluid).

It is of particular interest that microbes which are coated with the partially digested salivary mucoproteins and proteins can be "labeled for destruction" if they penetrate host tissue. One of the most important areas of oral biology research lies in exploring the specific nature of these partially digested proteins and mucoproteins, and the precise mechanism by which they activate the complement pathways. In a very broad sense, these modified salivary substances serve one of the same functions of the specific antibodies in marking or identifying for the host's complement system the presence of a foreign invader (from the oral cavity) which has penetrated host tissue. A summary of some of the more studied proteins in salivary secretions is shown in Table 3-2.

SALIVARY PROTEINS AND MUCOSAL DEFENSE MECHANISMS: NEW CONCEPTS

Mechanisms for Defense

While current concepts of how salivary antibodies function are touched upon in Chapter 15, certain aspects of these mechanisms will be presented here because of possible complementary interactions of these proteins with other salivary proteins in influencing micro-

TABLE 3-2. GENERAL CLASSIFICATION OF SOME WELL STUDIED PROTEINS IN SALIVARY SECRETIONS

Salivary Proteins	Probable Functions
Proline Rich Proteins	
Mucins	Because of their high proline content, these are rigid collagen like molecules
Acidic Proline Rich Proteins	designed to form a pseudomembraneous layer (via ionic reactions) on the
Basic Proline Rich Proteins	hard and the soft oral surfaces as well as on the oral flora.
and Glycoproteins	
Enzymatic Proteins	
Amylase	Starch digestion
Lysozyme	Microbial cell wall (peptidoglycan) degradation
Lactoperoxidase	Chemical modification and neutrilization of vital microbial components.
Aromatic Rich (Special Function) Proteins	
Gustin	Taste acuity (binds zinc)
Statherin	Reminerilization (binds calcium)
Lactoferrin	Retards bacterial growth (binds iron)
Albumin	Stabilizes molecular conformations at the air-liquid interface (binds aromatics)
Immunoglobulins	
Secretory IgA	Help protect mucosa against invasion of microorganisms; participate in oral
IgG	immune response (see text and Chap. 15).
IgM	

bial colonization and growth on the mucosal surfaces.

At least three possible broad categories of activities can be described by which salivary proteins and salivary antibodies help protect oral mucosal surfaces. These categories are not mutually exclusive, but may in fact be complementary.

Direct Agglutination of Bacteria

Direct agglutination of bacteria and microorganisms is produced in the laboratory be secretory IgA. In the mouth this may prevent adherence of bacterial cells to mucosal cells and enhance the potential of the normal secretory flow to wash away or clear from the mouth microorganisms by swallowing activity. With respect to viruses, specific salivary antibodies can bind directly to viral membranes and neutralize the physical mechanisms by which they bind to host cells and inject their genetic material. Thus, salivary antibodies are able to *directly neutralize viral infectivity* and replication on the oral surfaces.

Since secretory IgA tends to form complexes with other salivary proteins, and salivary proteins other than antibodies (specific salivary agglutinins) are also able to agglutinate microorganisms, it is possible that specific antibodies and other salivary agglutinins may act cooperatively or synergistically in the agglutination and disposal of microorganisms, as explained above.

Antibody Binding to Mucosal Cells

Evidence has been presented that salivary IgA and IgM, (but *not* IgG) bind to mucosal epithelial cells. If there are specific receptors for secretory IgA on oral epithelial cells it is conceivable that the binding of secretory IgA to these cells may play an important role in mucosal defense mechanisms. Exactly how this may work is not known, but there are several possible interesting roles for secretory antibodies in light of mucosal cell binding and the known peculiarities of the secretory immune system.

Most individuals have low levels of secretory antibodies to most of the microorganisms that can be isolated from their oral cavities. The secretory IgA located on mucosal cells probably represents a mixed population of salivary antibodies to normal oral flora. This would seem to suggest, provocatively, that the normal secretory defense mechanism includes a steady low level production of antibodies to "normal" flora that continually populate mucosal surfaces. The very presence and continued secretion of the antibodies suggests a continued low level of "pathogenicity" of these organisms or associated antigens. In the normal or healthy condition, however, frank breakdown of the epithelium and outright invasion and infection does not occur. Thus it would appear that the existing low levels of antibodies to normal flora represents a secretory "immune response" that *permits* the continued maintenance of normal flora on mucosal and other oral surfaces. In one sense this might even be viewed as part of an overall selective mechanism that favors surface populations of some types or species of microorganisms at the expense of other types.

If low levels of antibodies to normal flora do play a role in the mucosal protective response of glandular secretory systems, can this be reconciled with the frank elevation of antibodies found during outright mucosal infections, or with elevations of specific antibody levels by immunization procedures? It seems that these concepts can be reconciled and incorporated into a broad scheme of mucosal defense by glandular secretory systems. This concept emphasizes two important aspects. One is that an outright local microbial invasion (infection) primarily elicits an induction of specific antibodies of the secretory system *and* of the systemic immune system, *plus* a specific localized inflammatory response. The latter aspect includes a major increase in blood flow to the tissues surrounding the site of invasion, production of a serous exudate from the blood, and migration of phagocytes into the affected area. These homeokinetic responses to mucosal invasion allow the secondary mediators of the systemic immune defense mechanisms to be brought into play, acting in concert with both systemic and secretory antibodies. It has been proposed that this concerted mucosal defensive response occurs *at the specific site of invasion* to combat the developing threat to the host. Thus, one of the major mucosal defense mechanisms brought into play during frank invasion and breakdown of the mucosa is in large part a systemic response directed at the site of invasion.

The second point of emphasis is that a developing site of invasion or infection represents a noxious stimulus to local tissues and nerves within the mucosa and the effects of such stimuli are widely distributed. Through appropriate reflex arcs, the effects of any oral noxious stimuli are reflected in an increase in flow from minor mucosal glands in the area of the invasion *and* from the major salivary glands. The major effect of this response is a huge increase in output of secretory products including secretory IgA. In itself, the increase in fluid flow will help wash away proliferating microorganisms. However it should also be recognized that the increased output of secretory IgA from the major salivary glands represents an increased output of many different

specific antibodies including secretory antibodies to the normal flora. If such antibodies exert a subtle selective effect on mucosal flora as discussed above, they may help maintain normal flora on mucosal sites, *especially* those away from the site of primary invasion. We are suggesting then, that the elevated specific antibody levels to the invasive microorganisms is primarily an elevation that is manifested to a major extent at and near to the site of invasion. In other words, it is thought that the antibodies of the various classes are able to manifest their antimicrobial role against the invasive organisms largely because they act in concert with the secondary mediators of the inflammatory response (e.g., complement) which are present and being produced locally at these sites (largely by virtue of the continuous production of vascular serous exudate).

Other Possible Mechanisms

The third manner in which salivary antibodies may help protect mucosal surfaces incorporates certain facets of the different views already presented. While salivary antibodies that bind to mucosal epithelial cells may permit or favor, in a sense, mucosal population by a certain microbial flora, the entire system also seems geared to a definite general suppression of microbial activity acting at the mucosal surface.

Three salivary proteins have been discussed which have definite antimicrobial activity: lactoferrin, lactoperoxidase, and lysozyme. There is evidence that lactoferrin binds to antibodies and that this may result in a specific localization of this iron binding protein to the bacterial (antigenic) cell surface. It is interesting that lactoperoxidase and lysozyme are enzymes which are similar to those elaborated by the host's phagocytic cells. It would seem that the secretory immune defense system evolved in a manner which was similar to at least some aspects of the systemic immune defense system. Since the oral cavity and alimentary canal in general do not present a favorable environment for phagocytic cell activity, the secretory system seems to have evolved to directly produce antimicrobial enzymes similar to those utilized by phagocytes in combatting invasive bacteria. Thus, although the normal complex of secretory antibodies may favor mucosal colonization by certain species, the continued production and presence of other salivary antimicrobial substances would seem to present a system geared to supress this selected population to growth rates which are consistent with optimum oral health.

Another part of the overall picture which may be very significant is the normal, rather rapid half-life of the mucosal epithelial cell surface, an estimated 1- to 3-day surface turnover cycle. Such sloughed cells carry significant numbers of bacteria on their surface. This in itself may represent a part of the antigen disposal system, and the dynamics of cell surface turnover may be tied to the dynamics of bacterial growth or antigen-antibody interaction on the surfaces of these mucosal cells. Further, it is conceivable that the mucosal cells themselves produce substances which influence microbial growth or survival, and that the cell surface antigen-antibody reaction triggers such reactions.

In summary, it seems unlikely that secretory immunoglobulins participate in mucosal defense *solely* through agglutinating oral microorganisms directly in the secretory fluid in the open environment of the mouth. Interactions of salivary antibodies with other salivary antimicrobial proteins are likely events in an overall mucosal defense scheme, and it is possible that many of the molecular mechanisms involved occur on or near the surface of the mucosal cells.

Of further interest to the oral biologist and clinician is the fact that even in the presence of lactoperoxidase, lysozyme and lactoferrin many oral microorganisms obviously survive. Perhaps their survival can be partially explained by their adaptability. For example, lysozyme alone is ineffective in killing most oral microorganisms. One of the most intriguing questions in oral biology research is how pathogens are discriminated for elimination, apart from the many other "nonpathogenic" microbiota in the oral cavity. The answer to this question is related to the intrinsic "invasiveness" of the foreign organism and whether it invokes a sufficient host immune response. The potent immune factors can be grouped into two broad categories, the specific antibodies and cell-mediated immune factors. It is important to understand that in order to evoke an immune response on mucosal surfaces a critical degree of active microbial contact with host soft tissue (mucosa) must occur. Such an action provokes the local immunological machinery into producing specific antibodies. Specific secretory IgA is the predominant immunoglobulin secreted by the major and minor salivary glands in response to an active, local, oral, mucosal, microbial infiltration. However, IgG and IgM are also secreted. In individuals with IgA deficiency, these other immunoglobulins are elevated in the secretions and compensate for the missing IgA.

Only low levels of antibodies are produced against the "noninvasive" microbial residents in the oral cavity. It is important to realize that a mucosal secretory IgA booster response to microorganisms or their products is very difficult to generate and maintain. The host's controlled repression of a response to noninvasive microbes (substances) is reasonable, considering that oral mucosal surfaces contact thousands of foreign substances each day, (i.e., in the form of food). The host is programmed (repressed) not to use its powerful immune machinery against these noninvasive foreign substances. In a similar sense, noninvasive resident oral flora would not evoke the immune response. However, this pure situation does not exist because there is always a very limited invasiveness which evokes a very limited antibody (and cell-mediated immune) response. When mucosal invasiveness by a particular organism does occur, the specific salivary secretory IgA antibody (and IgG and IgM antibodies) levels rise, but only temporarily. The biological effects of increased salivary antibody deposited on the specific microorganism include direct paralysis and neutralization (if it is an extracellular virus), a direct localization of innate defense systems such as lactoferrin to the foreign cell surface, and fixation of complement which could arrive as a serous transudate from inflamed tissue. Therefore, the key to understanding why a particular organism survives is directly related to the host's immune system—a mucosal immune system which has a built-in repression to noninvasive substances.

CONCLUSION

The knowledge arising from recent investigations on the protein constituents of saliva has grown dramatically. While it has long been appreciated that desalivation resulting from excision, atrophy, defect or secondary to X-ray therapy of the head and neck region leads to diseases of the oral cavity, the exact mechanisms underlying these effects is still far from

CONTENTS OF WHOLE SALIVA

1. Parotid secretion
2. Submandibular secretion
3. Sublingual secretion
4. Minor salivary gland secretions
5. Lingual (Ebner) secretions
6. Gingival crevicular fluid (GCF)
   a. Serum proteins and protein fragments
   b. Degenerating polymorphonuclear leukocytes
7. Microbiota (predominantly bacteria)
8. Microbial digestive enzymes
   a. Proteases (broad spectrum)
   b. Glycosidases (broad spectrum)
9. Sloughed degenerating oral epithelial cells

resolved. However, the role of the salivary proteins in pellicle formation, enzymatic reactions, "nonimmune" antimicrobial activities, and other immunoglobulin based defense mechanisms points to the many avenues of possible action for these potent macromolecules. It is hoped that through an understanding of the biochemical aspects of salivary proteins a biologic basis for understanding their significance in oral health will evolve.

* We wish to thank Charles L. Smith for excellent editorial assistance.

GLOSSARY

Acrylamide gel. A porous gel of cross-linked polymer that has a specific pore size depending upon the concentration of the polymer. Under an electric current, proteins in a solution are separated by both their charge and size.

Agglutinin. An organic molecule having at least two binding sites for particulate substances.

Anode. The positive electrode or the pole that attracts negative ions.

Antigens. Any substance which, when introduced into a host system, will illicit a specific immune response.

Cathode. The negative electrode from which electrons are emitted. Attracts positive ions.

Glycosidase. A hydrolytic enzyme that attacks glycosidic linkages.

Histidine. An α-amino acid, beta-4-imidazolyl alanine. The only amino acid with an imidazole group.

Hydroxyapatite. An inorganic compound found in the matrix of bone and teeth that gives rigidity to these structures. It is a hydrated calcium phosphate.

Immunoglobulin. A glycoprotein composed of at least two heavy and two light polypeptide chains which functions as an antibody.

Isoelectric point. That pH at which the net charge of a molecule is zero; therefore, the molecule will not move in an electric field.

Lipoteichoic acids. A polymer of either glycerol or ribitol residues with phosphodiester links. Contained in the cell walls of many gram (+) bacteria.

Microbe. A microscopic organism such as a virus, bacterium, fungus, or protozoan.

Neuraminidase. An enzyme that catalyzes the hydrolysis of terminal neuramic acid (sialic acid) residues.

Peptidoglycan. The major constituent of most gram-positive bacterial cell walls, consisting of a backbone of alternating N-acetylglucosamine and N-acetylmuramate residues in β-1, 4 linkage, with tetrapeptide side chains that are cross-linked by peptide bridges.

Polymorphonuclear leukocytes. A phagocytic cell that has receptors for antibody and complement-coated foreign cells and contains a variety of hydrolytic enzymes within its many lysosomes.

Porphyrin. Any one of a group of iron-free or magnesium-free cyclic tetrapyrrol derivatives.

Proline. An amino acid with a secondary amino group, which when incorporated into a peptide bond prevents any flexibility around that bond.

Protease. An enzyme that catalyzes the degradation of proteins by hydrolysis of peptide bonds.

Secretory IgA. The predominant immunoglobulin class in mucosal secretions. The secretory IgA differs from serum IgA in that it is dimeric, consisting of two IgA molecules that are linked by the molecule's J chain and contain secretory component.

SUGGESTED READINGS

Armstrong WG: Characterization studies of the specific human salivary proteins adsorbed *in vitro* by hydroxyapatite. Caries Res 5: 215–227, 1971

Arneberg P: Partial characterization of five glycoprotein fractions secreted by the human parotid glands. Arch Oral Biol 19: 921–928, 1974

Azen EA: Salivary peroxidase (SAPX): genetic modification and relationship to the proline-rich (Pr) and acidic (Pa) proteins. Biochem Genet 15: 9–29, 1977

Azen EA: Genetic protein polymorphisms in human saliva: an interpretive review. Biochem Genet 16: 79–99, 1978

Azen EA, Denniston CL: Genetic polymorphism of human salivary proline-rich proteins: further genetic analysis. Biochem Genet 12: 109–120, 1974

Azen EA, Oppenheim FG: Genetic polymorphism of proline-rich human salivary proteins. Science 180: 1067–1069, 1973

Baig MM, Winzler RJ, Rennert OM: Isolation of mucin from human submaxillary secretions. J Immunol 111: 1826–1833, 1973

Balakrishnan CR, Ashton CC: Polymorphisms of human salivary proteins. J Hum Genet 26: 145–150, 1974

Baum BJ, Bird JL, Miller DB, Longton RW: Studies on histidine-rich polypeptides from human parotid saliva. Arch Biochem Biophys 177: 427–436, 1976

Beeley JA: Separation of human salivary proteins by iso-electric focusing in polyacrylamide gels. Arch Oral Biol 14: 559–561, 1969

Belcourt A: Etude d'une glycoproteine salivaire humaine precipitable par les ions calcium. Eur J Biochem 53: 185–191, 1975

Belcourt A, Klein JP: Immunological studies of a human calcium precipitable salivary glycoprotein. J Dent Res 55, Special Issue D: 156, 1976

Bennick A: Chemical and physical characteristics of a phosphoprotein from human parotid saliva. Biochem J 145: 557–567, 1975

Bennick A: The binding of calcium to a salivary phospho-protein, protein A, common to human parotid and submandibular secretions. Biochem J 155: 163–169, 1976

Bennick A: The binding of calcium to a salivary phospho-protein, protein C, and comparison with calcium binding to protein A, a related salivary phosphopro-tein. Biochem J 163: 241–245, 1977

Bennick A: Chemical and physical characterization of a phosphoprotein C, from human saliva and compari-son with a related protein A. Biochem J 163: 229–239, 1977

Bennick A, Cannon M: Quantitative study of the inter-action of salivary acidic proline rich proteins with hy-droxyapatite. Caries Res 12: 159–164, 1978

Bennick A, Connell GE: Purification and partial charac-terization of four proteins from human parotid sa-liva. Biochem J 123: 455–464, 1971

Boackle RJ, Caughman GB, Carsgo EA: The partial iso-lation and function of salivary factors which interact with the complement system. Adv Exp Med Biol 107: 411–421, 1978

Boackle RJ, Pruitt KM, Silverman MS, Glymph JL Jr: The effects of human saliva on the hemolytic activity of complement J Dent Res 57: 103–110, 1978

Boat TF, Wiesman UN, Pallavicini JC: Purification and properties of the calcium precipitable protein in sub-maxillary saliva of normal and cystic fibrosis subjects. Pediatr Res 8: 531–539, 1974

Boehm-Truitt M, Harrison E, Wolf RO, Notkins AL: Radioimmunoassay for human salivary amylase. Anal Biochem 85: 476–487, 1978

Caldwell RC, Pigman W: The carbohydrates of human submaxillary glycoproteins in secretors and non-se-cretors of blood group substances. Biochim Biophys Acta 101: 157–165, 1965

Caldwell RC, Pigman W: Disc electrophoresis of human saliva in polyacrylamide gel. Arch Biochem Biophys 110: 91–97, 1965

Carlson DM: Chemistry and biosynthesis of mucin glyco-proteins. Adv Exp Med Biol 89: 251–273, 1977

Chauncey HH: Salivary enzymes. J Am Dent Assoc 63: 360–364, 1961

Courts FJ, Boackle RJ, Fudenberg HH, Silverman MS: Detection of functional complement components in gingival fluid from humans with periodontal disease. J Dent Res 56: 327–331, 1977

D'Silva JL, Ferguson DB: Zone electrophoresis of human parotid saliva in various media. Arch Oral Biol 7: 563–572, 1962

Ellison SA: Proteins and glycoproteins of saliva. In Handbook of Physiology, Section 6, Alimentary Canal Washington DC, American Physiological So-ciety, 1967, pp 531–559

Ericson T, Carlen A, Dagerskog E: Salivary aggregating factors. In Stiles HM, Loesche WJ, O'Brien TC (eds): Microbial Aspects of Dental Caries. Washington DC, Information Retrieval, 1976 pp 151–162

Evans RT, Genco RJ, Emmings FG, Linzer R: Antibody in the prevention of adherence: measurement of anti-body to purified carbohydrates of Streptococcus mutans with an enzyme linked immunosorbent assay (abstr). Microbiology 2: 375, 386, 1976

Forstner G, Sturgess J, Forstner J: Malfunction of intesti-nal mucus and mucus production. Adv Exp Biol Med 89: 349–369, 1977

Forstner JF: Intestinal mucins in health and disease. Di-gestion 17: 234–263, 1978

Friedman RD, Karn RC: Immunological relationships and a genetic interpretation of major and minor acidic proteins in human parotid saliva. Biochem Genet 15: 549–562, 1977

Friedman RD, Merritt AD: Partial purification and char-acterization of a polymorphic protein (Pa) in human parotid saliva. Am J Hum Genet 27: 304–314, 1975

Greenspan JS, Boackle RJ: Oral and dental diseases. In Fudenberg HH, Stites DR, Caldwell JL, Wells JV (eds): Basic and Clinical Immunology, 2nd ed. Los Altos, Lange Medical, 1978, pp 673–689

Gugler E, Pallavicini CJ, Swerdlow H, di Sant'Agnese PA: The role of calcium in submaxillary saliva of pa-tients with cystic fibrosis. J Pediatr 71: 585–588, 1967

Hamon CB, Klebanoff SJ: A peroxidase-mediated, strep-tococcus mitis-dependent antimicrobial system in sa-liva. J Exp Med 137: 438–450, 1973

Hamosh M, Burns WA: Lipolytic activity of human lin-gual glands (Ebner). Lab Invest 37: 603–608, 1977

Hauptman SP, Sobezak G: Origin of immunoglobulin-albumin complexes. Nature 263: 64–67, 1976

Hay DI: The isolation from human parotid saliva of a tyrosine-rich acidic peptide which exhibits high affin-ity for hydroxyapatite surfaces. Arch Oral Biol 18: 1531–1541, 1973

Hay DI: Fractionation of human parotid salivary proteins and the isolation of an histidine-rich acidic peptide, which shows high affinity for hydroxyapatite. Arch Oral Biol 20: 553–558, 1975

Hay DI, Gibbons RJ, Spinell DM: Characteristics of some high molecular weight constituents with bacte-rial aggregating activity from whole saliva and dental plaque. Caries Res 5: 111–123, 1971

Hay DI, Oppenheim FG: The isolation from human parotid saliva of a further group of proline-rich pro-teins. Arch Oral Biol 19: 627–632, 1974

Henkin RI, Lippoldt RE, Bilstad J, Edelhoch H: A zinc protein isolated from human parotid saliva. Proc Natl Acad Sci USA 72: 488, 1975

Jacobsen N, Brennhovd I, Jonsen J: Human subman-dibular gland tissue in culture. 1. Sulphate incor-poration and tissue culture technique. J Biol Buccale 5: 159–167, 1977

Jacobsen N, Brennhovd I, Jonsen J: Human subman-dibular gland tissue in culture. 2. Nickel affinity to se-cretory proteins. J Biol Buccale 5: 169–175, 1977

Karn RC, Shulkin JD, Merritt AD, Newell RC: Evi-dence for post-transcriptional modification of human salivary amylase (AMY$_1$) isozymes. Biochem Genet 10: 341–350, 1973

Kashket S, Guilmette KM: Further evidence for the non-immunoglobulin nature of the bacterial aggre-gating factor in saliva. Caries Res 12: 170, 1978

Kauffman DL, Watanabe S, Evans JR, Keller PJ: The existence of glycosylated and non-glycosylated forms of human submandibular amylase. Arch Oral Biol 18: 1105–1112, 1973

Kauffman DL, Zager NI, Cohen E, Keller PJ: The isoenzymes of human parotid amylase. Arch Biochem Biophys 137: 325–339, 1970

Keller PJ, Kauffman DL, Allan BJ, Williams BL: Further studies on the structural differences between the iso-enzymes of human parotid alpha amylase. Biochemistry 10: 4867–4874, 1971

Kleinberg I, Kanapka JA, Craw D: Effect of saliva and salivary factors on the metabolism of the mixed oral flora (abstr). Microbiology 2: 433–464, 1976

Kondo W, Sato M, Sato N: Properties of the human salivary aggregating factor for *Leptotrichia buccalis* cells. Arch Oral Biol 23: 453, 1978

Krasse B: Adherence of bacteria to tooth surfaces. Swed Dent J 1: 253, 1977

Levine MJ, Ellison SA, Bahl OP: The isolation from human parotid saliva and the partial characterization of the protein core of a major parotid glycoprotein. Arch Oral Biol 18: 827–837, 1973

Levine MJ, Herzberg MC, Levine MS, Ellison SM, Stinson MW, Li HC, Van Dyke T: Specificity of salivary-bacterial interactions: role of terminal sialic acid residues in the interaction of salivary glycoproteins with *Streptococcus sanguis* and *Streptococcus mutans*. Infect Immunol 19: 107–115, 1978

Levine MJ, Keller PJ: The isolation of some basic proline-rich proteins from human parotid saliva. Arch Oral Biol 22: 37–41, 1977

Levine MJ, Weill JC, Ellison SA: The isolation and analysis of a glycoprotein from parotid saliva. Biochim Biophys Acta 188: 165–167, 1969

Magnusson I, Ericson T: Effect of salivary agglutinins on reactions between hydroxyapatite and a serotype C strain of *Streptococcus mutans*. Caries Res 10: 273, 1976

Mandel ID: Electrophoretic studies of saliva. J Dent Res 45: 634–643, 1966

Mandel ID: Dental plaque: nature, formation and effects. J Periodontal 37: 357–367, 1966

Mandel ID: Relation of saliva and plaque to caries. J Dent Res 53: 246–266, 1974

Mandel ID: Sialochemistry in diseases and clinical situations affecting salivary glands. In Critical Reviews in Clinical Laboratory Sciences. West Palm Beach, CRC Press (in press)

Mandel ID, Ellison SA: Characterization of salivary components separated by paper electrophoresis. Arch Oral Biol 3: 77–85, 1961

Mandel ID, Thompson RH, Ellison SA: Studies on the mucoproteins of human parotid saliva. Arch Oral Biol 10: 499–507, 1965

Martin F, Mathian R, Berard A, Lambert R: Sulfated glycoproteins in human salivary and gastric secretions. Digestion 2: 103–112, 1969

Masson PL, Carbonara AO, Heremans JF: Studies on the proteins of human saliva. Biochim Biophys Acta 107: 485–500, 1965

Mayo JW, Carlson DM: Protein composition of human submandibular secretions. Arch Biochem Biophys 161: 131–145, 1974

Mekel AH: The formation and properties of organic films on teeth. Arch Oral Biol 10: 585–599, 1965

Merritt AD, Karn RC: The human alpha-amylases. Adv Hum Genet 8: 135–234, 1977

Meyers TS, Lamberts BL: Use of coomassie brilliant blue R250 for the electrophoresis of microgram quantities of parotid saliva proteins on acrylamide gel strips. Biochim Biophys Acta 107: 144–145, 1965

Moreno EC, Kresak M, Hay DI: Adsorption of two human parotid salivary macromolecules on hydroxy-, fluorhydroxy- and fluorapatites. Arch Oral Biol 23: 525, 1978

Nungester WJ, Jourdonais LF, Wof AA: The effect of mucin on infections by bacteria. J Infect Dis 59: 11–21, 1936

Oemrawsingh I, Roukema PA: Isolation, purification and chemical characterization of mucins from human submandibular glands. Arch Oral Biol 19: 615–626, 1974

Oemrawsingh I, Roukema PA: Compositions and biological properties of mucins, isolated from human submandibular glands. Arch Oral Biol 19: 753–759, 1974

Oemrawsingh I, Roukema PA: Immunological characterization and detection of human submandibular mucins in saliva, dental plaque and submandibular glands. Arch Oral Biol 21: 755–759, 1976

Oppenheim FG, Azen EA: Genetic polymorphism of proline-rich human salivary proteins. Science 180: 1067–1068, 1973

Oppenheim FG, Hay DI, Franzblau C: Proline-rich proteins from human parotid saliva. I. Isolation and partial characterization. Biochemistry 10: 4233–4238, 1971

Patton JR, Pigman W: Electrophoretic and ultracentrifugal components of human salivary secretions. J Am Chem Soc 81: 3035–3040, 1959

Peters EH, Azen EA: Isolation and partial characterization of human parotid basic proteins. Biochem Genet 15: 925–946, 1977

Peters EH, Goodfriend T, Azen EA: Human Pb, human post-Pb, and nonhuman primate Pb proteins: immunological and biochemical relationships. Biochem Genet 15: 947–962, 1977

Pollock JJ, Iacono VJ, Vicker HG, MacKay BJ, Katona LI, Taichman LB: The binding, aggregation and lytic properties of lysozyme (abstr). Microbiology 2: 325–352, 1976

Pruitt KM: Macromolecular components of oral fluids at tooth surfaces. Swed Dent J 1: 225, 1977

Pruitt KM, Adamson M: Enzyme activity of salivary lactoperoxidase adsorbed to human enamel. Infect Immunol 17: 112, 1977

Revis GJ: Immunoelectrophoretic identification of lysozyme in saliva. Proc Soc Exp Biol Med 137: 90–96, 1971

Rölla G: Inhibition of adsorption. General considerations (abstr). Microbiology 2: 309–324, 1976

Rölla G: Formation of dental integuments—some basic considerations. Swed Dent J 241: 1977

Schachter H: Control of biochemical parameters in glycoprotein production. Adv Exp Biol Med 89: 103–129, 1977

Schlesinger DH, Hay DI: Complete covalent structure of statherin, a tyrosine-rich acidic peptide which inhibits calcium phosphate precipitation from human parotid saliva. J Biol Chem 252: 1689–1695, 1977

Schneyer LH: Amylase content of separate salivary gland secretions of man. J Appl Physiol 9: 453–455, 1956

Schrager J, Oates MDG: Isolation and partial characterization of the principal glycoprotein from human mixed saliva. Arch Oral Biol 16: 287–303, 1971

Skude G: Isoenzyme variation in human salivary amylase. Hum Genet 12: 255–256, 1971

Slowey RR, Eidelman S, Klebanoff SJ: Antibacterial activity of the purified peroxidase from human parotid saliva. J Bacteriol 96: 575–579, 1968

Spik G, Cheron A, Montreuil J, Dolby JM: Bacteriostasis of a milk-sensitive strain of Escherichia coli by immunoglobulins and iron-binding proteins in association. Immunology 35: 663, 1978

Steiner JC, Keller PJ: An electrophoretic analysis of the protein components of human parotid saliva. Arch Oral Biol 13: 1213–1221, 1968

Suddick RP, Staat RH, Malena DE, Burchfield DC: Attachment of IgA and IgM to oral epithelial cells (abstr). J Dent Res (Special Issue A) 57: 413, 1978

Tenovuo J, Valtakoski J, Knuuttila MLE: Antibacterial activity of lactoperoxidase adsorbed by human salivary sediment and hydroxyapatite. Caries Res 11: 257–262, 1977

Virella G, Goudswaard J, Boackle RJ: Preparation of saliva samples for immunochemical determinations of immunoglobulins and for assay of lysozyme. Clin Chem 24: 1421, 1978

Ward JC, Merritt DD, Bixler D: Human salivary amylase: genetics of electrophoretic variants. Am J Hum Genet 23: 403–409, 1971

Watkins WM: Blood group substances. Science 152: 172–181, 1966

4 Salivary Water and Electrolytes and Oral Health

RICHARD P. SUDDICK

ROBERT J. HYDE

RALPH P. FELLER

Introduction
Osmolality and the Four Major Osmolytes
   Sodium
   Potassium
   Bicarbonate
   Chloride
Functional Significance of Hypotonic Secretion
Other Salivary Factors
   Saliva pH
   Calcium and Phosphate
   Fluoride, Urea, Ammonia

   Magnesium, Iodine, Thiocyanate
   Tin, Iron, Zinc and Other Trace Metals
   Differences With Age, Sex, and Diet
Saliva Composition and Caries
Dentinal Tubule Fluid Movement
Relation of Salivary Components to Oral and Gastric Cancer
Saliva Composition and Taste
Saliva Composition and Systemic Disease
Summary
Glossary
Suggested Readings

INTRODUCTION

In the previous two chapters we spent a considerable amount of time discussing the hypothesized mechanisms underlying the secretion of saliva and some of the salivary proteins involved in the maintenance of oral health. In this chapter we will concentrate on salivary electrolytes and their role in the oral cavity.

OSMOLALITY AND THE FOUR MAJOR OSMOLYTES

The main constituent of pure glandular or whole saliva is water, constituting about 99 per cent of pure glandular secretions. Fluid from the major salivary glands is very hypoosmotic to all other body fluids and very hypotonic to plasma regardless of the rate of secre-

132

tion. Essentially all of the osmolality of saliva is accounted for by four ions: sodium, potassium, chloride, and bicarbonate, again regardless of the rate of secretion. However, the concentrations of each of these four osmolytes changes quite dramatically as flow rate increases.

Secretions from the human parotid gland have been studied more extensively than those from any other gland as far as constituents, including electrolytes. Figure 4-1 shows the concentrations of the four major osmolytes over the total physiologic flow rate range of the human parotid gland. These same electrolytes appear to behave in a very similar manner in secretions from human submandibular glands and from the major salivary glands from various mammalian species which have been studied. In short, there does not seem to be any reason to suspect that there are any major deviations from this *pattern* of concentrations of the major electrolytes in the secretions from any major salivary gland. Therefore, the pattern is extremely important with respect to fluid and electrolyte secretory mechanisms. Any plausible theory of fluid and electrolyte secretion must be able to account for the changes in the concentrations of the four major osmolytes as flow rate changes. A viable theory of fluid and electrolyte secretion must eventually be able to accommodate and explain these changes on the basis of transfer of ions and water across the secretory epithelium. However, until recently it has been generally believed that there is active ductal reabsorption of sodium and secretion of potassium with little or no concurrent transepithelial transfer of water. The viewpoint that considers a more rigid tie of major electrolyte concentration changes with the *actual secretory transfer mechanisms* has been largely overlooked. It is suggested here that this prevaling benign and flexible view of the major electrolyte concentration pattern vis-a-vis the generation of the primary secretion can no longer be justified. The alternative position follows directly from the newer views of fluid and electrolyte secretion presented in Chapter 2. We are suggesting, in other words, that *the pattern of changes in the major osmolytes at different rates of secretion, as shown in Figure 4-1, must represent a similar pattern which is occurring at the site of transepithelial fluid secretion.* Sodium reabsorption in the ducts undoubtedly occurs, but the degree of change

that this produces in the concentration pattern of the major osmolytes in the exiting fluid is relatively insignificant relative to the contributions to the total secretory output at the site of epithelial transfer (most likely in the secretory tubules). This is especially true at the higher rate of secretion. The individual patterns of each of the four osmolytes with respect to flow rate changes are thus very important with respect to implications concerning secretory mechanisms.

Sodium

In human parotid secretion under resting conditions (about .05 to 0.1 ml./min.) sodium concentration is minimal, about 2 to 5 mEq./l. Changes in concentrations at increasing flow rates have been studied by means of many different modes of physiological reflex stimulation. The concentrations at successively higher flow rates in figure 4-1 represent the best estimate of data derived from a great number of experiments conducted on over 1000 subjects. Data on sodium and the other electrolytes at the lowest flow rates (below 0.05) were obtained from experiments in which atropine was used to depress resting rates of secretion, or the resting rates were lowered by blindfolding or by another means of light deprivation. Thus changes in sodium and the other electrolytes are presented over the entire normal range of secretion.

Sodium and other electrolytes have been studied at flow rates higher than those shown in Figure 4-1, some data of this nature being derived from studies of pilocarpine stimulated secretion and some from individual subjects who have inherently higher rates of flow than most individuals. At flow rates of 3.0 ml./min./gland, sodium concentrations approach 100 m Eq/l. Thus, at the highest recorded rates of physiologic secretion sodium concentration remains well below plasma levels.

The most significant aspects of the sodium plot in Figure 4-1 is the very low, relatively constant values throughout the range of flow which varies from 0.01 ml./min. to 0.1 ml./min., and the abrupt increase in concentration between 0.1 and 0.2 ml./min. This indicates that at the onset of reflex stimulated secretion the increase in flow rate begins at this point to carry a constant high sodium primary secretion past ductal sodium transport sites at rates which do not permit maximal sodium extraction, *or* the sodium concentration of the primary secretion elicited by reflex stimulation increases steadily as the flow rate rises, which brings total sodium secretory output beyond the capacity of ductal sodium transport sites to achieve maximal sodium extraction. A significant contribution to the continuous elevation in sodium by the latter mechanism is suggested by the latest ideas about fluid secretory mechanisms.

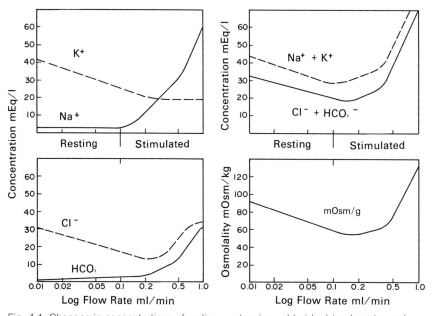

Fig. 4-1. Changes in concentrations of sodium, potassium, chloride, bicarbonate, and osmolality in human parotid secretion over the normal physiological range of flow rate (from a single parotid gland in 18–22 year old adults). Concentration curves compiled from experiments on over one thousand subjects.

The normal range of resting secretion extends from 0.01 to 0.1 ml/min. However, data was obtained throughout this range by examining the secretions from individuals with wide variations in their individual rates of resting secretion, and by experiments in groups whereby mean resting rates were depressed experimentally by administration of atropine or by placing the subjects in total darkness. Sodium and bicarbonate remain at a constant very low concentration, while potassium and chloride decline slowly over the range of secretion, 0.01 to 0.1 ml/min. When data is massed in this manner, it is necessary to rather arbitrarily select a value which signifies progression from the resting secretion to reflex stimulated secretion. However, in an individual, the resting secretion may be as low as 0.01 or as high (or higher) than 0.1, and progression to higher levels of secretion from that resting base *depends on* overt oral receptor stimulation; the subject would then be secreting, by definition, in the stimulated range.

Major ion changes which are characteristic of the stimulated secretion are: Marked increases in sodium, bicarbonate, and chloride concentrations. Potassium, in contrast, remains at a steady level (between 15–20 m Eq 1) which is substantially higher than plasma concentrations (normally, 4–5 m Eq 1). When sodium and potassium concentrations, and chloride and bicarbonate concentrations each are summed throughout the flow range, the total cation and anion concentration curves produced are strikingly parallel. In addition, the curve of experimentally obtained osmolality values plotted over this same flow range is strikingly similar to the sum of the cation and anion curves, both in shape and in apparent total ionic content at any given flow rate; this demonstrates that the osmolality of the secretion is almost entirely dependent on the concentrations of these four ions. Note also that osmolality throughout the full range of physiologic secretion remains substantially below that of plasma (about 290 m Osm/Kg) and other body fluids, and that the summed concentration curve for the cations, sodium and, potassium is at all times quantitatively greater than the summed concentration curve for chloride and bicarbonate.

Figure modified and redrawn from Shannon IL, Suddick RP, and Dowd FJ: *Saliva: Composition and Secretion. In* Myers, HM (ed): *In* Monographs Oral Science. vol. 2. Basel, S. Karger, 1974.

Potassium

At unstimulated flow rates potassium concentration ranges from 40 m Eq/l to about 30 m Eq/l which relatively speaking, is about midway between what is expected of a cellularly derived fluid and one that is derived from extracellular fluid sources (secretory potassium being about 6 to 7 times plasma levels, but only about $1/5$ of cellular potassium). Since the tubules of the entire secretory tree are lined by cells containing potassium at concentrations of 130–150 m Eq/l, it must be presumed that primary secretory fluid transfer involves a relatively low potassium fluid concentration (i.e., of extracellular fluid origin), and that steady cellular potassium leakage, probably throughout the tubules and ducts, contributes to the elevation of potassium observed at the lowest flow rates.

As was the case for sodium, the most significant point on the potassium curve begins just beyond 0.1 ml/min which marks the demarcation line between unstimulated and stimulated secretion. From this point potassium levels remain virtually constant as flow rates rise. Furthermore, in studies where concentrations have been measured up to flow rates of 3 ml/min this situation is maintained; potassium concentrations remain relatively constant and substantially higher than plasma values. This strongly suggests that the rate of fluid production (i.e., the mechanism of fluid secretion) is directly linked to the rate of potassium secretion. Furthermore, the source of secreted potassium must be from glandular cells since plasma concentrations are closely regulated to constant levels of 4 to 5 m Eq/l. One means by which the potassium linkage to fluid secretion may operate is presented in Chapter 2 in the most recent views of fluid and electrolyte secretion (i.e., the potassium channel concept for transepithelial fluid transfer). It is important to note that the constant high secretory potassium levels are difficult to reconcile with the more conventional views of fluid secretion that have been adopted by the salivary micropuncture investigators to explain their findings (see Chapter 2).

Bicarbonate

The bicarbonate levels in saliva generally follow closely the sodium levels. The bicarbonate curve in Figure 4-1 parallels the sodium curve for the most part, the main difference being that concentrations do not climb as high as sodium. In general however, the ratio of plasma bicarbonate to secretory bicarbonate is much lower than the corresponding ratio for sodium. One reason for this is the generation of bicarbonate in secretory cells creating a concentration gradient favoring rapid diffusion into the lumen. There has been a suggestion that ductal cells contain a metabolic energy requiring bicarbonate-chloride exchange pump which is active only during stimulated secretion resulting in bicarbonate secretion and simultaneous chloride uptake. Irrespective of this, the absolute concentration of the bicarbonate ion in the secretion during any given rate of stimulated secretion seems likely to be due primarily to diffusion from the intracellular compartment, and the proportion of secreted bicarbonate from this source probably matches the secretory potassium output from cellular stores. However, the situation changes with increasing duration of stimulation, and chloride tends to replace bicarbonate as the dominant anion as stimulated flow is maintained for longer periods. Therefore, the pH of the secretion decreases with increasing duration of stimulation (see below).

Chloride

At the lowest unstimulated flow rates chloride concentration ranges from about 30 m Eq/l to 20 m Eq/l and the curve shows a downward trend until the onset of reflex–stimulated secretion. Then chloride concentration begins to incease and the stimulated secretion portion of the concentration curve is very similar to that of bicarbonate. The force that underlies the secretory transport of both chloride and bicarbonate is total secretory cation distribution across the epithelium which is essentially to match the total output of sodium and potassium.

The steady source of secretory chloride is from the extracellular compartment (plasma). In that respect as well as others, the secretion of chloride greatly resembles the secretion of sodium. In terms of the most recent view of the energetics of fluid secretion the stimulated secretion of both must be viewed as passive phenomena in which the ions are entrained in the flow of extracellular fluid that is forced through the lateral channels and tight junctions by the vascular pressure gradient. These columns of fluid are modified in their sodium and chloride content as they pass alongside the lateral unit membranes of the epithelium, with sodium being reabsorbed down a generated concentration gradient and chloride tending to follow sodium into the cells (and finally back out at the basal pole; see Chap. 2 for details). However, the total amount of chloride that enters the lumen as secretory chloride depends to some extent on the amount of bicarbonate being generated. The total positive ion transfer across the epithelium can be as easily matched by bicarbonate as chloride, with the tendency simply to match total cation transfer by total anion transfer. From the evolutionary perspective, an optimum degree of secretion of the bicarbonate ion seems to be advantageous from the view of function in the oral cavity, and it also seems to be the preferential choice for a matching anion from the perspective of the plasma/secretory ratios of the two.

From the overall viewpoint of the concentration curves of the four main osmolytes, potassium stands out. Regardless of the rate of secretion, its concentration is always at least several times the plasma concentration, and at any rate of stimulated secretion its concentration remains constant. If we sum the concentrations of sodium and potassium and those of chloride and bicarbonate throughout the full flow rate range shown in Figure 4-1, a constant positive ion flow of about 10 m Eq/min. is evident regardless of the rate of secretion. When considered together these facts indicate that the ability of the salivary glands to secrete large quantities of fluid over extended periods of time depends on the ability of the secretory cells to continuously sequester potassium from the circulating blood. According to the concepts presented in Chapter 2 the generation of secretory fluid during physiologic stimulation depends in part on the release of potassium from the fluid secretory epithelial cells. The concept that some secretory lobules are "working" or secreting while others are not secreting in the stimulated gland at any given time allows us to explain how human parotid glands are able to continuously secrete at high (stimulated) flow rates for as long as three hours and still maintain constant high potassium levels in the secreted fluid (levels which remain significantly above plasma levels throughout).

FUNCTIONAL SIGNIFICANCE OF HYPOTONIC SECRETION

From the foregoing it is apparent that the major salivary glands have developed during evolution into organs capable of continuously delivering a very dilute solution of electrolytes, proteins, and mucins into the oral cavity. Although dramatic changes occur in the concentrations of three of the four major osmolytes as flow rate increases or decreases, the fluid remains very hypotonic to plasma or cellular fluids, and this may be the most significant aspect of the evolution of salivary gland secretory mechanisms. Through the evolutionary process over millions of years nature has engineered secretory organs which utilize the four most abundant electrolytes in the body to provide the necessary minimum osmotic pressure which still allows the glands to produce abundant quantities of water. Other than providing the solvent for the proteins, glycoproteins, and mucins that are so vitally important to maintaining the health of the oropharyngeal mucosa and teeth, this fluid also provides the medium for the secretion of many other ions, trace elements, and hormones. Many of these substances also may contribute to maintaining the vitality of the oral tissues. Most of the remainder of this chapter will be devoted to the remaining ions and trace elements which are found in these secretions, and to experimental evidence concerning their potential roles in oral physiology and dental disease. For the present, we would like to posit some ideas concerning the possible functional significance of the hypotonic fluid itself and the selective advantage that the capacity to produce such a fluid may have conferred during evolution.

The continuous bathing of the oral tissues by this very dilute, low salt fluid appears to be advantageous in a number of ways. With respect to the oropharyngeal mucosa it can be expected that water continuously diffuses from the saliva into the epithelium down the concentration gradient that is present (water is more concentrated in saliva than in the mucosa). Thus, solutes present in the fluid will be continually carried to the surface of the mucosal cells through normal diffusion in the thin finite layer of saliva which slowly washes over the surface and by entrainment in the water of the secretion as it diffuses into the epithelium itself. These processes provide a steady supply to the mucosal surface of the important protein and mucinous constituents of the secretions that appear to play important roles in mucosal defense mechanisms (as outlined in Chap 3.)

While there does not appear to be any experimental data that supports the notion that osmotic movement of water occurs into the mucosal epithelium from hypotonic saliva, rudimentary facts of physical chemistry seem to require water uptake into the mucosa (assuming that the oropharyngeal mucosa is permeable to water to some degree). The osmotic pressure differential between the *internal* plasma, cellular and extracellular fluids, and the *external* saliva is equivalent to a hydrostatic pressure differential on the order of 2500 torr. This would more than offset any possible derived hydrostatic pressure gradient in the opposite direction due to vascular pressures in subepithelial capillary beds. Since the mucosa is *continually* bathed (while we are awake) by a thin layer of hypotonic saliva, water uptake and solute entrainment could be expected.

A similar phenomenon may contribute to the rapid development of the pellicle on the tooth surface (see Chap. 5). While we might expect dental enamel to be less permeable to water than the mucosa, evidence exists for water permeation under physiological circumstances. When a tooth is isolated from the oral fluids by application of the dental rubber dam and dried, minute beads of fluid slowly accumulate on the enamel surface. This has been described as the "enamel weeping phenomenon." Undoubtedly, this simply represents the filtration of extracellular water through the enamel driven by the hydrostatic pressure head in the pulp chamber of the tooth. These pressures have been reported to be about 40 torr. Under the conditions of drying the enamel surface this hydrostatic pressure head probably drives fluid through the dentinal tubules and then around or through the crystalline lattice columns of hydroxyapatite in the enamel itself. However, the net pressure differential is dramatically reversed in the presence of normal hypotonic saliva, the osmotic pressure differential being at least two orders of magnitude greater than the hydrostatic pressure differential. Thus water from the saliva should continually penetrate enamel and in so doing carry its solutes to the outer surface. This may be the major mechanism involved in the development of the salivary pellicle on the enamel surface. Even more interesting is the potential significance of such

fluid transport on the etiology of dental caries. For example, sufficient depositions on the enamel surface of dental plaque with its own productive metabolism, and restrictions with accumulation on diffusion of its metabolic products, might be expected to eliminate the natural osmotic pressure differential at the enamel surface. When this occurs, it might then be expected that the internal hydrostatic pressure may force extracellular body fluids, which carry natural nutrients of plaque bacteria (such as glucose), outward from the pulp chamber into the mass of metabolically active, acidogenic plaque. Critical parameters which would be expected to influence such a reversal of the natural fluid dynamics involve both thickness of the deposits and the total surface area covered by the deposits, as well as any natural or induced deficiencies in the secretion of adequate quantities of saliva (xerostomia). These notions about the dynamics of fluid movement through the enamel may also provide a plausible basis for an unorthodox salivary endocrine theory of the etiology of dental caries proposed by two investigators (described later in this chapter).

The possibility that water is taken up by mucosa bathed by hypotonic saliva also has major implications. Some of the facets that relate to maintenance of mucosal epithelial integrity and mucosal defense have already been alluded to here and in Chapter 3. Other implications are obvious, (e.g., epithelial growth and differentiation). However, this cannot be generalized to other mucosal sites. There are a number of mucosal surfaces of the body which are also in continuum with the external environment that clearly are not bathed by significant quantities of hypotonic fluid. The epithelium of the nasal cavity, sinuses, and air passages fall in this category. These observations indicate that a critical examination of the dynamics of transepithelial fluid transfer in the different mucosal sites would be a helpful step at gaining an understanding of the mechanisms of mucosal defense.

Another major potential function of saliva that follows from its low osmolality and low salt content relates to taste. If the sodium and chloride content of saliva were equivalent to plasma, the salt content of the fluid would in all likelihood mask many flavors which are now detectable. The sodium chloride content itself would in fact be equivalent to or greater than that of many common sources of these minerals. It may well be that the evolutionary pressures that encouraged the emergence of mechanisms of low salt secretion are in part related to the selective advantage of being able to detect minimal levels of salt in ingested foods. Extracellular fluid volume regulation is closely tied to the regulation of sodium excretion in urine. The hormone aldosterone stimulates sodium extraction from the distal convoluted tubules of the kidney and thereby helps retain body water. Aldosterone also causes increased sodium extraction from salivary ducts by increased sodium pumping at the basal membrane. Since, at resting flow rates, water is reabsorbed in the ducts, this hormone may also reduce resting secretory rates. It is known that secretion is reduced during water deprivation correlating with the expected increase in aldosterone output that can be expected during this condition. The decrease in flow, in turn, is probably related to the increase in thirst that occurs during water deprivation. On the other hand, excessive fluid retention and the low salt content of saliva ensures that minimal levels of salt in water or foods are detectable. The very low content of all solids in saliva, in fact, is advantageous with respect to taste. Other small molecules in plasma, such as glucose, do not normally appear in saliva. Glucose at plasma concentrations is certainly tastable. From this perspective the salivary glands have evolved to provide abundant secreted water with the lowest possible salt content so that molecules which stimulate taste buds can be dissolved and distributed to these chemoreceptors.

Still another physiologic function of the hypotonic salivary secretions may be to adjust the osmolality of gastric contents after eating. Mixtures of foods, ingested liquids such as milk, and gastric secretions are often very hypertonic. The continued secretion of hypotonic saliva that is known to occur during the gastric phase of salivary secretion will dilute the hypertonic chyme in the stomach. This can be important. The stomach will not empty as long as the chyme is hypertonic and retention of a very hypertonic fluid in the stomach can cause a fall in blood pressure (the so-called "dumping syndrome").

OTHER SALIVARY FACTORS

Saliva pH

As mentioned earlier, the pH of saliva is determined primarily by the bicarbonate concentration. The partial pressure of carbon dioxide is about equal to that in blood and is relatively constant. Thus pH will vary according to the bicarbonate content in the following equation (known as the Henderson-Hasselbach equation): $pH = pK + \log \dfrac{[HCO_3^-]}{[H_2CO_3]}$.

The pK is about 6.1 and the carbon dioxide partial pressure is reflected in the carbonic acid concentration in the denominator ($CO_2 + H_2O \leftrightharpoons H_2CO_3 = 0.03 \times p_{CO_2}$), so that saliva pH increases with flow rate as bicarbonate levels increase. Saliva may be slightly acidic as it is secreted at unstimulated flow rates but it may reach a pH of 7.8 at high flow rates. As it is exposed to the atmosphere CO_2 will diffuse out (lowering the denominator of the equation, above) and pH will rise, often to 9 or more in saliva present as a thin film. A rise in pH of this magnitude may be sufficient for the solubility product of hydroxyapatite to be exceeded leading to precipitation of this mineral (see below).

Several other salivary components contribute to the ability of saliva to neutralize acid, particularly acids produced in dental plaque. Salivary phosphate and the salivary proteins contribute in a relatively minor way to the direct buffer capacity. However, together with ammonia, urea, and the recently described pH rise factor (termed sialin, an arginine peptide), and the antisolubility factors such as statherin (see Chapter 3), the salivary components may represent a surprisingly efficient antacid and antisolubity system that works best at the enamel saliva interface (as a function of the pellicle), as well as in the matrix of plaque. Sialin, for example, appears to rapidly clear glucose from plaque, increases base formation, and elevate pH in the plaque itself.

Calcium and Phosphate

Phosphate and calcium are among the most significant inorganic salivary constituents for oral health. Phosphate levels in parotid and submandibular saliva are similar, and decrease slightly when flow increases. About 80 per cent of the salivary phosphate is ionized and its various ionic species are pH dependent. At the normal pH of 6 or higher, saliva is supersaturated with respect to the hydroxyapatite which forms dental enamel (see Chap. 7). Apatite begins to dissolve below the "critical pH of 55" when sufficient PO_4^{3-} ions in saliva become HPO_4^{2-} and phosphate leaves the enamel surface in order to maintain chemical equilibrium which has shifted to the right:

$$PO_4^{3-} + H^+ \overset{pH\ 5.5}{\rightleftharpoons} HPO_4^{2-} + H^+$$
$$\overset{pH\ 3}{\rightleftharpoons} H_2PO_4^- + H^+$$

The level of calcium in submandibular saliva is twice that of parotid saliva and increases directly with flow rate, whereas calcium in parotid saliva is relatively independent of flow. Because the parotid glands contribute proportionately more fluid to stimulated whole saliva volume, the calcium levels paradoxically decrease with elevated flow rates. As much as 30–50 per cent of the calcium present in saliva is protein-bound and is released as pH falls. When saliva is collected under oil to prevent loss of carbon dioxide and the resulting increase in pH, calcium carbonate crystals are detectable by x-ray diffraction because equilibrium has shifted to the right (saturation):

$$H_2O + CO_2 = H_2CO_3 \rightleftharpoons HCO_3^- + H^+$$
$$\rightleftharpoons CO_3^{2-} + H^+ + CaCO_3$$

In theory, **critical pH** occurs when saliva ceases to be supersaturated and apatite subsequently dissolves in it. However, bicarbonate ions in saliva increase directly with flow rate and usually buffer against a critical fall in pH. Also, some macromolecules recently isolated from saliva specifically inhibit the precipitation of calcium phosphate salts. The most active inhibitor is a phosphopeptide called statherin, or "stabilizer", because of its major role in maintaining saliva in a stable supersaturated state and preventing the dissolution of apatite:

Apatite   Saliva

$$Ca_5(PO_4)_3OH + Ca^{++} + PO_4^{3-} + HPO_4^{2-}$$

Not Present in Saliva

$$\overset{Inhibitor}{\longleftarrow} Ca_3(PO_4)_2 + CaHPO_4$$

Because of the previously mentioned factors, carious lesions rarely occur at an enamel-saliva interface. Only when saliva is chronically absent (xerostomia) is there a consistent relation between saliva and caries. When xerostomia results from oral radiation therapy, salivary gland extirpation, disease, or use of medication that reduces flow rate, the buffering capacity and cleansing effects of saliva are lost and oral health degenerates. As noted above, it is also possible that reversal of the normal fluid flow pattern through the tooth

mineral itself may play a role in the rapid degeneration seen under those circumstances.

Dental plaque is the usual intermediary to caries, calculus, or inflammatory changes in adjacent tissue. In determining the relation of saliva composition to these processes, the plaque-saliva interface must be considered. Wherever plaque exists between saliva and tooth surfaces, critical pH and oral health may be affected indirectly through the action of saliva on bacteria or the fluid matrix of either the acquired pellicle or plaque. Direct salivary effects could be due either to the deposition in oral tissues of excreted heavy metals or to the general absence of saliva. In addition to glucose, sucrose, and lactic acid, unbound calcium, phosphate, and other free ions or trace elements also diffuse through the gelatinous matrix of plaque, although the diffusion probably is limited osmotically with increased plaque maturity. Extracts of dental plaque contain inhibitors for calcium phosphate precipitation as does saliva. However, plaque from light, moderate, or heavy calculus formers exhibits hydroxyapatite crystal formation, which never occurs spontaneously in saliva. Thus, the inorganic components of saliva, as well as salivary proteins, may influence plaque chemistry and hence, oral health.

Fluoride, Urea, Ammonia

Several major components of saliva remain to be described. Salivary components which show relatively constant or decreasing levels when flow rate increases usually are dependent on plasma concentrations (the major exception: potassium). Both ammonia and urea in saliva are related inversely to flow rate, and their concentrations in parotid saliva exceed those in submandibular saliva (for reported values here and in each of the categories below, see Table 4-1). Caries susceptibility does not appear to be related to the salivary levels of these constituents. Fluoride in stimulated parotid saliva is independent of flow rate, but is directly related to the amount ingested. However, the fluoride content in whole saliva shows a significant negative correlation to stimulated flow rate in caries-resistant subjects, while fluoride levels are higher in saliva from caries-prone individuals. The continuous bathing of teeth by salivary fluoride logically should exhibit a caries-protective function by enhancing the formation in enamel of a caries-resistant

TABLE 4-1. COMPARISON BETWEEN SERUM AND SALIVA FOR SELECTED CONSTITUENTS*

| | BLOOD | SALIVA† | | | | | | PLAQUE |
| | Serum, Plasma or Whole Blood (B) | Parotid | | Submandibular | | Whole (mixed) | | |
		U	(S)	U	(S)	U	(S)	
pH	7.35–7.45 (B)	5.8	(7.7)	6.5	(7.4)	6.7	(6.8–7.5)	6.5
Bicarbonate (mM)	23–32 (B)	1.0	(22–30)	2–4	(14–16)	5	(15–50)	
Sodium (mM)	135–145 a	1.5–2.5	(30–55)	3–4	(25)	4–6	(26)	35 (mM)
Potassium (mM)	3.5–5.5	24–28	(13–22)	14–15	(13)	22	(20)	20–28 (μg/mg)‡
Calcium (mM)	2–2.5	1.0	(1.0)	1–1.6	(1.6–2)	1.5–4	(1.5–3)	6–22 (μg/mg)
Magnesium (mM)	1–1.5	0.1–0.2	(0.02)	0.05–0.1	(0.035)	0.2	(0.15–0.2)	1–6 (μg/mg)
Chloride (mM)	95–105	17–22	(17–33)	11–12	(16–26)	15	(30–100)	
Phosphorus (inorg)	1–1.5	10	(3)	4–6	(2)	6	(4)	6–20 (μg/mg)
Glucose (mg%)	70–100 (B)	0.8	(0.2)	0.5		0.5–1.0	(1.0)	
Ammonia (mg%)	0.08–0.11 (B)	0.9	(0.06)	0.7	(0.04)	12	(4–8)	
Urea (mg%)	14–40 (B)	30	(22–27)	10	(5)	20	(13–22)	
Thiocyanate (mg%)	0.1–1.5		(3)			15	(7–16)	
Total Protein (mg%)	6.5–8.2 (g%)	250	(270–320)	110	(150)	225–350	(280–300)	330
Iodide (μg%)	3–8 (bound)	4–10	(2–15)	12	(6)	4–24	(15–180)	
Fluoride (μg%)	10–20	3	(2)			8–25	(2–20)	0.04
Iron (μg%)	50–150	(5–10)				0–60	(20)	
Zinc (μg%)	90–125		(5)			20	(14–80)	0.01–0.1
Copper (μg%)	106–114		(9)			0–10	(2–25)	0.01–0.1
Chromium (μg%)	0.014						(9)	
Lead (μg%)	5–20 (B)	(2–10)				1–30	(0.4)	0–0.01

* Means or ranges for means are given. No entry indicates lack of data.
† Values are for unstimulated (U), or stimulated (S) flow rates approximating 1.0 ml/min for pure secretions, usually exceeding 1.0 ml/min for whole saliva.
‡ All plaque values which follow the plaque fluid concentration given for sodium are in μg/mg plaque dry weight.

fluorapatite complex. Studies of pure glandular secretions are indicated for verifying these contradictory results.

Magnesium, Iodine, Thiocyanate

Magnesium levels in submandibular saliva are higher than those in parotid saliva and vary inversely with flow rate. This element exists in relatively high concentrations in subsurface enamel, and its levels in dental plaque (along with those of calcium, phosphorus, and fluoride) have been associated inversely with caries experience. However, the concentration in whole saliva of iodine and the four elements just mentioned does not differ with caries susceptibility. Iodine levels in saliva decrease with increased flow rate and are too low for bacteriocidal effects. However, the physiologic concentration of thiocyanate (SCN^-) ions in saliva, which varies inversely with stimulated parotid flow rate, is effective against bacteria. Smokers show significantly higher salivary levels of SCN^-, a detoxification product of cyanide, than nonsmokers. For whole saliva, smoking decreases the levels of iodine in proportion to the increase observed for SCN^-. This effect is greater in male than female subjects, and in general is directly dependent on the number of cigarettes smoked per day. Recently it was found that SCN^- and iodine in saliva are competitive in reactions involving iodide oxidation and iodination of tyrosine. The relation of SCN^- inhibition of iodine metabolism to oral health is unknown.

Tin, Iron, Zinc and Other Trace Metals

It has been found that the essential trace elements that are normally under strict biologic control, generally occur more frequently in human whole saliva than nonessential metals, which appear to be influenced by dietary composition. Tin (nonessential), iron, zinc and chromium are present in paraffin-stimulated whole saliva more consistently and in relatively higher concentrations than other trace metals studied. Manganese and molybdenum (both essential), and nickel and cadmium are found least frequently and in much lower concentrations. Found more frequently but in very low levels are copper (essential), lead,

aluminum and strontium. Cobalt, which is mostly protein-bound with cyanocobalamin, and selenium are in relatively low concentrations in whole saliva. Manganese in whole saliva and nickel in parotid saliva do not differ with caries susceptibility, while copper levels in whole saliva have been shown to vary directly with caries incidence in children. Molybdenum and strontium, like fluoride, probably are taken up by apatite to form a protective surface against decay, but only strontium levels in saliva have been studied in caries with no correlation in evidence. Except for zinc (see below), the salivary effects on oral health for the other trace metals mentioned are unknown, unless possibly when toxic levels occur.

Differences With Age, Sex, and Diet

The influence of age on saliva composition is also important. For stimulated parotid saliva, the pH, sodium, calcium, chloride, protein and amylase levels decrease significantly with advancing age, while urea increases. Flow rates, potassium, and bicarbonate remain constant. Results from an unpublished study indicate that whole saliva composition varies with age in a similar manner.

The zinc concentration in whole saliva is significantly lower in caries-prone adults. Ionic zinc levels in whole saliva from subjects in different age groups are independent of flow rate and lowest in youngsters, who normally exhibit greater caries experience. It is notable that supplementation with zinc, molybdenum, and chromium in a cariogenic diet fed to young rats significantly reduced caries incidence in direct proportion to the amount of the trace metals given. Human female subjects fed a zinc-deficient diet for three weeks exhibited a significant decline in whole saliva zinc levels, as did another group of female subjects who consumed a lacto-ovo-vegetarian diet for the same time period. Increased fiber intake with a vegetarian diet that should not be cariogenic, may decrease the absorption of minerals but probably will not increase tooth decay. As with most other salivary constituents, whole saliva zinc levels fluctuate in direct circadian relation to the percentage of solids found in the saliva. Much of salivary zinc may be protein-bound and a zinc binding protein called gustin may affect taste. In addition, a zinc-binding ligand that may facilitate zinc absorption recently was isolated from whole saliva. With respect to the lower levels of zinc found in the saliva of caries-prone individuals, it is notable that detection thresholds for the basic taste qualities as related to caries susceptibility were significantly lower for sucrose only in caries-prone adults. Perhaps gustin levels also were lower in these individuals.

SALIVA COMPOSITION AND CARIES

Consistent correlations between saliva composition and caries have not been demonstrated. Gross external measurements (usually pH) and pooled samples of plaque and saliva, although studied without precise knowledge of oral status at the location from which obtained, have demonstrated that several potentially significant phenomena occur at the plaque-saliva interface. It is likely that salivary components differentially influence plaque depending upon plaque's maturity. For example, as apatite-binding proteins from saliva initiate formation of the acquired pellicle, salivary phosphate tends to retard plaque growth by facilitating the desorbtion of adsorbed proteins. The ammonia in saliva, or ammonia liberated from salivary urea via bacterial activity, can directly neutralize the acid produced locally in bacterial plaque. Formation of ammonium carbonate should assist in preventing a critical fall in pH, especially since buffering in plaque fluid is greater at pH 5–6 and is attributed to salivary bicarbonate. In fact, the pH of early plaque has been found to be dependent largely on salivary pH. At pH 4–5, proteins and amino acids released by bacterial proteases become the principal buffers in plaque fluid.

Whole saliva in caries-resistant individuals appears to exhibit a higher buffer capacity. It was demonstrated that carbonic anhydrase activity is significantly lower in the whole saliva of caries-active children. Also, rinsing with glucose lowers the plaque pH below 5 only in subjects with extreme caries activity. The pH of plaque on lower anterior teeth drops less than the pH of plaque on opposing maxillary teeth due mainly to the pooling of saliva on mandibular surfaces. For the same reason, much higher levels of calcium and phosphate generally are found in plaque on mandibular teeth. Thus, a direct relation exists between saliva and plaque concentrations of calcium and phosphate. *This accounts for the significant negative correlation between calcium and phosphate levels in plaque and increasing incidence of caries when salivary levels apparently are unrelated to caries experience.*

A major factor in plaque metabolism is its thickness, which influences ionic diffusion bacterial effects, and in all probability, the direction and type of body fluid which moves into the mass due to osmotic or hydrostatic forces. Positive linear relationships exist between accumulated plaque and caries experience. Of particular significance to plaque chemistry and oral health is fluoride because of its relative abundance and demonstrable inhibitory action on bacterial growth and acid production. The thickness of plaque and the amount of viable plaque microorganisms are both reduced in direct proportion to increasing concentrations of stannous fluoride in a mouth rinse used over a period of days in the absence of brushing. A more refined study revealed that plaque is not freely permeable to aqueous fluoride when rinsed orally although plaque levels of fluoride were elevated for more than two hours, possibly in response to recirculation from saliva. To reach its high levels in plaque relative to saliva, fluoride probably is bound to inorganic cations. Plaque fluoride levels are shown to be strongly interdependent with calcium, a predominant plaque constituent also found in much higher concentrations than seen in saliva. *In vitro* studies indicate that fluoride may act to reduce the driving force for diffusion of calcium out of plaque regions and hydrogen ions into plaque regions. This would impede enamel dissolution and facilitate remineralization (see Chap. 19). It is notable that pellicle grown on fluorapatite *in vitro* exhibits greater ionic permselectivity than hydroxyapatite pellicle, such that diffusion of sulfate is retarded to a greater extent while water remains unaffected. Since plaque fluoride levels decrease as plaque accumulates, the significant diffusion and antibacterial effects of fluoride in plaque disappear accordingly. Chronic exposure to fluoride via dietary intake and salivary recirculation should help stabilize plaque growth, thereby increasing the potential for plaque uptake of fluoride. It should be noted that the relation of fluoride levels in saliva to oral health is unknown, although it may yet be proven significant that salivary fluoride bathes oral tissues continuously.

The evidence presently available indicates

that of the trace elements only zinc, and possibly copper, iron, and tin exist in sufficient concentration in saliva to influence oral health. Zinc and copper in concentrations equivalent to average plaque levels are known to inhibit acid and plaque production by several strains of oral streptococci. This agrees, in part, with the elevated salivary zinc levels in caries-resistant adults and the lower plaque zinc concentrations associated with plaque accumulation. However, enamel levels of zinc and copper are positively correlated with caries incidence. This evidence is in agreement only with the elevated levels of salivary copper found in caries-prone children, but is contrary to what would be expected for the antibacterial effects of both zinc and copper. In plaque, the levels of zinc, copper and lead are independent of calcium and phosphate, but not of one another. This supports the notion that bulk fluid flow mechanisms in plaque play a role in regulating its mineral content.

It generally is not known if trace element levels in oral tissues assume different roles, degrees of significance, or variance in concentration during human growth and aging. Zinc, for example, is actively accumulated in the dentin but not in the enamel of developing teeth in young rats, and shows lower concentrations in the saliva of children. There could be differences for salivary levels of other trace elements in children compared to adults. The plaque zinc content of adults is greater for males than females, which implicates endocrine involvement. The relation of iron levels in saliva to caries experience is not known, but lactoferrin, a salivary protein, exhibits bacteriostatic properties which are mediated by its ability to withhold iron from bacterial utilization. In addition, iron levels in tooth enamel are positively correlated to caries resistance, but plaque relationships are unknown. Salivary tin, whose concentration in whole saliva exceeds that of all the trace elements studied to date, may contribute to formation of ionic complexes with fluoride ions to facilitate their uptake by hydroxyapatite.

Saliva contains several enzymes (see Chap. 3) which may influence dental caries. Acid phosphatase could cleave enamel matrix-bound phosphate once it became established in plaque. The adsorption of acid phosphatase to enamel is increased markedly following incubation of the teeth in solutions of calcium, zinc or phosphorus; zinc-and calcium-treated enamel exhibits enhanced enzymatic activity, whereas phosphate treatment causes inhibition. Since magnesium- and fluoride-treated enamel also reduces acid phosphatase activity, and fluoride, magnesium, and phosphate are released when apatite dissolves, the antagonistic ionic environment which would result from activity of this enzyme on enamel eliminates its potential role in cariogenesis. Lactoperoxidase (LPO) adsorbed onto hydroxyapatite exhibits antibacterial activity in the presence of cofactors, hydrogen peroxide (which can be liberated by lactic acid bacteria) and SCN^- ions which can arise from saliva. This system also inhibits bacterial acid production in dental plaque. The ionic permselectivity of mature pellicle appears to be less restrictive of SCN^- diffusion between charged sites on the pellicle matrix than it is for the diffusion of divalent sulfate ions. Therefore, even accumulated plaque could be permeable to the influx of SCN^- ions from saliva. A possible mechanism proposed for the SCN^- inhibition of bacterial metabolism is the formation of hypothiocyanite ions following the LPO-catalysed oxidation of SCN^- in the presence of hydrogen peroxide. Hypothiocyanite could inhibit glycolysis in bacteria by reacting with the thiol groups in glycolytic enzymes. Clearly, additional studies are needed to understand the role of these and other salivary enzymes which may influence oral health.

DENTINAL TUBULE FLUID MOVEMENT

The previous discussion of plaque-saliva influences on dental caries assumed the validity of the acidogenic theory for cariogenesis (see Chap. 8). A potentially significant *endocrine* salivary gland-mediated phenomenon for the etiology of this disease that has been virtually ignored in caries research is that of dentinal tubule fluid movement. The evidence indicates that a hypothalamic factor stimulates the parotid gland to release a hormone directly into the circulation, which in turn promotes fluid movement in dentinal odontoblastic tubules. Hypothalamic and parotid extracts have both been shown to stimulate increased fluid movement, but the hypothalamic factor is effective only when the parotid glands are intact. The proposed "hypothalamic-parotid axis" remains functional in rats when all salivary ducts are ligated, and also remains functional in the absence of the submandibular-sublingual complex or pituitary gland. The endocrine axis is disrupted only after extirpation of the parotid glands. Subsequently it has been found that caries incidence decreases significantly in rats fed a cariogenic diet which is supplemented with substances, such as urea, that are known to increase dentinal fluid movement when administered systemically. These results may well attain future prominence.

RELATION OF SALIVARY COMPONENTS TO ORAL AND GASTRIC CANCER

It has recently come to light that nitrites may play a role in the etiology of some cancers. It could be of significance to the etiology of oral and gastric cancer that thiocyanate is a powerful catalyst of nitrosation reactions. The nitrate secreted by salivary glands is reduced to nitrite in the oral cavity by bacterial nitrate reductase. Nitrosamine formation in saliva already has been demonstrated for two tertiary amine drugs, aminopyrine and oxytetracycline, which react with salivary nitrite to yield a potent hepatocarcinogen, N-nitrosodimethylamine. Because the pH optimum for these reactions is 3.4, the nitrosative toxification of orally administered drugs probably occurs in plaque, in the presence of salivary SCN^- which catalyses nitrosation at near neutral pH conditions, or in the stomach where the pH range is 1–5. The higher levels of SCN^- in the saliva of smokers could facilitate nitrosamine formation and oral exposure to carcinogens, in addition to the irritative effects of cigarette smoke alone. The SCN^- found in gastric juice, which also contains nitrite, is attributed to swallowed saliva. However, ascorbic acid, glutathione, and other dietary antioxidants, such as various food additives, can inhibit drug-nitrite interactions. In addition, nitrosation reactions in saliva can be inhibited by tannic and caffeic acids, which are found in red wine, coffee, and tea.

SALIVA COMPOSITION AND TASTE

Saliva and its components influence taste perception. The potential importance of gustin, a zinc-binding protein found in parotid saliva,

was noted earlier. Abnormally low *salivary* zinc levels in patients with significantly impaired taste perception (**hypogeusia**) increase only in association with improved taste acuity. However, dietary zinc supplementation increases serum zinc levels irrespective of a patient's taste status. Zinc and copper ions, in concentrations that approximate physiologic levels of these elements in saliva, significantly affect rat chorda tympani taste nerve responses to various taste solutions. Saliva itself is essential for gustation. Phenylthiocarbamide (PTC) is a substance perceived as a bitter taste by a majority of the population, the remainder being "taste blind" to this compound. Tasters can perceive PTC only in the presence of their own saliva or saliva transferred from a nontaster, but not in the absence of saliva.

Significant reductions in saliva flow can occur in association with Sjögren's syndrome, radiation therapy for head and neck cancer, or experimental desalivation in rats. Taste perception often is altered in these situations. However, impaired taste for one or more of the basic taste qualities has been reported in cancer, cirrhosis, diabetes, and renal disease even though critical reductions in saliva flow were not observed in related studies. Calcium, which binds readily to protein, and total protein levels in the saliva of these patients often differed from normals. This suggests that the levels of certain protein constituents could be common denominators in altered taste perception. In addition to gustin, proteolytic enzymes in saliva could influence taste to some unknown degree. The application of proteolytic enzymes to the tongue in much higher concentrations than found in saliva decreases subjective taste acuity. Saliva also contains enzyme inhibitors which have not been studied in relation to taste. Because knowledge in this area is practically nonexistent, any gustatory influence that is proposed for salivary constituents at this time must be based on pure speculation.

SALIVA COMPOSITION AND SYSTEMIC DISEASE

The levels of many salivary constituents have been shown to vary in systemic disease. Differences often noted for total protein levels in saliva from Sjögren's patients are reflected in increased anode-migrating proteins when the protein components are separated electrophoretically. Salivary electrophoretograms reveal additional protein bands in cystic fibrosis, even though total protein levels are normal in some studies. The turbidity observed for saliva in this disease is attributed mainly to precipitation of a calcium-phosphoprotein in response to elevated salivary calcium levels. Abnormality in the properties of statherin, an inhibitor of calcium-phosphate precipitation in saliva, also has been postulated. Electrophoretic differences in salivary protein components have been demonstrated in other systemic disorders such as diabetes, which shows relatively normal total protein levels in saliva. It is significant that in normal rats, the pharmacologic manipulation of flow rate and total protein concentration of parotid saliva failed to demonstrate electrophoretic differences in the proportions of proteins secreted. Evidently, salivary proteins can be influenced by disease processes in response to hormonal, if not autonomic, effects. To support this contention, a salivary enzyme characteristic of ovulating women, and a parotid glycoprotein which is unique to late pregnancy and postpartum were discovered recently. Salivary electrolyte levels are not as potentially useful as electrophoresed protein components in depicting systemic disorder. They often exhibit inconsistencies which are related partly to variance with flow rate, a parameter which differs greatly even between normals. When consistent, electrolyte levels in saliva usually cannot provide a specific diagnosis. However, for monitoring digitalis toxicity in cardiac patients, the levels of calcium and potassium in unstimulated whole saliva have been shown to increase significantly in response to digoxin administration and exhibit a further significant increase whenever toxicity did occur. Even so, the use of salivary calcium/potassium ratios to monitor digitalis toxicity remains a point of controversy. Perhaps the most practical and reliable salivary test for systemic monitoring is the determination of whole saliva urea levels for diagnosis of uremia, a procedure that can be performed at bedside in a few minutes time.

SUMMARY

During the long process of evolution, the salivary glands have developed into major secretory organs which maintain homeostasis of the oropharyngeal mucosa and teeth. They do this by their capability to produce two distinct homeokinetic responses to appropriate stimuli which results in two levels of secretory activity. One level is the resting secretion which is produced continually while we are awake, providing a thin layer of hypotonic, low salt fluid that moves slowly and continuously over the mucosa and teeth. The other is the oral reflex-stimulated secretion which occurs when we eat. Evolutionary development of the major salivary glands has resulted in epithelial secretory mechanisms which produce this very low salt fluid over the great range of secretory flow encompassed by these two levels of gland activity. The homeostatic functions of the secretions may depend to a major extent on the capability to produce hypotonic fluid, as well as on the capability to secrete important proteins, glycoproteins, and mucins into this fluid.

Four ions contribute the overwhelming share of the osmotically active particles (being thereby termed "osmolytes") in the secreted fluid regardless of the rate of secretion: sodium, potassium, chloride, and bicarbonate. Individually, three of these—sodium, chloride, and bicarbonate—vary greatly with changes in flow. Potassium decreases slightly when going from the unstimulated to stimulated rates of flow but does *not* change at steadily increasing rates of stimulated secretion (in which flow rate may increase up to 30 times the highest resting rates). Potassium levels always remain substantially above plasma levels at any rate of secretion, and the constancy of its concentration suggests a relationship to the mechanism by which fluid is produced.

Overall, the glands demonstrate an ability to produce fluid at a relatively constant osmolality which is substantially below that of plasma and other body fluids. The glands maintain this over the entire range of secretion, even though three of the individual major osmolytes vary greatly in concentration. From the evolutionary perspective, we might view this as selective development of epithelial fluid transport mechanisms which enable the glands to produce abundant quantities of water with a necessary minimum, but low, salt content.

Secretion of this low salt fluid serves several major physiologic purposes. It provides the solvent into which macromolecular secretory products are transported by the secretory epithelium, (i.e., the proteins, glycoproteins, and mucins described in Chap. 3). It provides the solvent into which the necessary minerals, trace elements, and hormones are transported (while the secretory fluid is in transit along the secretory lumen). It provides the medium which carries these secretory products into the oral cavity and which further enables wide dispersal as a watery film covering the oral tissues. And, finally, this hypotonic fluid may also promote surface adsorption of the secretory products by virtue of entrainment in the secretory water as it is absorbed osmotically into oral tissues. From the perspective of these functions the relative changes in three of the four main osmolytes may be functionally insignificant, since they would appear to serve primarily to provide the necessary lowest osmotic salt content which permits water transport across the secretory epithelium. The secretion of these ions then are the necessary osmolar backdrop for water secretion, and the secretory water provides the solvent for the functionally important macromolecular constituents, minerals, and trace elements. Of the four major osmolytes, only bicarbonate has obvious potential functional significance

in and of itself. Thus, the salivary secretions may be viewed as a watery oropharyngeal palliative lubricant and nutrient fluid; its overall quality as such will depend on the overall quality of the health and nutritional status of the individual. A summary of the important mineral and trace element content of saliva of healthy individuals is presented in Table 4-1.

At the second level of homeokinetic secretory response the salivary glands deliver much greater quantities of fluid, but osmolality remains less than other body fluids, and concentrations of proteins, mucins, minerals, and trace elements remain virtually constant. The primary functional significance of the ability of the glands to produce this higher rate of delivery is twofold: to mix with relatively dry foods taken in which facilitates chewing and swallowing; and, to adjust the osmolality of swallowed foods to plasma like values. However, it is also significant that the glands are able to produce fluid at (ca.) 50 to 100 times the resting rate and still retain the most important functional characteristics of the resting secretions, (i.e., hypotonicity and relatively constant protein, mucin, mineral and, trace element content.

GLOSSARY

Chyme. The semifluid mass of partly digested food passed from the stomach into the duodenum.

Critical pH. The *p*H in the oral cavity, below which saliva ceases to be supersaturated relative to tooth mineral, causing apatite to dissolve.

Cystic fibrosis. A hereditary disease of children, adolescents, and young adults characterized by generalized dysfunction of exocrine glands. Whenever saliva flow in these patients is abnormal for the major salivary glands, parotid secretion is greater and submandibular secretion lower than normal.

Hypotonic. Denoting that one of two solutions possess the lesser osmotic pressure.

m Eg/l. Milliequivalents per liter

Osmol. The molecular weight of a solute, in grams, divided by the number of ions or particles into which it dissociates in solution.

Osmolarity. The osmotic concentration of a solution expressed as osmols of solute per liter of solution.

Osmotic. Relating to the net passage of fluid from the less concentrated to the more concentrated side of a membrane.

Pilocarpine. A parasympathomimetic agent used as a sialogogue and stimulant of intestinal motility.

Sialin. An arginine peptide found in saliva and described as a "*p*H rise factor."

Sjögren's syndrome. Predominantly an autoimmune disease of middle-aged women. It consists of the triad of xerostomia, keratoconjunctivitis sicca, and in 50 to 60 per cent of all patients, a connective tissue disorder, usually rheumatoid arthritis.

Statherin. A phosphopeptide found in saliva that is an active inhibitor of the precipitation of calcium phosphate salts.

Taste thresholds. Detection (or difference) threshold is the concentration of a tastant at which a subject can identify a difference in taste between stimuli. Recognition threshold is the concentration at which a specific taste (sour, salt, sweet, bitter) can first be recognized and is higher than detection levels.

SUGGESTED READINGS

Abe K, Dawes C: The effects of electrical and pharmacological stimulation on the types of proteins secreted by rat parotid and submandibular glands. Arch Oral Biol 23: 367–372, 1978

Ashly FP, Wilson RF: The relationship between calcium and phosphorus concentrations of human saliva and dental plaque. Arch Oral Biol 23: 69–73, 1978

Atkin-Thor E, Goddard BW, O'Nion J, Stephen RL, Kolff WJ: Hypogeusia and zinc depletion in chronic dialysis patients. Am J Clin Nutr 31: 1948–1951, 1978

Ben-Aryeh H, Gutman D, Hammerman H: Salivary

levels of calcium and potassium as indicators of digitalis toxicity. Chest 72: 131–132, 1977

Brown LR, Dreizen S, Rider LJ, Johnston DA: The effect of radiation-induced xerostomia on saliva and serum lysozyme and immunoglobulin levels. Oral Surg 41: 83–92, 1976

Brown WE, Chow LC: Mechanism of F⁻ cariostasis (abstr 444). J Dent Res 56 (SIA): A154, 1977

Burch RE, Sackin DA, Ursick JA, Jetton MM, Sullivan JF: Decreased taste and smell acuity in cirrhosis. Arch Intern Med 138: 743–746, 1978

Carson JS, Gormican A: Disease-medication relationships in altered taste sensitivity. J Am Diet Assoc 68: 550–553, 1976

Chauncey HH, Bell B, Kapur KK, Feller RP: Parotid fluid composition in a study of healthy aging males (abstr 51). J Dent Res 54 (SIA): 57, 1975

Chauncey HH, Feller RP, Henriques BL: Comparative electrolyte composition of parotid, submandibular and sublingual secretions. J Dent Res 45: 1230, 1966

Cohen J, Ogdon DP: Taste blindness to phenylthiocarbamide as a function of saliva. Science 110: 532–533, 1949

Curzon MEJ, Crocker DC: Relationships of trace elements in human tooth enamel to dental caries. Arch Oral Biol 23: 647–653, 1978

Dawes C: The effects of flow rate and duration of stimulation on the concentrations of protein and the main electrolytes in human parotid saliva. Arch Oral Biol 14: 277–294, 1969

Dawes C: Effects of diet on salivary secretion and composition. J Dent Res 49: 1263–1272, 1970

Dawes C: The effects of flow rate and duration of stimulation on the concentration of protein and the main electrolytes in human submandibular saliva. Arch Oral Biol 19: 887–895, 1974

Dawes C: Rhythms in salivary flow rate and composition. Int J Chronobiol 2:253–279, 1974

Dijken JV, Ericson T: Preliminary report on composition of saliva in patients with cystic fibrosis (abstr 163). J Dent Res 57(SIA): 229, 1978

Dreizen S, Levy BM, Niedermeier W, Griggs JH: Comparative concentrations of selected trace metals in human and marmoset saliva. Arch Oral Biol 15: 179–188, 1970

Ferguson DB, Thomas PD: Variability of calcium and phosphorus concentrations in dental plaque collected from human anterior teeth. Arch Oral Biol 23: 839–841, 1978

Finestone AJ, Schacterle GR, Pollack RL: The comparative analysis of diabetic and non-diabetic saliva. Study I. Protein separation by disc gel electrophoresis. J Periodontol 44: 175–176, 1973

Galili D, Maller O, Brightman VJ: Effects of drug-desalivation on feeding and taste preferences in the rat. Arch Oral Biol 23: 459–464, 1978

Gillard BK, Markman HC, Feig SA: Differences between cystic fibrosis and normal saliva-amylase as a function of age and sex. Pediatr Res 12: 868–872, 1978

Hay DI, Gron P: Inhibitors of calcium phosphate precipitation in human whole saliva (abstr). In (eds): Microbial Aspects of Dental Caries Stiles HM, Loesche WJ, O'Brian TC Washington DC Information Retrieval, Vol I, 143–150, 1976

Henkin RI, Schecter PJ, Freidewald WT, Demetes DL, Raff M: A double blind study of the effects of zinc sulfate on taste and small dysfunction. Am J Med 272: 285–299, 1977

Johnson AR: The effects of inorganic ions situated at the enamel surface on the adsorption and activity of acid phosphatase. J Dent Res 56: 1173–1178, 1977

Kleinberg I, Kanapka JA, Craw D: Effects of saliva and salivary factors on the metabolism of the mixed oral flora (abstr). In Stiles HM, Loesch WJ, O'Brien TC (eds): Microbial Aspects of Dental Caries, Washington DC, Information Retrieval Vol II 433–464, 1976

Leonora J, Steinman RR: Evidence suggesting the existence of a hypothalamic-parotid gland endocrine axis. Endocrinology 83: 807–815, 1968

Mandel ID: Relation of saliva and plaque to caries. J Dent Res 53: 246–266, 1974

Mandel ID, Baurmash H: Sialochemistry in Sjögren's syndrome. Oral Surg 41: 182–187, 1975

Picarelli A, Colasanti R: Comparative concentrations of zinc in the saliva of caries-resistant and caries-prone human subjects (abstr 45). J Dent Res 54: 671, 1975

Rao GS: Nitrosation of drugs by human salivary nitrite. Arch Oral Biol 23: 749–750, 1978

Schamschula RG, Bunzel M, Agus HM, Adkins BL, Barmes DE, Charleton G: Plaque minerals and caries experience: associations and interrelationships. J Dent Res 57: 427–432, 1978

Shannon IL: Reference table for human parotid saliva collected at varying levels of exogenous stimulation. J Dent Res 52: 1157, 1973

Shannon IL, Feller RP, Chauncey HH: Fluoride in human parotid saliva. J Dent Res 55: 506–509, 1976

Shannon IL, Feller RP, Eknoyan G, Suddick RP: Human parotid saliva urea in renal failure and during dialysis. Arch Oral Biol 22: 83–86, 1977

Shannon IL, Suddick RP, Dowd FJ: Saliva: composition and secretion. In Myers HM (ed): Monographs in Oral Science, Vol 2. Basel, Karger, S 1974

Smith QT, Shapiro BL Hamilton MJ, Biros M: A parotid salivary protein present during late pregnancy and postpartum. Proc Soc Exp Biol Med 153: 241–246, 1976

Steinman RR, Leonora J: Relationship of fluid transport through the dentin to the incidence of dental caries. J Dent Res 50: 1536–1543, 1971

Szabo I: Carbonic anhydrase activity in the saliva of children and its relation to caries activity. Caries Res 8: 187–191, 1974

Tannenbaum PJ, Posner AS, Mandel ID: Formation of calcium phosphates in saliva and dental plaque. J Dent Res 55: 997–1000, 1976

Tatevossian A: Buffering capacity in human dental plaque fluid. Caries Res 11: 216–222, 1977

Tatevossian A: Distribution and kinetics of fluoride ions in the free aqueous and residual phases of human dental plaque. Arch Oral Biol 23: 893–898, 1978

Tenovuo J: Inhibition by thiocyanate of lactoperoxidase-catalysed oxidation and iodination reactions. Arch Oral Biol 23: 899–903, 1978

Tuompo H, Raeste AM, Nuuja T: Ionic zinc in normal human mixed saliva (abstr 188). J Dent Res 56(SIA): A89, 1977

Turtola LO: Salivary fluoride and calcium concentrations, and their relationship to the secretion of saliva and caries experience. Scand J Dent Res 85: 535–541, 1977

Wrobel WL, Catalanotto FA, Walter RG: Taste thresholds in caries-free and caries-active naval recruits. Arch Oral Biol 23: 881–885, 1978

5 Nonmineralized Coverings of the Enamel Surface

CLYDE W. MAYHALL

Introduction
Classification of Surface Coverings
   Coverings of Embryologic Origin
   Coverings Acquired after Eruption
     of the Teeth
      Food Debris
      Materia Alba
      Dental Plaque

Acquired Pellicle
   Introduction and Definition
   "Natural" Pellicle
   "Experimental" Pellicles
   "Function" of the Pellicle
Summary
Glossary
Suggested Readings

INTRODUCTION

It is generally agreed that dental caries begins at the surface of the enamel and that the etiologic agent is dental plaque (see Ch. 14). It is also generally accepted that any organic covering intervening between plaque and the enamel surface could influence the initiation of the caries process. There is, however, much disagreement concerning the types and composition of the surface coverings of enamel, partly because several of the coatings can coexist as layers on the enamel surface, giving rise to extreme difficulty in distinguishing the physical limits of each. Historically, many different terms have been used to describe the coverings found on the enamel. In fact, there is still no general agreement today on a universal classification of these surface coatings, or even about which coverings actually exist. Many of the descriptions and definitions of surface coatings have been based on histologic and histochemical observations. The advent of electron microscopy (transmission and scanning) and advances in understanding optic phenomena and histochemistry have now made questionable many of the observations based on light microscopy accepted in the past. The purpose of this chapter is to introduce the student and clinician to the classification, structure, composition, and function of the surface coatings of the teeth in an understandable way based on our most current knowledge. This discussion is limited to the coverings of the enamel surface of the clinical crown since these have been studied more and are better understood. The surface coating of enamel when it is covered by epithelium is not discussed.

CLASSIFICATION OF SURFACE COVERINGS

It is both convenient and logical to divide the organic surface coverings of enamel into those of embryologic origin and those acquired after eruption of the teeth.

Coverings of Embryologic Origin

Historically, the embryologic coverings of the enamel have been described as a "primary enamel cuticle" covered by the reduced enamel epithelium. The primary enamel cuticle was described as an organic layer that was the final secretory product of the ameloblasts (after the formation of enamel was completed). Those structures were also called the "inner acellular and outer cellular layers of

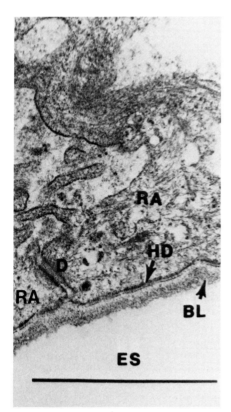

Fig. 5-1. Reduced ameloblasts (**RA**) joined by desmosome (**D**) are attached to enamel by hemidesmosomes (**HD**) and a basal lamina (**BL**). **ES,** enamel space. (Listgarten, MA: J Periodontol 47: 139, 1976) (×45,000)

Nasmyth's membrane." With the electron microscope, no organic structure corresponding to a primary enamel cuticle or to the dark layer seen between ameloblasts and enamel by phase-constrast microscopy was ever observed. The absence of a "primary enamel cuticle" in sections studied with electron microscopy suggests that the appearance of a cuticle with light microscopy is probably an artifact due to an optical phenomenon.

It has also been reported that the enamel of unerupted human teeth is covered by a collagenous layer. But electron microscopic and chemical studies by other investigators have found no evidence of a collagenous covering of enamel.

The embryologic covering of enamel is now considered to be the reduced enamel epithelium and a basal lamina. Postsecretory ameloblasts are attached to the enamel surface by hemidesmosomes and a basal lamina (Fig. 5-1). The peripheral portion of the reduced enamel epithelium consists of cells derived primarily from the stratum intermedium (Fig. 5-2). Although it is generally agreed that the structures of embryologic origin are lost with, or soon after, eruption of the teeth, the exact sequence of events accompanying the loss of the embryologic covering of enamel and the acquisition of an acquired coating is not known.

Coverings Acquired after Eruption of the Teeth

The eruption of the teeth is usually accompanied by some hemorrhage, as well as by profuse salivation, and components from the blood might be important first contributors to an acquired enamel coating. But most investigators reject the hypothesis that blood constituents contribute the major portion of the acquired covering of mature teeth.

While the embryologic covering of enamel is mostly of academic interest, the acquired coatings are of very real clinical interest since they are what we deal with every day in the mouths of our patients. The four coatings acquired after eruption of the teeth (but not in the sequence of acquisition) are food debris, materia alba, dental plaque, and pellicle. This classification is admittedly clinical but in accord with the objectives of this chapter.

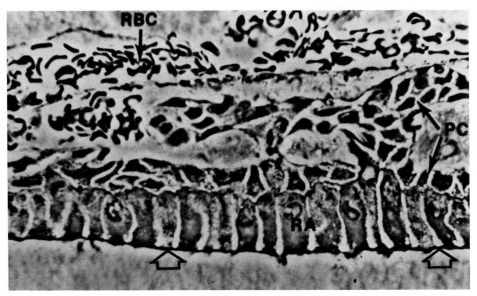

Fig. 5-2. Reduced enamel epithelium floated off the surface of a demineralized enucleated human premolar. **Large arrows** point to a dense line at the distal end of the reduced ameloblasts (**RA**). This line, which probably results from a "summation effect" (see text) of the basal lamina has been interpreted in the past as a "primary enamel cuticle." **PC,** papillary layer of external cells of the reduced enamel epithelium. **RBC,** erythrocytes due to surgical hemorrhage. Phase-contrast. (Listgarten, MA: Arch Oral Biol 11: 999, 1966) (×600)

Food Debris

Clinically, the acquired coverings of the teeth may be subdivided into those that can and those that cannot be removed with a stream of water or by vigorous mouth rinsing by the patient. In the first category are food debris and materia alba. Unless impacted between the teeth or retained by dental defects or prostheses, food debris can be removed with a stream of water (e.g., dental water syringe or home irrigation device). Of course, foods vary in their ability to stick to the teeth and therefore in the difficulty of their removal with rinsing. It is, however, essential that the clinician be able to identify food debris in the mouth of the patient and know the importance, or relative lack of importance, of that finding. Unfortunately, many patients have the misconception that food debris is the cause of dental caries. That fallacy has been perpetuated by the dental profession's support of slogans such as "brush after every meal to prevent dental decay." It seems obvious now that it is dental plaque that we should be teaching our patients to remove completely once a day to prevent dental caries. All too often a patient presents for oral hygiene instruction with a defense such as "You're going to find a lot of junk on my teeth because I didn't get a chance to brush since eating." The clinician must be firm and certain in conviction in teaching patients that, while food debris is unsightly and can contribute to mouth odor, it in itself does not cause caries. Actually, large particles of food are not the source of available nutrients for cariogenic bacteria. Also to be stressed is that home irrigation devices, which may be pleasant to use and do remove loose food debris, do not "clean" the teeth and do not, therefore, replace the toothbrush and dental floss for plaque removal.

Materia Alba

Materia alba, which means "white matter," is an old term in the dental literature and was often used to include dental plaque and food debris. Because of poor definition, a lack of understanding, and inaccurate application, the term *materia alba* has been dropped from many classifications of tooth coverings. From a clinical point of view, however, the term has some validity and is useful when specifically defined and correctly used. For our purposes, **materia alba** is defined as a soft, white mixture of bacteria, salivary components, desquamated epithelial cells, and disintegrating leukocytes that adheres loosely to the surface of the tooth (actually the pellicle), dental plaque, or the gingiva. Although materia alba is composed largely of bacteria, it does not possess a specific architecture, in contrast, as we shall see, to dental plaque. Moreover, although the relative distribution of classes of microorganisms is essentially the same in materia alba and dental plaque, materia alba contains fewer living microorganisms and significantly lower bacterial counts than dental plaque does. From a research point of view materia alba may be considered of trivial import or simply as a part of dental plaque. Clinically, however, the presence of materia alba indicates a total lack of oral hygiene in the area of its occurrence. In truth, there is some danger in considering such a loosely bound covering as an integral part of dental plaque, especially when one is discussing and educating patients to the problems of mechanical removal of plaque. The low level of viability of the microorganisms and the location of materia alba on the surface of dental plaque, away from the tooth surface, strongly suggest that materia alba plays little or no role in caries. (Materia alba may, however, play a role in the inflammatory periodontal diseases.)

Dental Plaque

Whereas food debris and materia alba are relatively easily removed from the tooth surface, dental plaque and the acquired pellicle are tenaciously attached to the enamel and are not removed by vigorous rinsing or with a stream of water. The importance of plaque lies in its role as the etiologic agent of dental caries (and the inflammatory periodontal diseases). **Dental plaque** may be defined as a soft, concentrated, adherent mass of microorganisms colonizing on the surface of the tooth. Plaque is composed mainly of microorganisms, which are embedded in an intercellular matrix that is mostly of microbial origin. In mature stages, plaque is characterized histologically by a palisading arrangement of microcolonies perpendicular to the tooth surface (Fig. 5-3). Since other sections of this book deal with dental plaque in great detail (see Chaps. 11, 13, 14), the objective here is to present a more general picture of dental plaque.

One basic concept that must be understood at the outset is that plaque is not a homogeneous entity. In other words, "plaque is not plaque is not plaque." It is now accepted that

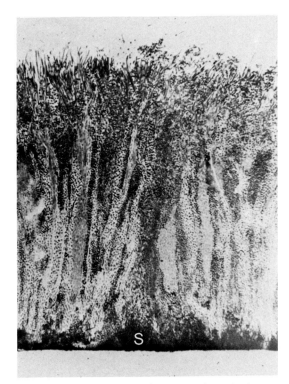

Fig. 5-3. One-week plaque. Columnar microcolonies are still well-defined. Note numerous filaments attached to the surface of this predominantly coccal plaque. **S**, epon surface. (Listgarten, MA: J Periodontol 46: 10, 1975) (×860)

the bacterial composition of plaque not only varies between individuals, between different areas of the same mouth, between surfaces on the same tooth, between supragingival and subgingival locations, but also with time. It is therefore misleading to speak of "plaque" as if it were an entity with a defined bacterial composition and pathogenic potential. Clinical observations of patients who have severe periodontal disease and no carious lesions, or the converse, make it clear that the pathogenic potential of plaque (perhaps coupled with host resistance and other variables) produces different results in different patients. We still do not, however, understand why some plaque formation leads to caries and other plaque has the ability to accumulate mineral and become dental calculus, or why calculus can sometimes form in an existing carious lesion. In many respects, caries and calculus are the opposite results of the presence of "dental plaque." In spite of these questions, one sound clinical conclusion for the practicing dentist to accept is that control of dental plaque is a vital factor in the prevention of dental caries (and the periodontal diseases).

Acquired Pellicle

Introduction and Definition. It should be remembered, of course, that the acquired coverings of enamel can, and often do, occur simultaneously on the same tooth surface. The single coating most likely to be found on any enamel surface is the pellicle. Although many names have been used for this covering, "pellicle" seems preferable to "cuticle" or any of the other terms. **Pellicle** means "a thin skin or film," and indeed the enamel pellicle meets that definition, having been described as a fraction of a micrometer to several micrometers in thickness. The pellicle (Fig. 5-4) is generally described as acellular, structureless, bacteria free, and of salivary origin. The pellicle may occur as the only enamel covering or it may underlie dental plaque, materia alba, or food debris.

The discovery of the pellicle may be attributed to Alexander Nasmyth. Although there were many errors in his conclusions, he observed "a membrane floating on the surface of a solution in which human teeth had been submitted to the action of acid." Indeed that description has been the basis of the definition of the pellicle since Nasmyth first gave it in 1839.

With no intention of adding to the already enormous clutter of terminology in this field, studies related to two types of pellicle are discussed—"natural" and "experimental" pellicles.

"Natural" Pellicle. The term *natural pellicle* was chosen because the material was obtained from extracted, erupted, permanent human teeth. To the practicing dentist this material should be interesting because it is what we deal with in the mouths of our patients.

The advent of the electron microscope has renewed interest in the histologic study of the enamel integuments and has raised as many questions as it has answered. Various investigators have observed surface, subsurface, and suprasurface pellicles. It is very difficult to correlate the results reported by different investigators. Often a new name is introduced because of the inability to be certain whether the structure observed is the same as that reported and named by another investigator. Although "stained pellicle" has sometimes been described as a separate entity, many investigators think it may result from a thicker accumulation of pellicle that has acquired additional constituents that impart the color. In fact, the apparently colorless pellicle from

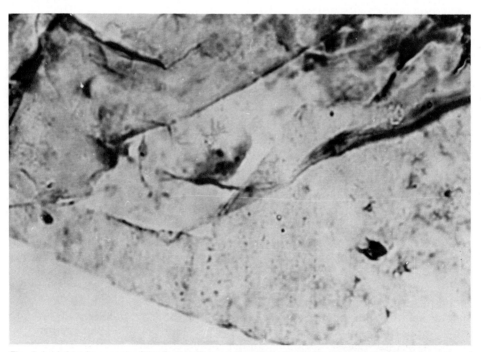

Fig. 5-4. Light micrograph of the "natural" enamel pellicle illustrating the structureless character of the pellicle. In portions of the micrograph the pellicle may be seen folded back upon itself. (gram stain, bright field × 1600)

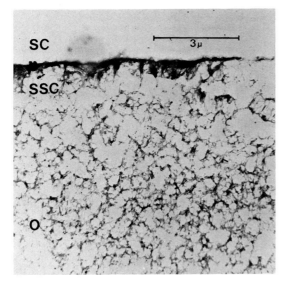

Fig. 5-5. Electron micrograph of the organic deposit on the labial surface of a freshly extracted upper central incisor. Demineralized cross section. **SC** = surface cuticle. **SSC** = subsurface cuticle. **O** = organic residue of enamel. (Meckel AH: Arch Oral Biol 10: 585, 1965)

nonstained enamel normally has a slight brownish color.

Many investigators have reported the presence of a thin organic surface pellicle (some still call it a "cuticle"), as seen in Figure 5-5. Several investigators have also observed a subsurface pellicle—a penetration of organic material from the surface pellicle into the superficial enamel. The inward projection of the organic material that is confluent with the surface pellicle is perpendicular to the enamel surface and is "dendritic" in appearance (Fig. 5-6). The subsurface pellicle was originally described as closely interwoven fibrils deposited within the surface layer of slightly damaged enamel only. Subsurface pellicle has since been reported in sound enamel and in unerupted teeth, indicating that its formation is not always the result of early carious activity. Of course, there may be different origins of materials that appear similar in electron micrographs. Moreover, different histologic situations may be observed on different areas of the same tooth.

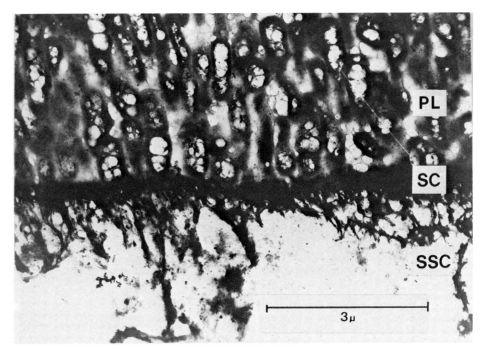

Fig. 5-6. Cross section through an organic film floated off in 2% HCl from the buccal surface of an extracted molar. **PL** = plaque. **SC** = surface cuticle. **SSC** = subsurface cuticle. Electron micrograph, approximately 0.08 μ section. (Meckel AH: Arch Oral Biol 10: 585, 1965)

Another histologic observation of interest is the deposition of mineral within different pellicles. The possible importance of this observation is discussed with respect to the "function" of the pellicle.

A suprasurface (or stained) pellicle has been found on areas of the tooth that were not self-cleansing or subject to toothbrushing (Fig. 5-7). It has been suggested that the suprasurface pellicle results from the binding of salivary proteins to the surface pellicle and that the suprasurface pellicle is not as condensed as the surface pellicle.

An amorphous pellicle has also been described overlying dental plaque, but its origin and importance are unclear and discussion of it is outside the scope of this chapter.

There are many possible contributors to the composition of organic material on the surface of extracted teeth, including saliva, bacteria, epithelium, gingival crevicular fluid, hemorrhage from extraction, and exogenous materials such as the diet, oral hygiene agents, and dental materials and restorations. Any organic film formed on the enamel surface could be affected to some extent by each of these contributors and by the "enamel fluid" that apparently flows from the pulp to the enamel surface.

One area of particular interest and debate is the relationship of the acquired pellicle to the overlying dental plaque (Fig. 5-6). Some investigators consider pellicle formation to be the first stage of plaque formation (i.e., part of a continuum). Others consider the pellicle to be a product of the plaque. Several investigators have demonstrated pellicles with scalloped borders (Fig. 5-8), which apparently represent remnants of the cell walls of bacteria. Others have shown plaque bacteria in direct contact with the enamel mineral (no underlying pellicle). These observations have led to speculation that the bacteria may either metabolize the pellicle or physically displace it. The same histologic observations have led others to speculate that the pellicle is a product of the plaque bacteria. That speculation is not generally accepted, since it is well known that pellicles exist on enamel surfaces that have not been covered by plaque. The pellicle underlying dental plaque may have constituents from more than one source. In other words, it is possible (and even probable) that "pellicle is not pellicle is not pellicle."

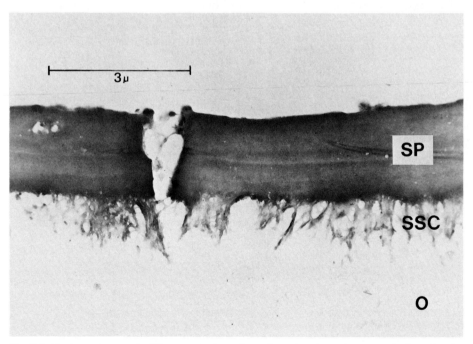

Fig. 5-7. Electron micrograph of the organic deposits on lingual surface of an upper incisor. Demineralized cross section. **SP** = stained pellicle. **SSC** = subsurface cuticle. **O** = organic residue of enamel. (Meckel AH: Arch Oral Biol 10: 585, 1965)

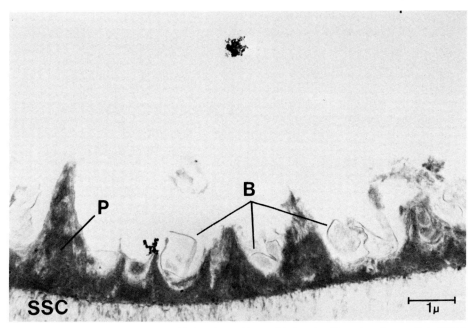

Fig. 5-8. Section of pellicle from the labial surface of lower third molar. The subsurface cuticle (**SSC**) is continuous with the overlying pellicle (**P**). Lysed bacteria (**B**) occupy recesses in the scalloped pellicle surface). (Armstrong WG, and Hayward AF: Caries Res 2: 294, 1968) (×8500)

Histochemical studies have demonstrated the presence of protein, carbohydrate, and lipid constituents in the pellicle. The protein-carbohydrate has generally been considered, at least in part, a glycoprotein. There has been disagreement whether the lipid was actually a pellicle component or was due to remnants of dental plaque that had covered the pellicle.

In an effort to determine more about the nature and source of the "natural" pellicle, several investigators have analyzed its chemical composition. In most studies of the composition of the natural pellicle, the material was collected by decalcification of the enamel with hydrochloric acid (HCl) solutions of 0.6 to 2.0 N and exposure times of 2 to 5 minutes (conditions very similar to those described by Nasmyth in 1839). The teeth were always first brushed thoroughly in an attempt to remove any dental plaque and surface debris. Stained, carious, and restored areas and soft tissue attachments were purposely eliminated from the collection materials. Because of the sparsity of pellicle on a single tooth, the pellicle analyzed was pooled material from at least several, and as many as 70, teeth.

Until recently the material that could be seen separating from the enamel surface upon acid decalcification was considered to be the pellicle and was collected with a glass rod or by filtering. One investigator who collected the pellicle by centrifuging down the visible film (the pellicle sediment) also collected and analyzed the supernate solution (the pellicle supernate) resulting from the centrifugation.

One method of characterizing the pellicle is by chemically analyzing its amino acid constituents. The results of the amino acid analyses of the total natural pellicle and the pellicle supernate and sediment are presented in Figure 5-9.

From the heights of the bars in Figure 5-9, it is apparent that the pellicle supernate and sediment differed markedly in composition. The abbreviations *DAP* and *Mur* represent diaminopimelic acid and muramic acid, respectively, and are amino acids characteristic of bacterial cell wall. The total natural pellicle and both its fractions were characterized by a high content (about 22%) of the acidic amino acids (aspartic and glutamic), which was more than twice the level of the basic amino acids (lysine, histidine, and arginine). Some investigators have attributed the ability of the pellicle to adhere to the enamel surface to the apparent acidic nature of the pellicle. Because the composition of the total natural pellicle was midway between the supernate and sediment compositions, it has been suggested that the total pellicle was composed of approximately equal proportions of the relatively acid-soluble and acid-insoluble fractions. Stated another way, it appears that about half the total pellicle dissolved in the collection acid.

Figure 5-10 compares some of the amino acids of a sample of 3-day-old dental plaque with the natural pellicle. There are obvious differences in some of the constituents, exemplified by serine, glycine, alanine, lysine, and the bacterial markers muramic acid and diaminopimelic acid. This data indicates that, although dental plaque obviously contributed part of the amino acids, plaque was not the primary contributor to the composition of the natural pellicle.

Studies of the carbohydrates of the total natural pellicle indicated the presence of fucose, mannose, glucosamine, galactosamine,

rhamnose, and of equal quantities of glucose and galactose. Rhamnose is a typical component of the cell walls of many oral bacteria.

There are obviously many problems involved in studying the organic material that comes from the surface of extracted teeth of unknown and varied history. Several conclusions may, however, be reached from the studies of the chemical composition of the "natural" pellicle:

1. There is a definite contribution of bacterial cell walls to the composition of "natural" pellicle.
2. A substantial portion of the organic material from the enamel surface of extracted teeth is soluble in the acid used to collect the pellicle.
3. The relatively soluble and insoluble fractions of the natural pellicle, the supernate and sediment, differ considerably in amino acid composition.
4. In discussing the organic integuments of the enamel surface, it seems, therefore,

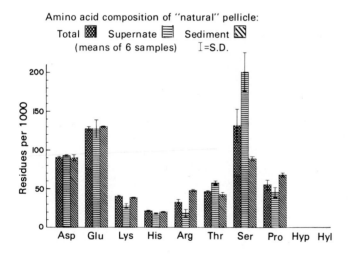

Amino acid composition of "natural" pellicle: Total Supernate Sediment (means of 6 samples) I=S.D.

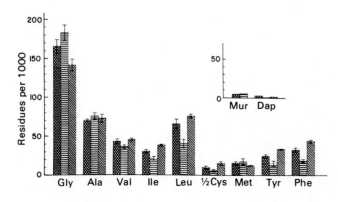

Fig. 5-9. Comparison of the amino acid composition of the total natural pellicle, pellicle supernate, and pellicle sediment.

pertinent to consider the total pellicle, as well as its fractions that differ in acid solubility and composition.

"Experimental" Pellicles. In an effort to eliminate some of the variables operating in the formation of the "natural" pellicle, model systems were designed for the formation of "experimental" pellicles. The basic idea was to study the initial enamel pellicle to gain insight into the composition, properties, source, and "function" of the pellicle. No model system is perfect, of course, and there may well be false assumptions involved in the use of any such system. G. V. Black was apparently the first to attempt the formation of experimental pellicles. He described a comparatively bacteria-free "agglutinin" that was deposited on glass slabs held intraorally opposite the parotid salivary duct by means of a dental applicance.

Morphologic and compositional studies of various types of experimental pellicles have been conducted by separate groups of investigators in recent years. Although the pellicle is usually described as "structureless," recent studies have indicated that the pellicle formed on synthetic hydroxyapatite may be globular, fibrillar, or granular in appearance when viewed with electron microscopy. (The presence of lamination lines within the "natural" pellicle, approximately parallel to the enamel surface, had previously been reported.)

Two different model systems have been used rather extensively to study the chemical composition of the early or initial pellicle. One model system uses a palatal appliance to hold enamel slabs for the formation of an *in vivo* pellicle (Fig. 5-11). The *in vivo* pellicle is formed under conditions intended to resemble the formation of the initial acquired pellicle as it occurs *in situ*. The *in vitro* pellicles

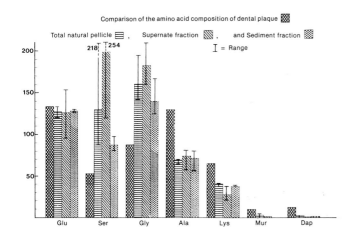

Fig. 5-10. Representative comparison of the amino acid composition of 3-day-old plaque with the total natural pellicle, pellicle supernate, and pellicle sediment. (Mayhall CW: Ala J Med Sci 12: 252, 1975)

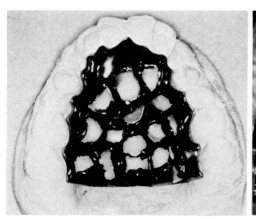
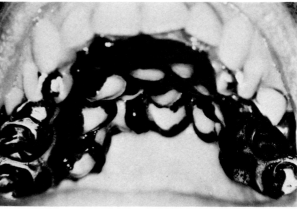

Fig. 5-11. Palatal appliance for the formation of *in vivo* experimental pellicle, on a stone model (**left**) and in the subject's mouth (**right**). (Mayhall CW: Ala J Med Sci 12: 252, 1975)

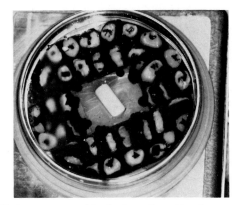

Fig. 5-12. Apparatus used for the formation of *in vitro* experimental pellicles. (Mayhall CW: Ala J Med Sci 12: 252, 1975)

are formed on similar enamel that is exposed only to saliva, which had been ultrafiltered to remove any bacteria (Fig. 5-12).

In each instance the pellicle is collected by decalcification of the superficial enamel in dilute HCl. Since preliminary studies indicated that much of the organic material from the enamel surface was soluble in the dilute HCl used to collect the pellicle, these studies dealt only with the total pellicle, which included both the acid-soluble and acid-insoluble fractions. Comparison of the two types of experimental pellicles is intended to provide information concerning the composition and source of the initial pellicle and the reliability

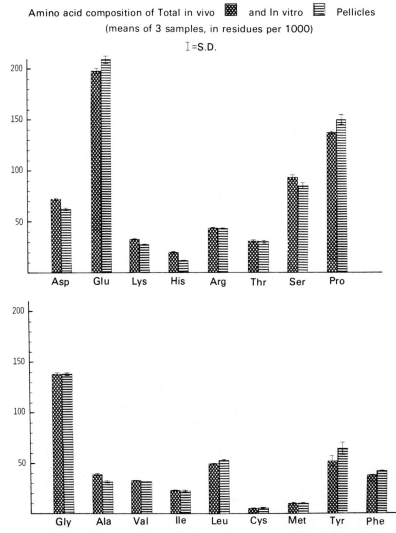

Fig. 5-13. Comparison of the amino acid composition of total *in vivo* and *in vitro* pellicles. (Mayhall CW: J Periodontol 48: 78, 1977)

of the *in vitro* model system to duplicate that process. The results of these studies, presented in Figure 5-13, indicate that the total *in vivo* and *in vitro* pellicles were quite similar in amino acid composition. These experimental pellicles were characterized by large amounts of glutamic acid, proline, and glycine, these three amino acids accounting for almost one-half of the total. The content of the acidic amino acids was almost four times that of the basic amino acids. The absence of hydroxyproline and hydroxylysine indicated that the pellicles did not contain collagen. In addition there was no trace of the bacterial marker amino acids in the experimental pellicles.

The high degree of similarity between the two types of experimental pellicles was surprising. The *in vivo* pellicle was formed in a somewhat controlled oral environment, whereas the *in vitro* pellicle was formed in a closed system in which the enamel was exposed to saliva alone. With the *in vivo* pellicle a flow of fresh saliva was continuously passing over the enamel. In the *in vitro* system, however, the enamel was exposed to a limited quantity of saliva free from oral microorganisms for a similar period of time. The similarity in chemical composition indicates that the process of formation of the two types of experimental pellicle was similar despite the differences in the conditions under which they were formed and that saliva contains all the constituents necessary for the formation of short-term pellicles.

The similarity between the experimental pellicles also indicated that bacteria were not essential to the formation of a short-term pellicle, since the influence of bacteria was absent in the formation of the *in vitro* pellicle. Although bacteria in the saliva and on the oral surfaces could have influenced the formation of the *in vivo* pellicle, there was no bacterial plaque present on the enamel surfaces of the crown sections.

In a subsequent study the composition of the total mixed (submandibular-parotid) salivary pellicle was compared with the pellicle supernate and sediment. Those data suggested that there was a representative dissolution of the total mixed salivary pellicle in the collection acid, rather than a preferential dissolution of a part of the total pellicle material. A mixture of stimulated submandibular and parotid salivas was analyzed for comparison with the mixed salivary pellicle (Fig. 5-14). Comparison of the composition of the experimental pellicles with the salivas from which they were formed should indicate whether certain salivary components are selectively involved in the formation of the acquired pellicle or whether the pellicle is simply a layer of dried saliva, as has been suggested by some investigators. The amino acid composition of the experimental pellicles differed markedly from the salivas from which they were formed, indicating that formation of the short-term pellicles from saliva is a highly selective process.

Carbohydrate analyses (Figs. 5-15 and 5-16) of the total and fractionated *in vivo* and *in vitro* pellicles support some of the conclusions reached from the amino acid analyses, (i.e., that the pellicles were remarkably similar in composition and that the *in vitro* model system was reliable in producing a pellicle similar in composition to that produced in the *in vivo* model system). The data (Fig. 5-15) also suggest that the *in vivo* pellicle fractions that differ in acid solubility (the supernate and sediment) also differ in carbohydrate composition and support the conclusion that pellicle formation from saliva is a highly selective process. The same conclusions were reached concerning the *in vitro* pellicle (Fig. 5-16). The most remarkable finding with respect to the carbohydrate composition of the experimental pellicles is the relatively high levels of glucose, which is not normally present in large quantities in glycoproteins. The data suggest, therefore, that the pellicle is, at least in part, composed of an unusual glucose-rich glycoprotein.

The *in vitro* model system was subsequently used to study the composition of the total and fractionated pellicles formed from isolated submandibular saliva and isolated parotid saliva. Knowledge of the chemical composition of the various salivary pellicles was intended to make possible a meaningful comparison of the pellicles formed in salivas that differ in composition, to provide a more precise biochemical definition of the initial salivary pellicle and to supply information concerning the precise origin of the pellicle from the saliva.

The most remarkable finding of these studies was the striking similarity in composition of the pellicles formed from the isolated salivas, even though the compositions of submandibular and parotid saliva differ widely. The total submandibular salivary pellicle and both its fractions were remarkably similar in amino acid and carbohydrate composition to

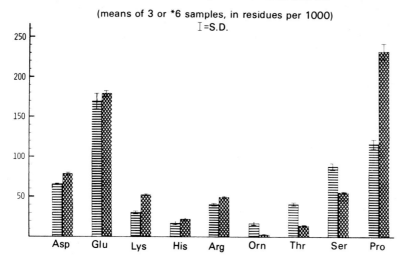

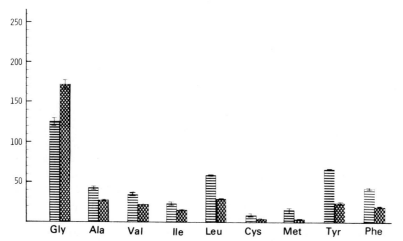

Fig. 5-14. Comparison of the amino acid composition of the total mixed salivary pellicle and the saliva mixture from which it was formed. (Mayhall CW: J Periodontol 48: 78, 1977)

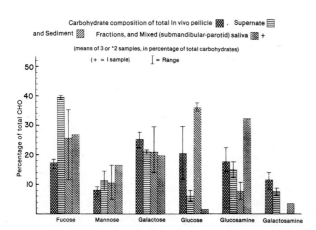

Fig. 5-15. Comparison of the carbohydrate composition of the total *in vivo* pellicle, the *in vivo* pellicle supernate, the *in vivo* pellicle sediment, and mixed (submandibular-parotid) saliva. (Mayhall CW, and Butler WT: J Oral Path 5: 358, 1976)

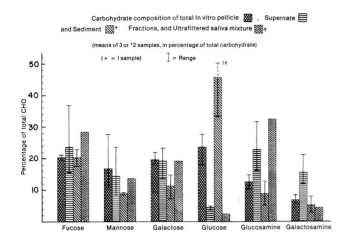

Carbohydrate composition of total In vitro pellicle ▦ , Supernate ▤
and Sediment ▨* Fractions, and Ultrafiltered saliva mixture ▦+

(means of 3 or *2 samples, in percentage of total carbohydrate)

(+ = I sample) ⏱ = Range

Fig. 5-16. Comparison of the carbohydrate composition of the total *in vitro* pellicle, the *in vitro* pellicle supernate, the *in vitro* pellicle sediment, and mixed (submandibular-parotid) saliva that had been ultrafiltered. (Mayhall CW, and Butler WT: J Oral Path 5: 358, 1976)

their counterparts formed from isolated parotid saliva. Figure 5-17 exemplifies this similarity and the observation that the mixed salivary pellicle differs in composition from the pellicles formed in submandibular and parotid salivas. Submandibular and parotid saliva, on the other hand, are quite different in amino acid and carbohydrate composition. The data strongly suggest that there are present in both submandibular and parotid salivas similar glycoproteins that are selectively deposited onto etched enamel as the initial pellicle.

Relatively high levels of glucose were found in the submandibular and parotid salivary pellicles, again suggesting that at least one pellicle component is an unusual glucose-rich glycoprotein. The carbohydrate and amino acid data also suggest that the salivary pellicle is probably composed of fractions of differing composition that also differ in solubility in the dilute acid used to collect the pellicle material. The differences in composition between the supernates and sediments also suggest that the total pellicle is composed of more than one component. The less soluble component may be bound to the mineral phase of enamel more tightly than the more soluble component, or it may be denatured in the removal of the pellicle and thereby rendered insoluble. It has been suggested that the organic material on the enamel surface may consist of relatively loosely and tightly bound components. One group of investigators has suggested that many different proteins may be associated with the stable portion of the pellicle. A model is thus emerging of the pellicle as consisting of a stable portion bound to the enamel surface and a labile portion that may vary in composition owing to changes in con-

ditions at the pellicle surface. The clinical implications of such a model are many.

Whenever the acquired pellicle is collected by decalcification of enamel, some contamination of the pellicle by enamel protein is to be expected. Since there is no consensus concerning the composition of enamel protein, it is not possible at this time to evaluate the extent of its contribution to the pellicle analyses. This is definitely an area for future research.

To elucidate further the chemical composition of "primary" pellicle, another group of investigators conducted their studies on pellicles formed *in situ*. Because of the probable contamination by enamel protein and the partial solubility of the pellicle in dilute acid, they avoided the use of acid and collected the total pellicle material removable from the enamel surface with a dental scaler. The pellicle material they analyzed was that formed *in situ* in 2 hours after the teeth of dental student volunteers were brushed with pumice and rinsed with water. The rate of deposition of pellicle material was studied by taking samples at various time intervals after pumicing (Fig. 5-18). An insignificant amount of material was removable immediately after the teeth were brushed with pumice, which indicated that most of the organic material investigated in their study was deposited in the interval between pumicing and pellicle removal. The amount of removable material increased during the first 60 to 90 minutes, the difference in amount between 60 and 90 minutes being only slight, and no qualitative differences were detected among the various samples.

When the pellicles obtained from the buccal surfaces of teeth from various areas of the

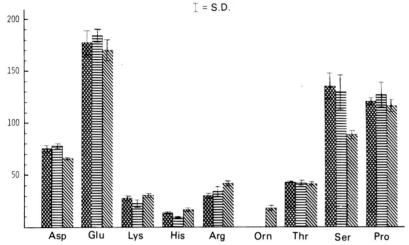

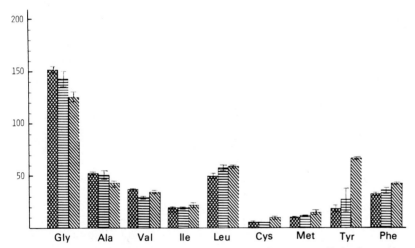

Fig. 5-17. Comparison of the amino acid composition of the total pellicles formed from isolated submandibular, isolated parotid, and mixed (submandibular-parotid) salivas. (Mayhall CW: J Periodontol 48: 78, 1977)

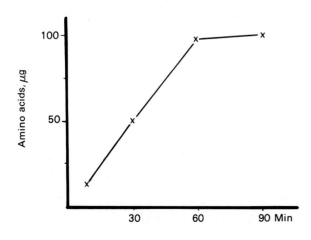

Fig. 5-18. Rate of formation of pellicle material as indicated by the total amount of amino acids at various time intervals between pumicing and pellicle removal. (Sönju T, and Rölla G: Caries Res 7: 30, 1973)

mouth were compared (Fig. 5-19), it was concluded that there were no differences in the amino acid composition. That observation supports the results of the *in vitro* studies discussed earlier, that a selective adsorption of salivary proteins takes place in the formation of the pellicle (regardless of the area of the mouth or the source of the saliva). The same group reported on the carbohydrate composition of their 2-hour *in situ* pellicle (Fig. 5-20). The glucose:galactose ratio in their 2-hour

pellicle was more then 6:1. No sialic acid or fucose was consistently present. No difference in the carbohydrate composition between secretor and nonsecretor pellicle material was found.

From the data presented it is obvious that the results of the *in vivo* and *in vitro* experiments discussed earlier do not agree completely with the results of the *in situ* experiments. There are several possible explanations for the divergent results, the most probable

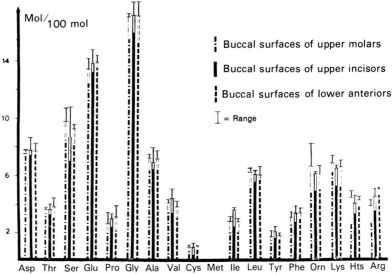

Fig. 5-19. Amino acid composition of pellicle material obtained from various tooth surfaces. Averages and ranges. (Sönju T, and Rölla G: Caries Res 7: 30, 1973)

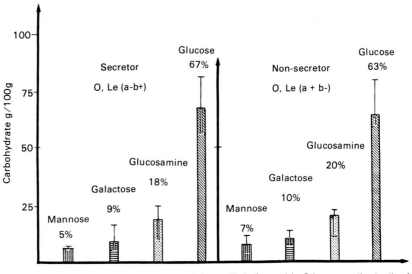

Fig. 5-20. Carbohydrate composition of the pellicle formed in 2 hours on the teeth of secretors and nonsecretors (with ranges). (Sönju T *et al.*: Caries Res 8: 113, 1974)

being that differences in the experimental techniques of pellicle formation, collection, and analysis produce pellicles of somewhat different composition.

"Function" of the Pellicle.   Almost everyone has had the experience of "having an edge" on his teeth. This sensation of a "gritty feeling" when the teeth are in occlusal contact results from the removal of the enamel pellicle (e.g., after one accidentally draws acid into the mouth while pipetting in a chemistry laboratory, drinks a cola or citrus drink that was too "sour," or regurgites stomach acid). The "edge" disappears rapidly owing to the formation of another acquired enamel pellicle. This common experience probably demonstrates one of the functions of the pellicle—to form a lubricating medium between opposing surfaces of enamel hydroxyapatite.

Hydroxyapatite (see Chap. 7) has long been known to be a very reactive substance. Organic chemists have used columns of hydroxyapatite for partition chromatography of protein mixtures for many years. It is no surprise, therefore, that many substances react with and adhere to the enamel surface. In the acid-etch composite technique of dental restorations, the manufacturers direct that, after the enamel surface has been "conditioned" with acid (i.e., etched), the surface must be kept isolated from the saliva. The reason is simply that exposure of the etched enamel to the saliva will result in the immediate formation of a pellicle (similar to the "experimental" pellicles) and interfere with the physical bonding of the composite to the etched enamel.

If one completely removes the pellicle *in situ* by using dental prophylaxis abrasives (and there is disagreement whether this occurs normally), one can ask what sequence of events follows. Owing to incompletely understood physicochemical reactions, the highly mineralized enamel reacts with the proteinaceous fluid, saliva, and pellicle formation is initiated. It is generally accepted that the formation or deposition of pellicle is an *ad*sorption phenomenon, (i.e., a surface phenomenon). We now know that specific components of the saliva are apparently selectively adsorbed onto the enamel surface. The formation of the initial pellicle occurs rapidly, and the quantity of pellicle seems to level off at about 1 hour after the enamel surface is cleaned.

"Naked" enamel does not, therefore, exist in the mouth for any length of time. The cleaned enamel surface is soon covered by a pellicle, certainly in a matter of minutes. Pellicle exists, therefore, before plaque formation simply because of the chronology associated with the physicochemical conditions that result in pellicle formation.

Several studies have shown that, after the formation of pellicle, bacteria begin to attach to the surface of the pellicle. These bacteria reproduce and are joined by other adherent bacteria from the oral cavity. If these are left undisturbed, the formation of dental plaque has begun. Because of this sequence of events, some have considered the pellicle to be the beginning of plaque formation and therefore to have a detrimental function. However, *in situ* there is really no such thing as a "clean" tooth, (i.e., a tooth devoid of some bacterial colonization). The outgrowth of microorganisms from defects and protected areas of the tooth is probably of greater importance than the colonization of newly acquired pellicle.

Since the insolubility of the pellicle in acid led to its discovery by Alexander Nasmyth, it has been suggested that the presence of an organic membrane on the enamel surface may offer some protection against acid demineralization of the underlying enamel. Any organic covering of the enamel mineral could be a diffusion barrier to slow the acid demineralization of caries. There is some evidence to support this protective function of the pellicle, but it is an area that requires further research.

Another question concerning the "function" of the pellicle is its relationship to fluoride. It has been customary in dentistry to perform a thorough prophylaxis by using abrasives before the topical application of fluoride. It has long been known that the concentration of fluoride is highest in the outer layer of enamel, which is partly removed by an abrasive cleaning. The question is now being asked whether the teeth should indeed be "polished" before topical fluoride application or whether the removal of plaque with brush and floss is not only adequate but preferable. This is still a very controversial area, but dentists and dental students should be aware that changes in the traditional method of preventive dental practice may be coming with increasing knowledge concerning the function of the pellicle. On the other hand, it has also been suggested that the pellicle may organically bind topically applied fluoride and prevent its ionic interaction with the enamel mineral. Others think that fluoride organically bound by pellicle would constitute a reservoir for the gradual release of fluoride for a longer and more beneficial reaction with the enamel. Obviously, further research is needed to answer these questions.

The deposition of mineral in the pellicle has been reported by several investigators and has been suggested as a possible mechanism whereby the remineralization (see Chap. 19) of damaged enamel might occur. On the other hand, the mineralization of pellicle has been suggested as the "seeding" mechanism whereby the calcification of dental plaque (the formation of dental calculus) begins. Without getting into a teleologic discussion, it should be apparent that the pellicle may have various influences under differing circumstances. There may not be a single answer concerning the "function" of the pellicle, (i.e., the function of the pellicle may depend on the circumstances existing at the surface of the enamel at a particular time).

Future research with respect to the pellicle will be oriented toward a more nearly complete understanding of the morphology, composition, source, function, and relationship to fluoride, plaque, and the organic matrix of enamel. The ultimate goal of workers in this area is to learn to use or modify the acquired pellicle to increase the resistance of the patient to dental caries and the inflammatory periodontal diseases.

SUMMARY

The reader should have the impression at this point that the nonmineralized coverings of the enamel surface are a complex but very important area of study and research. The surface of the tooth is where the most common diseases of man begin with the formation of dental plaque. It is obvious from this discussion that there are still more questions than answers concerning the nonmineralized coverings of the enamel surface and their relationship to dental caries. It is hoped that this chapter has prepared the reader with an understanding of the basic concepts about the organic coverings found on teeth, that this knowledge will enable the dentist to read and understand developments as new information is gained and disseminated, and that this knowledge will be applied to the prevention of oral disease in patients.

GLOSSARY

Adsorption. The attachment of one substance to the surface of another.

Basal lamina. A structure, identified by electron microscopy, consisting of an electron-dense and electron-lucent areas, the lamina densa and lamina lucida, respectively, and generally considered to be epithelial in origin.

Dental plaque. A soft, concentrated, adherent mass of microorganisms colonizing the surface of the tooth.

Electron microscope. An instrument that is used to obtain greatly enlarged images and that uses electrons as the source of illumination.

   Transmission electron microscope. An electron microscope in which the electron beam passes through the sample to form the image.

   Scanning electron microscope. An electron microscope in which the electron beam is reflected from the surface of the sample to form a three-dimensional image.

Hemidesmosome. Half a desmosome, a method of attachment of epithelial cells to the tooth surface, observed in electron micrographs.

Materia alba. A soft, white mixture of bacteria, salivary components, desquamated epithelial cells, and disintegrating leukocytes that adheres loosely to the surface of the tooth, dental plaque, or the ginviva.

Primary enamel cuticle. Light microscopic term for an apparent organic layer present on the enamel surface of unerupted teeth and considered to be the final secretory product of the ameloblasts. Electron microscopic observations have failed to substantiate the existence of the primary enamel cuticle.

Reduced enamel epithelium. A few layers of flat cuboidal cells that are the remains of the epithelial enamel organ after the formation of enamel is complete.

Secretor. An individual whose saliva contains a glycoprotein with the A, B, H (O), Le antigens (blood group substances).

   Nonsecretor. An individual whose saliva contains only the Le(a) substance.

Subsurface pellicle. A concentration of organic material within the surface enamel that is confluent with the surface pellicle and observed with electron microscopy.

Suprasurface (stained) pellicle. A thicker pellicle structure found on areas of the tooth that are not self-cleansing or subject to toothbrushing.

SUGGESTED READINGS

Armstrong WG, Hayward AF: Acquired organic integuments of human enamel: a comparison of analytical studies with optical, phase-contrast and electron microscope examinations. Caries Res 2: 294–305, 1968

Lie T: Scanning and transmission electron microscope study of pellicle morphogenesis. Scand J Dent Res 85: 217–231, 1977

Listgarten MA: Structure of the microbial flora associated with periodontal health and disease in man. A light and electron microscopic study. J Periodontol 47: 1–18, 1976

Listgarten MA: Structure of surface coatings on teeth. A review. J Periodontol 47: 139–147, 1976

Mayhall CW: Concerning the composition and source of the acquired enamel pellicle of human teeth. Arch Oral Biol 15: 1327–1341, 1970

Mayhall CW: Studies on the composition of the enamel pellicle. Ala J Med Sci 12: 252–271, 1975

Mayhall CW: Amino acid composition of experimental salivary pellicles. J Periodontol 48: 78–91, 1977

Mayhall CW, Butler WT: The carbohydrate composition of experimental salivary pellicles. J Oral Pathol 5: 358–370, 1976

Meckel AH: The formation and properties of organic films on teeth. Arch Oral Biol 10: 585–597, 1965

Salkind A, Oshrain HI, Mandel ID: Materia alba and dental plaque. J Periodontol 45: 489–490, 1974

Schwartz RS, Massler M: Tooth accumulated materials: a review and classification. J Periodontol 40: 407–413, 1969

Sönju T, Christensen TB, Kornstad L, Rölla G: Electron microscopy, carbohydrate analyses and biological activities of the proteins adsorbed in two hours to tooth surfaces in vivo. Caries Res 8: 113–122, 1974

Sönju T, Rölla G: Chemical analysis of the acquired pellicle formed in two hours on cleaned human teeth in vivo. Rate of formation and amino acid analysis. Caries Res 7: 30–38, 1973

Tinanoff N, Glick PL, Weber DF: Ultrastructure of organic films on the enamel surface. Caries Res 10: 19–32, 1976

B. Tooth Composition

6 Biochemistry of Tooth Proteins

WILLIAM T. BUTLER

WILLIAM S. RICHARDSON III

Introduction
Protein Constituents of Connective Tissues
  Why Study Components of Connective
    Tissues
  Collagen
    Organizational Levels
    Collagen Types
    Other Collagen-like Chains
    Biosynthesis
    Fibril Formation
    Cross Linking of Collagen Chains
    Catabolism of Collagen
    Some Methods Used to Study Collagen
Proteoglycans of Connective Tissues
  Introduction
  The Glycosaminoglycans
  Glycosaminoglycan-Protein Linkage
  Core Protein

  Aggregation
  Heterogeneity of Proteoglycans
  Metabolism
  Significance of Proteoglycans
Tissues of the Tooth
  Dentin
    Introduction
    Dentin Collagen
    The Proteoglycans of Predentin and
      Dentin
    The Phosphoprotein of Dentin
    The Formation of Dentin by Odonto-
      blasts (Dentinogenesis)
    Cementum
    Periodontal Ligament
    Enamel
Glossary
Suggested Readings

INTRODUCTION

The tooth and its surrounding tissues are specialized forms of connective tissues adapted for the masticatory process. Connective tissues are defined as those that provide strength, support, and form; they literally allow organisms to "hang together" and withstand the forces and pressures imposed by movement and weight. The main structural elements of a connective tissue are fibers, proteoglycans, and other proteins (e.g., glycoproteins). Of course, cells and vascular elements are also present, nurturing and rebuilding the tissues.

In recent years a great deal of information has been obtained about the biochemistry of these constituents of connective tissues. The purpose of this chapter is to detail the available knowledge with reference to the individual organic components of the tooth and its suspensory apparatus. This discussion should provide the reader with an appreciation for the molecular basis of normal tooth structure, a foundation for understanding the biochemistry of dental caries, and a basis for appreciating future advances in research in dental decay and periodontal disease.

PROTEIN CONSTITUENTS OF CONNECTIVE TISSUES

Why Study Components of Connective Tissues

In order to comprehend the molecular structure of dentition and of the physical properties vested in these structures, one must understand the nature of the individual constituents in connective tissues and how these components relate to one another. This approach might be likened to that of an architectural engineer who computes the stresses and strains of the foundation materials to be used in building a skyscraper. By analyzing the properties of individual constituents in the foundation, it is possible to ensure the durability and safety of the building.

In the case of the dental organ the major protein to be considered is collagen, a tough fibrillar material. Another major constituent in connective tissues, the proteoglycans, are polymers with acidic polysaccharides attached to a core protein. We now have a thorough knowledge of the molecular structures of collagen and proteoglycans and of the basis for the physical properties they impart to tissues. An understanding of the organization and metabolism of the constituents of connective tissues is necessary to comprehend the properties of normal oral tissues as well as the pathological basis of dental caries and periodontal disease. In this section we will examine the various constituents of connective tissues and the levels of organization involved in forming these tissues.

Collagen

Organizational Levels

The fibrillar material found in almost all connective tissues is collagen. At the microscopic level collagen is composed of numerous fibers that are layered and arranged within the connective tissue (Fig. 6-1E). This array of fibers differs from tissue to tissue, so that some tis-

sues contain adjacent layers of fibers lying perpendicular to one another, while in others the fibers swirl in all directions with no apparent orderly arrangement. An example of the former is the fibrillar arrangement in the cornea, and of the latter, that in dentin.

At the submicroscopic level collagen fibrils are made of thousands of rod-like collagen molecules aggregated in a staggered, overlapping fashion (Fig. 6-1D). These individual collagen moieties are thin, elongated molecules which are stiff and rod-like. These physical properties, inherent in the substructure, are important to the functions which the molecules ultimately perform. At an even lower level of organization, a collagen molecule is triple-stranded with a length of approximately 300 nm. and a width of about 1.5 nm. (Fig. 6-1C). Each of the three polypeptide alpha (α) chains found in a collagen molecule is composed of slightly over a thousand amino acids. The general form of the amino acid sequence throughout the triple helical portion is (Gly-X-Y-)$_n$; that is, glycine occurs as every third amino acid (Fig. 6-1A). Almost 40 per cent of the X positions of this repeating sequence are occupied by the amino acid proline (Pro) and about 30 per cent of the Y positions have hydroxyproline (Hyp). The occurrence of the large amounts of glycine, proline, and hydroxyproline in the α chains is the most important feature in determining the spatial conformation of the three chains to form the triple-stranded collagen molecule (see below).

The three α chains of collagen exist in an ordered conformation often referred to as a "coiled coil." An individual α chain is coiled in the left-handed sense to form a minor helix (Fig. 6-1B) and three minor helices are twisted about each other in the right-handed sense, giving rise to the major helix (Fig. 6-1C). The minor helix repeats, or makes a complete turn, about every 0.9 nm (Fig. 6-1B). Since the length spanned by a single amino acid residue in this helix is 0.29 nm, there are slightly over three residues per turn. The major helix repeats about every 9 nm and has approximately 30 residues per turn. The triple helix is stabilized by numerous hydrogen bonds formed by sharing the hydrogens of the NH groups of one chain with the oxygen atoms of C=O groups on an adjacent chain.

The three chains assembled in this coiled coil fashion are closely packed leaving little room in the interior. The side chain of every

A   Gly-Pro-Hyp-Gly-Pro-Y-Gly-X-Y-

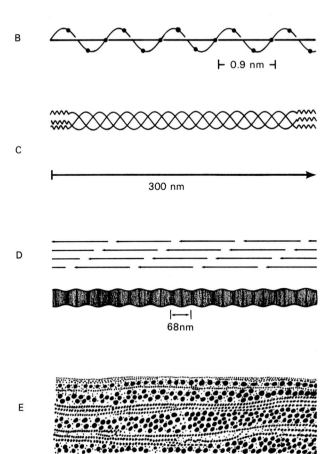

Fig. 6-1. The different organizational levels of collagen.

A. Amino acid sequence—the general form of the amino acid sequence found in a helical portion of an α chain is (Gly-X-Y)n. **B.** Minor helix— this diagram illustrates the fact that an individual α chain twists into a helix with three amino acid residues (represented by balls) per repeat. **C.** Major helix—three polypeptide α chains are coiled about each other to form the triple helix. Each end of all three chains is nonhelical. Single collagen molecules of this form are represented by elongated arrows about 300 nm. long. **D.** Collagen fibrils—a large number of collagen molecules aggregate in a staggered way to form a fibril large enough to be seen by electron microscopy. The staining procedure reveals that bands in the fibril repeat about every 68 nm. **E.** Connective tissue—collagen fibrils are laid down into bundles to form networks of stable fibers in extracellular spaces. The fibers are large enough to be seen by light microscopy. The tissues also contain other interfibrillar materials such as proteoglycans.

third amino acid (glycine) is projected toward the inside of the major helix while the other two are pointed outward. The ones facing inward *must* be glycine, an amino acid with no bulky sidegroups (Fig. 6-2), because there simply is no room to accomodate larger groups. Prolyl and hydroxyprolyl residues are ring structures (Fig. 6-2) and therefore do not allow as much freedom of rotation of a polypeptide chain as the other amino acids. The large numbers of prolines and hydroxyprolines distributed throughout the three collagen chains thus impose steric restrictions which force the polypeptide α chains into the minor helices and ultimately into the triple-helical conformation.

With this background we can begin to understand some of the biologic properties which are "written into" these molecules. For example, native collagen is highly resistant to attack by most proteases, a property which

can be attributed to the close packing of the three chains wrapped about each other in a coiled coil. Additionally, the ability of the rod-like molecules to interact with each other to form fibrils resides in the presence of amino acid sidegroups radiating outward from the central axis of adjacent triple helices (see below).

Another point of interest in the chemistry of collagen molecules is that the extreme ends of the three molecules do *not* have a Gly-X-Y sequence and thus do not exist in the triple-helical conformation. For the NH₂-terminal end of an α chain this encompasses 10 to 16 amino acids, while at the COOH-terminal end usually 25 to 27 residues exist without a helical structure. These regions are extremely important as they serve as sites for cross linking, the process of chemically binding molecules together in the fibrillar state. This aspect will be discussed in detail later.

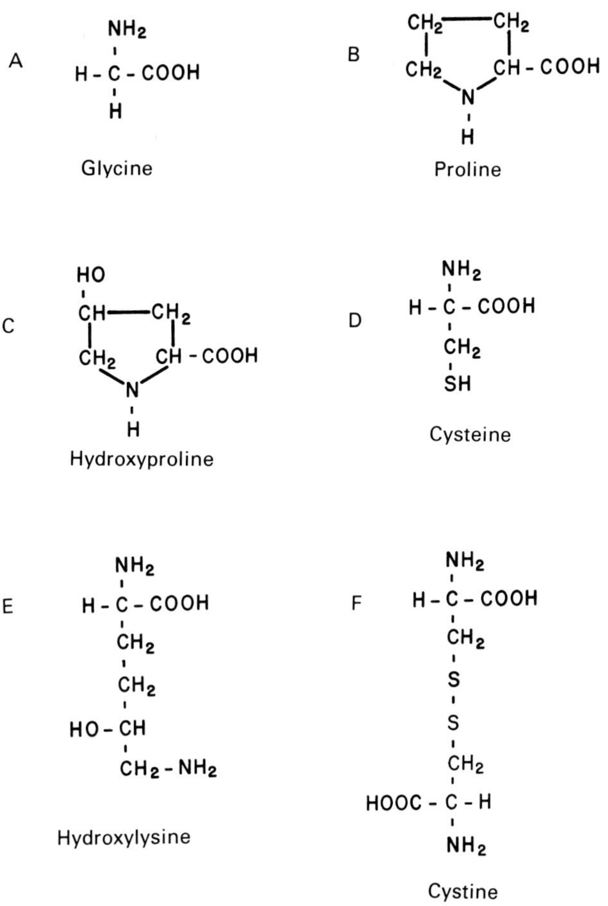

A

NH$_2$
|
H - C - COOH
|
H

Glycine

B

CH$_2$————CH$_2$
| |
CH$_2$ CH - COOH
      \   /
        N
        |
        H

Proline

C

HO
|
CH————CH$_2$
| |
CH$_2$ CH - COOH
      \   /
        N
        |
        H

Hydroxyproline

D

NH$_2$
|
H - C - COOH
|
CH$_2$
|
SH

Cysteine

E

NH$_2$
|
H - C - COOH
|
CH$_2$
|
CH$_2$
|
HO - CH
|
CH$_2$ - NH$_2$

Hydroxylysine

F

NH$_2$
|
H - C - COOH
|
CH$_2$
|
S
|
S
|
CH$_2$
|
HOOC - C - H
|
NH$_2$

Cystine

Fig. 6-2. The molecular structures of some amino acids important in the structure of collagen. **A.** Glycine (Gly)—note that the sidegroup is a hydrogen. **B.** Proline (Pro)—contains a five-membered ring. **C.** Hydroxyproline (Hyp)—the same structure as proline except with a hydroxyl group at position 4. Hyp is fairly unique for collagen and has been used as a measure of the amounts of collagen in tissues. **D.** Cysteine (1/2 Cys)—an amino acid with a reactive sulfhydryl (SH) group. **E.** Hydroxylysine (Hyl)—the same structure as lysine except with a hydroxyl group on carbon 5 (also called the δ carbon). Hyl is found almost exclusively in collagen. **F.** Cystine (Cys)—formed from two 1/2 Cys residues in formation of a disulfide (S-S) bridge. Disulfide bridges form cross bridges between two polypeptide chains, as well as between two 1/2 Cys residues on the same chain.

Collagen Types

For many years scientists thought that the collagen in all fibrils was the same. During the past decade more detailed analyses of collagen have revealed that this concept is incorrect and that several molecular forms of collagen exist. Within extracellular spaces, at least three *major types* of collagen are recognized (Table 6-1) and several minor collagenous structures are under investigation. In this discussion we will concentrate on the type I, type II and type III collagens because these three make up the majority of collagen fibrils in the body and because the knowledge of their chemistry and molecular properties is further advanced.

Although the three collagen types have distinctly different chain compositions, their overall properties are very much alike. In fact, even though the amino acid sequence of the α chains found in these collagen types do *differ*, they are strikingly *similar* and are said to be

homologous (Fig. 6-3). All three have the (Gly-X-Y) repeating sequence that continues for over a thousand residues with high levels of proline and hydroxyproline in the X and Y positions. Likewise, all four chains of the three types have nontriple-helical NH$_2$ and COOH-terminal ends.

Type I collagen is the most abundant form as it is found in virtually all connective tissues. In fact it was the only collagen recognized until 1969, when type II was identified in cartilage by Miller and Matukas (see Suggested Readings). Type I is the only type comprised of two different kinds of α chains with two α1(I) chains (alpha one, type one chains) and a single α2 chain making up the triple helix (Table 6-1).

Type II collagen is the major form of collagen in cartilage, but it is also found in other tissues such as intervertebral discs and notocord. Its triple helix is comprised of three identical α1(II) chains (Table 6-1). Two unusual features of this collagen are that it con-

TABLE 6-1. THE CHAIN STRUCTURE AND
DISTRIBUTION OF THE COLLAGENS
FOUND IN INTERSTITIAL SPACES

Collagen	Molecular Structure	Tissue Distribution
Type I	$[\alpha1(I)]_2\alpha2$	The most abundant collagen in tendons, dermis, bone, dentin and many other connective tissues.
Type II	$[\alpha1(II)]_3$	Hyaline cartilage, fibrocartilage, intervertebral disc; notocord.
Type III	$[\alpha1(III)]_3$	A minor component of many soft connective tissues and a major one in aorta, fetal skin and uterine wall.
Type I trimer	$[\alpha1(I)]_3$	Made by certain connective tissue cells; present as a minor component in dentin and in embryonic tendon and bone.

tains more than ten times as much carbohydrate attached to hydroxylysine residues (Fig. 6-2) as does type I collagen and that it forms relatively small fibers *in vivo*.

Type III collagen is found as a minor component in most connective tissues. In adult skin, for example, it accounts for about 20 per cent of the collagen, the rest being type I collagen. In a few tissues type III collagen does occur in relatively high amounts; for example, it makes up about half the collagen in the aorta and in fetal skin. The three $\alpha1(III)$ chains of the triple helix are covalently bonded together near the COOH-terminal extremes by disulfide bonds formed from two cysteines in each chain (see Fig. 6-2). This arrangement does not occur in the other two types.

A minor collagen only recently discovered is referred to as the type I trimer because it has three chains apparently identical to the $\alpha1(I)$ chains found in type I collagen. Collagenous structures with the type I trimer were first found by culturing connective tissue cells and determining the nature of the collagens they produce. Later type I trimer was discovered in embryonic bone and tendon and in dentin.

The chemical differences between the types of collagen may help explain their physical differences and the molecular basis for their functions. The fine network in reticular fibers has been shown to contain type III collagen, but type III collagen may be found in other tissue structures as well.

Other Collagen-like Chains

In addition to fibrillar collagen, nature appears to utilize the GLY-X-Y structure to produce stiff, rodlike portions of other proteins as well. Basement membranes contain long Gly-X-Y sequences which undoubtedly fold into triple-helical structures, but may not form fibrils within the tissues. One collagen-like component from basement membranes (e.g., from the glomerulus and from certain membranes of the eye) has been isolated and shown to have three identical chains in a triple helix (as do type II and type III collagens). These chains, classified as $\alpha1(IV)$ chains, appear to be slightly longer than those in the three interstitial collagens. They also contain a considerably higher amount of hydroxylysine-linked carbohydrate. In the basement membrane within the glomerulus of the kidney, the rod-like conformation of this collagen-like protein must be important in forming structures necessary to form filtration barriers during passage of waste materials from blood into kidney spaces.

Another protein with a collagen-like sequence is the blood protein C1q, which is one of the first components acting in the comple-

```
                  405              410              415
α I(I)    Gly-Phe-Hyp-Gly-Pro-Lys-Gly-Ala-Ala-Gly-Glu-Hyp-Gly-Lys-Ala-

α 2       Gly-Phe-Hyp-Gly-Pro-Lys-Gly-Pro-Thr-Gly-Glu-Hyp-Gly-Lys-Hyp-

α I(II)   Gly-Phe-Hyp-Gly-Pro-Hyl-Gly-Ala-Asn-Gly-Glu-Hyp-Gly-Lys-Ala-

α I(III)  Gly-Phe-Hyp-Gly-Pro-Lys-Gly-Asn-Asp-Gly-Ala-Hyp-Gly-Lys-Asn-
```

Fig. 6-3. Amino acid sequences of short segments (amino acids 403 to 417) near the center of the four α chains found in type I, type II and type III collagens. Note the similarity of the sequences in this region, showing that the four chains are homologous polypeptide chains. Numbering begins with the first glycine of αl(I) which is in the triple helix of type I collagen.

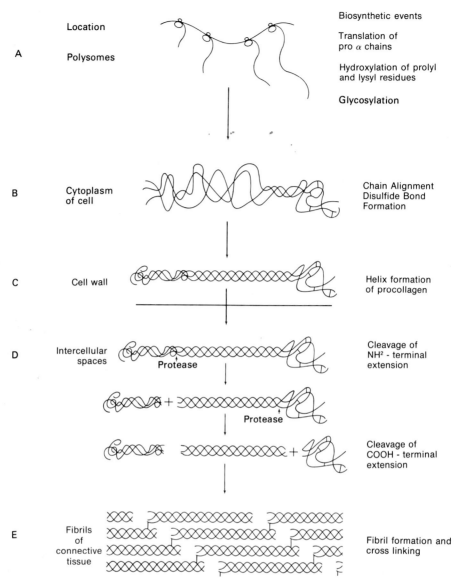

A	Location		Biosynthetic events
	Polysomes		Translation of pro α chains
			Hydroxylation of prolyl and lysyl residues
			Glycosylation

B — Cytoplasm of cell — Chain Alignment Disulfide Bond Formation

C — Cell wall — Helix formation of procollagen

D — Intercellular spaces — Protease — Cleavage of NH² - terminal extension

Protease — Cleavage of COOH - terminal extension

E — Fibrils of connective tissue — Fibril formation and cross linking

Fig. 6-4. An overview of the steps in the biosynthesis of collagen.
A. Cytoplasmic biosynthesis of polypeptide chains—the procollagen α chains are synthe-sized on ribosomes of the rough endoplasmic reticulum within the cytoplasm of cells in the usual way. While these polypeptide chains are being formed, many of the prolines and some lysines are enzymatically hydroxylated to form hydroxyproline and hydroxylysine. Addition-ally, carbohydrate is attached to some of the hydroxylysines. **B.** Chain association—after being released from ribosomal complexes, the three procollagen α chains associate, disul-fide bonds are formed at one end, and the chains begin to entwine to form the triple-helical conformation. **C.** Formation of the triple helix—the triple helix is completed and the complex is now referred to as a procollagen molecule. Note that there are polypeptide "extensions" on both ends of procollagen, not found in collagen molecules. **D.** Conversion of procollagen to collagen—after being transported out of the cell the two ends are removed stepwise by the action of at least two proteolytic enzymes. The extension at the NH_2-terminus is removed first and then that at the COOH-terminus is excised. **E.** Fibril formation—collagen molecules have the inherent capacity to interact with each other to form large aggregates in which molecules are staggered relative to one another. This array produces some areas which are unfilled, the "hole zones," and other areas where the ends of molecules overlap, the "overlap zones." The latter are important for it is here that covalent cross links form, binding the collagen mole-cules together. The cross linking process might be likened to putting mortar between bricks.

ment cascade of reactions. This protein has a much shorter Gly-X-Y triple-helical sequence (only 75 amino acids per chain), adjacent to a globular, noncollagenous portion (one that does not have a Gly-X-Y sequence). The rod-like portions of C1q position the complement protein in such a way that interaction with antibodies triggers the complement cascade. The two examples cited here illustrate how specialized molecular structures are formed from collagen-like, Gly-X-Y amino acid sequences.

Biosynthesis

Collagen is synthesized in the cytoplasm of blast cells. The linkage of amino acids in the proper order of the polypeptide chains takes place on ribosomes and is directed by messenger RNA's. This phase of collagen synthesis is thus similar to that for other proteins, the message for proper alignment of amino acids being derived from the genetic information in DNA.

However, the formation of collagen molecules by connective tissue cells has several unusual features (Fig. 6-4). The α chains are synthesized in an elongated fashion called pro α chains; thus as the chains leave the ribosomes they have extensions on both the NH_2-terminal and COOH-terminal ends of the completed polypeptide chains. When three of these pro α chains assemble and form the triple helix, the molecule is known as procollagen. This type of phenomenon (i.e., the initial synthesis in a precusor form) is not uncommon for proteins destined to be exported from a cell. Since procollagen does not spontaneously aggregate to form fibrils, as does collagen, there is no danger that irreversible precipitates will form within cells thus preventing the external transport of the molecules. The peptide extensions of procollagen are also thought to initiate the rapid formation of the triple helix by bringing three chains into juxtaposition shortly after synthesis.

Prior to formation of the triple helix, while the polypeptide chains are being formed on the ribosome, certain enzymatic steps known as posttranslational modifications take place. These modifications are peculiar to collagen. Prolyl and lysyl residues are hydroxylated (Figs. 6-4 and 6-5) by prolyl hydroxylase and lysyl hydroxylase to form hydroxyproline and hydroxylysine, respectively. Both of these enzymes require as cofactors molecular oxygen, ferrous iron, α-ketoglutarate, and ascorbic acid. Experiments which prevent these reactions from occurring, such as chelating the iron with α, α'-dipyridyl, have shown that unhydroxylated collagen accumulates in cells because it is transported from cells at a low rate. Many of the pathologic symptoms of scurvy can thus be explained by the lowered production of collagen due to the absence of ascorbic acid necessary for these hydroxylation reactions leading to impaired secretion from cells.

After hydroxylation of lysyl residues, sugars are attached to a few hydroxylysines by glycosyl transferases (Fig. 6-5). Shortly after the hydroxylation and glycosylation reactions take place and the procollagen chains are released from their ribosomal attachments, they spontaneously fold into triple-helical structures. Simultaneous with this helix formation, disulfide bonds in the COOH-terminal extensions are formed, and stabilize the structures. Now the protein is ready to be transported from the cell.

Detailed information about the manner in which collagen gets out of cells is unknown. However, some clues have been provided by electron microscopic examination of structures inside the cytoplasm of collagen producing cells. Apparently, procollagen is "packaged" into saccules that appear as flattened, membrane bound structures. After moving to the periphery of the cell, the packages empty their contents into the extracellular spaces. Shortly thereafter, procollagen is converted to collagen by the action of at least two proteases (Fig. 6-4). The NH_2-terminal extension is excised first by a proteolytic enzyme (or protease), and then the COOH-terminal portion is cleaved from the molecule by another protease. The liberated molecules aggregate spontaneously. Note that the ability to form fibrils is inherent in the molecular structure of collagen but not in procollagen.

Fibril Formation

As described earlier, the collagen molecules are rods with many amino acid side chains radiating outward from the axis of the major helix. Unlike globular proteins, even the hydrophobic groups are facing the aqueous environment when the molecules are in solution. Collagen molecules interact spontaneously through lateral interactions involving certain combinations of these projecting amino acids

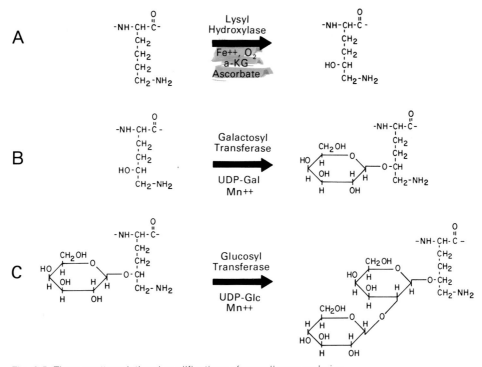

Fig. 6-5. Three posttranslational modifications of procollagen α chains.
A. The formation of hydroxylysine from lysine residues—this reaction is similar to the formation of hydroxyproline from proline residues. The enzyme lysyl hydroxylase catalyses oxidation at carbon 5 of certain lysines to convert them to hydroxylysine. The enzyme requires ferrous iron (Fe^{++}), α-ketoglutarate (α-KG), molecular oxygen, and ascorbic acid, as cofactors. In forming the hydroxyl group, O_2 is split, supplying an atom of oxygen for the reaction. **B.** Attachment of galactose to hydroxylysine—the reaction is a transfer of galactose from the nucleotide sugar UDP-galactose to the hydroxyl group of some hydroxylysine groups in the procollagen α chains. The enzyme is like other sugar transferases and requires a metal cofactor. **C.** Attachment of glucose to galactose—in this reaction glucose is transferred from UDP-glucose to the hydroxyl at position 2 of the galactosylhydroxylysine (Gal-Hyl). The disaccharide (Glc-Gal-Hyl) is found in a few sites of type I and type III collagens but in many areas of type II collagen.

to form a fibril. One type of bond that forms is electrostatic, that is, between neighboring positively and negatively charged amino acids. Another type of interaction involves adjacent hydrophobic amino acids which cluster to provide even more thermoenergetically favorable stability to the structure. These interactions result in a fibrillar array with continual staggering of molecules relative to each other (Fig. 6-4). The length of this stagger is slightly less than ¼ the distance of a molecule and is known as D. This D stagger is equal to that repeat of 68 nm seen in the electron microscopic presentation of stained collagen fibrils (see Fig. 6-1D).

One result of the precise way molecules align is that two molecules in the same row do not butt up against each other; that is, the COOH-terminal end of one molecule is never adjacent to the NH_2-terminus of the next one. The resultant cavities are known as the "hole zones." Another consequence of the alignment is that the ends of molecules in adjacent rows are overlapped forming "overlap zones," regions vitally important to the formation of a stable fibrillar complex because it is here that covalent cross links form (see below). Once again we see that the higher order of molecular organization is dependent on the substructure. The ability to form fibrils is vested in the physical projection of the amino acid side groups of individual collagen molecules, that is in turn a result of the amino acid sequence.

Cross Linking of Collagen Chains

The fibrillar arrangement of collagen fibrils does not of itself produce a structure with the high tensile strength found in mature collagen. The tensile strength of this protein is derived from the formation of cross links between the ends of adjacent molecules. This process occurs after fibrils are formed, and begins by the conversion of some of the lysines or hydroxylysines found in the nontriplehelical portions into amino acids containing aldehydic groups (Figs. 6-6A & 6-6B). These newly formed amino acids are called allysine and hydroxyallysine, respectively. The conversion is catalyzed by the enzyme lysyl oxidase which requires copper and molecular oxygen as cofactors. The aldehydes thus formed are reactive and form aldimine bonds with the NH_2 groups of the side chains in adjacent molecules (Figs. 6-6C and 6-6D). These bonds are located for the most part in the overlap zones, and literally tie the ends of collagen molecules together (Fig. 6-4). The allysine (or hydroxyallysine) groups located in the NH_2-terminal, nonhelical regions, bind to hydroxylysines located in the triple helical portion near the COOH-terminus of α chains.

Likewise, cross links are known to form between allysine (or hydroxyallysine) in the COOH-terminal nonhelical region and a hydroxylysine in the triple-helical portion near the NH_2-terminal end. The cross linking process thus forms a continuum of elongated molecules tied together by stable bonds and results in structures with enormous tensile strength. The most stable cross links form from hydroxyallysine molecules since the double bond between the carbon and nitrogen shifts to produce the more stable keto form (Fig. 6-6D).

Catabolism of Collagen

All proteins produced by the body are in a dynamic state; they are in a continual state of renewal, being synthesized and degraded constantly. In general, the rate at which collagen is renewed, or "turned over," is much slower than that of other proteins (i.e., blood proteins). The rate of collagen turnover also varies from one tissue to another.

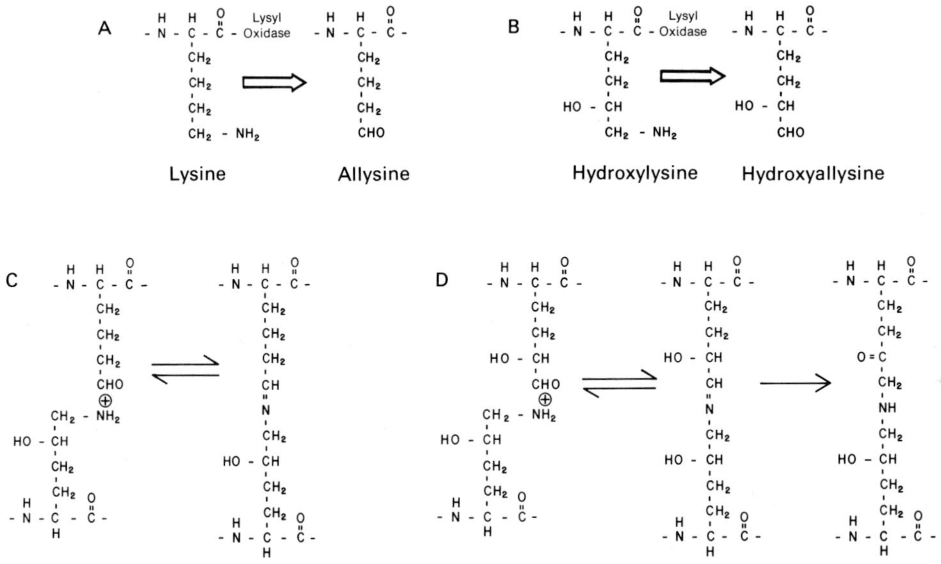

Fig. 6-6. The formation of covalent cross links in collagen.
    A. Allysine—certain lysine residues in the nontriple-helical ends are oxidized to the aldehyde-containing residue allysine. The enzyme lysyl oxidase catalyzes this reaction on fibrillar collagen, requires copper, and is inhibited by β-aminopropionitrile (βAPN). **B.** Hydroxyallysine—this reaction is the same as for allysine except the enzyme is acting upon hydroxylysine residues. **C.** Formation of cross links involving allysine—the reactive aldehyde of allysine on one chain, interacts with the -NH_2 group on another chain to form an aldimine covalent bond (i.e., an —N=C— bond). **D.** Formation of cross links involving hydroxyallysine—the aldehyde of hydroxyallysine forms a bond with the -NH_2 group of an adjacent hydroxylysine residue. The hydroxyl group of hydroxyallysine now allows the double bond of the aldimine to shift forming a keto (—C=O) group and a more stable —N—CH_2— bond.

The destruction of collagen is begun by collagenase. This enzyme, which is produced by a number of cell types, cleaves collagen molecules at a specific place about $^3/_4$ of the distance from the NH$_2$-terminus. Collagenase is one of the few proteases known which can cleave collagen peptide bonds located in the triple helix region. Recall that the triple-helical structure confers resistance to attack by proteases. The scission by collagenase takes place across all three α chains at the same place. As a result the chains begin to unravel (denature) and can then be attacked by other proteases or engulfed by phagocytosing cells.

It is obvious that if the amount of collagen present in a mature connective tissue is constant, the rate at which it is synthesized must exactly equal the rate of destruction. The two processes are intricately regulated, but the mechanisms which maintain this homeostasis in connective tissue cells are not understood at this time.

However, some clues as to the way collagenase is controlled are available. The enzyme appears to be largely found in an inactive, or latent form, and must be activated before it will begin the process of collagenolysis. The cells would then regulate the breakdown of collagen by controlling the conversion of the latent form to the active form of collagenase.

One possible way that the enzyme might be controlled is by being synthesized as a proenzyme, in which case it would be necessary to cleave a fragment from the latent form to convert it to active collagenase. The process would then be similar to that for other proteases. For example, the proenzyme chymotrysinogen is inactive and is converted to the active protease chymotrypsin after a small segment is cleaved from it.

A second possible mechanism for controlling collagenase might be the synthesis of inhibitors of the enzyme that would prevent its action until the enzymatic collagen degradation is necessary. Although evidence has been found for each of the two mechanisms, the details of how collagenase activity and collagenolysis are controlled are incomplete.

If the balance between synthesis and degradation is not maintained, a loss or accumulation of collagenous material in connective tissues will result. Ascorbic acid has already been cited as lowered biosynthesis of collagen because ascorbic acid is necessary for hydroxylation of proline and lysine. Thus an im-

portant area for the future understanding of diseases which adversely affect the properties of connective tissues is the manner by which cells regulate the levels of collagen.

Some Methods Used to Study Collagen

In order to fully comprehend some of the experiments designed to elucidate the nature of the collagens in tooth structures, one must understand some of the methods and approaches specifically designed to study collagen.

Most proteins are soluble, or can be rendered soluble in aqueous solvents. In contrast, collagen is largely insoluble and since the complete chemical characterization requires a soluble form, methods have been devised to solubilize some or all the collagen of a given tissue. One of the earliest methods employed was the extraction of tissues first with neutral buffered NaCl solutions to remove the newly synthesized collagen prior to its conversion to a cross linked form. This was then followed by extraction with dilute acids. The amount of neutral salt soluble material obtained is small but that amount extracted by acid is somewhat greater. The latter procedure is now known to break aldimine cross links since some of these bonds are acid labile. Furthermore, some tissues yield little or no soluble collagen; for example, the collagen of dentin is totally insoluble. Therefore this approach has serious limitations.

Another method used to render collagen soluble is to feed laboratory animals the drug β-aminopropionitrile (βAPN), which interrupts the cross linking process. The drug produces a disease called lathyrism, resulting in generalized weakness of all connective tissues. Until recent times this disease afflicted some human beings who consumed foods high in lathyrogens. →sweet peas. The drug acts by inhibiting the enzyme lysyl oxidase (Fig. 6-6). After feeding to laboratory animals for several weeks, βAPN produces a collagen which is readily extracted. Many of the early ideas about the structure of collagen came from fundamental studies on lathyritic collagen. However, the limitation of this approach lies in the fact that the collagen of certain tissues is unaffected by lathyrism and remains insoluble. It is possible that βAPN is simply not taken up by these tissues. In addition this procedure can only be used for small laboratory animals.

Two more recent approaches that have ren-

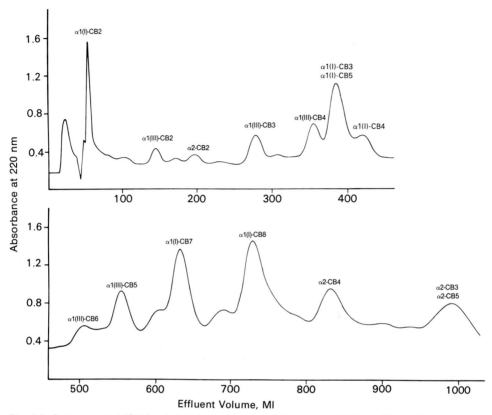

Fig. 6-7. Carboxymethyl (CM-) cellulose chromatography of collagen CNBr peptides—the connective tissue from the dermis of a rat contains both insoluble type I and type III collagens. After cleavage with CNBr, a number of peptides from known areas of α1(I), α2, and α1(III) chains can be visualized.

dered valuable information and have found wide application are the use of pepsin and cyanogen bromide (CNBr) in the production of soluble fragments derived from insoluble collagen. Pepsin is a protease which cleaves a variety of peptide bonds in acidic media. When soft tissue collagens are incubated with pepsin at low temperatures (the triple-helical configuration remains intact) certain peptide bonds in the nontriple-helical extremities containing the cross-links are cleaved, rendering the collagen soluble. The resultant helical portions of collagens can then be studied. This approach has proven invaluable in studies designed to establish collagen types. Since the solubilities of the collagen types differ considerably, they can be separated from one another by raising the salt concentration of the mixture. Type III collagen, the least soluble, precipitates in 1.5 M NaCl, type I collagen in 2.5 M NaCl and type II in 4.5 M NaCl. Unfortunately, not every collagen is solubilized by limited pepsin digestion; the solubilities of bone and dentin collagens appear unaffected by this treatment.

CNBr is a chemical reagent which cleaves polypeptide chains at the amino acid methionine converting these chains to smaller CNBr peptides. Collagen chains contain relatively few methionines, and thus treatment of a collagen chain will produce only a small number of CNBr peptides. In recent years extensive work has been completed on the isolation, characterization, and alignment of the CNBr peptides from the type I, type II and type III collagens of several species. The principal advantage of the CNBr peptide approach is its broad applicability. Insoluble collagens from a number of sources can be converted to soluble fragments which can then be isolated by chromatography. An example of the kind of results obtained by chromatography of a tissue containing a mixture of type I and type III collagen is shown in Figure 6-7. Since the positions of methionines differ in the α chains, the resultant CNBr peptides have different sizes and chemical characteristics reflected by differing behavior on chromatography. The chromatogram is thus a map indicating the presence and even the amounts of collagen types within a tissue.

PROTEOGLYCANS OF CONNECTIVE TISSUES

Introduction

The proteoglycans are a family of unusually large macromolecules found primarily in the extracellular spaces of vertebrate connective tissues including the predentin and dentin of the tooth. Their unusual size and polycationic character have led to much speculation about the role that the molecules play in connective tissue. Before that role is discussed, we should first examine their molecular structure with emphasis on the carbohydrate portion.

Proteoglycans consist of two major polymeric components and a protein core to which are attached carbohydrate side chains, the glycosaminoglycans. The glycosaminoglycans are long, unbranched polysaccharides containing many carboxylate and sulfate functional groups that provide the unusually acidic nature of these macromolecules. The nature of the glycosaminoglycans will be discussed in more detail below.

The glycosaminoglycans of cartilage proteoglycans are not uniformly distributed along the backbone of the core protein but are distributed by pairs in closely spaced groups. Charge repulsion between the carbohydrate moieties favor an expanded structure with the

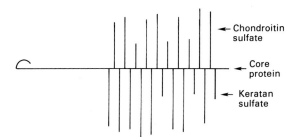

Fig. 6-8. The general structure of proteoglycan molecules. Chondroitin sulfate and keratan sulfate glycosaminoglycans are attached covalently to a core protein. One end of the protein is globular and relatively free of glycosaminoglycans. This arrangement is referred to as the "bottle brush" model.

chains extending perpendicularly from the core protein. This structure has been referred to the "bottle-brush" model for the proteoglycans (Fig. 6-8). Electron micrographs of proteoglycans, as well as their hydrodynamic behavior in solution, support the concept of this structure. The molecular weights of the proteoglycans range from 100,000 to 4 million, but all preparations are polydisperse. Thus, the material with an average molecular weight of 2.5 million may contain molecules with sizes of one to four million daltons.

The Glycosaminoglycans

The general properties of proteoglycans are largely determined by the carbohydrates of the glycosaminoglycans attached to the protein core. Seven different types of glycosaminoglycans are found in vertebrate tissues. These long, unbranched polysaccharides are composed of repeating disaccharides units containing hexuronic acid and a hexosamine which is usually acylated (Table 6-2). Keratan sulfate is an exception and contains galactose in place of the hexouronic acid. The presence of carboxylate and/or sulfate functional groups on each repeating unit of the polysaccharide results in a strongly polyanionic molecule with physical and chemical properties dominated by the negative charges. The interaction of glycosaminoglycans with other macromolecules is particularly influenced by the polyanionic character. Close examination of Table 6-2 and Figure 6-9 as you read the following section will aid your understanding of the structures of the glycosaminoglycans.

Hyaluronic acid is found in most connective tissue and is particularly abundant in cartilage and embryonic tissues. It is the only nonsulfated glycosaminoglycan. The repeating disaccharide unit contains a D-glucuronic acid residue linked to N-acetyl-D-glucosamine. The basic units are linked in turn to form the continuous carbohydrate polymer. The molecular weight of hyaluronic acid ranges from 100,000 to 10,000,000 and depends on the source as well as the degree of degradation suffered by the polysaccharide during isolation. Thus, it is approximately ten times larger than the other glycosaminoglycans. In addition, hyaluronate apparently is not associated with a core protein and electron microscopy indicates that the undegraded molecule is a separate, single chain.

TABLE 6-2. REPEATING DISACCHARIDE UNITS OF THE GLYCOSAMINOGLYCANS FOUND IN THE PROTEOGLYCANS OF CONNECTIVE TISSUES

Glycosaminoglycan	Tissue Location	Monomeric Units	Structure in Figure 6-9
Hyaluronic Acid	Most Connective Tissue; Abundant in Cartilage and Embryonic Tissue	D-Glucuronic Acid N-Acetyl-D-Glucosamine	A
Chondroitin-4-Sulfate	Cartilage, Skin, Cornea, Blood Vessels	D-Glucuronic Acid N-Acetyl-D-Galactosamine	B
Chpmdrotom-6-Sulfate	Same as Chondroitin-4-Sulfate	D-Glucuronic Acid N-Acetyl-D-Galactosamine	C
Dermatan Sulfate	Skin, Cardiovascular Tissue, Scar Tissue	L-Iduronic Acid* N-Acetyl-D-Galactosamine	D
Keratan Sulfate	Cornea, Cartilage, Spinal Tissue	D-Galactose N-Acetyl-D-Glucosamine	E
Heparan Sulfate	Blood vessel walls, Skeletal Tissues	D-Glucuronic Acid* N-Acetyl-D-Glucosamine	F

* See text for Variations in Monomeric Unit.

The chondroitin sulfates are the most abundant glycosaminoglycans with very large amounts being found in cartilage. They are also broadly distributed in other connective tissues such as skin, cornea, and blood vessels. The repeating disaccharide unit is similar to that of hyaluronic acid except that N-acetyl-D-galactosamine replaces N-acetyl-D-glucosamine in the chondroitin sulfates. The galactosamine contains sulfate on either the 4 or the 6 hydroxyl group, giving rise to two distinct glycosaminoglycans, chondroitin-4-sulfate and chondroitin-6-sulfate. The molecular weight of these glycosaminoglycans varies from 10,000 to 60,000 daltons. In addition, the degree of sulfation varies within single preparations as well as from tissue to tissue. The condroitin-4- and 6-sulfates occur in tissues independently of each other and as mixtures. There is also some evidence for copolymeric 4- and 6-sulfate disaccharide units occurring in the same chain.

Dermatan sulfate is an isomer of the chondroitin sulfates in which 10 to 40 per cent of the D-glucuronic acid is replaced by L-iduronic acid. The structure of the dermatan sulfate illustrated in Figure 6-9 contains L-iduronic acid to provide the reader with the structure of this acid for comparison with D-glucuronic acid. Large amounts of dermatan sulfate are found in skin as well as other connective tissues such as blood vessels, heart valves, umbilical cord, and scar tissue. Patients with Hurler's and Hunter's syndromes, two inherited diseases, excrete large amounts of dermatan sulfate.

Keratan sulfate is unique among the glycosaminoglycans because its disaccharide repeat unit contains no uronic acid, but is composed of dimers consisting of D-galactose bound to N-acetyl-D-glucosamine. The absence of uronate is not the only feature that distinguishes keratan sulfate from the other glycosaminoglycans. This polysaccharide is limited in its distribution, being found only in cornea, cartilage, and spinal tissue. The genetic disorder called Morquio's disease is characterized by defects in these tissues; abnormal amounts of dermatan sulfate are also excreted in the urine of patients with this disease. In addition, the molecular weight of keratan sulfate is relatively low when compared to that of the other glycosaminoglycans. On the basis of its link-

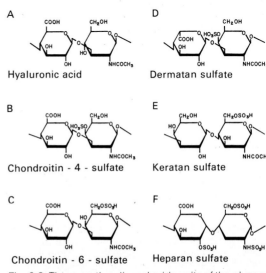

Fig. 6-9. The repeating disaccharide units of the glycosaminoglycans. Refer to Table 6-2 and the text for details.

age to the protein core, keratan sulfate is divided into two types: KS-I found in cornea and KS-II found in cartilage and spinal tissue. KS-II is the form of keratan sulfate that is linked to the same protein as some chondroitin sulfate in cartilage proteoglycans. In a later section we will examine the nature of the carbohydrate-protein linkages that allows the subdivision of keratan sulfate into two types.

Heparin and heparan sulfate are closely related structurally but differ in distribution and function. The disaccharide repeat unit is composed of D-glucuronic acid or L-iduronic acid and N-acetyl-D-glucosamine. Heparin is found in most connective tissue not as a structural component, but as an intracellular component in mast cells. Skin and lung contain heparin and there is a particularly large amount in the liver capsule and gastric mucosa. Approximately half the dimeric units contain L-iduronic acid and the glycosaminoglycan is highly sulfated. Most of the glucosamine residues are N-sulfated but there is a smaller amount that is N-acylated. About 30 per cent of these residues have an additional sulfate at the six position. Additional sulfate is found at the two position of half the uronic acid residues, primarily in L-iduronate. Therefore, up to three sulfate groups per disaccharide unit may be found in heparin. However, there is considerable variation in the degree of sulfation of heparin prepared from different tissues.

Heparan sulfate, found in blood vessel walls and in skeletal tissue, is basically composed of the same disaccharide repeat unit as heparin but the units differ to a large extent in sulfate content. There is the same amount of N-sulfate and N-acetyl substitution in the glucosamine residue but much less 0-sulfate on both sugars, such that each disaccharide unit contains about one sulfate.

Glycosaminoglycan-Protein Linkage

As was noted earlier, the glycosaminoglycans are linked to a core protein by a covalent bond forming the proteoglycan molecule. The carbohydrate-protein linkage in the chondroitin sulfates, dermatan sulfate, heparin, and heparan sulfate is illustrated in Figure 6-10A. Xylose, a pentose residue, is involved in an 0-glycosidic bond to a serine residue of the core protein. To this two galatose residues are attached. The Gal-Gal-Xyl trisaccharide thus joins the repeating dimeric units of the glycosaminoglycan with the polypeptide by covalent bonds.

As noted earlier, keratan sulfate does not contain a typical carbohydrate-protein linkage region and the glycosaminoglycan may be classed in two types, KS-I and KS-II, by two types of linkages. KS-I is bound through a glycosylamine linkage (i.e., an N-glycosyl linkage) from glucosamine to asparagine or gluta-

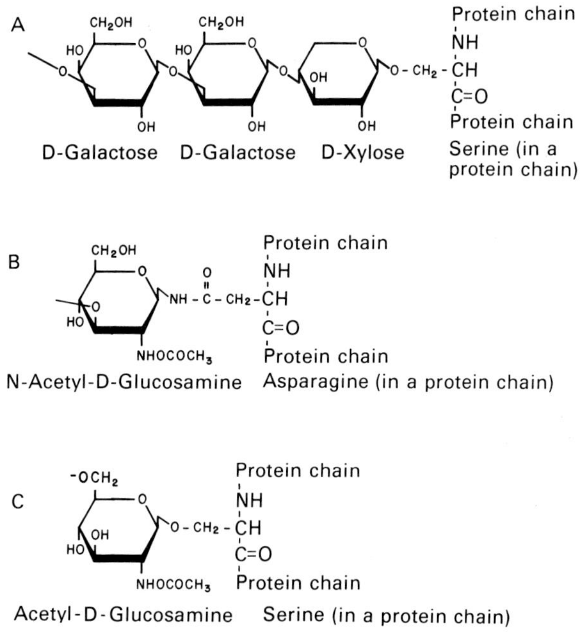

Fig. 6-10. Structure of the region linking glycosaminoglycans to the protein core.
A. Most glycosaminoglycans are attached to serine residues of the protein. The first sugar in this attachment region is the pentose xylyose which is attached glycosidically to the hydroxyl of serine. Two galactose moieties link the xylose to the repeating disaccharide units of the glycosaminoglycans. **B.** The linkage of KS-I chains to protein—this bond is an N-glycoside linking the disaccharide repeats to the NH of asparagine (or glutamine) on the protein. **C.** The linkage of KS-II chains to protein—this bond is an O-glycosidic bond linking the repeating units of keratin sulfate to serine residues.

mine (Fig. 6-10B) while KS-II consists of an 0-glycosyl linkage between glucosamine and serine (Fig. 6-10C). The linkages may be distinguished by the fact that the glycosylamine linkage in KS-I is stable to alkali but the KS-II glycosyl bond is labile in mild alkaline conditions.

Core Protein

The core protein of proteoglycan molecules is complex in structure (see Figs. 6-8 and 6-11). Recent evidence from proteoglycans found in cartilage indicates that there are three distinct regions of the protein that differ in amino acid composition. One region, a globular polypeptide located at one end of the protein, is the binding site to hyaluronic acid in the high molecular weight aggregate that we will examine in the section below. The second region, called the polysaccharide attachment region, is an extended conformation (i.e., nonglobular) containing the attachment sites for proteoglycans such as the chondroitin sulfates. It has been suggested that this region is variable in length and that this variability may be one reason for the polydisperse molecular weights observed with the molecules. The third region of the core protein found in cartilage is the area rich in keratan sulfate sidechains.

Aggregation

Proteoglycans found in cartilage form very large aggregates with molecular weights as high as 30 million. This phenomenon is illustrated in Figure 6-11. The aggregation does not represent self-association of proteoglycans with each other, but results from the noncovalent association of many proteoglycans to a single hyaluronic acid chain. The ratio of proteoglycan to hyaluronate under optimum conditions indicates that there is only one binding site for hyaluronic acid on the proteoglycan.

Two low molecular weight proteins are also components of the structure. These proteins are called link proteins since they add stability to the association by binding both to the proteoglycan and to hyaluronic acid. The association of hyaluronic acid, proteoglycans, and link proteins into a stable aggregate results in a structure with unusual biological properties (discussed below). It should be pointed out

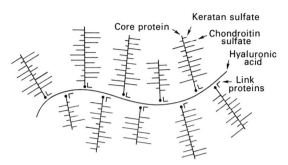

Fig. 6-11. The structure of Proteoglycan—Hyaluronic acid aggregates—a number of proteoglycan molecules are noncovalently bound to an elongated hyaluronic acid molecule. The association is stabilized by the link proteins which bind to both the globular end of proteoglycans and to hyaluronic acid.

that although aggregates of this kind have only been demonstrated in cartilage, they probably exist in other connective tissues as well.

Heterogeneity of Proteoglycans

Proteoglycans are heterogeneous in composition and polydispense in size. As we have seen in the above discussion, they differ with respect to length of the protein and polysaccharide chains, composition of the protein and polysaccharide chains, and, positions and amounts of glycosaminoglycans attached to the core protein. The proteoglycans are not extremely heterogenous but rather they fall into a range of sizes which can be viewed as **microheterogeneity**—a term we may use in describing macromolecules in which the finer details of structure are in varying degrees of completion or in which minor modifications of structures are observed. These differences probably reflect variations brought about by biosynthetic processes rather than by genetic differences. An excellent example of microheterogeneity is seen with heparin in which some of the glucosamine residues have a sulfate group on the position six and some do not.

Metabolism

Proteoglycans are made by connective tissue cells such as fibroblasts, osteoblasts, and chondroblasts and are secreted by the cells into the extracellular matrix of the connective tissue. They are also manufactured and stored within certain specialized cells such as platelets and leucocytes. Although there is a continuous and quite rapid turnover of proteoglycans in the matrix of connective tissue, a steady state is maintained by continual formation of the molecules by healthy tissue.

The unique structure of the proteoglycans with the carbohydrate extending from the central core protein makes the molecules especially susceptible to attack by proteolytic enzymes. One such enzyme found in polymorphonuclear leucocytes degrades proteoglycans, and its action may be important in tissue breakdown during inflammation. It is interesting that the same protease has been extracted from cells found in rheumatoid synovial fluids. Degradation of cartilage proteoglycans by the fluid is largely due to this enzyme.

As we shall see in the next section, the intact proteoglycans are trapped in the collagenous matrix of connective tissue. However, once degraded their components may diffuse out into the circulation, be degraded further in the liver, and then excreted as polysaccharides in the urine. Alternately, the components may be engulfed by phagocytic cells and degraded by lysozomal enzymes.

Significance of Proteoglycans

Now that we are familiar with some specific structural features and physical characteristics of the proteoglycans, we are in a position to examine the affect of the molecules on the tissues in which they are found. As we have seen the proteoglycans are primarily molecules of extracellular space and are most abundant in soft connective tissues such as cartilage and skin.

Following their biosynthesis, proteoglycans are secreted into the extracellular spaces of connective tissues where they may interact with available hyaluronic acid macromolecules, along with link proteins, to form the huge aggregates discussed previously. The presence of sulfate and carboxyl groups on each dissacharide unit of the proteoglycans makes the molecules strong polyanions. This characteristic is one of the dominant properties of the proteoglycans. Because of the large number of negatively charged groups which form repulsive forces, the polysaccharides are fully extended, stiffened rods occupying a very large amount of space. These large and expanded molecules become entangled and immobilized in the collagen network and impede the flow of interstitial water when an external pressure is applied. Thus, the tissue is elastic yet resiliant to compressive forces. At the same time, the hydrophilic character of the proteoglycan-hyaluronic acid aggregate, coupled with the binding of high concentrations of counterions, such as Na^+, K^+, and Ca^{++}, creates a swelling effect. Thus, the higher the proteoglycan concentration in the tissue the more swelling and turgor is observed. These properties are particularly evident in cartilage.

The extended network of proteoglycan aggregates also serves as a molecular sieve that excludes molecules with a size larger than the pores of the network. This exclusion might offer protection for the matrix in the sense that it prohibits the diffusion of macromolecules (such as proteases) through the connective tissue spaces.

Proteoglycans are also found in lesser amounts in certain cells, organelles, and membranes. They are much smaller in size than those of extracellular spaces and seem to function as binders and carriers of cationic materials.

TISSUES OF THE TOOTH

Dentin

Introduction

Most of a tooth's mass and overall shape can be attributed to **dentin,** consisting largely of collagen fibers onto which inorganic crystals of apatite (see Chap. 7) have been deposited. Only about 20 per cent of the weight of dentin is organic material, the remainder being inorganic mineral. However, the organic phase takes up most of the space of this tissue. This arrangement of inorganic crystals laid onto an undergirding of organic, fibrillar material produces a stable concretion ably suited to withstand the forces of mastication. Our attention will now focus on the available information concerning the physical and chemical properties of the organic constituents of dentin, including an overview of the dynamics of the formation of dentin by odontoblasts.

Dentin Collagen

About 85 to 90 per cent of the organic material of dentin is collagen. This collagen is completely insoluble using the previously described laboratory techniques, even after removal of the inorganic phase. Decalcification of dentin can be achieved by extraction with dilute acids (e.g., 0.5 M acetic acid) or with EDTA (ethylenediamine tetraacetic acid, a strong calcium chelator) solutions. After decalcification and removal of any remaining soluble proteins, the insoluble matrix left behind is almost exclusively dentin collagen. The amino acid composition of such a preparation is similar to that of skin collagen, except that the amount of hydroxylysine is 2 to 3 times higher (Table 6-3). The reason for this elevated level of hydroxylysine is unknown; perhaps it occurs because the process of hydroxylation of lysines by lysyl hydroxylase (see Fig. 6-5) is simply more efficient in odontoblasts than in fibroblasts.

Despite the overall similarities of composition, dentin and skin collagen display certain differences in physical and chemical properties. When suspended in dilute acid solutions, soft tissue collagen swells and expands until it occupies 7 to 8 times its original volume. The acid causes a disruption of the close contacts of adjacent molecules in the fibrillar lattice

TABLE 6-3. AMINO ACID COMPOSITION* OF COLLAGENS AND DENTIN PHOSPHOPROTEIN FROM THE RAT

Amino Acid	Skin Collagen	Dentin Collagen	Incisor Phosphoprotein
Hydroxyproline	93	96	0
Aspartic acid	46	45	359
Threonine	19	18	12
Serine	43	41	104
Phosphoserine	0	0	443
Glutamic acid	71	72	29
Proline	121	119	0
Glycine	331	334	31
Alanine	106	102	9
Valine	24	23	0
Methionine	8	7	0
Isoleucine	11	10	0
Leucine	24	24	0
Tryosine	3	4	0
Phenylalanine	12	14	0
Hydroxylysine	5	15	0
Lysine	29	20	8
Histidine	4	4	5
Arginine	51	52	0

* The composition is given in residues per thousand amino acids (i.e., the numbers are *relative* values).

and results in the filling of the spaces by solvent. Insoluble dentin (or bone) collagen does not display this property, but retains its original volume even in the presence of acidic solutions. This matrix contains covalent cross links not only between the ends of molecules but also in other locations (see below).

The determination of the nature of collagen in dentin rests mainly upon the nature of CNBr peptides liberated from the insoluble matrix. Attempts to solubilize dentin collagen molecules by the use of lathyrogens or with limited pepsin digestion have been unsuccessful. The chromatography, chemical composition, and partial amino acid sequence of the CNBr peptides show that dentin collagen is type I collagen, since CNBr peptides from both α1(I) and α2 have been found in dentin. It should be emphasized that, while most soft connective tissues contain type III collagen in addition to type I, the three calcified tissues with collagenous fibers (dentin, bone, cementum) contain largely or exclusively type I collagen. This finding suggests that type I collagen might promote mineralization while the presence of type III collagen in a tissue might deter this process. As noted earlier, dentin contains a small amount of type I trimer collagen but the physiologic significance of its presence is not understood.

Unlike most soft connective tissues, dentin collagen contains cross links that connect two triple-helical segments of adjacent molecules. These cross links occur in addition to those involving nontriple-helical portions at the ends of molecules. The cross links of dentin collagen almost entirely involve hydroxyallysines, the most stable variety of cross links (see Fig. 6-6D).

From this tentative description of dentin collagen, one can see that the physical stability of dentin collagen goes beyond that of soft tissue collagens, not because of differences in the initial polypeptide chains that are biosynthesized, but due to posttranslational modifications (i.e., hydroxylation of lysines and additional cross links).

The Proteoglycans of Predentin and Dentin

The glycosaminoglycans represent less than 0.5 per cent of the weight of dentin matrix or about 2.5 per cent of the organic material in the tissue. These glycosaminoglycans are protein bound and in the form of polydisperse proteoglycans, as described earlier. Chondroitin-4-sulfate is the predominant component accounting for 70 per cent of the glycosaminoglycans while chondroitin-6-sulfate accounts for 10 to 15 per cent of the material. It also appears that the ratio of the 4-isomer to the 6-isomer may vary with age so that there may be a loss of the 6-isomer with age.

In addition to the chondroitin-4- and 6-sulfates, hyaluronic acid (3 to 6 per cent), dermatan sulfate (2 to 3 per cent), keratan sulfate (1 per cent) and some nonsulfated galactosaminoglycan are also present as minor proteoglycan constituents of dentin. Thus aggregates of proetoglycans and hyaluronic acid similar to the ones found in cartilage might exist in certain areas of dentin or predentin. Despite the low amount on a weight basis, the extended structure of aggregates of proteoglycans and hyaluronic acid would occupy a considerable amount of space within the tissue.

Predentin contains significantly more glycosaminoglycans than dentin and, in contrast to dentin, chondroitin-6-sulfate predominates in the tissue. Since the amount of chondroitin-4-sulfate is the same in both tissues, the predominance of the 4-isomer in dentin may reflect the biodegradation of the chondroitin-6-sulfate upon transformation of predentin to dentin (see below).

The Phosphoprotein of Dentin

An unusual constituent present in dentin but not in bone or other connective tissues is a **phosphoprotein.** This protein is polyanionic with about 36 per cent of its amino acids being aspartic acid and greater than 40 per cent being phosphoserine (Table 6-3). The phosphoprotein accounts for 3 per cent of the weight of the organic material of human dentin and more than 10 per cent of that in the continuously erupting rat incisor. It is formed by odontoblasts, and it is in some way transported to the site where the mineralization of dentin takes place (that is, at the predentin/dentin junction) where it binds to the surface of collagen fibrils. Although the exact role which this unusual protein plays in the process of mineralization is unknown, several facts stand out. Most of the phosphoprotein can be readily extracted from demineralized dentin by aqueous solvents. However, it is nonextractable unless mineral is first removed. Therefore, the phosphoprotein is trapped, or encased within the mineralized matrix. Another relevant factor is the protein's ability to bind calcium. The large number of negatively charged groups of the phosphoprotein make it especially effective in binding large numbers of metal cations, such as Ca^{++}, with a relatively high affinity. This property may reflect its role in the mineralization of the tissue. An understanding of the role played by the phosphoprotein in the deposition of mineral will undoubtedly be a major thrust in comprehending the process of dentinogenesis.

The Formation of Dentin by Odontoblasts (Dentinogenesis)

Dentin is produced by a single row of elongated cells, the **odontoblast,** which line the pulp cavity (Fig. 6-12). The organic matrix of dentin, consisting primarily of dentin collagen fibrils and proteoglycans, is laid down outside the periphery of these cells in an uncalcified form called **predentin.** As the cells produce this organic matrix, they are moved pulpally in a direction away from the material they have secreted. Odontoblastic processes are left behind, providing cellular communication with the tissue. As more and more predentin matrix is amassed, older predentin is transformed to dentin at a site several microns from nascent predentin. This transformation of predentin to dentin involves the laying down of mineral onto the collagen fibrils of the tissue, a process which is not as yet well understood. Since the mineralization process is one of the keys to understanding dentinogenesis, let us focus for a moment on what is known about the events transpiring at the predentin-dentin (P-D) junction.

A method used in the study of these events is **radioautography.** These experiments involve injection of radioactive precursors of the substance to be studied followed by localization of the isotope in the tissue by overlaying a microscopic section with photographic film. The emission of particles by the radioisotope develops the film and the positions within tissues where the radioisotope label is located is indicated by dots on the film. If animals are sacrificed at different intervals after injecting the radioactive precursors, the kinetics of formation and of deposition of various constituents that contain the radioisotopes in the tissues can be studied.

The classic experiments of Weinstock and Leblond, (see Suggested Readings) using ra-

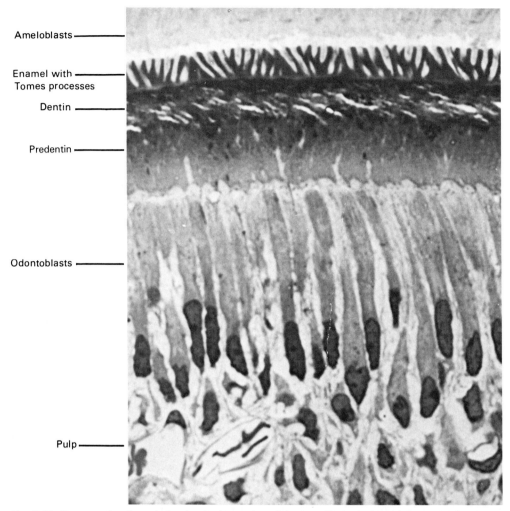

Ameloblasts

Enamel with Tomes processes

Dentin

Predentin

Odontoblasts

Pulp

Fig. 6-12. Cross section through the developing region of the mandibular incisor of the rat. Light micrograph (× 1350). (Courtesy Dr. James W. Simmelink, Case Western Reserve University, Cleveland, Ohio)

dioautography have shown that collagen labeled with [³H]-proline was laid down just outside the odontoblasts in the predentin and found in dentin only 30 hours later. In contrast, the phosphoprotein, labeled with [³³P]-phosphate, quickly moved through predentin and was deposited at the P-D junction in 1–4 hours after its synthesis. These experiments indicate that one of the events in the conversion of predentin to dentin is the binding of phosphoprotein to the surface of collagen fibrils at the P-D junction.

Another process occurring when predentin is transformed to dentin is the degradation and removal of some of the proteoglycans. As mentioned earlier, the proteoglycans of dentin are not only smaller in quantity from those of predentin but also differ in their quality. It

is therefore, speculated that the presence of proteoglycans in predentin may prevent the formation of a phosphoprotein-collagen complex. Thus, the biodegradation of proteoglycans at the P-D junction may be an important prologue to transformation of predentin to dentin.

Though the exact mechanism of dentinogenesis is not completely understood, the foregoing discussion illustrates some extracellular steps which may form part of a series of reactions in this process. We know that the formation of dentin is a finely controlled process occurring at a finite distance from the cells. A number of other important biologic processes are controlled by involvement of a series of cascading reactions terminating in the desired end result or product. For example, a blood clot forms as the result of a series of proteolytic enzymes interacting stepwise to convert inactive substances to active products. In the final step fibrinogen is converted to fibrin and a blood clot ensues. The series of reactions does not take place until some necessary activating event occurs, and thus blood clots do not normally occur at undesirable locations. In an analogous fashion, the location and speed of the deposition of mineral onto collagen fibrils must correlate with the production of predentin by odontoblasts and the molecular events must act in a controlled, stepwise manner.

Cementum

Cementum consists of a thin layer of calcified tissue which covers the root surface of teeth. Like dentin and bone, the organic material of cementum is largely insoluble collagen. Relatively few studies have been performed with cementum collagen because of the paucity of material available for biochemical studies. After treatment of bovine cementum with CNBr, peptides from $\alpha 1(I)$ and $\alpha 2$ collagen chains are obtained. In addition peptides from the $\alpha 1(III)$ chain are found in small quantities. When human cementum is used only peptides from type I collagen are found. These findings are similar to those using bone and dentin, and emphasize that calcified connective tissues contain almost exclusively type I collagen and little or no type III collagen. The collagen of cementum appears to be highly cross linked and resistant to pepsin cleavage. The major cross link is the one formed from hydroxylysine and hydroxyallysine (see Fig. 6-6). In this respect cementum also resembles bone and dentin.

Periodontal Ligament

The fibers which connect alveolar bone to the cementum, known collectively as the **periodontal ligament,** are collagenous fibers. Studies on the ultrastructure of the periodontal ligament have shown two different types of fibers which differ in size and orientation. The so called indifferent fibers are small and course in many directions, but often are joined with the larger principal fibers. Such an arrangement, obviously important to the functional properties of the ligament, must be reflected in the molecular structures from which the fibers are composed.

To discover the nature of the collagens of periodontal ligament, this tissue has been subjected to the standard laboratory procedures previously described. CNBr peptides originating from both type I and type III collagen were obtained. The relative amounts of CNBr peptides showed that about 20 per cent of periodontal ligament collagen was type III and 80 per cent was type I collagen. The presence of these two collagen types was also shown by pepsin digestion and then separation by differential salt precipitation.

The presence of two collagen types in a tissue suggests that they perform separate functions. It is known that type III collagen forms small fibers *in vivo*, while larger fibers are attributable to type I. A logical conclusion, therefore, is that the smaller indifferent fibers are composed of type III collagen while the larger principal fibers are type I. It should be emphasized that the proper experiments to test this hypothesis have not been performed.

One unusual aspect of the collagenous fibers of the periodontal ligament is the high turnover rate. Recall that all tissues are in a dynamic state and that the proteins and other macromolecules are continually being broken down, or biodegraded, and replaced by biosynthesis. For the adult rat, the rate of turnover of periodontal ligament collagen is five times faster than that in gingiva, six times that of bone collagen, and fifteen times faster than skin collagen. The half life of periodontal ligament collagen, that is the length of time necessary for half to be degraded and replaced, is about one day. Similar studies have not been done for the tissues of man, but we can be assured that the finding of a rapid turnover of the fibers of periodontal ligament is generally true.

Enamel

Unlike the other calcified structures of the body, enamel crystals are *not* deposited onto a fibrillar collagen matrix. However, proteins do play an important role in the formation of the enamel.

Enamel is laid down by a single row of cells, the **ameloblasts.** In the initial stages of enamel formation the ameloblasts secrete matrix proteins (so called fetal enamel proteins, or amelogenins) and, as the cells move periph-

TABLE 6-4. AMINO ACID COMPOSITION OF THE
MIXTURE OF ENAMEL PROTEINS FROM
TWO STAGES OF DEVELOPMENT*

Amino Acid	Fetal Enamel	Mature Enamel
Asparitic acid	33	88
Threonine	27	53
Serine	49	108
Glutamic acid	159	134
Proline	253	80
Glycine	54	161
Alanine	22	73
Cystine	0.2	11
Valine	38	45
Mathionine	55	1
Isoleucine	34	31
Leucine	95	71
Tyrosine	47	13
Phenylalanine	26	40
Hydroxylysine	1	1
Lysine	16	42
Histidine	73	16
Arginine	19	33

* The composition is given in residues per thousand
amino acid residues.

erally, they leave behind ribbon-like enamel crystals within the preenamel. Gradually the protein matrix is removed and replaced by the inorganic apatite crystals as they grow in size. In the early stages of development, when the preenamel is soft and "cheese-like," the tissue contains about 30 per cent protein. Gradually the inorganic content increases and the protein content falls to about 1 per cent or less. This loss represents a selective loss of high molecular weight proteins. Consequently the quality of the protein material left behind is different from that present in the early stages, as shown by a dramatic difference in the overall amino acid composition of the two (Table 6-4). Other biochemical experiments have also demonstrated that certain high molecular weight proteins are lost as more and more mineral is deposited.

The proteins of fetal enamel have been studied in several laboratories. They consist of 10 to 20 proteins which seem to be related. For example, bovine enamel proteins act as a single antigen when injected into the rabbit. Furthermore, several of the purified fetal enamel proteins are similar in amino acid con-

tent. These proteins found in developing enamel are probably derived from one or two common high molecular weight proteins, and when they are isolated are simply in the process of being degraded.

About 20 per cent of the weight of fetal enamel proteins consist of two closely related proteins with molecular weights of about 6000 daltons. These proteins have a small amount of phosphoserine residues, leading some scientists to believe that this phosphate is involved in the initiation of the mineralization process in enamel.

The apatite crystals of enamel are much larger than those in dentin and bone and exhibit a high level of orientation. In order for crystals of this nature to form, special conditions permitting their growth and orientation must be achieved. It is believed that such conditions are created by the properties of the enamel proteins and the subsequent events which transpire relative to these proteins. The protein matrix probably initiates formation of small elongated crystals, and as the proteins are gradually degraded by proteases, the crystals grow in an orderly fashion. By the time the complete removal of fetal enamel proteins has taken place, the gradual, controlled growth results in the formation of unusually large apatite crystals with the proper orientation. That protein which is not degraded but is left behind may then be located on the periphery of the apatite crystals. This process is one of many ways nature utilizes proteins to form a tissue with unusual properties destined to perform a specialized function.

As more information is gained about the nature of the organic components of enamel, we can expect this information to draw us closer to an understanding of how the large apatite crystals in enamel are formed. However, the present knowledge already tells us that ameloblasts control the process by formation and degradation of extracellular proteins.

With this understanding of the biochemistry of tooth proteins, we are now, hopefully, more prepared to appreciate the clinical entity of dental caries.

GLOSSARY

Aldimine bond. The covalent bond formed when an aldehyde (—CHO) reacts with an amino (—NH₂) group.

Allysine. Amino acid derived from lysine by removal of the —NH₂ group and oxidation of the carbon to an aldehyde. Allysine plays an important role as a precursor of collagen cross-links.

Alpha (α) chain. An individual polypeptide chain in the collagen molecule. There are three α chains in a molecule and the three are wound around each other to form the triple chain collagen helix.

Amelogenins. The group of proteins found in embryonic enamel, or preenamel, that are removed as the apatite crystals of mature enamel are formed.

β-Aminopropionitrile (βAPN). A chemical reagent that causes lathyrism by inhibiting lysyl oxidase, thus blocking collagen cross-linking.

Chondroblast. A cartilage-forming cell that arises from the mesenchyme.

Chondroitin sulfate. A glycosaminoglycan containing repeating dimeric units of D-glucuronic acid and N-acetyl-D-galactosamine that is partially sulfated; a major constituent of bone and cartilage.

Chymotrypsin. A protease that is one of the enzymes involved in the normal digestion of food within the small intestine.

Chymotrypsinogen. The inactive precursor of chymotrypsin that is formed by the pancreas. The activation process involves the proteolytic removal of a small segment from chymotrypsinogen, thus converting it to chymotrypsin.

Clq. The first component of the complement cascade. This protein interacts with the antigen-antibody complex and then activates the next protein in the cascade.

Collagen fiber. The structure seen by light microscopy and composed of a number of bundles of collagen fibrils.

Collagen fibril. The structure seen with an electron microscope that is composed of thousands of collagen molecules.

Collagen molecule. The elongated, triple-stranded molecule that can interact to form fibrils.

Collagenase. The proteolytic enzyme responsible for beginning the degradation of collagen. The latter process is a normal part of the turnover of collagen.

Collagenolysis. The process of collagen breakdown brought about by collagenase and other proteases.

Column chromatography. A method of separating and analyzing mixtures of chemical constituents. The mixture is washed onto a column, or tube, filled with some type of absorbent material. The mixture is then separated by selecting conditions which sequentially wash the constituents from the column. These constituents are detected as they elute from the column.

Complement cascase. The series of biologic reactions taking place when complement, a group of serum proteins, is activated. Activation may occur when antigen-antibody complexes are formed.

Connective tissue. A tissue which binds or supports portions of the body. The tissue usually contains fibrillar elements, proteoglycans, and cells.

Core protein. The central protein in the proteoglycan molecule that covalently binds the glycosaminoglycans.

Cross links. The covalent bonds formed between the chains of different collagen molecules.

Cyanogen bromide (CNBr) cleavage. Chemical cleavage of protein chains at methionine residues.

D stagger. The dimension by which collagen molecules are laterally staggered relative to one another when they form fibrils. The D stagger is about 1/4.4 times the length of the collagen molecule and is about 68 nm in length (see Figure 6-1E).

Dermatan sulfate. A glycosaminoglycan containing repeating dimeric units of either L-iduronic or D-glucuronic acid and N-acetyl-D-galactosamine that is partially sulfated. Formerly called chondroitin sulfate B, which is mostly found in skin.

Dissacharide. A carbohydrate consisting of two covalently bound monossacharides.

Electrostatic interaction. The association of oppositely charged chemical groups. For example, the side groups of arginine residues bearing positive charges, interact with the negative groups of glutamic acid residues.

Extracellular matrix. The area outside the cells of connective tissue.

Fibrin. An insoluble protein which forms a blood clot.

Fibrinogen. The precursor of fibrin.

Glycosaminoglycan. A long, straight chain polysaccharide containing many carboxylate and sulfate functional groups and hexosamines that are N-acylated or N-sulfated. Formerly called mucopolysaccharide.

Glycosidic linkage. The bond between the anomeric carbon of a carbohydrate and another atom or molecule.

Heparan sulfate. A glycosaminoglycan very similar to heparin but containing less O-sulfate.

Heparin. A glycosaminoglycan containing repeating dimeric units of D-glucuronic acid and N-sulfate-D-glucosamine that is additionally sulfated on both dimeric units. It is found mostly in the liver and lung, and exhibits anticoagulant activity.

Homologous. Two proteins are said to be homologous if their amino acid sequences are more similar than could have arisen by chance mutations. Thus two homologous polypeptide chains are presumed to have arisen from a common ancestral gene.

Hyaluronic acid. A glycosaminoglycan containing repeating units of D-glucuronic acid and N-acetyl-D-glucosamine. It is found in most connective tissue.

Hydrophobic interactions. The property of certain chemical groups with low water solubility to self associate in an attempt to remain shielded from the aqueous environment. This force is a major factor in the folding of globular proteins into their native conformation.

Hydroxyallysine. Similar to allysine excepting its derivation from hydroxylysine.

Kertan sulfate. A glycosaminoglycan containing repeating dimeric units of D-galactose and N-acetyl-D-glucosamine that is partially sulfated. It was formerly called keratosulfate.

Latent collagenase. An inactive form of collagenase.

Lathyrism. A disease characterized by general weakening of connective tissues. Lathyrism is caused by blocking of the normal cross linking process.

Macromolecule. A large polymeric molecule with a high molecular weight (above 2,000 daltons).

Major helix. The conformation into which three collagen α chains fold. The major helix repeats about every 9 nm and has approximately thirty residues per turn.

Mast cells. A connective tissue cell that contains heparin and functions in hypersensitivity.

Microheterogenity. A property of some preparations of macromolecules in which the molecules exhibit slight differences in charge, location of functional groups, completeness of synthesis, or some other property.

Minor helix. The spiral into which a single collagen α chain folds. This helix repeats about every 0.9 nm and encompasses three amino acid residues per repeat.

Pepsin. A proteolytic enzyme involved in food digestion within the stomach. The enzyme acts at acidic pH and has been useful in cleaving nontriple-helical ends of insoluble collagen where cross links are found. The action does not degrade the helical portion of collagen.

Phosphoserine. An amino acid in which the sidegroup has a phosphate moiety attached to a hydroxyl.

Polyacrylamide gel electrophoresis. A method used to separate and analyze mixtures of macromolecules such as proteins. The mixture is placed on the top of a small column (about the size of a pencil) of a gel support. Separation is attained by passing an electrical current through the gel. The molecules migrate to differing degrees because of differences in weight and charge. They can then be seen by staining the polyacrylamide gels.

Polydisperse. Variation of some macromolecules with respect to their size or molecular weight.

Polysaccharide. A carbohydrate consisting of a large number of covalently bound monossacharides.

Posttranslational modification. Any modification of a polypeptide chain taking place after the polypeptide linkages are formed on the ribosomal complexes. Recall that this latter process is referred to as translation, since chemical information specifying the amino acid sequence is "translated" from messenger RNA to the polypeptide chain.

Procollagen molecule. The triple-stranded molecule synthesized by cells which contains the segment destined to be a collagen molecule with extensions on both ends of all three pro α chains.

Protease (or proteolytic enzyme). An enzyme which catalyzes the hydrolysis of peptide bonds, thus cleaving proteins into smaller fragments, or peptides.

Proteoglycans. A family of unusually large macromolecules consisting of numerous and varied glycosaminoglycans covalently bound to a core protein.

Radioautography. The experimental method of visualizing a radiolabeled substance in a tissue section. After introduction of the radioisotope, histologic sections of the tissue are made and placed next to photographic film. The areas within the section where the isotope is located are denoted by development of the film by the radioactive substance.

Reticular fibers. A network of thin, collagenous fibers which stain with substances known to detect carbohydrate-rich macromolecules.

SUGGESTED READINGS

Bailey AJ, Robins SP: Current topics in the biosynthesis, structure and function of collagen. Sci Prog 63: 419, 1976

Butler WT, Munksgaard EC, Richardson WS: Dentin proteins, chemistry, structure and biosynthesis. In Nylen MU Termine JD (eds): Tooth Enamel III, Its Development, Structure, and Composition. J Dent Res 58(B): 817–824, 1979

Campo RD: Protein-polysaccharides of cartilage and bone in health and disease. Clin Orthop 68: 182, 1970

Fessler JH, Fessler LI: Biosynthesis of procollagen. Annu Rev Biochem 47: 129, 1978

Jones IL, Leaver AG: Glycosaminoglycans of human dentine. Calc Tiss Res 16: 37, 1974

Miller EJ: Biochemical characteristics and biological significance of the genetically-distinct collagens. Molec Cell Biochem 13: 165, 1976

Muir H, Hardingham TE: Structure of proteoglycans. In Whelan WJ (ed): Biochemistry of Carbohydrates, Vol 5. London, Butterworths, 1975, p 153

Munksgaard EC, Butler WT, Richardson WS: Phosphoprotein from dentin. New approaches to achieve and assess purity. Prep Biochem 7: 321, 1977

Ramachandran GN, Reddi AH (eds): Biochemistry of Collagen New York, Plenum Press, 1976

Robinson CR, Lowe NR, Weatherell JA: Changes in amino-acid composition of developing rat incisor enamel. Calcy Tissue Res 23: 29, 1977

Rosenberg L: Structure of cartilage proteoglycans. In Burleigh PMC, Poole AR (eds): Dynamics of Connective Tissue Macromolecules. New York, American Elserior, 1975, p 105

Roden L, Horowitz MI: Structure and biosynthesis of connective tissue proteoglycans. In Horowitz MI, Pigman W (eds): The Glycoconjugates, Vol II. New York, Academic Press, 1978

Shackleford JM: The indifferent fiber plexus and its relationship to principal fibers of the priodontium. Am J Anat 131: 427, 1971

Sodek J: A comparison of the rates of synthesis and turnover of collagen and non-collagen proteins in adult rat periodontal tissues and skin using a microassay. Arch Oral Biol 22: 655, 1977

Weinstock M, Leblond CP: Radioautographic visualization of the deposition of a phosphoprotein at the mineralization front in the dentin of the rat incisor. J Cell Biol 56: 838, 1973

7 Enamel, Apatite, and Caries-A Crystallographic View

HOWARD M. EINSPAHR

CHARLES E. BUGG

Introduction
Levels of Structure in Dental Enamel
  Enamel Crystallites
  Structure of Enamel Rods
  Chemical and Structural Composition of
    Enamel Mineral

Effects of Ionic Substitutions on the
  Structural Properties of Apatites
Crystallographic Aspects of Dental Caries
Summary
Glossary
Suggested Readings

INTRODUCTION

Dental enamel is a highly mineralized system. More than 95 per cent of the mass of enamel is inorganic material, most, if not all, of which is in the crystalline state. A detailed knowledge of the crystalline structure of enamel permits a better understanding of the physical, chemical, and biological properties of teeth, and sheds some light on the etiology of dental caries.

Dental enamel, with its unusual chemical composition and highly ordered structure, is the densest material in the vertebrate system. Mature enamel is acellular and practically devoid of organic material, but it is far from being the inert system that might be expected of a mineral constituent in the oral cavity. On the contrary, enamel is an active chemical system that participates in a variety of reactions, including solute and ion transport from saliva to dentin, ion-exchange reactions with saliva, and demineralization-remineralization processes. Further consideration of the many surface reactions that occur between enamel and the organic and bacterial components of saliva reinforces the concept that enamel is a dynamic component of the oral cavity.

The structure of enamel and its chemistry have been subjects of persevering research. However, several features of enamel structure remain to be clarified, and many aspects of the available data remain open to interpretation. Several models of enamel structure have been postulated; each has its proponents. To present all of the viewpoints would require a whole volume rather than a single chapter. Consequently, many of our conclusions about the pertinent features of enamel structure must be regarded as subjective choices. We shall attempt to summarize some of the results that have been obtained with electron microscopy, light microscopy, X-ray diffraction, spectroscopic investigations, and chemical analyses. Building on these results, we shall offer specific models for the structure of dental enamel, for the changes that occur with the formation of carious lesions, and for the mechanisms by which specific agents, particularly fluoride, alter the chemical and physical properties of enamel.

LEVELS OF STRUCTURE IN DENTAL ENAMEL

The organization of the mineral in dental enamel follows a hierarchy of structural levels from the macroscopic down to the atomic. The largest structural elements encountered are the rods (or prisms). Enamel is composed of a densely packed and intertwined assembly of rods that extend from the enamel-dentin junction toward the outer surface. The rods are of the order of 10,000 angstroms (Å) thick and up to 3 millimeters (mm.) in length. Many of the bulk properties (e.g., density, hardness) of enamel stem from the structural characteristics of the composite arrangements of these rods. A closer inspection reveals that the rods are composed of millions of small, elongated crystallites (length of the order of 1,000 Å), arranged in characteristic patterns within the rods. Each crystallite, in turn, is composed of thousands of subunits called unit cells (dimensions of the order of 10 Å), which are stacked together like building blocks. Examination of the internal structure of the unit cell reveals a highly ordered arrangement of atoms. In this chapter each structural level will be discussed in some detail, and we shall attempt to correlate a few of the chemical and physical properties of enamel with what is known about enamel structure.

Enamel Crystallites

In the early stages of enamel biosynthesis, the first mineral appears in the form of long, thin ribbons. Figure 7-1 is an electron micrograph of these ribbons, or precursor crystallites, as found in human enamel. The average length of the ribbons, about 1000 Å, is of the order of that of the final crystallites, but the ribbons lack the thickness acquired with maturity. These incipient crystallites appear to be somewhat disordered. They follow undulating paths suggestive of stacking faults and lack the straight edges and planar faces characteristic of well-ordered crystals. Furthermore, many of the ribbons are only about 15 Å thick (scarcely more than 10 to 15 atoms in width) and lack the long-range atomic interactions that would stabilize an ordered structure.

Figures 7-2 and 7-3 are electron micrographs of the crystallites in mature rat enamel. Similar observations have been made in mature human enamel. The mature crystallites are well developed, elongated plates of hexagonal cross section. It is probable that they have developed by slow thickening of ribbons that are similar to those shown in Figure 7-1.

It is apparent that, as the crystallites mature and thicken, they become more ordered. Nevertheless, it is likely that some defects (misalignments of atoms or missing atoms) present in the ribbons remain trapped in the cores of the mature crystallites. Any remaining defects are likely to influence the stability of the crystallites, and the acid dissolution patterns of enamel.

Table 7-1 compares some of the physical properties of mature enamel and bone. For crystal size the table shows a range for each dimension that is thought to encompass the majority of crystallites in mature tissue. Individual crystallites within a given tissue vary both in size and shape for various reasons, but the columnar shape shown in Figures 7-2 and 7-3 seems to be characteristic. It should be pointed out that because of procedures necessary to prepare samples for electron microscopy, there is some uncertainty as to what are representative dimensions for crystallites in enamel and bone. There is always the possibility that procedures such as sectioning or polishing may have distorted the observed size distributions of crystallites. The problem is further complicated by a variety of other variables involved in sampling, such as portion of tooth used, type of tooth sampled, age, and dental history of donor. It is nevertheless clear that crystallites in enamel are, on the average, 5 to 10 times larger in each dimension than those in bone. Enamel is almost completely

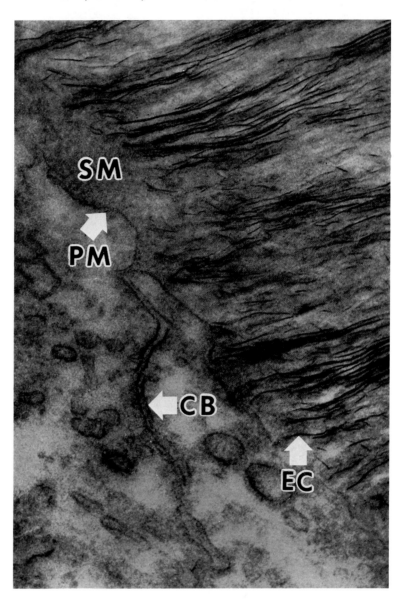

Fig. 7-1. Crystallite precursors.
Electron micrograph of earliest observable crystallites (EC) in human enamel. The initial crystallites (upper right) are ribbon-shaped and oriented approximately perpendicular to the mineralization front, which runs diagonally from upper left to lower right. (approx. ×300,000) (Ronnholm E: J Ultrastruct 6: 268, 1962)

mineralized, and experimental evidence suggests that it contains only about 3 per cent water and less than 1 per cent organic material. Bone is only about 72 per cent mineral and is much less dense than enamel. The larger size of enamel crystallites is undoubtedly an important factor in maintaining the structural integrity of enamel and in enhancing the resistance of enamel to the variety of chemical and physical challenges in the oral cavity. Another structural feature that is a major factor in adapting the mineral to the oral environment is the characteristic pattern in which the large crystallites of enamel are packed together.

Structure of Enamel Rods

In mature enamel crystallites are incorporated as members of larger structures that are referred to as rods or prisms. Each rod is an elongated assembly of millions of crystallites laid end-to-end and packed into a staggered bundle many crystallites thick. Figure 7-4 is an image of a typical section of enamel that

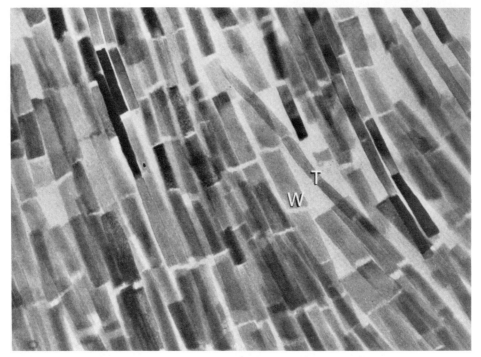

Fig. 7-2. Mature crystallites.
Electron micrograph of crystallites in mature rat enamel. The enamel sample was sectioned parallel to the long axes of crystallites. Long dimensions vary from 1600 to 2000 Å. The width (W) and thickness (T) of crystallites are about 400 and 200 Å, respectively. (approx. ×175,000) (Nylen MU, Eanes ED, Omnell K-Å: J Cell Biol, 18: 117, 1963)

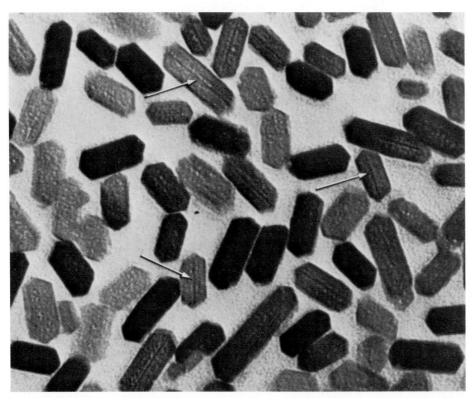

Fig. 7-3. Mature crystallites in cross section.
Electron micrograph of crystallites in mature rat enamel. The enamel sample was sectioned perpendicular to the long axes of crystallites. The hexagonal form of the crystallite cross section is apparent. (approx. ×350,000) (Nylen MU, Eanes, ED, Omnell K-Å: J Cell Biol, 18: 119, 1963)

TABLE 7-1. PROPERTIES AND COMPOSITION OF
MATURE ENAMEL AND BONE

	Enamel	Bone
Density (g/cc)	2.9–3.0	2.1–2.2
Mineral Content (Wt. %)	96	72
Crystal Size (Å)		
Length	1,000–10,000	300–500
Width	300–600	100–300
Thickness	100–400	25–50

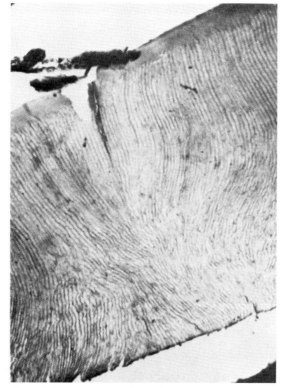

Fig. 7-4. The arrangement of rods in enamel.
A light micrograph of a transverse section through the crown of an erupted human tooth showing the composite organization of enamel rods. The surface of the tooth is in the upper left of the figure. (approx. × 350) (Gustafson G, Gustafson A-G: Microanatomy and histochemistry of enamel. In Miles AEW (ed): Structural and Chemical Organization of Teeth. vol 2., p. 101. New York, Academic Press, 1967)

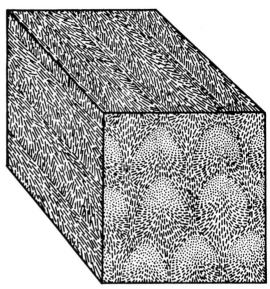

Fig. 7-5. Enamel rods.
A schematic drawing of a block of enamel illustrating the packing of rods and the arrangements of crystallites. The upper and left faces of the block represent longitudinal sections of the rods, and the front face is a cross section. (Carlstrom D: Adv Oral Biol 1: 266, 1964)

displays the composite arrangement of rods. The average rod is about 4 to 6 micrometers (µm) (40,000–60,000 Å) in diameter. The rods follow undulating paths that span the distance from the enamel-dentin junction to the tooth surface in most cases, although some rods terminate before reaching the surface and a few may form branches or fuse with neighbors. The length of an average rod is thus limited by the thickness of the enamel layer, usually about 1 to 3 mm. Despite the twisted pathways seen in Figure 7-4, the rods tend to be roughly perpendicular to both the enamel-dentin junction and the tooth surface.

Figure 7-5 is a schematic drawing of a block of enamel that contains several rods, each running parallel to the long dimension of the block. In cross section these rods have a peculiar keyhole shape, as depicted by the ends of the central rods. The alignment of the crystallites relative to the rod axis varies in different regions of the keyhole cross section. Within the central region of the head of the keyhole, the long axes of crystallites are aligned almost parallel to the rod axis but incline with increasing angles to this axis as the tail region of the keyhole is approached. The greatest inclination of crystallites is observed in the extremes of the tail regions and in the regions bordering the heads. The crystallites that border the heads are somewhat larger than those at other locations in the keyhole.

Figure 7-6 shows a model of a cylindrical core through the head of a rod. A large portion of the central head region (in the upper part of the cylinder) has been cut away. The crystallites in this region are approximately parallel to each other and have their long axes

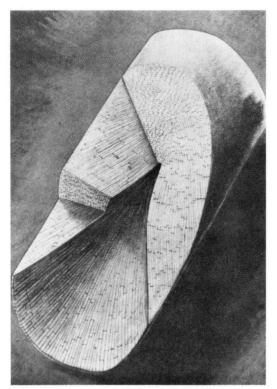

Fig. 7-6. Crystallite orientation in the enamel rod.
A schematic representation of a cylindrical core taken down the rod axis and comprising the head region of an enamel rod. The artful use of cut-aways depicts the variation in crystal orientation within the rod. (Helmcke J-G: Atlas der menschlichen Zahnes im elektronenmikroskopischen Bild, Part I: Histologie des normalen Zahnes. Berlin, Transmare Photo, 1953)

been described. The rods are the largest structural subunits of enamel and it is the assembly of rods that produces the shape and the bulk properties of the mineral of the tooth. In the following sections we shall reverse the course of our discussion and examine what is known of the composition and substructure of the enamel crystallite.

Chemical and Structural Composition of Enamel Mineral

The crystallites in enamel display X-ray diffraction patterns that are characteristic of apatite structures. Apatite is a generic name for a class of minerals with a characteristic crystalline arrangement. Chemically, apatites have compositions that are variants of the formula D_5T_3M, where D is a divalent cation (Ca^{+4}, Ba^{+4}, etc.); T is a trivalent, tetrahedral, compound anion (PO_4^{-3}, AsO_4^{-3}, etc.); and M is a monovalent anion (OH^-, F^-, Cl^-, etc.). The basic building block (unit cell) of apatite crys-

nearly parallel to the long axis of the rod. Away from this head region, toward the lower part of the cylindrical segment, the crystallites deviate from alignment with the rod axis. These deviations increase toward the lower part of the segment.

Figure 7-7 is a schematic drawing of a rod sliced along the longitudinal axis. This view illustrates how the crystallites tilt away from the rod axis in the tail region. The resultant configuration is one in which the long axes of crystallites (labelled c in the drawing) are inclined over a fairly wide angular range, but tend to be preferentially aligned roughly parallel to the rod axis, particularly in the center of the head region.

Thus far, we have considered the structural levels of enamel that are accessible by microscopy methods. The general properties of the crystallite (the smallest subunit so far discussed) and its organization into rods have

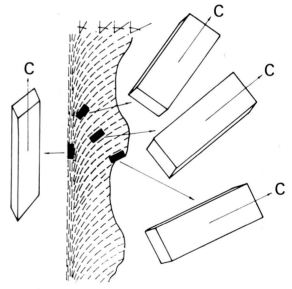

Fig. 7-7. Crystallite orientation in the enamel rod.
Schematic representation of the crystallite orientation pattern in a longitudinal section through an enamel rod. The head region of the rod is on the extreme left, the tail region on the right. Blow-ups of crystallites in different portions of the section are shown and c-axis directions are indicated. The variation in inclination angle with increasing distance from the head region is shown across the top of the section. For simplicity, the enlarged crystallites are depicted with quadrangular rather than hexagonal cross sections. (Helmcke J-G, Schultz L, Scott DC: Deutsche zahnärztliche Zeitschrift 18: 574, 1963)

tals contains two of the D_5T_3M formula units and thus has the formula $D_{10}T_6M_2$. Since ionic substitutions can take place at various sites within the unit cell, the stoichiometry of apatite structures is conveniently expressed in terms of the contents of a complete unit cell.

The mineral components of enamel and bone are often described as impure forms of hydroxyapatite, $Ca_{10}(PO_4)_6(OH)_2$. The arrangement of atoms within the unit cell of hydroxyapatite (Fig. 7-8) corresponds to that of all other apatites with respect to the relative dispositions of the D, M, and T species. The shape of the unit cell of hydroxyapatite is also characteristic of apatite unit cells in general. This shape is termed hexagonal in that the *a* and *b* axes of the cell (Fig. 7-8) intersect at an angle of 120° and have equal lengths, and the *c* axis is perpendicular to both *a* and *b*. (For our purposes, we will ignore the existence of a number of closely related apatite structures that are pseudohexagonal in a crystallographic sense.) Each apatite crystallite is an ordered aggregate of many unit cells. Figure 7-9 is a schematic drawing that shows the apatite crystallite as an assembly of unit cells. The long dimension of an apatite crystallite in enamel corresponds to the *c* axis of the apatite unit cell (Fig. 7-7). Thus, the average enamel crystallite is many more unit cells long than it is wide or thick. Since the lengths of the *a* and *c* axes of the enamel unit cell are about 10 and 7 Å, respectively, a representative crystallite might be about 300 unit cells long, 40 wide, and 20 thick.

Hydroxyapatite is only one example from the class of apatite minerals. Table 7-2 describes several other examples of apatites, some that occur naturally or have been synthesized, others that may be purely hypothetical. Biological apatite samples are often characterized by their calcium/phosphorous

molar ratios. For pure hydroxyapatite, the first entry in Table 7-2, the Ca/P molar ratio is 1.67. The second entry in Table II shows the chemical formula of fluorapatite, wherein the two hydroxyl groups of hydroxyapatite are replaced by fluoride ions. The third entry corresponds to pure chlorapatite, which contains chloride ions in place of the hydroxyl groups. Apatites of intermediate compositions are also found. An example of this type is described by the fourth entry, which defines apatites that have various compositions of monovalent anions, with each value of x between 0 and 2 representing a stable, mixed species intermediate between pure hydroxyapatite and fluorapatite. Noninteger values of x may be thought of as expressing the overall average composition of apatites that vary from unit cell to unit cell with respect to the composition of the monovalent species. Variation in the monovalent anion composition does not affect the Ca/P molar ratio.

Entry 5 of Table 7-2 represents the substitution of another divalent cation for calcium. Substitutions of this type lower the Ca/P molar ratio. Entry 6 is an example in which a divalent hydrogen-phosphate anion replaces a trivalent phosphate ion. Both of these anions have tetrahedral geometries. However, for charge balance, a monovalent potassium ion has replaced one of the calcium ions thereby lowering the Ca/P molar ratio. Entry 7 describes one of the proposed mechanisms by which carbonate ions may be incorporated in apatite. In this example, a divalent, planar carbonate anion replaces a trivalent, tetrahedral phosphate, and charge balance is maintained by replacing a calcium ion with the monovalent sodium cation. Sodium, potassium, hydrogen phosphates, and carbonate ions are found in naturally occurring apatites, including enamel, but are seldom present in concentrations that correspond to formulae as simple as entries 6 or 7. Entries 8 and 9 are idealized formulae for synthetic and naturally occurring apatite compounds, respectively, that give some idea of the extremes of compositional variety that can be accommodated by the apatite structure.

Chemical analyses indicate that enamel has an exceedingly complex composition. The concentrations of certain ions that are especially prevalent in enamel are shown in Table 7-3 and are compared with concentrations that would be expected for three homogeneous apatites. Both the calcium and the

TABLE 7-2. EXAMPLES OF APATITES

	Composition	Ca/P Molar Ratio
1.	$Ca_{10}(PO_4)_6(OH)_2$	1.67
2.	$Ca_{10}(PO_4)_6(F)_2$	1.67
3.	$Ca_{10}(PO_4)_6(Cl)_2$	1.67
4.	$Ca_{10}(PO_4)_6[(OH)_x(F)_{2-x}]$, $0 \leq x \leq 2$	1.67
5.	$Ca_9Mg(PO_4)_6(OH)_2$	1.5
6.	$Ca_9K(PO_4)_5(HPO_4)(OH)_2$	1.5
7.	$Ca_9Na(PO_4)_5(CO_3)(OH)_2$	1.8
8.	$Ca_6Al_4(PO_4)_4(AlO_4)_2(F)_2$	1.5
9.	$Ca_{10}(SiO_4)_3(SO_4)_3(OH)_2$	∞

TABLE 7-3. COMPARISON OF ENAMEL COMPOSITION WITH THAT OF PURE APATITES (WT. %)

Ion	Enamel	Hydroxy-apatite	Chlor-apatite	Fluor-apatite
Ca	33.6–39.4	39.9	38.5	39.7
P	16.1–18.0	18.5	17.8	18.4
CO_3	1.95–3.66			
Mg	0.25–0.56			
Na	0.25–0.90			
K	0.05–0.30			
Cl	0.19		6.81	
F	0.006–0.3			3.77
Ca/P (Molar Ratio)	1.48–1.67	1.67	1.67	1.67

phosphorus contents of enamel are usually lower than those found in pure calcium phosphate apatites, but it is the lower Ca/P molar ratio usually found for enamel that is responsible for the characterization of enamel apatite as "calcium deficient." While the bulk of the phosphorus content of enamel is due to the presence of the trivalent phosphate ion, the content of divalent monohydrogen phosphate ion, HPO_4^{-2}, in sound human enamel is about 5 per cent by weight. It is likely that requirements of charge balance as a result of this substitution are at least in part responsible for less than ideal Ca/P molar ratios in enamel. A number of plausible substitution mechanisms that would contribute to "calcium deficiency" in enamel have been proposed, but the correct mechanisms have yet to be confirmed experimentally.

As may be seen in Table 7-3, enamel contains appreciable amounts of carbonate. It is because of this carbonate content that some authorities prefer to characterize enamel mineral as a carbonate apatite, thereby also avoiding implications of simplicity and homogeneity of composition that might be mistakenly conveyed by referring to enamel mineral as hydroxyapatite. The composition of enamel mineral is even more complex than suggested in Table 7-3, and a number of components, principally cations, that have been detected in enamel in trace quantities are not listed. Also missing from the list is a value for the amount of chemically bound water. Water is a significant component of enamel, but little is known about the sites that water molecules occupy.

It is important to realize that no single unit cell can exhibit so complex a composition as that described above. Enamel must therefore be composed of unit cells with a variety of simpler compositions. The nonuniformity of enamel composition extends over much broader ranges than unit cell to unit cell or crystallite to crystallite. Actually, the chemical composition of enamel varies considerably from individual to individual, from tooth to tooth, and even shows variations within a single tooth, and within a given section of enamel. Apparently, the elemental composition of mature enamel is dependent upon the concentrations of ions present at the various stages of development, and upon the environmental history of the mature tooth. Concentrations of several of the components vary at different distances from the tooth surface. For example, fluoride concentration is usually highest in samples obtained from the external regions of enamel, and the concentration diminishes in moving from the tooth surface toward the enamel-dentin junction. Carbonate concentration follows a reverse pattern. It is lowest in regions at the tooth surface and increases toward the enamel-dentin junction. Some other ions, such as strontium, appear to be uniformly distributed through the depth of enamel.

Crystallographic data also attest to the nonhomogeneity of dental enamel. Table 7-4 shows the average lengths of the unit cell edges for the apatite phase of enamel, along with the corresponding values for pure fluor-, hydroxy-, and chlor-apatites. Variations in unit cell parameters within such a simple series may be related to the differing sizes of the constituents, F^-, OH^-, and Cl^-. However, enamel apatite is characterized by unit cell parameters that cannot be explained by any such simple pattern. The unit cell parameters of enamel apatite in Table 7-4 represent the dimensions of an average enamel unit cell. These dimensions reflect the effects of all substitutions, including those that are at present immeasurable by chemical analysis. Thus, both chemical and crystallographic data

TABLE 7-4. UNIT CELL DIMENSIONS OF SOME APATITIC MINERALS

Material	a	c
Fluorapatite	9.367(1) Å	6.884(1) Å
Hydroxyapatite	9.418(1)	6.880(1)
Chlorapatite	9.647(2)	6.771(2)
Enamel	9.442(3)	6.885(3)

* The a and b unit cell parameters are of equal length. Estimated standard deviations (included in parentheses) refer to uncertainties in the final decimal place.

strongly indicate that dental enamel is not a simple substance, but rather contains a large variety of minor constituents that are distributed in various patterns within the mineral.

Effects of Ionic Substitutions on the Structural Properties of Apatites

The arrangement of ions in the hydroxyapatite unit cell (Figure 7-8) is the structural pattern common to all apatites. This pattern is the framework into which ionic substitutions are inserted, and it can accommodate a variety of substitutions without drastic alteration. The primary structural effects that result from the simpler ionic substitutions, such as replacing calcium ions with other divalent cations, replacing phosphate ions with other tetrahedral, trivalent anions, or replacing hydroxyl

groups with other monovalent anions are perturbations of the atomic arrangement that stem mainly from differences in ionic radii. Although the apatite structure is preserved, the chemical and structural perturbations that accompany such ionic substitutions can substantially affect the chemical and physical properties of the mineral and influence the stability, chemical reactivity, and hardness of enamel. One such substitution, the replacement of some of the hydroxyl groups of hydroxyapatite by fluoride ions, has been extensively studied and is of special importance to dentistry.

The hydroxyl groups in hydroxyapatite are arranged in columns parallel to c that are surrounded by channels formed by triangles of calcium ions. These triangles are defined by dotted and dashed lines in the lower left corner of Figure 7-8. In this region of the unit cell

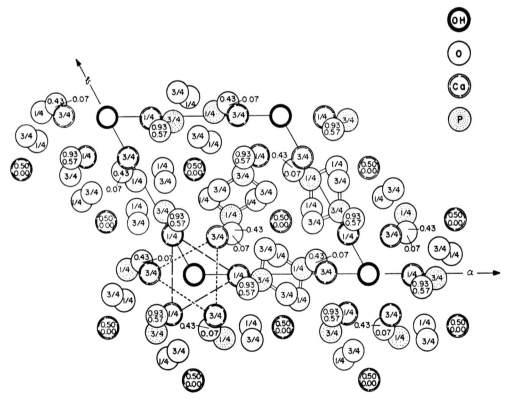

Fig. 7-8. The hydroxyapatite crystal structure.

A representation of the crystal structure of hydroxyapatite, viewed down the c axis, which shows the details of the atomic arrangement. The solid lines drawn between hydroxyl positions outline the edges of the unit cell. The centers of circles representing atoms (see legend at upper right) define the x and y coordinates of the atoms; z coordinates, expressed as fractions of the c-axis length, are the numbers written within the circles. Hydroxyl groups are superimposed in this projection; the z coordinates of hydroxyl groups are approximately 1/4 and 3/4. Hydrogen atoms have been omitted for clarity. (Young RA, Elliott JC: Arch Oral Biol 11: 700, 1966) there are two calcium triangles that lie perpendicular to the crystallographic c axis. One triangle is located ¼ of the way up the c axis and the second one is situated ¾ of the way along c. These triangles are twisted 180° relative to each other. The calcium triangles are repeated along c from unit cell to unit cell, resulting in cylindrical arrays of calcium ions that, in the absence of dislocations or other defects, run throughout the length of the crystals in the c direction. Further definition of these channels is added by triangles of oxygen atoms from phosphate groups arranged around the channels (at $z = 0.07$, 0.43 and $z = 0.57$, 0.93 in Fig. 7-8). The calcium ions that form the c-axis channels are coordinated to oxygen atoms from hydroxyl groups and from phosphate groups. Phosphate groups occupy the bulk of the space between the calcium channels in the structure (for our purposes, we will ignore the calcium ions along the major cell diagonal at $z = 0$ and ½). The hydroxyl groups are lined up along the central axes of the channels of calcium ions, thereby forming columns running in the c direction. The individual hydroxyl groups are slightly displaced from the planes of the calcium triangles; however, a single hydroxyl group is closely associated with each triangle, and is oriented with its hydrogen atom directed away from the triangle along the channel axis.

X-ray evidence indicates that for about half the calcium triangles the hydroxyl group is above the plane of the triangle, and for the other half it is below. The most reasonable model to explain the X-ray evidence has the hydroxyl groups within a given column generally pointing hydrogens in the same direction. However, the orientation varies in a random fashion from column to column, with half the columns having hydroxyls pointed in the $+c$ direction, and half having hydroxyls pointed in the $-c$ direction. Figure 7-9 shows the ordering of columns found for pseudohexagonal hydroxyapatite. In this form, adjacent columns are oriented in the same direction along a, but in opposite directions along b. This form has not been found in enamel. The hexagonal form of hydroxyapatite, which corresponds to enamel mineral, lacks this order and the orientation of columns varies randomly in the ab plane.

As mentioned earlier, the c axis of the apatite unit cell corresponds to the long axis of the enamel crystallite, and the crystallites are

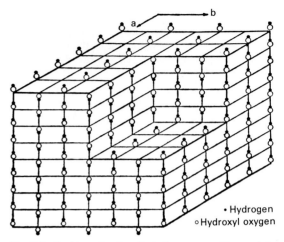

Fig. 7-9. Packing of unit cells to form an apatite crystal. This is a schematic representation of the arrangement of unit cells in hydroxyapatite. The c axis corresponds to the vertical direction. Columns of hydroxyl groups are shown; the rest of the ions, calcium and phosphate, are omitted for clarity. The ordered alignment of hydroxyl columns, which is found in the pseudohexagonal form of hydroxyapatite, is replaced by a random arrangement in the hexagonal form. (Elliott JC, Mackie PE, Young RA: Science 180: 1056, 1973)

aligned so that their long axes are roughly parallel to the rod axis. Since the rods tend to extend from the enamel-dentin junction toward the enamel surface, the channels containing hydroxyl groups are generally pointed roughly perpendicular to the outer surface of enamel. Hence, if viewed from the surface, the apatite unit cells of enamel would present a view of the atomic arrangement much like that shown in Figure 7-8, which is a view down the c axis.

Fluoride ions become incorporated into hydroxyapatite by substituting for hydroxyl groups; these ions then occupy positions along the columns of hydroxyl groups within the channels formed by the calcium triangles. X-ray diffraction studies of fluorapatite show that fluoride ions, in contrast to the hydroxyl groups, are situated in the planes of the calcium triangles equidistant from the three calcium ions. Figure 7-10 shows the site that is occupied by fluoride ions.

Incorporation of fluoride ions into the columns of hydroxyl groups can exert several substantial effects on the chemical and physical properties of hydroxyapatite. By occupying a position at the center of the calcium triangle, the relatively small fluoride ion is able to form stronger Coulomb interactions with the calcium ions than the hydroxyl group

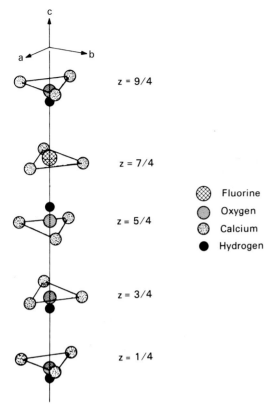

Fig. 7-10. The calcium triangles along the c axis.
A column of calcium triangles along the c axis is shown together with the positions of monovalent anions. Note the alternating orientation of the triangles. Hydroxyl groups are slightly displaced either above or below the triangles and hydrogen atoms point away from the calcium planes to which the oxygens are bound. The fluoride ion, on the other hand, assumes a position exactly in the center of the triangle, equidistant from the three calcium ions. (Young RA, Elliott JC: Arch Oral Biol 11: 701, 1966)

TABLE 7-5. CALCIUM-TO-CALCIUM AND CALCIUM-TO-ANION DISTANCES ASSOCIATED WITH CALCIUM TRIANGLES IN FLUOR- AND HYDROXY- APATITES

Material	Ca ⋯ Ca	Ca––Anion
Fluorapatite	3.975(1) Å	2.295(1) Å
Hydroxyapatite	4.084(1)	2.389(1)

Z	A	B	C
1/4	O H	O H	O H
3/4	O H	O H	O H
5/4	O H	—F—	—F—
			H O
7/4	O H	O H	
			H O
9/4	O H	O H	

Fig. 7-11. Fluoride substitution in the hydroxyl columns.
A representation of possible arrangements of hydroxyl groups within c-axis channels with or without the presence of fluoride. The horizontal bars at increments of 1/2 in z represent calcium triangles viewed edge-on. (A) Ordering in an uninterrupted hydroxyl column; (B) the formation of a single O—H⋯F hydrogen bond. The fluoride ion is shown as slightly displaced from the plane of the calcium triangle toward the hydrogen atom. (C) The formation of two hydrogen bonds. Note the reversal of hydroxyl-group orientations in part of the column. (Young RA, Van der Lugt W, Elliott JC: Nature 223: 729, 1969)

can form, as evidenced by calcium-fluoride contact distances that are appreciably shorter than those of calcium-hydroxyl contacts. Additional evidence of these stronger interactions is the shrinkage of the calcium triangle, with the calcium ions actually pulled in closer to the fluoride ion despite the increase in repulsive forces between cations. The calcium-calcium and calcium-anion distances at the calcium triangle in fluorapatite are compared with the corresponding values for hydroxyapatite in Table 7-5.

Substituted fluoride ions may also affect the chemical and physical properties of apatites by establishing hydrogen-bonding interactions with neighboring hydroxyl groups. Within the columns, adjacent hydroxyl groups are separated by a spacing of 3.44 Å;

this distance is too great to permit hydrogen bonding. However, the distance between fluoride ions (which are in the center of the calcium triangles) and neighboring hydroxyl groups (which can be displaced toward the fluoride substituents) is short enough to permit strong O—H⋯F hydrogen bonds within hydroxyl columns that contain fluoride. The types of interactions that are possible can be seen from Figure 7-11. The column at the left in Figure 7-11 shows an example of the hydroxyl-group arrangement that might be expected in the absence of fluoride. The middle column shows how a fluoride ion within one of the calcium triangles would be in a position to hydrogen-bond to one of the hydroxyl groups adjacent to it. The third column at the right in Figure 7-11 shows an alternate arrangement that permits hydrogen bonding on both sides of the fluoride ion by reversing the direction of the hydroxyl column below the fluoride ion; Figure 7-10 shows this type of arrangement in greater detail.

Spectroscopic data confirm the importance of O—H···F hydrogen bonds within fluoride-substituted apatites. Such hydrogen-bonding interactions, together with the enhanced ionic effects, are probably responsible for most of the increased stability of fluoride-substituted apatites relative to pure hydroxyapatite. Even trace amounts of fluoride have dramatic effects on the stability of enamel, as reflected by lower acid solubility, decreased rates of demineralization, and enhanced rates of remineralization. All of these features can be attributed to the stabilizing effects that fluoride exerts on the apatite of enamel, and it is likely that all of these factors contribute either directly or indirectly to the cariostatic activity of fluoride.

The effects that are induced by other types of substitutions are not so obvious. We have already noted that enamel contains appreciable amounts of carbonate ion, and spectroscopic data indicate that at least part of this carbonate is incorporated within the enamel crystallites. The problem of carbonate substitution is a perplexing one. For one thing, it violates the geometrical constraints of the apatite structure. Carbonate is a polyatomic anion, but it is planar, not tetrahedral. Furthermore, it is divalent and its substitution must be coupled with other substitutions to maintain charge balance. There have been suggestions that carbonate substitution might be accompanied by replacement of calcium ions with monovalent cations (see entry 7 of Table 7-2). To this date, the available evidence is inconclusive with respect to the site or sites at which carbonate substitution occurs, although disordered occupation of the phosphate site seems to be favored as the major component of the substitution scheme.

Apparently, substitution of carbonate ions within apatite tends to disrupt a number of the interactions that are responsible for stabilizing the apatite structure. Carbonate-substituted apatite is considerably less stable than normal apatite, as reflected by several physical properties including the increased susceptibility of the former to acid dissolution. It is likely that carbonate substitution also increases the susceptibility of enamel to carious lesions. In any case, the nature of carbonate substitution and its effect on enamel remains an unsolved problem in the study of enamel mineral.

CRYSTALLOGRAPHIC ASPECTS OF DENTAL CARIES

As the authors of other chapters in this volume show, many complicated factors are involved in the formation of carious lesions. However, chemical analyses indicate that the main process occurring in caries attack is one of demineralization, followed by replacement of the dissolved mineral with loosely bound water. For the purposes of our discussion, we shall assume that dental caries is simply a result of acid dissolution of enamel.

One of the most notable features of enamel dissolution patterns is the relationship to the enamel rods. Figure 7-12 shows a typical electron micrograph of a section of enamel that was sliced perpendicular to the long axes of the rods and then etched with acid. It is immediately obvious that the dissolution process is most advanced in the head regions of the rods. The tail regions and the periphery of the head regions appear to be relatively resistant to acid attack.

Why are crystallites from the head regions the first to be dissolved when enamel surfaces are etched with acid? The increased susceptibility of these crystallites to acid attack seems to be correlated with the orientations of their c axes. As stated earlier, the crystallites in the head region of a rod are aligned so that their long dimensions (that is, their c axes) are nearly parallel to the rod axis, and hence, roughly perpendicular to the enamel surface. The crystallites away from the head fan out in increasing degrees of oblique orientation. These oblique crystals appear to be the ones that are most resistant to acid dissolution. The importance of orientational factors is further apparent from electron micrographs of acid-etched enamel samples that have been sliced in directions oblique to the rod axes. For example, Figure 7-13 shows an electron micrograph of an acid-etched enamel section that was prepared so that in both the head and tail

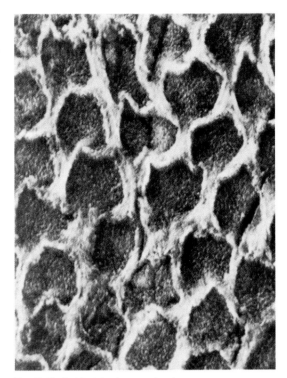

Fig. 7-12. Acid-etched enamel rods.
Electron micrograph of a section of human enamel after etching with acid. The section was prepared so that rods were cut almost in cross section. Rods are preferentially dissolved in the head region, where crystallites are oriented perpendicular to the surface. (approx. ×6000) (Scott DB, Simmelink JW, Nygaard V: J Dent Res 53:169, 1974)

regions crystallites are sliced at about the same angle. In this case, both head and tail are etched at equal rates. The periphery of the head, which is composed of larger crystallites, appears to be relatively resistant to acid demineralization.

Thus far it has been difficult to pinpoint the mechanism responsible for the correlation of c-axis orientation with the susceptibility of an enamel crystallite to acid attack. However, if access of the acid to the reactive hydroxyl groups of the apatite crystallites is an important factor, than one might expect that acid dissolution of the crystallites would proceed faster in the c-axis direction than in other directions. As suggested in Figure 7-8, the columns of hydroxyl groups are shielded by the surrounding material in directions perpendicular to the c axis, but are relatively unprotected from frontal attack in the c direction. The calcium triangles are stabilized in part by interactions with the hydroxyl groups, so that acid reaction of hydroxyl groups to form water

would weaken the calcium configuration and thus destabilize the environment around the reaction site.

Perhaps the most remarkable feature of fluoride-substituted enamel is the effect that small amounts of fluoride exert on caries susceptibility. As shown in Table 7-3, enamel contains only trace amounts of fluoride, even from geographical regions of rather high fluoride content. The content of fluoride found in samples of enamel is always far less than would be expected for pure fluorapatite. Therefore, any physical model to explain the cariostatic effects of fluoride must be able to account for the fact that trace amounts of fluoride in the partially-substituted apatite component of enamel greatly enhance the resistance of enamel to acid demineralization processes.

Assuming that acid attack down the columns of hydroxyl groups is an important mechanism for enamel demineralization pro-

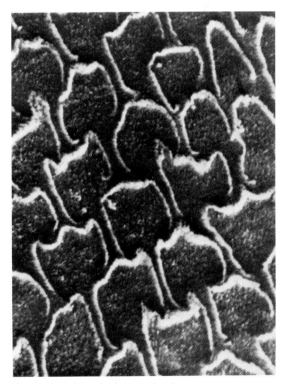

Fig. 7-13. Acid-etched enamel rods.
Electron micrograph of a section of human enamel after etching with acid. The section was prepared so that crystallites in the head and tail regions were cut at approximately the same angle. Both head and tail regions were equally damaged by acid treatment. (approx. ×6000) (Scott DB, Simmelink JW, Nygaard V: J Dent Res 53: 169, 1974)

cesses, one can appreciate how substitution of small amounts of fluoride near the tooth surface might enhance the stability of enamel. From Figure 7-11, it can be seen how a few fluoride ions that are substituted in the hydroxyl columns could impede acid attack down the c-axis channels. As discussed in the preceding sections, the fluoride ions should make significant contributions to increased structural stability. When substituted for a hydroxyl group, the fluoride ion is held more strongly by the calcium triangle. It occupies the center of the triangle, where it forms short calcium-fluoride contacts. Its hydrogen-bonding potential further contributes to the stabilizing influence. The net result of these stabilizing factors is that fluoride ions may act as "plugs" in the otherwise reactive hydroxyl columns. Acid attack down a given channel, and the resulting destabilization of its surroundings, would be relatively unimpeded until a fluoride ion was encountered, whereupon further attack at that locus would be retarded. When viewed as barriers along the c-axis channels, fluoride ions (even at fairly low concentrations) might be expected to impede acid demineralization processes, and hence caries attack.

Although preferential attack down the hydroxyl columns may be a significant mechanism for acid dissolution of enamel, it is not the only factor relevant to the observation that enamel crystallites are dissolved more rapidly in the direction of their long axes than in the lateral directions. High-magnification electron micrographs of acid-etched enamel (Figures 7-14 and 7-15) indicate that the first step in the destruction of an individual crystallite is the dissolution of its central core. It is evident from these micrographs that, while the outer regions of the crystallites in these preparations are relatively unaffected, the central portion of each crystal has been dissolved. The initially dissolved core often runs almost the entire length of the crystallite in the c direction, but generally covers only a limited area in the a and b directions. One may conclude that the apatite crystallites of enamel contain central cores that are considerably less stable to acid attack than the outer regions.

One explanation for the instability of these cores may be that they contain higher proportions of dislocations and imperfections than the surrounding material. Studies of synthetic apatite crystals tend to corroborate this sug-

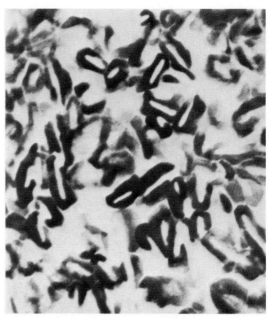

Fig. 7-14. Acid-etched enamel crystallites.
Electron micrograph of acid-etched human enamel crystallites. Centers of crystallites have been dissolved. (approx. ×250,000) (Scott DB, Simmelink JW, Nygaard V: J Dent Res 53: 172, 1974)

gestion. Acid dissolution patterns of poorly formed synthetic crystals mimic the dissolution patterns of enamel crystallites, whereas synthetic crystals that have been annealed to remove defects display uniform dissolution patterns without formation of central holes. It is known that strains induced by dislocations and other irregularities can markedly increase local rates of dissolution within crystals. Referring back to Figure 7-1, the thin ribbons of apatite that are first laid down in developing enamel contain many imperfections. The crystallites of mature enamel appear to be formed around these irregular ribbons by a process of lateral growth that may entrap irregularities in the central core. Since lateral growth is a relatively slow process, it is likely that the outer regions of the crystallites are more highly ordered and are thus less susceptible to acid dissolution. Investigations of the nature and distribution of defects in enamel is an active area of research at present.

SUMMARY

We have presented an abbreviated review of what is known about the structure of enamel, including the pattern of initial development

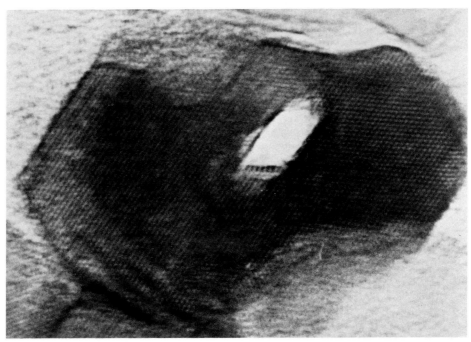

Fig. 7-15. Carious enamel crystallite.
   Electron micrograph of a cross section of a caries-damaged crystallite of human enamel. The c axis of the crystallite is perpendicular to the micrograph surface. Caries attack has apparently produced a hole in the center of the crystallite. The periodic striations in the surface of the crystallite reflect the hexagonal crystal-packing arrangement. Note also the shape of the hole with its suggestion of the 60° and 120° angles characteristic of hexagonal symmetry. (approx. ×1,750,000) (Voegel JC, Frank RM: J Biol Buccale 2: 47, 1974)

and the detailed substructure of the mature mineral. We have discussed enamel mineral at several structural levels that range from the packing of polycrystalline rods down to an image of the atomic arrangements in the hydroxyapatite crystal structure. We have attempted to highlight the physical, chemical, and biological features that are pertinent to the properties of enamel and its behavior in the oral cavity. The view that we have presented includes the following major points:

1. The first mineral to appear in developing enamel is in the form of thin ribbons that are about the same length as the mature crystallites. These ribbons are oriented approximately perpendicular to the mineralization front and to the enamel-dentin junction. The ribbons lack the degree of order that is found in mature crystallites.

2. The enamel crystallites probably develop though lateral growth of these ribbons. This growth is relatively slow, and the resultant crystalline material is highly ordered. The apatite crystallites in mature enamel are most often observed as elongated narrow plates, the long dimensions of which correspond to the c axis of the apatite lattice.

3. The crystallites are arranged in discrete, intertwining bundles known as rods or prisms. The rods follow undulating paths extending from the enamel-dentin junction toward the outer surface of enamel. In the head region of the rod the c axes of the crystallites are nearly parallel to the rod axis. Toward the tail region, the crystallites fan out in a featherlike array and deviate from parallel alignment with the rod axis. Thus the c axes of the crystallites in the head region are directed approximately perpendicular to the outer surface of enamel whereas the c axes of the crystallites toward the tail region are positioned obliquely to the enamel surface.

4. Electron micrographs of acid-etched enamel sections indicate that the rods are preferentially dissolved in regions where the crystallites are situated with

their *c* axes perpendicular to the surface that is exposed to acid. These findings suggest that the crystallites are most susceptible to acid dissolution down their *c* axes.

5. The crystallites of enamel belong to the general class of minerals known as apatites. Apatites are characterized by a particular spatial arrangement of ions, and this arrangement can accomodate a wide variety of chemical substitutions. Chemical analyses suggest that the apatite of dental enamel may be described as a partially substituted hydroxyapatite. A major feature of the hydroxyapatite crystal structure is the presence of columns of hydroxyl groups threading through channels formed by calcium ions. These columns run parallel to the *c* axis of the apatite crystallite, and hence, lie more or less perpendicular to the outer surface of the enamel. The columns of hydroxyl groups should be most susceptible to acid attack down the direction of the *c* axis.

6. Fluoride ions can substitute for hydroxyl groups in the *c*-axis channels. Chemical analyses indicate that, although only a small percentage of the hydroxyl sites are occupied by fluoride ions in mature enamel, the majority of the fluoride substitutions are concentrated near the enamel surface. Chemical and crystallographic evidence suggests that substituted fluoride ions can enhance the stability of the apatite structure particularly in the region of the *c*-axis channels, and thereby impede acid attack down the *c* axis direction. The result would be protection of the crystallites against the demineralization processes involved in caries attack by curbing the rate of demineralization and enhancing the rate of remineralization.

7. Electron micrographs of individual crystallites from partially demineralized enamel sections show that the crystallites are preferentially dissolved along their cores, parallel to the *c* axes. The susceptibility of the cores is probably due to the presence of trapped imperfections. These imperfections would increase the dissolution rate of the cores relative to that of the surrounding material.

GLOSSARY

Angstrom (Å). A measure of length customarily used for crystal dimensions and interatomic distances; 10^{-10} meters (m), 10^{-7} millimeters (mm), 10^{-4} micrometers (μm), 0.1 nanometers (nm); exactly one two-hundred-and-fifty-four-millionth of an inch.

Apatite. The name of a general class of minerals characterized by close similarities of stoichiometry (D_5T_3M; where D = divalent cation; T = trivalent, tetrahedral, compound anion; and M = monovalent anion) and crystal structure.

Caries. A disease of tooth mineral involving lesion formation characterized by progressive demineralization.

Crystallographic axis. A direction parallel to the direction of one of the unit cell edges, *a*, *b*, or *c*.

Enamel. The dense mineral unique to the outer layer of the teeth of higher vertebrates, usually 1–3 mm thick.

Enamel crystallite. The structural subunit of the enamel rod; a small (about $2000 \times 400 \times 200$Å) crystal of substituted hydroxyapatite.

Enamel-dentin junction. The narrow transition zone between enamel and dentin.

Enamel rod (or prism). The largest organizational subunit of enamel structure. An elongated composite of millions of mineral crystallites that follows an undulating pathway from the enamel-dentin junction toward the tooth surface, with a diameter about 4–6 μm and variable length (roughly 1–3 mm).

Hydroxyapatite. The pure apatite mineral that most closely resembles the mineral components of bones and teeth; $Ca_{10}(PO_4)_6(OH)_2$.

Ionic substitution. The replacement of one or more of the normal ionic constituents of certain crystalline materials by similar, but foreign, ionic impurities without major changes in the crystal structure.

Micrometer (μm). A measure of length commonly used for the dimensions of microscopic objects; 10^{-6} meters (m), 10^{-3} millimeters (mm), 10^3 nanometers (nm), or 10^4 Å. It is often referred to as a micron.

Stoichiometry. As used here, the relative proportions of the various elements of which a compound is composed.

Unit cell. Ideally, the smallest subunit of a crystal that retains all the characteristics of composition and structure of the crystal; a quadrangular prism enclosing a particular arrangement of atoms that represents the smallest building block of which, with thousands of identical blocks packed together in an orderly fashion, the crystal is composed. (The compositional complexity of crystalline materials such as enamel requires a pragmatic definition of unit cell in which the compositional identity requirement is achieved by ascribing to the unit cell an artificial average composition that reflects the composition of the mineral as a whole.)

Unit cell parameters. A set of six measurable values (three lengths a, b, and c; and three angles, α, β, and γ) needed to describe the exact size and shape of the unit cell; also called lattice constants. The six values for hydroxyapatite are 9.418, 9.418, and 6.880 Å; and 90°, 90°, and 120°, respectively.

X-ray diffraction. A technique for determining the unit cell parameters and the detailed arrangements of atoms of a crystalline material. The structural information that results is the average over all unit cells in the sample.

SUGGESTED READINGS

Miles AEW (ed): Structural and Chemical Organization of Teeth, Vols I, II. New York, Academic Press, 1967 (These two volumes, though in need of revision, represent the most exhaustive presentation and discussion available from one source. Volume II is especially pertinent to this chapter).

Scott DC, Simmelink JW, Nygaard V: Structural aspects of dental caries. J Dent Res 53: 165–178, 1974 (This article is a detailed account of some of the structural aspects of enamel rods and crystallites that relate to enamel dissolution patterns observed *in vitro* and in carious lesions. It contains some excellent examples of the ingenious use of EM techniques that characterizes recent ultrastructural studies of enamel).

Young RA: Implications of atomic substitutions and other structural details in apatites. J Dent Res 53: 193–205, 1974 (A comprehensive review of what is known regarding ionic substitutions in apatite by the person most responsible for our present understanding of the subject.)

PART TWO

The Disease

8 Definition, Etiology, Epidemiology and Clinical Implications of Dental Caries

DONALD W. LEGLER

LEWIS MENAKER

Introduction
Definition
Historical Considerations
Etiology
  Bacteria
  Acid Dissolution
  Carbohydrates
Epidemiologic Considerations
  Correlation with Civilization
  National Origins
  Geographical Differences
  Family Differences
  Sex
  Age

Intraoral Patterns of Occurrence
Root Surface Caries
Host Factors
  Salivary Flow
  Tooth Morphology
  Tooth Composition
  Fluoride Experience
The Clinical Course of Dental Caries
  Implications for the Dental Profession
  Implications for Society
Summary
Glossary
Suggested Readings

INTRODUCTION

Dental caries ranks among the most significant of human diseases simply because of its frequency of occurrence. In this country over 95 per cent of the population is affected, ranking dental caries first among the chronic diseases affecting humankind in terms of the numbers of people involved.

Although the severity of the disease in terms of its life-threatening potential is limited except in rare instances, certain important consequences must be stressed.

Dental caries is costly. Dental treatment by its very nature demands high levels of manpower, and is time consuming and exacting. Therefore, dental caries is costly both in terms of time lost and money spent. The man-hours lost from work, school, or home attributable to dental diseases and treatment is incalculable. It is also expensive in terms of dollar flow. Fees paid by patients through the private sector account for the greatest cost, but considerable sums are also expended for dental services through various governmental agencies and public health programs. Added to this is the expense involved in educating the large numbers of health professionals required to cope with this disease in terms of prevention, treatment and oral rehabilitation.

Dental caries and its sequellae often involve pain. This may range from the sharp sensations arising from ingestion of sweets, to the deeper, more throbbing pain associated with thermal hypersensitivity and pulpal inflammation. In fact, the pain experienced by one suffering from a common toothache can be excruciating, as recognized by cartoonists through the years.

Another notable characteristic of the disease is its effect on esthetics. Dental caries is a disfiguring disease since the dentition is integrally related to one's smile, speech, and total personality. Furthermore, dental caries has implications relative to overall health. Not only is the dentition essential to the proper mastication of food for deglutition and proper digestion, but diseases of the teeth can have systemic effects as in the case of subacute bacterial endocarditis.

On balance, dental caries must be recognized as a significant disease process in the life history of man. True, its mortality and morbidity rates are low, but the disease remains a universal and costly problem facing dentistry. Its uniqueness stems from its progressive character, cost, discomfort, and its effects on health and personality.

DEFINITION

Dental caries can be defined in various ways. From the standpoint of a histopathologist, the disease can be described in terms of the stages of the lesion viewed microscopically (see Chap. 9). The chemist describes the caries process in terms of the interrelationship between pH, mineral flux, and solubility at the tooth-saliva interface (see Chap. 19). The microbiologist defines caries primarily in terms of the interactions involving oral bacteria and dental tissues (see Chap. 13). The dentist in an office setting describes the disease more in terms of its clinical appearance and the progress of the gross lesion.

Dental caries is fundamentally a microbial disease which affects the calcified tissues of teeth, beginning first with a localized dissolution of the inorganic structures of a given tooth surface by acids of bacterial origin, and leading to a disintegration of the organic matrix. It is normally a progressive disease and, if unchecked, the lesion will expand in size and progress pulpally resulting in increasing degrees of pain and pulpal inflammation. Ultimately, pulpal necrosis and loss of tooth vitality results.

Looking at dental caries more broadly, it can be seen as a multifactorial disease. Bacterial mediation occurs through the production of organic acids by oral microorganisms which utilize locally available carbohydrates as substrates. The diet of the host provides the chief source of such carbohydrates, so that diet may be viewed as a primary factor in determining susceptibility to the disease (see Chap. 16). A number of factors indigenous to the host also determine susceptibility and severity of the disease. These include saliva composition and flow rate (see Chap. 2 and 4), tooth form, arch alignment, and the physicochemical nature of the tooth surface. The latter can be influenced by the intake of various trace elements in the diet, or through a surface effect by elements such as fluoride (see Chap. 19 and 20). Finally, the composition of the bacterial plaque (see Chap. 11) is a primary factor. A number of different oral bacteria have been implicated in the caries process. Therefore, oral hygiene procedures which effectively remove plaque or which alter plaque metabolism (see Chap. 14 and 18) tend to inhibit dental caries. It is the combination of all these factors, superimposed upon the basic mechanism of bacterial acid dissolution of the tooth surface, that determines susceptibility to dental caries and the ultimate course of the disease.

HISTORICAL CONSIDERATIONS

The complexity of the caries process has awakened a liberal measure of intellectual, philosophical and research interest down through the centuries. Aristotle, Hippocrates, and Shakespeare all commented on dental caries in their writings. Concepts relative to the etiology of dental caries have ascribed the problem at various times in history to worms as causative agents, to an imbalance of the body humours, or to the internal disintegration of the tooth (the Vital Theory). Beginning with the observations of L. S. Parmly, in 1819, however, current understandings of the carious process began to take shape. Parmly noted that caries began on the enamel surfaces of teeth at sites where food stagnated and that the lesion progressed inward toward the pulp. He further speculated that a chemical agent was involved in the process.

Building on the observation by Pasteur that certain microorganisms convert sugars to lactic acid through fermentation, Emil Magitot in 1867 showed *in vitro* that fermentation of sugars caused dissolution of tooth structures. In his experiments he covered sound teeth with wax leaving only a small window. The teeth then were exposed to fermentation mixtures or dilute acids for varying periods of time with the result that artificial carious lesions developed.

The work of W. D. Miller (ca. 1890) involved a series of experiments that resulted in the elucidation of the chemoparasitic theory of caries etiology. This theory, with some refinement, can now be considered factual since supportive evidence has continued to mount over the past eighty years. Miller showed that certain dietary foodstuffs such as bread and sugar could decalcify the crown of a tooth in the presence of saliva when incubated at 37°C. Specifically, he noted that lactic acid was one identifiable reactant in mixtures of saliva and carbohydrates. He also noted that a wide variety of oral bacteria could produce acids in sufficient quantities to be implicated in the caries process and that certain of them could be found in carious dentin. Miller concluded that "dental decay is a chemoparasitic process consisting of two stages—decalcification or softening of the tissues, and dissolution of the softened residue." He concluded that no single species of microorganism caused caries, and he suggested that the process could be mediated by any microorganism capable of acid production and protein digestion.

Other theories for the etiology of dental caries have attributed the initiation of lesions to proteolysis, proteolysis-chelation, or to certain bacterially mediated mechanisms for removing phosphate from dental enamel. The proteolytic theory held that the organic elements of tooth structure provide the initial pathways for invasion by microorganisms or their products. Initial destruction of the protein matrix by hydrolytic enzymes was considered to precede loss of the inorganic phase. Gottlieb, for example. suggested that proteolytic enzymes first attack the lamellae, rod sheaths, tufts, and finally the walls of the dentinal tubules. Acid dissolution of the mineral phase was considered as a secondary phenomenon.

The proteolysis-chelation theory also considers dental caries to be a bacterial destruction of teeth wherein the initial attack essentially involves the organic components of enamel. It is suggested that the breakdown products of this organic phase have chelating properties that lead to dissolution of enamel minerals. A chelating agent is a molecule which can grasp a metal ion in a claw-like configuration (from the Greek *chele*: claw) to form a heterocyclic ring. Citrate is a commonly recognized chelator capable of binding calcium. A number of other chelates are found in biologic systems. Chelation has been proposed in the proteolysis-chelation theory as a process by which the inorganic components of enamel can be removed at a neutral or even an alkaline *p*H. This theory, as set forth by Schatz and Martin, is of historical interest. Very little corroborative evidence has surfaced in support of this theory as an explanation of the major events involved in the initiation of the caries lesion.

Evidence suggests that phosphates in the diet contribute toward a reduction in experimental dental caries as noted in a rodent model. Relative to this, various investigators have suggested that phosphate may be removed from dental enamel as a sequel to certain phases of plaque metabolism. For example, it has been noted that phosphoprotein phosphatase releases phosphate from tooth enamel *in vitro*. It was suggested that this enzyme might participate in the caries process by breaking down enamel phosphoproteins. At this time, however, supportive evidence for such a mechanism as the primary etiologic factor in the caries process is meager.

While chelation, proteolysis, and phosphatase activities may contribute to the caries process in varying degree, it seems clear that the major underlying process involves the acid dissolution of calcified tooth structure. Other mechanisms, if viable, are secondary to this. Therefore, the acidogenic or chemoparasitic theory has advanced from the status of theory to that of fact in the light of current understandings of the caries process. Detailed evidence for these current concepts follows.

ETIOLOGY

Dental caries is a multifactorial disease. Numerous authors have recognized and described the caries process as one which is dependent upon the interrelationships of three main groups of factors. These groupings involve microbial, substrate, and host factors (see Fig. 8-1). It should be noted that for the disease process to be initiated, all three factors must exist simultaneously.

Bacteria

Definitive evidence for regarding dental caries as a bacterially mediated disease process has come from gnotobiotic studies. Orland, in 1955, conducted an experiment involving three groups of young, caries susceptible rats. One group was maintained under germfree conditions on a cariogenic diet. No caries resulted. A second group, which included littermates of those in the first group, was also maintained under germfree conditions, but these were infected with a strain of *enterococci* in conjunction with the cariogenic diet. Caries developed. The third group involved a control group raised in a normal environment with the same diet. Caries occurred in this group as well. It seemed clear that specific strains of bacteria were, in fact, involved in the caries process and that their cariogenic potential was interrelated with dietary factors. This same type of experiment has been repeated on numerous occasions in various other laboratories. From such experiments the role of certain oral streptococci in dental caries has been more clearly defined, as well as the cariogenic activity of other groups of bacteria such as the lactobacilli and actinomyces (see Chaps. 11 and 13).

More recently, attention has focused on the role of dental plaque in the initiation of the caries lesion at specific sites on the tooth. By definition, **plaque** is an adherent bacterial mass which preferentially develops on the tooth surface. It is easily stainable by using certain disclosing agents and it is not removable by rinsing or a water spray. Plaque generates bacterial metabolites. These, along with certain exogenous materials, are concentrated within plaque. It is this bacterial ecosystem which enables the destructive influences of cariogenic bacteria to be focused on specific tooth surface sites. (See Chapters 11, 12, and 13).

Acid Dissolution

The fact that teeth are decalcified in the presence of acid is well established. A number of *in vitro* experiments have shown that dental enamel will demineralize when suspended in a test tube containing acid buffered at a pH of 4.0 to 5.5. Calcium and phosphate from the dissolved tooth can be recovered in the buffer solution.

The acid producing (**acidogenic**) properties of a number of oral bacteria have been documented. These organisms are also **aciduric** in that most can grow and multiply best in an acid environment. These bacteria create an acid environment by converting carbohydrates to organic end products such as lactic, pyruvic, acetic, butyric, and propionic acids. The organic acids produced by plaque bacteria are capable of lowering the pH at the plaque-enamel interface to levels at which demineralization can take place. This has been

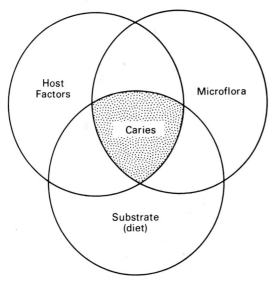

Fig. 8-1. The major etiologic factors involved in the dental caries process.

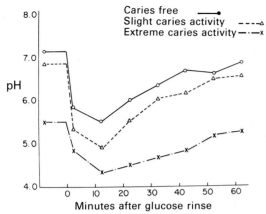

Fig. 8-2. *p*H recordings at the plaque-enamel interface of upper incisor teeth following a glucose rinse. (Stephan RM: J. Dent. Res. 23, 257–266 1944)

confirmed experimentally. Microelectrodes have been placed at the tooth surface beneath a layer of plaque in human subjects and, following rinsing with a sugar solution, *p*H ranges of 4.0 to 5.5 and below have been recorded. Recordings of the *p*H were much lower beneath the plaque of extremely caries active subjects as compared to caries free individuals, presumably reflecting differences in composition of the bacterial plaques (Fig. 8-2). These low *p*H levels have been shown to persist for periods of over one hour. The plaque layer also shields the tooth surface from the washing and buffering action of saliva.

Recent research indicates that when plaque is systematically removed from the tooth surface by closely controlled oral hygiene procedures and biweekly professional prophylaxis caries incidence can be markedly reduced to a level approaching zero.

All of these pieces of evidence fit together logically to portray the role of bacterial acids as prime mediators of the caries process.

Carbohydrates

For centuries it has been recognized that persons who ingest diets containing appreciable quantities of sugars and starches tend to experience tooth decay. Populations such as the Eskimos, who subsisted on diets heavy in fats but low in carbohydrates, historically have tended to have little or no tooth decay. Similarly, the natives of Tristan de Cunha with a simple diet low in fermentable carbohydrates

historically exhibited only minimal caries experience. With the recent encroachment of Western customs and a diet rich in fermentable carbohydrates, caries incidence in both of the above populations has increased. This strong direct correlation between intake of fermentable carbohydrates and caries seems to prevail on a worldwide basis.

The need for carbohydrates, especially sugars, in the caries process has been shown experimentally through a number of mutually supportive observations. First, as previously noted, oral bacteria which have been shown to be cariogenic in gnotobiotic experiments have also been shown to utilize fermentable carbohydrates preferentially as an energy source *in vitro*. Secondly, animal experiments involving caries susceptible rats inoculated with known cariogenic organisms fail to show the development of dental caries unless sugar is added to the diet.

A number of other formal experiments have illustrated the role of fermentable carbohydrates in the caries process, a role which is primarily a local one occurring at the plaque-tooth surface interface. The first of these experiments involved an animal study utilizing two groups of caries susceptible rats. Each group was fed a high carbohydrate diet, except that the test group was fed by stomach tube so that the dietary carbohydrate was excluded from the oral cavity. The control group was fed in the normal manner. Results showed that the thirteen rats in the test group developed no caries lesions during the course of the study as compared to an average of 6.7 lesions in the control group. This illustrates that the influence of carbohydrates is due primarily to the local effects during passage through the oral cavity.

Another classic experiment, this time involving human subjects, was the Vipeholm dental caries study, a comprehensive investigation which involved 436 adult patients housed in a mental institution in Sweden. Basically, this population was divided into several groups, each receiving a different diet. The control group was given a basic diet relatively low in refined carbohydrates for two years (Carbohydrate Study I). During the final two years the diet of the control group more closely resembled the typical Swedish diet (Carbohydrate Study II). A second group was given the same basic diet with the addition of sugar in solution at mealtime during the four year period (sucrose group). A third

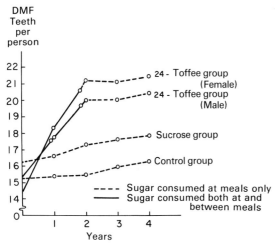

Fig. 8-3. Observations on the effects of sugar intake on dental caries incidence (Modified from BE Gustafsson, et al.: Acta. Odont. Scand. 11, 206–231 1954)

group received the basic diet plus twenty four pieces of chewy toffee which was eaten at various times throughout the day for two years. As can be noted (Fig. 8-3) the caries incidence of patients in the sucrose group exceeded that of patients in the control group. The caries experience of patients in the toffee group, expressed in DMF teeth per person, greatly exceeded that of patients in the sucrose and control groups. In fact, patients in the control group exhibited less than 10 per cent of the caries incidence noted in the toffee group over a two year period. Thus the importance of the frequency of sugar intake as well as consistency of the sugar containing foods was underscored (see Chap. 16).

Another set of observations, recorded in Australia, involved the orphaned children at Hopewood House. These children were raised on a diet which was essentially vegetarian and low in fermentable carbohydrates. Thirteen year old children raised on this dietary regime exhibited approximately 90 per cent fewer carious teeth (DMFT) than did similar aged children attending state schools in Australia. Viewed from a different perspective, for each ten carious teeth that a typical thirteen year old child would have, his counterpart at Hopewood House would have only one.

The common conclusion of these studies is to underscore the vital role that fermentable carbohydrates, especially sugars, play in the etiology of dental caries. The etiology of dental caries involves an interplay between oral bacteria, local carbohydrates, and the tooth surface that may be shown diagrammatically as follows:

$$\text{Bacteria} + \underset{\text{(Substrate)}}{\text{Sugars}} \rightarrow \underset{\text{Acids}}{\text{Organic}} \rightarrow \text{Caries}$$

This simplified explanation will be elaborated upon in several of the following chapters.

EPIDEMIOLOGIC CONSIDERATIONS

Epidemiology may be defined as the study of the frequency or patterns of occurrence and distribution of a disease as it is seen in population groups. Dental caries experience is usually estimated by means of a **caries index,** a measurement system designed to record the number of teeth or tooth surfaces in an individual that have been attacked by dental caries. The most commonly used system involves a determination of the number of decayed (D), missing (M) and filled (F) teeth or surfaces. This index is more fully discussed in Chap. 23. In addition, dental caries can be widely seen throughout the animal kingdom with its occurrence generally paralleling access to fermentable carbohydrate foods. Carious lesions have been noted in bears, dogs, horses, monkeys, and of course laboratory animals such as the hamster and the rat.

Correlations with Civilization

As previously noted relative to the indigenous populations of Northern Alaska and Tristan de Cunha, the incidence and frequency of dental caries in humans seems to parallel the degree of "civilization." Skulls of prehistoric man exhibit caries lesions very infrequently. Rough natural foods which probably constituted the diet were primarily responsible for this observation through their abrasive action and low cariogenic potential. Today, dental caries is virtually a universal disease as civilization has penetrated to almost all areas of the world. Even so, it is generally true that caries experience is higher in those highly industrialized nations with high annual intakes of sugar and easy access to processed foods, refined carbohydrates, soft drinks, and snack foods.

More remote areas of the world generally host populations with lower caries rates.

National Origins

Variations in caries rates between persons living in different countries have been observed. Higher caries rates can be noted in England, Norway, and Denmark, for example, than is the case in Spain or the countries of North Africa. These differences are probably attributable to different dietary habits, variance in access to cariogenic foodstuffs, cultural differences, and climatic conditions.

Differences in dental caries rates between countries may also be carried over to second and third generation descendants in the United States. Examinations of World War II recruits disclosed such differences. Recruits from Chinese and Russian backgrounds tended to exhibit fewer caries lesions than those from English or Irish backgrounds (Fig. 8-4).

Geographical Differences

Dental caries in the United States also exhibits a geographic pattern. Studies conducted on World War I and II recruits showed that individuals from New England, the Middle Atlantic states and the Northern Pacific states tended to have the greatest caries experience. Recruits from the Central and Southeastern regions followed, and those from the

Rocky Mountains and Southwestern states had the lowest caries experience.

Since artificial water fluoridation was not widespread at the time of the two World Wars, it may be assumed that these differences were due in part to regional differences in natural fluoride levels of water supplies. Concentration of different ethnic groups in certain geographic areas of the United States, variations in water intake between warmer climes and cooler ones, and a greater tendency toward snacking for energy purposes in cooler areas may also constitute factors underlying these geographic differences. Finally, variation in the content of other trace minerals in the water supply or foods may also be partially responsible for this variation.

Family Differences

A familial pattern of caries experience seems to hold true. Siblings of individuals with high caries susceptibility are also generally caries active, whereas siblings of caries immune individuals generally also exhibit low caries rates. Similarly children of parents with a low caries experience tend also to have a low caries rate, whereas the converse is true for children whose parents have a high caries rate. Although genetic factors such as tooth morphology may play a part, these patterns are attributable primarily to the emphasis placed upon oral hygiene in certain families as compared to others, the receipt of routine dental care, and the dietary habits of the family.

Sex

Girls consistently show a higher caries experience than boys of the same chronological age, at least into the early teens (Figure 8-5). Girls exhibit, in particular, a greater number of filled (F) teeth. This is attributable largely to the fact that the teeth of girls erupt at an earlier age than do the teeth of boys. Therefore, girls' teeth are at risk relative to dental caries at an earlier age.

This time differential is particularly significant during the formative years because teeth have been shown to be maximally susceptible to dental caries immediately after eruption. This is due to the fact that the chemical structure of teeth in the immediate posteruptive stage is suboptimal in terms of caries resist-

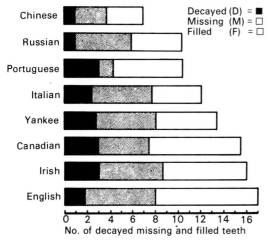

Fig. 8-4. The relationship between the incidence of dental caries and nationality. (N Eng J Med vol. 20: P 509, 1944)

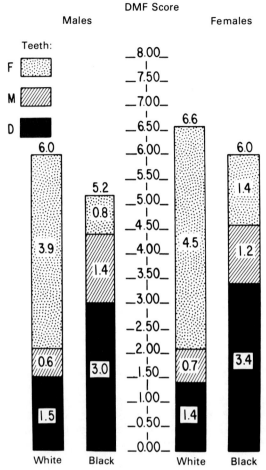

DMF Score

Males   Females

Teeth:

F

M

D

Fig. 8-5. Caries experience of individuals aged twelve to seventeen according to sex and age (Kelly, JE Vital Health Stat [11], no. 144. United States Public Health Service, 1974)

ance. As teeth are exposed to saliva and constituents in the diet, the outer layers of the tooth take up additional minerals (see Chap. 19) from the environment in a process known as posteruptive maturation. This maturation process confers on the tooth a greater resistance to dental caries.

Age

At approximately age six exfoliation of the primary teeth starts and the permanent teeth begin to erupt. By age twelve this process is usually complete with the exception of the third molars. Several studies have shown that even at age six, about 20 percent of children have experienced dental caries in their perma-

nent dentition, and a decayed, missing and filled teeth (DMFT) rate of 0.5 can be expected (Fig. 8-6). By age twelve over 90 per cent of children have experienced dental caries and a DMFT rate of approximately 5.5 can be noted in some areas of the United States. The generalization can be made that during the period of tooth eruption one new carious permanent tooth develops each year. The DMFS accelerates at a greater rate than the DMFT beyond the age of eight; so that by age twelve a DMFS of 7.5 can be taken as an average figure in the United States.

The most frequently involved tooth of the child of 6–12 years of age is the first permanent molar, or six year molar. By age 12, 70 per cent of the lower first permanent molars are carious, and 55 per cent of the upper first permanent molars are involved (Fig. 8-7). As the age of the individual advances the number of unaffected tooth surfaces at risk to dental caries is reduced, since carious teeth are either restored or extracted with time.

Intraoral Patterns of Occurrence

Pits and fissures are the most caries susceptible areas of teeth. Such sites provide protective niches for the entrapment of food debris and a sheltered environment for bacterial growth (Fig. 8-8).

Lesions which involve the buccal, lingual,

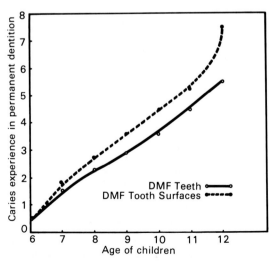

Fig. 8-6. DMF teeth and DMF tooth surfaces in the permanent dentition of 6 to 12 year old children. (Finn, in Toverud et al.: Survey of the Literature of Dental Caries. National Academy of Sciences-National Research Council, 1953)

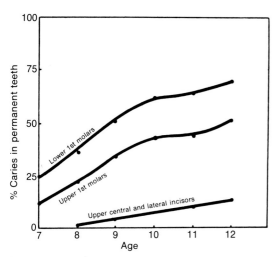

Fig. 8-7. Dental caries in selected permanent teeth. (Klein, et al.: The Epidemiology of Dental Disease. U.S. Public Health Service, 1974)

mesial, or distal surfaces of the tooth are referred to as smooth surface caries (Fig. 8-9). There is a differential susceptibility to caries on various smooth surfaces. Interproximally, a prime site for the initiation of caries is in the contact area. On the buccal and lingual surfaces, lesions tend to occur most frequently on that portion of the tooth surface which is gingival to the point of greatest convexity. Therefore, lesions tend to occur in the most inaccessible places which by definition are relatively protected from the normal self cleansing effect of the cheeks, tongue, and saliva as well as being more difficult to reach with a toothbrush.

There is a typical hierarchical pattern to caries attack. As previously noted the most frequently involved sites for coronal dental caries are the pit and fissure areas. The second most frequently involved sites are the interproximal smooth surfaces of the posterior teeth and the maxillary anterior teeth. The least frequently involved sites are the interproximal surfaces of the mandibular anterior teeth and the labial surfaces of the twelve anterior teeth. The occurrence of buccal and lingual smooth surface lesions is independent of the above scheme. One practical sequel of this observation, of course, is that if one notes caries involvement of the mandibular anterior teeth, one can assume that there is widespread involvement of the occlusal and interproximal areas elsewhere in the mouth. Caries also tends to occur bilaterally. In approximately 75 per cent of the cases, if caries is in evidence on a given posterior tooth it can also be noted in the same tooth on the contralateral side. Four out of five times this bilateral involvement will involve the same surface.

Root Surface Caries

Dental caries is often characterized as a disease of children and young adults. With the increasing life span of individuals in the United States, however, there is a marked increase in the percentage of elderly persons in our society. With advance in age, there is increased opportunity for gingival recession to occur due to a number of factors. With such gingival recession, the root surfaces become exposed leading to the possibility of caries attack. Root surface lesions exhibit a different pattern of destruction, as compared to enamel caries, in that the lesion usually presents as a broad, shallow defect which is usually noted in the area of the cemento-enamel junction (Fig. 8-10). Studies have indicated that as many as 60 per cent of individuals in the age group of 50 to 60 years have experienced root surface caries.

Host Factors

One of the fascinating aspects of dental caries as a disease is the variant picture of the appearance of the lesion itself and its progress with time. A caries lesion may appear clinically to be soft and mushy, brown and hard, or white and chalky. It may progress to a clini-

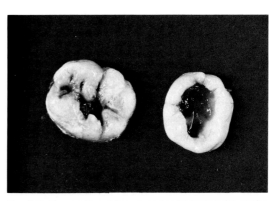

Fig. 8-8. Gross pit and fissure caries involving the occlusal surfaces of the teeth.

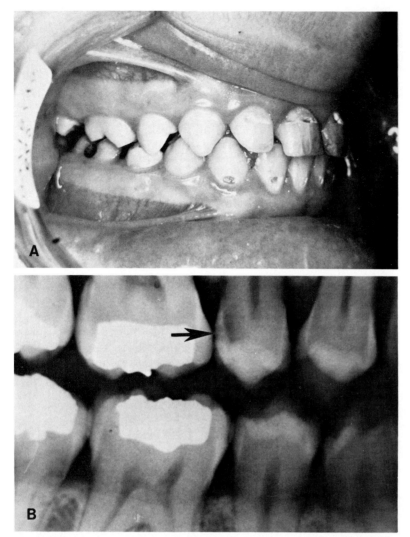

Fig. 8-9. Smooth surface caries involving (**A**) labial surfaces of teeth and (**B**) the interproximal surface as seen on a radiograph.

cally detectable cavity in less than three months, or it may display a slow progress extending over a period of years. Many incipient lesions never develop into clinical cavities, since they can be arrested (see Chaps. 19 and 20) in an early stage of development. Furthermore, sometimes even large clinical lesions can become hardened and shiny indicating arrestment following collapse of undermined tooth structure and the exposure of the lesion to the self cleansing forces of mastication or following changes in the local chemical and microbiologic environment (Fig. 8-11).

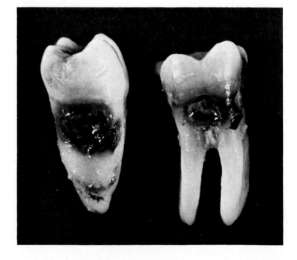

Fig. 8-10. Examples of root surface caries.

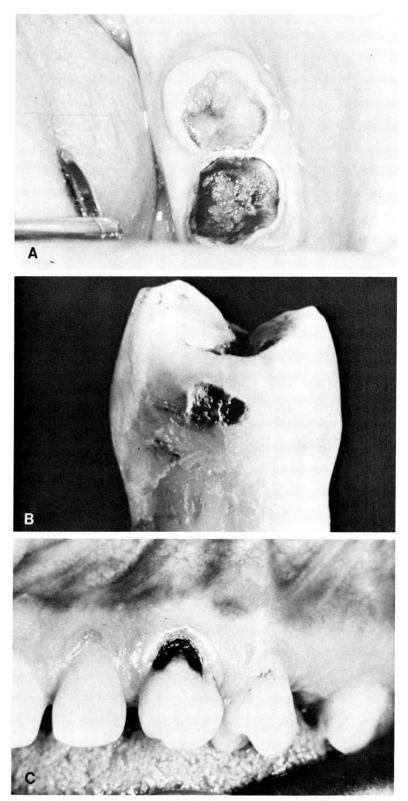

Fig. 8-11. Examples of arrested caries. (**A**) A large occlusal lesion; (**B**) an interproximal lesion; (**C**) a buccal smooth surface lesion. (Courtesy Dr. WR Bodden)

Of interest also is the individual with **rampant caries.** This is a relative term used to describe a condition characterized by an extremely high caries attack rate and rapid progression of lesions. Frequently, the labial surfaces of anterior teeth are involved as well as the interproximal surfaces of the lower incisor teeth (Fig. 8-12).

Others fall into the two per cent of the population in the United States which are **caries immune.** Such individuals exhibit no evidence of dental caries even though in many cases they display customary dietary habits. The absence of dental caries may be due to tooth morphology, type of oral flora, presence of immune factors in saliva, fluoride intake, dietary influences, or a combination of these and other host factors.

It can be seen therefore that the initiation, progress and clinical appearance of the lesion is influenced by a number of host factors which vary in impact according to the individual.

Salivary Flow

Salivary composition and flow (see Chap. 2, 3, and 4) is a determinant in the caries process. Individuals with xerostomia, a failure to form saliva, commonly exhibit rampant caries. Conversely, a liberal flow of saliva bathes tooth surfaces and acts to clear carbohydrates from the oral cavity. Immunoglobulins, nonspecific immune factors, minerals, and other substances present in saliva also have an impact on the caries process.

Tooth Morphology *High Risk*

Tooth contour is also a determinant in the dental caries process. Teeth with broad, flat cuspal inclines and shallow cuspal fossae are less likely to trap food than those with deep fossae and an abundance of accessory grooves. Similarly teeth with rounded, tight contact points interproximally are less prone to harbor plaque and debris interproximally than those with broad, flat contact areas. The degree of curvature of the buccal and lingual surfaces of the tooth and the height of contour relative to the gingival margin are also host factors which have an impact on the caries process. Teeth with diastemas, for example, are less apt to exhibit interproximal caries than are those with the usual contact relationship, since the interproximal surfaces are in self cleansing areas.

Tooth Composition

The composition of the mineralized portion of the tooth is another important variable in the caries process. Fluoride incorporated into developing teeth as fluorapatite affords a marked tooth resistance to acid dissolution. Other elements incorporated into tooth enamel are also known to alter the caries rate. Evidence also indicates that the outermost layers of enamel change in composition following tooth eruption through a process of maturation. **Enamel maturation** is the process by which a newly erupted tooth takes up

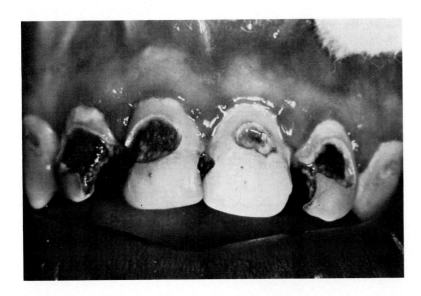

Fig. 8-12. Rampant caries.

additional minerals and trace elements from its environment while simultaneously increasing in surface hardness and acid resistance. In addition, evidence suggests that the preeruptive nutritional status, particularly as regards protein intake, may play a role in determining the caries resistance of teeth.

Fluoride Experience

Given the operation of other factors previously noted, the history of the individual relative to fluoride intake in the diet is an important variable in the development of dental caries. Individuals reared in an area containing optimal amounts of fluoride in the water supply can normally be expected to exhibit approximately 60 per cent fewer caries lesions than their counterparts living in non-fluoridated areas. The reduction in carious interproximal surfaces is most notable, approaching 80 per cent, whereas the reduction in pit and fissure lesions is considerably less than 60 per cent. Exposure to systemic fluoride tablets, office applied topical fluorides, fluoride dentifrices, and fluoride mouthwashes also modify caries experience (see Chap. 20). Clinically, one can still anticipate some pit and fissure caries in the patient who has grown up in a fluoridated community, but the reduction in smooth surface lesions is usually dramatic (see Chap. 21).

THE CLINICAL COURSE OF DENTAL CARIES

A definitive discussion of the caries lesion is presented in several chapters that follow. The clinical implications of the caries lesion should be recognized, however, since progress of the lesion results ultimately in need for treatment. As the caries lesion develops, the area of cavitation normally proceeds both laterally and pulpally. Varying amounts of functional tooth structure are lost and, if left untreated, eventually pulpal necrosis occurs (Fig. 8-13). The patient often presents with pain, sensitivity upon chewing on the affected side, and perhaps swelling. Periapical pathology usually follows as a sequel to pulpal pathosis. Ultimately, in the absence of restorative treatment, the disease requires extraction of the offending tooth or root canal therapy.

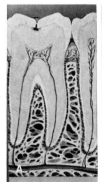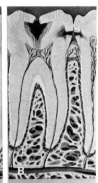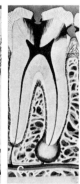

Fig. 8-13. A diagrammatic illustration of the progress of the gross clinical caries lesion: (**A**) an occlusal lesion penetrating into the dentin; (**B**) the occlusal lesion extending laterally along the dentinoenamel junction and extending pulpally through the dentin. Proximal smooth surface lesions are also depicted; (**C**) extension of the occlusal caries lesion to the pulp with ensuing pulpal necrosis and periapical abscess formation.

Implications for the Dental Profession

The treatment of dental caries is accomplished by the general dentist through restorative treatment of the lesion. This normally involves the removal of carious tissue and restoration with an amalgam, gold or plastic filling material. Advanced lesions may require endodontics or oral surgery performed either by the generalist or an appropriate specialist. Loss of the tooth results in the need for a fixed bridge or a removable partial denture. Alternatively, many patients choose to allow the area to remain edentulous. This process is frequently repeated over and over as successive teeth are neglected and eventually extracted due to dental caries. The end result of this chain of neglect is usually treatment with a removable complete denture.

By far, the vast majority of caries lesions involving the 40 per cent of the population who receive routine dental care are treated by restorative measures. Thus the disease of dental caries has determined in large part the character of dental practice in the United States. The average general dentist is essentially a restorative specialist who devotes the major portion of his or her professional efforts to the placement of amalgam, gold, or plastic filling materials. Oral diagnosis, radiology, treatment planning, and anesthesiology are all oriented toward this principal activity.

The remaining 60 per cent of the population who do not seek routine dental care find themselves in this category due to fear, lack of dental education, economics, inability to gain access to the dental care delivery system, or sheer apathy and neglect. These individuals demand emergency care, usually extractions, or they seek restorative care on an episodic basis. Proper replacement of missing teeth lost because of advanced dental caries involves removable or fixed prosthodontic treatment, with costs resulting which are much higher in comparison to those involving preventive or early restorative treatment.

Implications for Society

It can be seen that dental caries is indeed a costly disease. It monopolizes the attention, skills and time of the majority of dentists. Over one billion unfilled cavities are said to exist within the population of the United States. Approximately 15 per cent of the health care dollars spent each year in the United States involves dental treatment. The majority of this financial outlay is directly referrable to dental caries. Dental caries is a serious disease and a major public health problem which touches virtually every member of society in terms of personal involvement, cost, pain, and discomfort. When these factors are considered, along with the multifactorial nature of the disease, dental caries emerges as one of the most fascinating diseases affecting mankind.

SUMMARY

Dental caries is a complex, multifactorial disease. It occurs across a wide spectrum of the animal kingdom with incidence closely correlated with the dietary intake of fermentable carbohydrates. The etiology of dental caries is directly traceable to the action of certain oral microorganisms which produce organic acids through metabolism of carbohydrate substrates. The acids, in turn, attack the tooth surface resulting in dissolution of the inorganic structure of the enamel. Although caries is noted clinically as a cavitation in the tooth surface, this stage is preceded by a series of reactions at the biochemical level which involves the tooth surface and the surrounding medium especially at the plaque-tooth interface. There are correlations in population groups between caries experience and such factors as age, sex, national origin, geographic location, degree of civilization, and family influences. In addition, the occurrence of caries lesions within the oral cavity exhibits certain predictable patterns. The disease is of major impact on society because of its widespread, almost universal occurrence, and because of its progressive character, costs, and effects on health and personality. This situation is further underscored by the fact that dental caries, while the most widespread chronic disease known to mankind, is virtually 100 per cent preventable.

GLOSSARY

Acidogenic bacteria. Those bacteria which produce acids as metabolites through metabolic action on suitable substrates.

Aciduric bacteria. Those bacteria which grow and multiply best in a low pH environment.

Arrested caries. Carious areas in which the progression of the lesion has ceased. Frequently this is accompanied by a clinically detectable hardening of the lesion. Such arrest may follow the collapse of undermined enamel which allows exposure of the sheltered area to the cleansing activities of saliva and mastication, or to changes in dietary or host factors.

Caries immune. This term is applied to individuals comprising about 2 per cent of the population who have had no evidence of dental caries despite the fact that they seemingly conform to usual dietary standards. This may be due to tooth morphology, type of oral flora, presence of salivary immune fac-

tors, fluoride intake, dietary influence, or a combination of these and other host factors. The term is also used to describe certain areas of teeth such as lingual surfaces of lower anterior teeth which are seldom involved in the caries attack.

Dental caries. A microbial disease which affects the calcified tissues of the teeth, beginning first with a localized dissolution of the inorganic structures of a given tooth surface by acids of bacterial origin and leading to a secondary disintegration of the organic matrix. It is also a multifactorial disease in that the presence of fermentable carbohydrates which act as bacterial substrates, and a number of variable host factors combine to influence the disease process.

Dental plaque. A bacterial mass which preferentially develops and adheres to the tooth surface. It is easily stainable by using suitable disclosing agents and it is not removable by a water spray or rinsing.

Epidemiology. The study of the frequency, or pattern of occurrence and distribution, of a disease as it occurs in population groups.

Etiology. The sum of the known causative factors of a disease.

Fermentable carbohydrates. Those carbohydrates such as starch, sucrose, or the simple sugars which are easily metabolized as an energy source by appropriate bacteria leading to the production of acid metabolites.

Gnotobiotic Animals. Those experimental animals, such as rats or mice, which are raised in a germ-free or controlled environment and which harbor a known bacterial flora.

Multifactorial Disease. A disease that results from a combination of many different factors acting together to produce conditions which favor inception of the disease process.

Optimal Fluoridation. A situation in which the water supply of a community is adjusted to the ideal level, usually one part per million, by adding fluoride supplements to the water supply. Alternatively, in the limited number of communities which have an overabundance of fluoride in the water, it can involve the removal of fluoride in order to attain an appropriate level.

Rampant Caries. A relative term which describes a condition characterized by an extremely high caries attack rate with rapid progression of lesions. Frequently facial and lower anterior interproximal surfaces are involved.

Root Caries. Also termed senile or cemental caries in the literature, such lesions occur in older age groups secondary to gingival recession. Lesions develop on the root surface usually as a broad, shallow defect.

Tooth Maturation. The process by which a newly erupted tooth takes up additional minerals and trace elements from its environment while simultaneously increasing in surface hardness and acid resistance.

Vital Theory. A theory, prevalent during the eighteenth century, that ascribed the etiology of dental caries to an internal disintegration of tooth structure.

Xerostomia. A condition in which the flow of saliva is markedly reduced or absent. This condition is encountered in certain systemic diseases as well as in patients receiving heavy doses of radiation to the oral region in association with cancer therapy.

SUGGESTED READINGS

Axelsson P, Lindhe J: Effect of fluoride on gingivitis and dental caries in a preventive program based on plaque control. Commun Dent Oral Epidemiol 3: 156–160, 1975

Banting DW, Ellen RP: Carious lesions on the roots of teeth: a review for the general practitioner. J Can Dent Assoc 10: 496–504, 1976

Curzon MEJ, Losee FL: Dental caries and trace element composition of whole human enamel: Eastern United States. J Am Dent Assoc 94: 1146–1150, 1977

Fisher FJ: A field survey of dental caries, periodontal disease and enamel defects in Tristan de Cunha. Br Dent J 125(10): 447–453, 1968

Gibbons RJ, Van Houte J: Dental caries. Anna Rev Med 26: 121–136, 1975

Goldsworthy NE: The biology of the children of Hopewood House. Aust Dent J 3(5): 309–330, 1958

Gustafsson BG, Quensel CE, Swenlander LL, Lundquist C, Granen H, Bonow BE, Krasse B: The Vipeholm dental caries study. The effect of different levels of carbohydrate intake on caries activity in 436 individuals observed for five years. Acta Odontol Scand 11: 232–364, 1954

Hyde RW: Socioeconomic aspects of dental caries. N Engl J Med 230: 506–510, 1944

Kelly JE, Harvey CR: Decayed, missing and filled teeth among youths 12–17 years of age in the United States. United States Public Health Service. Vital Health Stat 11 144: 1–11, 1974

Kite OW, Shaw JH, Sognnaes RF: The prevention of experimental tooth decay by tube feeding. J Nutr 42: 89–103, 1950

Klein H: The epidemiology of dental disease. Collected papers 1937–47. Federal Security Agency, US Public Health Service, Washington DC, 1948

Kreitzman SN, Irving S, Navia JM Harris RS: Enzymatic release of phosphate from rat molar enamel by phosphoprotein phosphatase. Nature 223: 520–21, 1969

McPhail CWB, Grainger RM: A mapping procedure for the geographic pathology of dental caries. Int Dent J 19: 380–392, 1969

Menaker L, Navia JM: Effect of undernutrition during the perinatal period in caries develpment in the rat. J Dent Res 52: 680–687, 1973

Moore WJ, Corbett E: The distribution of dental caries in ancient British populations. Caries Res 7: 139–153, 1973

Orland FJ, Blayney JR, Harrison JW, Reyniers JA, Trexler PC, Ervin RF, Gordon HA, Wagner M: Experimental caries in germ-free rats innoculated with enterococci. J Am Dent Assoc 50: 259–292, 1955

Poulsen S, Horowitz HS: An evaluation of the hierarchical method of describing the pattern of dental caries attack. Commun Dent Oral Epidemiol 2: 7–11, 1974

Schatz A, Martin JJ: Speculation on lactobacilli and acid as possible anticaries factors. NY State Dent J 21: 367–379, 1955

Stephan RM: Intra-oral hydrogen ion concentrations associated with dental caries activity. J Dent Res 23: 257–266, 1944

Toverud G, Finn SB, Cox GJ, Bodecker CF, Shaw JH: Survey of the literature of dental caries. Publication 225. National Academy of Sciences-National Research Council, Washington DC, 1953

Volker JF: The effect of fluorine on the solubility of enamel and dentin. Proc Soc Exp Biol Med 42: 725–727, 1939

9 Histopathology of Caries Lesions

SEYMOUR HOFFMAN

Introduction
General Comments on Caries Infection
Microanatomy of Sound Enamel
    Surface Topography
    Subsurface Structures and Diffusion Pathways
Enigma of the Intact Surface Zone in Noncavitated White Spot Enamel Lesions
Pulpodentinal Complex and the Microanatomy of Sound Dentin

Microscopic Features of Active Dentinal Caries Lesions
Microscopic Features of Arrested Dentinal Caries Lesions
Caries of Cementum
Indirect Pulp Capping
Summary
Glossary
Suggested Readings

INTRODUCTION

While the chapter entitled "Clinical Cariology" was concerned primarily with the clinical and gross pathologic aspects of the caries process, the objectives of this chapter will be to concentrate on the microscopic alterations. In this regard, the microanatomic characteristics of sound dental tissues will be reviewed briefly. The subsequent discussions will deal with those histologic alterations which occur in early, noncavitated white spot enamel lesions and in advanced caries lesions of dentin and cementum.

As defined previously (see Chap. 8), "Caries is an infectious disease of the dental structures resulting in the dissolution of enamel or dentin, caused by microbial action;" (i.e., a lysis and demineralization of the basic structural components of the tooth. Keyes has referred to this disease as an odontolytic process.

GENERAL COMMENTS ON CARIES INFECTION

Caries infection usually is an intermittent process which may evolve through repeated phases of remissions and recurrances that ultimately will result in complete destruction of the involved tooth, if unchecked. Remissions may be short, long, or permanent. In the latter case the infectious process is considered to have been arrested and the remaining dental tissues remineralized (see Chap. 19).

In *any* infectious disease, the rate of tissue destruction is dependent upon any or all of several major factors. These factors include:

1. the local structural ability of the tissues to resist destructive forces (see Chap. 19);
2. the ability of systemic defenses or immunologic factors (see Chapter 15) to cope with the infection; and

3. the virulence of the etiologic microorganisms (see Chap. 13).

When tissues under attack are deficient structurally or chemically, or systemic resistance is low, tissue breakdown will be rapid. Conversely, when these tissues are not structurally or chemically deficient and systemic resistance is high, tissue breakdown will be slow or completely prevented. Of course, these are the extremes. In the general population there are many individual variations to the rate and pattern of tissue breakdown due to the wide gradation of structural deficiencies and resistances encountered on a person to person basis. Thus, the range of local tissue reactions to infectious processes is wide and varied among individuals. These same features are true of infections affecting the dentition. Structurally or chemically defective enamel will be destroyed more rapidly by a virulent cariogenic infection than enamel without such defects. On the other hand, if systemic defense factors are strong and efficient, and the enamel is well structured, it may be relatively immune to destructive virulent cariogens. Dental infection therefore may be clinically classified into acute, chronic, and arrested caries.

The acute phase is rapidly progressive and occurs generally among young individuals where the teeth are less mature and therefore more susceptible to attack. The chronic phase of dental caries is slow and intermittent and usually occurs in adults where the dentition is more mature. In both instances the structural integrity of the enamel, dentin, and systemic defense mechanisms undoubtedly are significant factors governing the rate of dental tissue destruction by virulent pathogens. Clinical acute cariogenic infection rapidly reduces sound dentin into a soft, necrotic, bacterial infected, yellowish-white mass. The dark brown affected zone (see Chap. 10) may be so narrow as to be not clinically recognizeable. However, it is still present. Chronic cariogenic infection slowly converts sound dentin into a leathery, brownish-black structure as seen on clinical examination. The third type of cariogenic disease affects a relatively small percentage of the young in the general population and is referred to as arrested dental caries. In this phase the destructive, active bacterial cariogens have been arrested and the pathologically softened, but structurally intact dental tissues have been remineralized (see Chap. 10).

This remineralization is probably the result of the deposition of mineral salts, either from the pulp, saliva or both, the saliva being considered to be a super saturated solution of calcium salts. Teeth with arrested caries lesions may remain functional for many years.

MICROANATOMY OF SOUND ENAMEL

Surface Topography

As with *all* disease conditions, one must know the gross and histiologic anatomy of sound tissues before one can understand and diagnose pathologic conditions in diseased structures, especially those in the intial phases of the disease. The same holds true for dental pathology. Thus, it is expedient that a brief review of the microanatomy of sound dental tissues be presented. Only through an understanding of the microstructures of sound dental tissues, the microscopic changes which occur under pathologic conditions, and the biologic potential of the pulp, can the clinician fully understand the mechanical and therapeutic aspects of his professional operations. The degree to which the dentist comprehends these relationships will be reflected in the quality of the dental health services provided.

As with all biologic mineralized structures, enamel is a mixture of inorganic and organic components, with the former comprising over 98 per cent of mature enamel. The major inorganic component is calcium hydroxyapatite, a hydrated calcium phosphate crystal (see Chap. 7).

The topographic morphology of the smooth surfaces of teeth (buccal, labial, lingual, and interproximal surfaces) which have not been exposed to abrasive masticatory forces for long periods of time are characterized by alternating concentric ridges, the perikymata, and narrow grooves. In unerupted and newly erupted teeth, the perikymata appear as sharply discreet, ridgelike bands, the occlusad edges of which terminate abruptly in an overlapping relationship with the upper contiguous ridge (Fig. 9-1). These ridges are narrower and in greater numbers per unit area in the cervical region of the enamel. They tend to broaden as they come closer to the buccal inclined planes of the cusps (Fig. 9-2). As

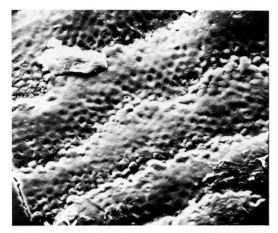

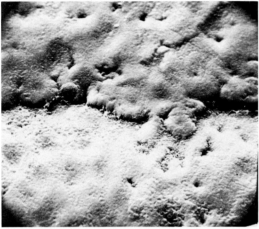

Fig. 9-1. Top: Scanning electron microscope view of overlapping perikymata in sound enamel from unerupted molar. (×600). Bottom: Higher power view of overlapped site rotated 180 degrees (×2300).

fuse organic matrix. The organization of these crystallites is one of outstanding consistency and orderliness. They are arranged in small packets of columns or prisms which comprise the structural units of the enamel. In the developing stages these crystallites are suspended in and separated from each other by the organic enamel matrix (intercrystallite matrix). The peripheral borders of immature prisms are partially or completely surrounded by a thin, noncrystalline zone of this matrix continuum, which is called the **prism sheath** (Fig. 9-4). These sheaths delineate the enamel prisms. Therefore, one may consider enamel as being a mineralized matrix composed of separate and distinct crystallites which are packaged into aggregate masses forming the prisms. Enamel prisms in the mature human dentition have been reported to be interdigitating structures possessing a "keyhole" configuration (Fig. 9-5A, B & C).

In the formation of enamel prisms, ameloblasts secrete minute membrane bound granules which coalesce extracellularly to form an amorphous, noncrystalline organic matrix. Shortly afterward, crystallites begin to form within this matrix. These crystallites are at first very thin. As they mature, they grow in

posteruptive maturation of enamel continues, resulting in increasing mineralization at the surface, these sharply discreet, overlapping ridges eventually are transformed into uninterrupted, smoothly continuous, undulating patterns of surface ridges and valleys (Fig. 9-3). Eventually, these topographic characteristics flatten out due to the abrasive forces of mastication and this distinctive enamel topography becomes obscured. However, the overlapping features appear to be retained into adulthood in the cervical region of the crown.

Subsurface Structures and Diffusion Pathways

As noted earlier, enamel is composed of hydroxyapatite crystallites dispersed within a dif-

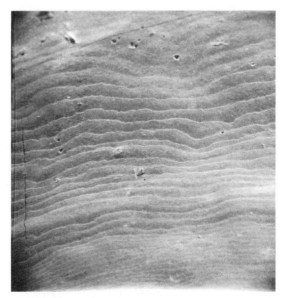

Fig. 9-2. Scanning electron micrograph illustrating the distribution of the overlapping type of perikymata on a sound enamel surface from a partially erupted third molar. Note the transtitional changes in the widths from narrow, concentric rings in the cervical area of the enamel to broader rings in the more occlusal areas (×18).

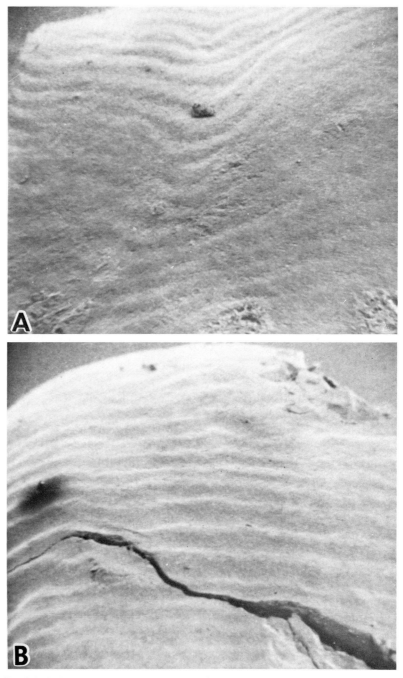

Fig. 9-3. **A, B.** The undulating topography of more mature enamel surfaces than seen in Figures 9-1 and 9-2 is illustrated above. These samples were obtained from teeth which had been in function for some time (×60).

length and in width at the expense of the surrounding and separating amorphous intercrystallite matrix, the excess matrix being forced outwardly by the growing, widening crystallites. During the process of enamel maturation, the earliest formed crystallites are always the longest and widest, with those forming subsequently being smaller and thinner until growth and maturation are completed. Thus, at the time of tooth eruption, the hydroxyapatite crystallites at the surface (the most recently formed crystallites) are much less mature than those in the subsurface regions and therefore are surrounded by a greater volume of matrix material. This material is continuous with the membrane which covers the surface of newly erupted teeth and probably represents what Gottlieb termed the primary enamel cuticle or what Listgarten identified as the basement membrane lamina of ameloblasts. During the years following the eruption of the tooth, the crystallites in this immature surface continue to mature by deposition of calcium and phosphate ions from the saliva until the surface becomes hypermineralized relative to its subsurface counterparts. This is referred to as the period of posteruptive maturation. During this period, teeth are usually highly susceptible to cariogenic attack, as evidenced by the high incidence of caries lesions which occur in children and adolescents, when compared to those in adults. From these observations it is conceivable to hypothesize that minute channels exist in this immature surface which may link it to subsurface regions. Many years ago, Darling reported that approximately 0.1 per cent of sound enamel was composed of minute spaces which increased in size and number with the progression of early enamel caries (see Chap. 10). It is conceivable that these microporosities may serve as diffusion pathways. Other more recent interpretations have suggested that bacterial acid diffusion can occur via intercrystallite spaces and prisms sheaths as described above, which are parts of the organic matrix continuum. Thus, structures are present in enamel which are not mineralized and which appear to be potential diffusion pathways for spread of the caries lesion.

There are other larger structures within enamel which may also serve as diffusion and/or invasion pathways to the subsurface areas. They are organic structures and are re-

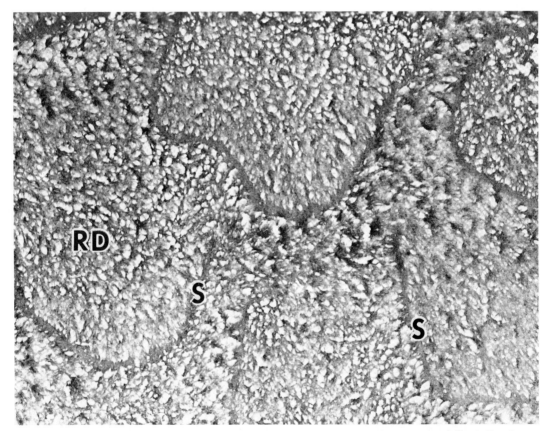

Fig. 9-4. Transmission electron photomicrograph of demineralized immature human enamel illustrating the organic matrix continuum in developing enamel. The empty spaces represent crystallite sites prior to demineralization. Note the matrix continuity of prism sheath substance (S) with that of the matrix lying between the crystallite spaces (intercrystallite matrix) RD. (Frank R, Nalbandian J: Structural and Chemical Organization of the Teeth. New York, Academic Press, 1967)

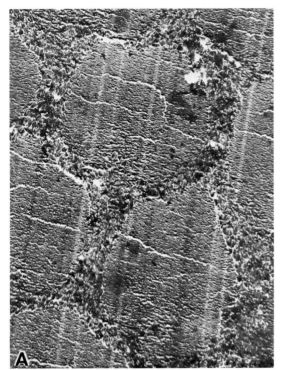

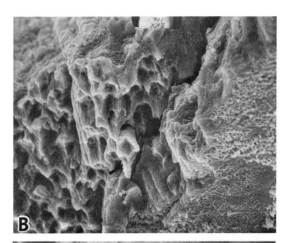

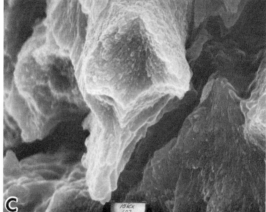

Fig. 9-5**A.** Transmission electron photomicrograph of mature enamel prisms in cross section illustrating the interdigitating "keyhole" pattern of prism relationships (approximate magnification ×20,000). (Meckel AH: Arch Oral Biol 10: 775–783, 1965) **B. C.** Scanning electron photomicrographs of prisms from sound enamel fractured perpendicularly to their long axes. These photomicrographs illustrate the full-dimensional appearance of the "keyhole"-like features of enamel prisms. (Top ×2000; Bottom ×10,000)

ferred to as **enamel lamellae.** These structures appear to be faults in the formation of enamel, extending from the surface (where they are attached to the embryologically derived enamel cuticle) into the subsurface regions for varying distances, sometimes reaching the dentinoenamel junction (Fig. 9-6). At times, they even have been found to extend well into dentin. The exact nature of these faults has not been definitively determined. Some believe them to be due to focal failures of the calcification process within or between developing prisms. Others believe them to be entrapped ameloblasts or portions thereof and their products (Fig. 9-7). The role these lamellae play in caries has long continued to be controversial. There are those who refer to these structures as major inroads for caries producing bacteria (Fig. 9-8). Others completely discount this possibility, while still others take a middle of the road attitude feeling that lamellae should not be overlooked as possible routes for toxin diffusion or bacterial invasion, but still believe that the "cracks" can be filled in and that subsequent secondary mineralization of these structures can occur. In any event, the experimental demonstration by Bergman of a fluid flow from the dentin to the enamel surface which appears to be related to enamel spindles and lamellae, accords well with the view of many investigators that these structures do constitute important pathways for the passage of substances into the enamel both from within and from without. Detailed microscopy studies have indicated that a very close relationship exists between enamel lamellae and the surrounding contiguous prism sheaths, (Fig. 9-9), a significant feature in relation to the spread of destructive cariogenic toxins.

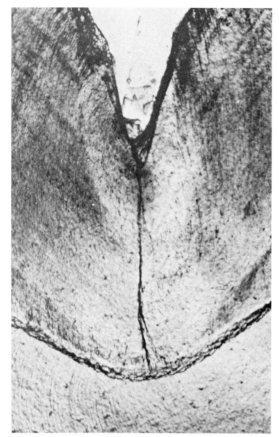

Fig. 9-6. Ground sections of mature human enamel through the occlusal fissure illustrating extension of a lamella from the surface to the dentino-enamel junction. (Hodson JJ: Oral Surg, Oral Med, Oral Pathol. 6: 305–317, 1953)

Rising for short distances into the enamel substance at the dentoenamel junction (DEJ) are the *enamel spindles*. These structures represent the terminal segments of odontoblastic processes within the enamel above the DEJ (Fig. 9-10). They may serve to link up diffusion lanes from enamel into the dentin. Thus, there would appear to be a vast network of intercommunicating organic structures dispersed throughout the enamel, perfusing every conceivable organic area from the surface cuticles to lamellae to prism sheaths to intercrystallite spaces and microporosities to spindles, right down into the pulp via the dentinal tubules. One may readily perceive how these ramifying organic networks may link up pathologic environmental disturbances originating on the enamel surface and subsequently transmit them to the pulp, inciting biochemi-

cal and structural changes and reactions all along the way.

Another microstructure of enamel, and one considered to be of major significance as a potential diffusion pathway, are the *Striae of Retzius* or incremental lines of prism growth. These "lines" may also serve as pathways for the subsurface diffusion of bacterial plaque toxins or for the transfer of ions from beneath the surface to the surface as in mineral losses due to acid attack. Darling has demonstrated by microradiography that in late white spot lesions, just prior to surface breakdown, radiolucent lines parallel to the Striae of Retzius and continuous with those in the body of the lesion could be seen passing through the surface under the "lips" of overlapping perikymata, which until that time have been totally radiopaque (Fig. 9-11).

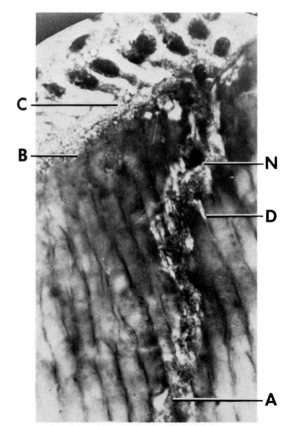

Fig. 9-7. High power view of an enamel lamella in developing enamel illustrating origin from the ameloblastic layer "A". An "entrapped" nucleus is seen at "N". A rod surface is shown at "B". "D" = interrod opening; "A" = part of an entrapped ameloblast. (Hodson JJ: Oral Surg, Oral Med, Oral Pathol, 6: 305–317, 1953)

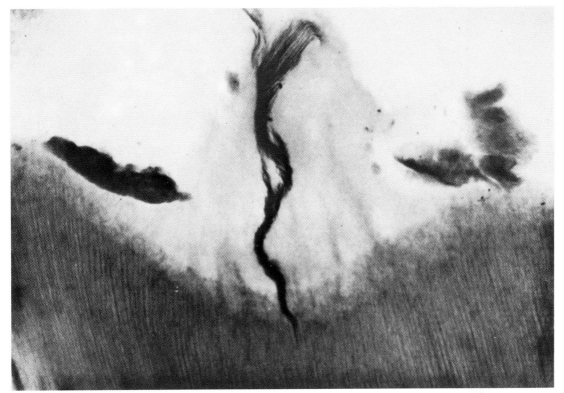

Fig. 9-8. Demineralized section of human tooth illustrating bacterial invasion through a lamella. (dark areas). Note the persistence of the enamel matrix adjacent to the lamella (×110.) (Pindborg JJ: Pathology of the Dental Hard Tissues. Philadelphia, WB Saunders, 1970)

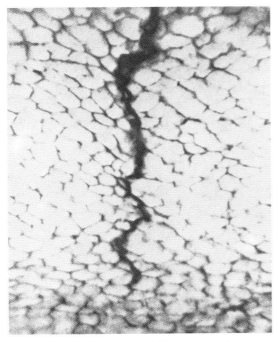

Fig. 9-9. Section from the decalcified enamel of a human molar showing the intimate relationship between a lamella and the surrounding organic interprismatic substance (prism sheaths). (×1000). (Sognnaes RF: J Dent Res 29: 260, 1950)

Additional support for this concept of the relationship of the perikymata-Retzius diffusion pathways was provided in scanning electron microscope studies on the variations in enamel surface resistance to demineralization *in vitro*. The results obtained graphically illustrated surface demineralization changes resulting in an undermining destruction of the overlapped edges of the perikymata (Fig. 9-12A). Additionally, it was seen that the undulating pattern was more resistant to subsurface toxin penetration suggesting a more effective inhibition of toxin diffusion by this variety of topography than the overlapping type (Fig. 9-12B).

In order to better understand the role of the Striae of Retzius as potential pathways for extending subsurface attack, a brief discussion of its position in the scheme of enamel structure would be helpful at this point. The Striae of Retzius, or incremental lines of growth of enamel prisms, are seen as arcuate, concentric, brownish lines in ground sections of enamel. They arise at the DEJ and terminate on either the enamel surface or on the DEJ at another site (Fig. 9-13). In other words, the latter type arch radiates from one point

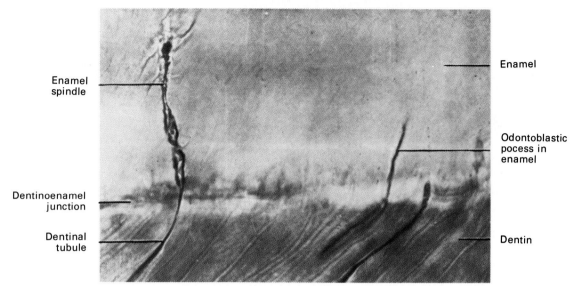

Fig. 9-10. Ground section of human tooth at the dentino-enamel junction illustrating terminal portions of odontoblastic processes extending across the DEJ into enamel as the enamel spindles. (Bhaskar SN: Orban's Oral Histology and Embryology. ed 8. St. Louis, CV Mosby, 1976).

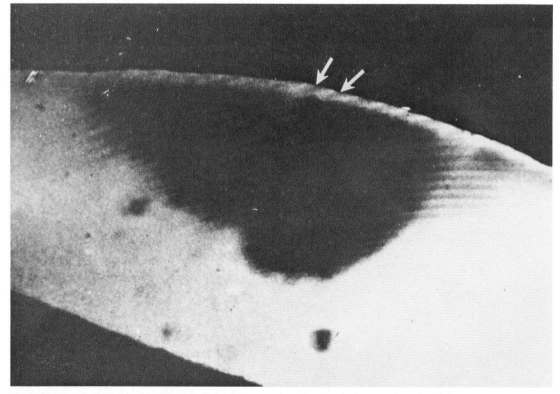

Fig. 9-11. Microradiograph of a white spot lesion in human dental enamel prior to surface breakdown. There is extensive subsurface demineralization as evidenced by the large area of radiolucency (Body of the Lesion) which underlies a relatively intact surface layer. Note that the surface entry sites, identified by radiolucent areas (**arrows**) apparently are undermining the edges of convex segments of perikymata (×140). (Darling Al: Br Dent J, *105*: 119, 1958)

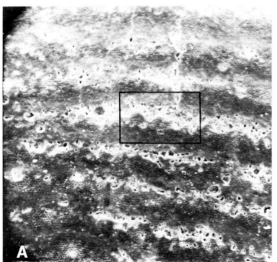

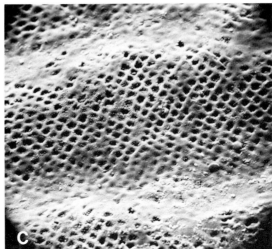

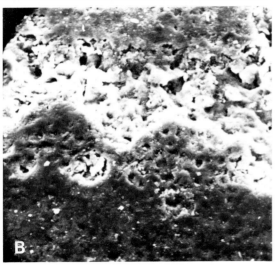

Fig. 9-12**A.** Acid effects on the overlapping type of topography on enamel surfaces; (×115). **B.** A higher power view of the rectangle marked in the TOP figure. Note the undermining demineralization occurring at the bordering edge of a perikymata. Compare with Fig. 9-11. (×570). (US Navy Med 62: 15–19, 1973) **C.** The pattern of acid attack on a more mature surface than seen in Figure 12A is illustrated above. This SEM reveals a "punch-board" type of demineralization which is occurring along the slopes and crests of undulating perikymata. Note that there is no overlapping topography here and that the grooves or "valleys" are more resistant to the acid with no evidence of the undermining destruction seen in Fig. 12A (×600).

on the DEJ to another around the cuspal prominences, without appearing to reach the surface. The former terminate on the smooth surfaces of the teeth between the cemento-enamel junction and the outer surfaces of the cusps. These structures, which represent

phases in prism growth, originate during amelogenesis. They are considered to represent the alignment of segmental alterations in prism mineralization. When amelogenesis starts, the first group of prisms to be formed are those arising around the tip of embryonic cusp. The second groups to form are those on either side of these primitive cuspal prisms. Subsequent groups of prisms begin to form more cervically at later stages, the last formed groups being located close to the cemento enamel junction (CEJ). Thus, the oldest and longest prisms are cuspal, and the youngest (i.e., most immature) and shortest are in the cervical region of the enamel crown. During the growth of each individual prism there occur periodic interruptions in the normal process of maturation. Since these growth interruptions appear to occur in all prism groups which are developing at that time, and since the groups are staggered due to the time lag for commencement of each group (from cuspal region to CEJ), a stepped alignment of interrupted segments is formed ranging from the oldest prism groups (cuspal) to the youngest groups growing at that moment (Fig. 9-14). These interrupted maturation intervals are probably related to refractory periods in ameloblastic function, and thus form segments within the prisms which contain fewer mineral components, (i.e., physiologically hypomineralized segments). When longitudinal ground sections of mature enamel are viewed with the light microscope these hypomineralized prism segments fall into alternating parallel alignments, thereby giving rise to the

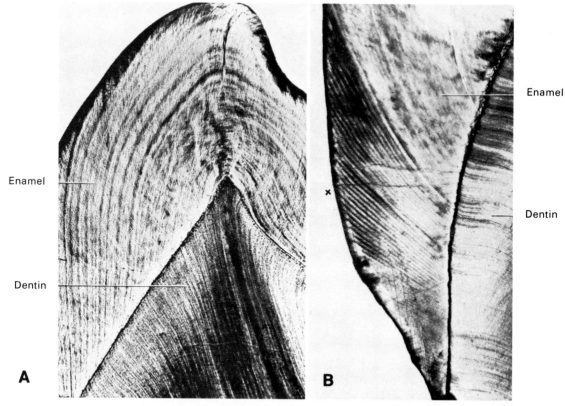

Fig. 9-13. Ground sections of human dental enamel illustrating two patterns of Retzius lines: **A.** Long sweeping concentric arcs radiating around the cuspal prominence, arising and terminating at different sites on the dentino-enamel junction; **B.** Shorter segments of parallel arcs arising at the dentino-enamel junction and terminating at the surface in the cervical region of the crown. (Bhaskar SN: Orban's Oral Histology and Embryology. ed. 8. St. Louis, CV Mosby, 1976)

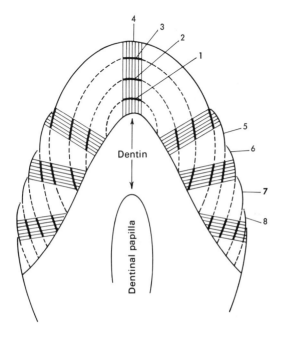

Fig. 9-14. This is a schematic representation of the origin of the Striae of Retzius. The numbers refer to the chronology of subsequently developing prisms and their arc forming segments at progressively advancing stages in amelogenesis. As the numbers increase in value, additional groups of new prisms commence development, with continuing growth of new segments in prisms which have previously formed. Thus, segment #1 shows the prisms which started to grow around the cuspal prominence and represents the first group of prisms. The arcuate segment labeled #2 shows the commencement of growth for the second group of prisms and the continuation of segmental growth in the first groups. With each higher number one can see that new prisms are commencing to grow at more cervical regions and the Striae of Retzius become more prominent. Note that from #5-8 the arcuate segments terminate at the surface in an overlapping configuration, whereas the arcuate segments included in #1-4 originate at the DEJ and terminate at the DEJ.

arcuate, concentric features of the matrix-rich, mineral-poor Striae of Retzius. In the newly erupted tooth the topographic configurations of concentric, convex ridges, the perikymata, represent the terminal surface extensions of the Striae of Retzius. With time, the posteruptive maturation process completes the mineralization of the surface crystallites and eventually forms a hypermineralized surface with respect to the subsurface crystallites.

Thus, in considering the overall features of enamel microstructure it becomes obvious that enamel is not really a solid, impermeable structure, but rather an efficiently mineralized, sieve-like "membrane" containing microporosities and organic pathways for fluid diffusion and ionic exchanges. If the equilibrium between enamel structure and its external environment is maintained, the structure remains unaltered chemically and morphologically. However, if this equilibrium is disturbed, a disease state is initiated with destructive alterations occuring at the microanatomic level which eventually progresses to the clinical level.

Bearing these histologic features in mind, the pathologic changes occuring in enamel white spot lesions may be better understood.

ENIGMA OF THE INTACT SURFACE ZONE IN NONCAVITATED WHITE SPOT ENAMEL LESIONS

Based on studies of noncavitated white spot lesions, Darling delineated four zones of pathologic alterations in enamel: the translucent zone, the dark zone, the body of the lesion, and the intact surface zone. This subject was discussed in detail in the chapter by Dr. Ostrom and therefore, will not be repeated here. Instead, this part of the chapter will be concerned with brief summaries of the current thinking which attempts to explain the enigma of the intact surface zone. The retention of this zone in the presence of a significant amount of demineralization immediately below it presents a most complex phenomenon which stubbornly eludes satisfactory scientific explantions. However, there is no dearth of hypotheses and several credible concepts have been suggested:

Bypassing of Surface Crystallites by Bacterial Toxins. It has been suggested that when the enamel surface becomes saturated with diffusing bacterial toxins, the more resistant surface crystallites may be bypassed, the toxins diffusing down microporosities, intercrystallite pathways, lamellae, or the overlapped edges of the perikymata. In the latter case such action would provide access to the underlying Striae of Retzius. Darling has suggested that toxic bacterial products attack hydroxyapatite crystallites located at the prism peripheries in those segments of prisms within the Striae of Retzius. He further hypothesizes that they then course into the prisms via the cross striations and proceed to dissolve crystallites within the cores of those prisms. This would tend to explain subsurface demineralization with minimal effects on the surface crystallites.

Another consideration relating to this bypassing phenomenon may be the efficiency of crystallite packing at the enamel surface. It has been reported that there exists a prismless zone at the surface, (i.e., that prism delineation terminates below the surface zone and that hydroxyapatite crystallites diffusely cover the enamel surface overlying the prisms, their long axes parallel to each other and aligned perpendicularly to the enamel surface). Thus, prismatic structures do not extend to the enamel surface. This would mean that the prism sheaths are not present at the surface and only the matrix areas between crystallites and an occasional lamella would provide the only pathways to the subsurface regions.

The Presence of High Concentrations of Fluorides in the Surface Crystallites and/or Intercrystallite Matrix Areas. It has been reported that fluorides are most heavily concentrated within the first 15 to 20 microns of the enamel surface. This would serve to increase the resistance of surface crystallites to dissolution, thereby helping to preserve the integrity of the surface zone.

Transport of Internal Minerals During Dissolution. Another possible explanation of the intact surface is that before subsurface pathologic porosities can develop the mineral dissolved must be transported from the internal tissues entirely out to the tooth surfaces. Such transport probably depends largely upon a slow ionic diffusion via the previously described pathways. It has been suggested that in passage to the enamel surface, some of this ionic mineral redeposits within the surface zone thereby helping to preserve its integrity.

Thus, there appear to be several feasible hypotheses to explain the enigma of the intact surface zone in white spot lesions. The truth probably will eventually be found in a combination of these factors.

We have endeavored to summarize currently held concepts which attempt to explain the complex pathologic alterations that occur in white spot lesions. Intact enamel has been likened to a semipermeable membrane, or a sieve-like structure, which allows a selective diffusion of materials into and out of its internal compartments. Visualization of such a structure may help to more clearly elucidate this sieve-like morphology. Figure 9-15 illustrates enamel surface alterations at the interface of an indigenous plaque environment that had been physically displaced by cleaning prior to scanning electron microscope (SEM) examination. These alterations present a diffuse, reticulated pattern of microporosities which had been covered by a bacterial plaque-like environment, foci of which still can be seen. The diameters of these minute openings range from 3000 to 5000 Å (⅓ to ½ a micron). Thus, the openings are large enough to permit the bacterial toxins saturating the plaque-enamel interface (but not the bacteria) to easily diffuse into the subsurface regions and attack the structures present therein. This morphologic pattern graphically illustrates the sieve-like structure in early pathologic alterations.

Evidence in support of the concept of toxin diffusion and attack by way of these various organic pathways is circumstantial and controversial. However, it would be most difficult to explain the occurrences of pulp responses to these incipient, noncavitated white spot lesions if these organic ultrastructures did not function as potential diffusion pathways.

PULPODENTINAL COMPLEX AND THE MICROANATOMY OF SOUND DENTIN

Before considering the subject of caries in dentin, it is important that one understand the microstructure of sound dentin and its relationship to the pulp. The concept that dentin and pulp comprise a single tissue with dentin representing the mature end product of pulp cell differentiation and maturation is gradually gaining recognition. It is most essential that the clinician keep this relationship in mind in the treatment of caries or in abut-

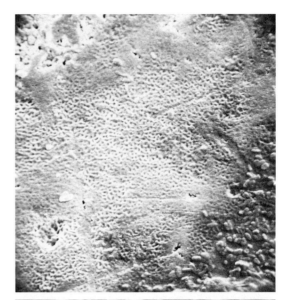

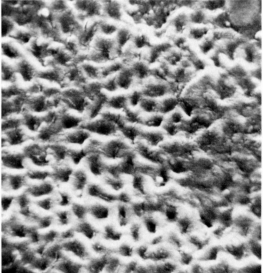

Fig. 9-15. **Top:** The enamel sample in this scanning electron micrograph was vigorously cleaned to remove all exogenous surface coatings so that "naked" enamel could be viewed. In the lower right hand corner the edge of a plaque-like aggregate of rod shaped microorganisms can be seen. The remaining surface shows a reticulated lace-like pattern of minute porosities from which this colonial aggregate apparently had been removed (× 1,170). **Bottom:** A higher magnification of the reticulated area seen in the TOP photomicrograph. Note the microporosities which characterize this surface, graphically demonstrating the sieve-like ultrastructural morphology of enamel. In the upper right hand corner there is an oval shaped structure consistent with a bacterium. Comparison of the diameters of these microporosities with the diameter of the bacterium provides some indication as to how small these openings really are (× 11,300). (Top photograph: Hoffman, S. 50: 1355, 1971)

ment tooth preparations. Embryologically, the pulp originates from the undifferentiated mesenchyme of the dental papilla of the developing tooth germ. Mature odontoblasts are derived from this structure. The **dentin** is the end product of odontoblastic activity. Thus, both structures (dentin and pulp) develop from a common antecedent tissue, the undifferentiated cells of the dental papilla.

The structure of the mature, mineralized portion of dentin is characterized by a highly organized network of microtubules or canals arising radially at the pulp and terminating at the dentinoenamel junction. These canals provide a honeycombed pattern to mature dentin housing the odontoblastic processes

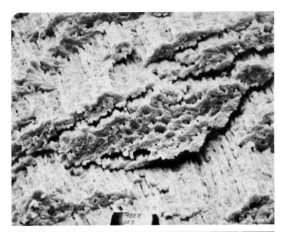

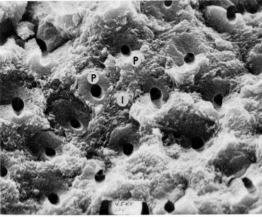

Fig. 9-16. Composite of low and high power scanning electron micrographs of dentin fractured perpendicularly to the dentinal canals illustrating peritubular (P) and intertubular dentin (I). Note the smooth, dense, compact characteristics of the peritubular dentin which forms the walls of the dentinal canals in contrast to the rough, porous, intertubular dentin located between the canals. P = peritubular dentin; I = intertubular dentin. (**Top:** × 900; **Bottom:** × 4,500).

and pulpal fluids. The walls immediately surrounding these canals are known as **pericanalicular** (or peritubular) **dentin.** That portion of dentin which lies between these canals and provides the solid substance of dentin is referred to as **intercanalicular** (or intertubular) **dentin** (Fig. 9-16). Pericanalicular dentin differs from intercanalicular dentin in that it is a hypermineralized component of the intercanalicular dentin, forming a collar or sleeve around the tubular lumen and its contents. This fact has been established through microradiographic studies of dentin in which the increased radiopacity of pericanalicular dentin over that of intercanalicular dentin has been demonstrated.

Histologically, there exists an inseparable relationship between dentin and pulp. The **odontoblasts,** located at the periphery of the pulp at their junction with the predentin, consist of a cell body and a long tapering cytoplasmic process or tail (Tomes' fiber). The cell body is cylindrical or columnar in shape and contains the nucleus and major organelles. The long, tapering tail-like processes are contained within mineralized canals and course through the dentin to terminate at the dentinoenamel junction, occasionally crossing this barrier to extend for short distances into the enamel as enamel spindles (Fig. 9-10). As long as the pulp remains vital, any irritation in dentin induces a pulpitis of varying degrees of intensity with resultant stimulation of reparative (secondary) dentin formation and sporadic intratubular calcifications. Thus, the relationship of odontoblasts and their processes to dentin is very intimate and may be compared with that of osteoblasts to bone. It is apparent that embryologically and histologically, as well as physiologically and pathologically, dentin and pulp are two inseparable components of one tissue.

The odontoblastic processes should not be considered as sealed off, separated components isolated within these narrow channels, but rather as intercommunicating, anastomotic networks. Many secondary branches are given off in all directions near the DEJ which communicate with secondary branches of other adjacent processes. Additionally, it has been observed in scanning electron microscopy studies that the walls of dentinal canals have scattered minute foramina not only in the vicinity of the DEJ but all along the length of the dentinal canals (Fig. 9-17). It is presumed that these foramina probably provide the channels for anastomotic linkups of secondary branches from odontoblastic processes. Thus, it may be understood how physical, thermal, chemical or bacterial stimuli may travel from odontoblastic processes in the direct path of such irritations to adjacent processes that are not in direct contact with these irritants via the secondary branches. Thus, pulpal dissemination of irritating stimuli is more extensive than had these processes been in separately, sealed—off isolated channels. In view of such pulpodentinal relationships, these structures should be considered and treated as a single entity.

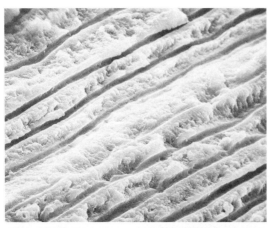

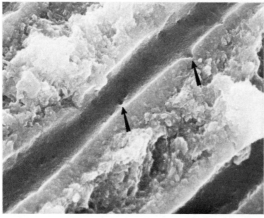

Fig. 9-17. Composite of low and high power scanning electron micrographs of dentin fractured parallel to the longitudinal axes of the dentinal canals. Note the presence of minute foramena (*arrows*) in the peritubular walls of the canals which probably serve as channels for the passage of anastomozing secondary branches from odontoblastic processes. (**Top:** ×3,250; **Bottom:** ×13,000)

MICROSCOPIC FEATURES OF ACTIVE DENTINAL CARIES LESIONS

In the cariogenic process, long before enamel cavitation occurs, there is evidence of dentin involvement. Plaque toxins diffusing down the enamel ultrastructural pathways previously described, initiate biochemical reactions within the dentin which result in compositional alterations. As the infectious process in intact enamel progresses in depth, mineral loss and matrix changes occur in dentin. By the time of enamel cavitation dentinal mineral losses and matrix changes may be quite extensive. When the advancing front of the infectious process in enamel reaches the DEJ, lateral spread (as well as extension in depth) may occur with secondary involvement of enamel at new sites along the junction. It is generally accepted that at least a partial demineralization of the dentin is necessary before bacterial invasion occurs. Thus, the extent of demineralization is always greater than the area of bacterial involvement seen in histologic preparations.

The histopathology of active and arrested dentinal lesions has been well described by Massler and his coworkers (see Chap. 10). In active, deep cariogenic infections the following pathologic zones have been identified:

Pathologic Zones in Active Deep Cariogenic Infections
  Infected Dentin
    Necrotic Zone
    Superficial Portion of Demineralized Dentin Zone
  Affected Dentin
    Deep Portion of Demineralized Dentin Zone
    Hypermineralized Zone
      Sclerotic Layer
      Reparative Dentin Layer

The infected zone in deep active lesions consists of a necrotic region and the superficial portion of the demineralized dentin. Affected dentin is that remaining mass of dentin "affected," but not destroyed, by the carious process. It consists of the deep portion of the demineralized zone, the sclerotic zone, and the reparative dentin layer.

In the *necrotic zone* of the active lesion

few, if any, intact tubular structures can be found. This zone consists mostly of disintegrating dentinal tubules, masses of mixed bacterial flora, and a granular, structureless material. It has recently been reported that when the dentinal tubules become completely filled with bacteria, the pericanalicular walls become eroded and cleavages appear which extend into the intertubular dentin. These cracks occur at right angles to the course of the dentinal tubules. The cleavages, which contain bacteria and necrotic masses, coalesce to create the necrotic zone, a large clinical cavity in the dentin. This consists of a mass of wet, soft, mushy debris which has no consistency and which can be easily spooned out with excavators and mashed over a hard surface. The superficial *zone of demineralization* comprises the deeper portion of the infected zone. The dentinal tubular morphology here is distorted by massive demineralization, but generally the organic matrix remains intact so that its tubular morphology is retained. The lumina of the softened tubules are markedly dilated and engorged with bacteria (Fig. 9-18).

The *deep portion* of the demineralized zone reveals intact, well formed tubular matrices and comprises the first portion of affected dentin. There is minimal evidence of tubular alterations and no evidence of clefting. Occasionally a few bacteria may be found, but this is rare. The major difference between this and sound dentin is depletion of mineral components. The clinical appearance at this point is that of a dry, leathery dentinal structure.

Depending on the depth and rate of progress of the lesion, there may or may not be a sclerotic zone present beneath the deep demineralized zone. If present, the sclerotic zone generally occupies a narrow area in which the tubular lumens may be narrowed or occluded by fine, precipitated hydroxyapatite crystallites leached out during the earlier phases of caries demineralization. It is also possible that the lumens may have been occluded by a recrystallization brought on by

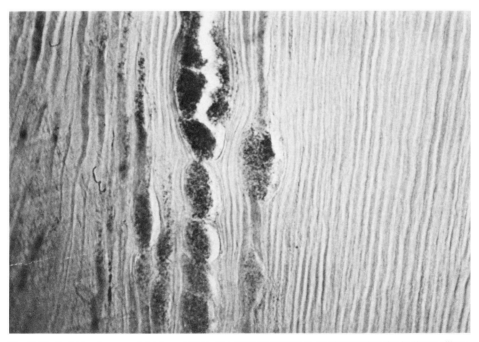

Fig. 9-18. A photomicrograph from a section of a carious human molar illustrating the bulbous dilatations in pathologically softened, infected dentin. This area is from the superficial portion of the demineralized zone in an active lesion. The distorted tubules are engorged with bacteria. Note the intact morphology in the adjacent, uninfected canals which were not in the direct path of invading organisms but were probably demineralized by bacterial toxins diffusing from an overlying infectious process, or via secondary anastomozing branches of odontoblastic processes. Thus, infected and affected dentin are in a side-by-side relationship. (× 1,000).

odontoblastic action during periods of cariogenic remission. In electron microscopy studies it has been reported that bacterial invasion along dentinal tubules occurs when the cariogenic process is reactivated. This is accomplished either after destruction of the material occluding the lumens via irregular spaces caused by deformities along the odontoblastic processes, or following the partial destruction of the peritubular matrix. Reparative dentin produced in response to irritations arriving in the pulp from the toxic products of the caries process (or from other irritations) usually is formed as a protective, walling—off response to the infectious processes. The reparative dentin may contain as many tubules as the circumpulpal dentin, fewer tubules, or it may be atubular.

MICROSCOPIC FEATURES OF ARRESTED DENTINAL CARIES LESIONS

Pathologic Zones in Long Arrested Cariogenic
    Infections
    Infected Zone—absent
    Affected Zone
        Demineralized Dentin Zone
        Sclerotic Layer
        Reparative Dentin Layer

As noted above, arrested dentinal lesions do not have *necrotic zones* nor *superficial demineralized zones*, the bulk of the remaining structures being composed of *sclerotic dentin* with occasionally a thin surface layer comparable to the deep demineralized zone of active lesions. Arrested lesions are characterized clinically by deep pigmentation and a leathery or a hard polished surface. Histologically, dentinal canals in the sclerotic zone are almost completely closed off by intraluminal calcification, and have been found to be impermeable to a number of dyes in contrast to the situation found in active dentinal caries. Increased pigmentation of the lesion is associated with a decrease in permeability. Studies from the literature have revealed an absence of bacteria in these regions. In chronic caries the pulp responds by building up dense, compact, well formed layers of reparative dentin underlying the sclerotic zone. It has been implied that a reciprocal relationship may exist between the process of tubular sclerosis and reparative

dentin formation that may be of clinical significance in therapeutically induced arrest of deep, active dentinal lesions.

Thus, in the long arrested caries lesion there is no infected zone, the necrotic and superficial demineralized zones being absent. The lesion is composed of affected dentin only. There may be a thin layer of the deep demineralized zone present along the surface or it may be completely absent. The major portion of the remaining dentin is sclerotic with most of the lumens occluded by calcification. Generally, there is a dense, compact region of reparative dentin underlying the sclerotic zone.

In this section, we have endeavored to delineate structural changes in dentin within the various pathologic zones of the caries process for both active and arrested dental infection. Of major interest to the clinician is the integrity of the "affectd zone" in active advanced carious lesions. It is significant that the basic dentinal structures in this zone (i.e., the dentinal tubules), although partially softened by mineral losses, are intact morphologically and can still receive mineral ions from pulp tissues or therapeutically via $Ca(OH)_2$. Thus they have the potential either to remineralize under proper conditions or remain in an inactive state with no further lesional progress. In other words, isolated from pathogenic bacterial plaque, vital dental tissues, like vital tissues elsewhere in the body, have the potential to heal themselves.

CARIES OF CEMENTUM

Cemental caries seem to begin as a superficial softening of exposed cementum close to the margin of receded gingiva. Relatively little has been written on this subject, but it is generally accepted that there is an initial and progressive softening of the cementum and later of the underlying dentin. The cavities that first develop are saucer shaped but become deeper as the dentin becomes involved. Superficially, they tend to follow the outline of the gingival contour, and if they lie close to the cervical margin of the enamel, it may become undermined.

When gingival recession has occurred the cementum becomes covered by an organic cuticle which must be disintegrated before the carious attack can begin. Micrographs of initial caries lesions in cementum have shown subsurface demineralization and the frequent occurrence of a densely mineralized surface layer wider than that observed in exposed, noncarious cementum, suggesting the possibility of remineralization at the plaque-cementum interface.

INDIRECT PULP CAPPING

Indirect pulp capping has long been a controversial issue among researchers and clinicians. In pediatric dentistry the issues have been less emotional. In fact, the technique is being taught in nearly all dental schools, and pedodontists use it routinely. However, with regard to indirect pulp capping procedures for the permanent dentition of young adults, the issues appear to be irreconcilable at this time.

Indirect pulp capping is a philosophy advocating a conservative approach to the management of deep caries lesions. It involves removal of the necrotic layer and most of the deep demineralized zone of dentin in active lesions. A floor of dry, leathery dentin is left at the base of the cavity preparation as close to the pulp as possible without actually exposing it. This approach is used in those conditions where the complete removal of soft, stained dentin would result in pulp exposure. A thin layer of calcium hydroxide is spread over the residual softened dentin and a restoration is placed which can insure a good marginal seal, thus minimizing or preventing leakage. In children, the pedodontist generally fills the tooth so treated immediately with a permanent restoration. However, this approach in the treatment of deep lesions in adults is controversial and not completely accepted. Where it is performed, a zinc oxide and eugenol base is generally placed over the layer of calcium hydroxide, the remaining cavity preparations being filled with oxyphosphate cement. The tooth is checked periodically for 6 months to a year before a final restoration is inserted. This is done to insure that no adverse developments occur during this period. The philosophy of this procedure is based upon the biologic potential of vital injured tissue to heal when isolated from etiologic factors. The pulp, being a highly specialized connective tissue, as noted earlier, possesses the same potential to heal as does connective tissue in any other part of the body. Pathologi-cally softened dentin, which is considered to be a part of the pulp, has the potential to remineralize or reharden if infectious or toxic irritants are removed for long enough periods of time. However, certain clinical criteria must be met before using this technique. The tooth involved must have no evidence of periapical pathology, must be vital and asymptomatic, and must have sufficient remaining structure to allow for good retention of a permanent restoration.

In discussing the histopathology of advanced active caries lesions, it was brought out that the deep demineralized zone of dentin was morphologically intact and contained little or no bacteria. Clinically, such dentin has a leathery consistency and will remain dry when isolated with a rubber dam. It has been reported by a number of investigators that remineralization of this softened dentin can occur under such circumstances and that it is mediated by odontoblastic activity. Thus, by indirect pulp capping procedures the etiologic cariogens will be removed, or at least so attenuated as to become ineffective as tooth destroying agents. In this way, the biologic potential of the pulp is harnessed by the clinician. It is believed that the temporary restoration, or "dressing," provides protection from the environment so long as it remains intact, allowing for repair of the affected dental tissues by intratubular remineralization. After a sufficient period of time has elapsed, the "dressing" is removed and a permanent restoration inserted. Many have questioned the efficacy of this technique since it has not been unequivocally resolved as to what happens to the vital tissues in the pulp chamber and canals or to the residual cariogenic microorganisms which may be left at the base of the cavity preparation. Endodontists have found that in some teeth so treated there is obliteration of pulp canals by dystrophic calcification, rendering subsequent definitive endodontic therapy difficult or impossible to perform. Well controlled clinical research trials are needed to further evaluate and develop this therapeutic philosophy.

SUMMARY

In the preceding pages the histopathologic alterations which occur in white spot enamel lesions, in deep dentinal lesions, and in cemental lesions has been discussed. In addition, the concept of a conservative clinical management of deep caries in adult dentitions (i.e., indirect pulp capping) was commented upon.

In considering how major microscopic changes occur in the incipient enamel lesion, potential ultrastructural pathways for diffusion of bacterial toxins were described. Emphasis was placed on enamel surface topography containing the overlapping type of perikymata and the related, subsurface, hypomineralized prism segments, the Striae of Retzius. Other high organic content structures were also considered such as intercrystallite matrix areas, microporosities in enamel, prism sheaths, enamel lamellae, and enamel spindles. To account for the enigmatic retention of the surface zone in white spot lesions (while significant demineralization occured in the subsurface region represented as the "body of the lesion") the concept of ionic transfer into and out of enamel via these organic pathways was discussed.

In prefacing the section concerned with dentin and dentinal lesions, the importance of the pulpodential complex as a single unit tissue was stressed. Considered from the aspect of embryology, histology, physiology, and response to irritants, the pulpodential complex must be considered as a single, highly differentiated connective tissue which responds to stimuli or injury just as does connective tissue in any other part of the body, (i.e., it has the potential to react and to heal itself). This concept was stressed in regard to the therapeutically induced remineralization of deep caries lesions.

Pathologic zones in advanced dentinal lesions were described and emphasis placed upon the retained morphologic integrity of the softened dentinal tubules. Active and arrested lesions were compared on the basis of their histopathologies. The philosophy of indirect pulp capping was summarized with a brief review of some of the pros and cons concerning this procedure.

The added dimensions contributed to the science of cariology by multidisciplinary research efforts have helped to increase our understanding of this very complex disease process. The talents of oral microbiologists, biochemists, oral pathologists, biophysicists, electron microscopists, epidemiologists, etc. (see Suggested Readings) have contributed significantly to our knowledge of the mechanisms involved in this odontolytic disease. All the answers are not in yet, but through the efforts of scientists from multiple disciplines we are more rapidly progressing to a more complete understanding and an eventual conquest of this infectious disease.

GLOSSARY

Arrested caries. Chronic caries is characterized by alternating periods of active attack and remission or arrested activity. During remission the vital pulp tissues attempt to repair caries damage. This is possible where demineralized dentinal matrix is still intact. In children, and on occasion in young adults, if the infectious process is permanently arrested, complete remineralization ensues.

Cariogens. Those microorganisms which are considered to be the destructive agents in cariogenic infections (i.e., polysaccharide producing streptococci, S. mutans and possibly S. sanguis).

Dental papilla. The primitive mesenchymal component of the tooth germ which gives rise to odontoblasts and subsequently dentin.

Enamel lamellae. "Cracks" or defects in enamel extending from the surface to various distances into the subsurface regions. These "cracks" contain portions of ameloblasts or other cellular debris. They may serve as pathways for plaque toxin diffusion.

Enamel spindles. Terminal extensions of the odontoblastic processes which have crossed the dentinoenamel junction and extend for short distances into the enamel.

Intercanalicular (intertubular) dentin. The solid component of dentin compromising those areas between the dentinal canals (or tubules).

Lamina dura. The thin cortical plate of bone lining the alveolar processes and serving as the bony attachment site for the periodontal fibers.

Lysis. The digestion or liquefaction of tissue; odontolysis, the digestion of dental tissues.

Percanalicular (Peritubular) dentin. A hypermineralized collar of dentin which immediately surrounds and forms the walls of the dentinal canals (or tubules).

Perikymata. Concentric ridges which circumscribe the enamel surface in a roughly horizontal plane.

Posteruptive maturation. The continuing process of tooth maturation after its eruption. At the time the tooth erupts into the oral cavity, the enamel surface and root apex are incomplete. For several years following its eruption, enamel continues to mineralize and the root apex continues to elongate with concomitant narrowing of the apical foramen.

Prisms (Rods). The unit of structure of enamel.

Prism (Rod) sheaths. A thin "sleeve" of organic matrix which partially or completely surrounds the peripheral borders of the prisms.

Reparative dentin. Sometimes referred to as irritation dentin or, incorrectly as secondary dentin. It is a continuous process of dentin build-up by odontoblasts at the expense of the pulp. It is a less perfect product than primary or circumpulpal dentin and is stimulated by irritations. It is an attempt to wall off and protect the pulp from irritating stimuli.

Striae of retzius. These are subsurface, concentric lines seen in ground sections of enamel and they represent incremental lines of prism growth. They terminate on the smooth surfaces of recently erupted teeth as the perikymata.

Tomes' fibers. Long, slender tail-like processes of odontoblasts which extend into the dentinal canals from the pulp to the dentinoenamel junction.

Toxin. A product of cellular metabolism, generally of bacterial origin, which may be located intracellularly or extracellularly or which may be combinations of both types. Such metabolic "toxins" are complex molecules whose compositions are only partially known. Their precise natures in the carious process are not fully known. It is clear that the hydrogen ion's effect on solubility of hyroxyapatite plays an important part, but it is also probable that other products such as proteolytic enzymes and/or chelators may also contribute to the destruction of dental structures. For this reason "toxin" is considered the word of choice in the present chapter.

White spot enamel lesions. The first and earliest clinical manifestations of an active cariogenic process. They develop as a result of biochemical changes which occur at the plaque-enamel interface.

SUGGESTED READINGS

Applebaum E: Tissue changes in dental caries. Ann Dent 7: 1, 1948

Applebaum E: The arrangement of enamel (rods). NY State Dent J 26: 185, 1960

Aponte AJ, Harsock JT, Crowley MC: Indirect pulp capping success verified. J Dent Child 2nd quarter, 33: 164–166 1966

Bergman G: Microscopic demonstration of fluid flow through human dental enamel. Arch Oral Biol 8: 233, 1963

Black GC: The peritubular translucent zones in human dentine. Br Dent J. 104: 57, 1958

Brand F, Helmcke JG, Neubauer G, Rau R: Sprunge und lamellen i normalen und kariosen schmelz menschlicken zahne. Bull Group Eur Rech Sci Stomatol Odontol 11: 279, 1968

Brannstrom M, Lind PO: Pulpal response to early dental caries. J Dent Res 44: 1045, 1965

Crabb H: Structural patterns in human dental enamel revealed by the use of microradiography in conjunction with two-dimensional microdensitometry. Caries Res 2: 235, 1968

Darling AI: The distribution of the enamel cuticle and its significance. Proc R. Soc Med 36: 499, 1943

Darling AI: Studies of the early lesions of enamel caries with transmitted light, polarized light and radiography. Br Dent J 101: 289, 329, 1956

Darling AI: Microstructural changes in early dental caries. In Sognnaes RF (ed): Mechanisms of Hard Tissue Destruction. Washington DC, American Association for the Advancement of Science 78, 1963

Darling AI: Ultrastructure of enamel in relation to mineralization, demineralization, and remineralization as revealed by microradiography, polarized light and plane light microscopy. Int Dent J 17: 648, 1968

Eastoe JE: Chemical aspects of the matrix concept in calcified tissue organization. Calci Tissue Res 2: 1, 1968

Eidelman E, Finn SB, Koulourides T: Remineralization of carious dentin treated with calcium hydroxide. J Dent Child 4th quarter, 32: 218–225, 1965

Frank RM: The ultrastructure of caries-resistant teeth. In

Wolstenholme GEW, O'Connor N (eds): Caries-Resistant Teeth, Ciba Foundation Symposium. London, JA Churchill, 1965, 169–91

Frank RM: The ultrastructure of the tooth from the point of view of mineralization, demineralization and remineralization. Int Dent J 17: 661, 1968

Frank RM, Brendel A: Ultrastructure of the approximal dental plaque and the underlying normal and carious enamel. Arch Oral Biol 11: 883, 1966

Frank RM, Nalbandian J: Ultrastructure of amelogenesis. In Miles AEW (ed): Structural and Chemical Organization of Teeth, Vol I. New York, Academic Press, 1967, p 399

Furseth R, Johansen E: A microradiograph comparison of sound and carious human dental cementum. Arch Oral Biol 13: 1197, 1968

Fusayama T, Okuse K, Hosoda H: Relationship between hardness, discoloration and microbial invasion in carious dentin. J Dent Res 45: 1033, 1966

Gottlieb B: Aetiology und prophylaxe der tzahnkaries. Dtsch Stomat 19: 129, 1921

Gottlieb B: Dental Caries. Philadelphia, Lea & Febiger, 1947

Gray JA, Francis MD: Physical chemistry of enamel dissolution. In Sognnaes RF (ed): Mechanisms of Hard Tissue Destruction. Washington DC, American Association for the Advancement of Science, 1963, p 213

Hals E, Morch T, Sand HF: Effect of lactate buffers on dental enamel in vitro observed in polarizing microscope. Acta Odontol Scand 13: 85, 1955

Held-Wydler E: Natural (indirect) pulp capping. J Dent Child 31: 107, 2nd quarter, 1964

Hodson JJ: An investigation into the microscopic structure of the common forms of enamel lamellae with special reference to their origin and contents. OS OM OP 6: 305, 383, 495, 1953

Hoffman S: Tubular diameters in sound and carious dentin. Washington DC, 45th General meeting International Assoc. for Dental Research. 303: 112. 1967

Hoffman S: Histopathologic response of the human dental pulp to indirect pulp capping procedures in adults. Great Lakes, Naval Dental Research Institute 68–02, 1968

Hoffman S: Variations in surface resistance to enamel etching. J Dent Res 51: 795, 1972

Kato S, Fusayame T: Recalcification of artificially decalcified dentin in-vivo: J Dent Res 49: 1060, 1970

Kerckeart GA: Electron microscopy of human carious dental enamel. Arch Oral Biol 18: 751, 1973

Kerebel B: Les Structures organiques del l'email et les theories proteolytiques des caries. Arch Oral Biol 4: 107, 1961

King JB, Crawford JJ, Lindahl RL: Indirect pulp capping: a bacteriologic study of deep carious dentin in human teeth. OS OM OP 20: 663, 1965

Lenz H: Ultrastructure of the tooth in respect to mineralization, demineralization and remineralization. Int Dent J 17: 693, 1968

Listgarten MA: Phase contrast and electronmicroscopic study of the junction between reduced enamel epithelium and enamel in unerupted human teeth. Arch Oral Biol 11: 999, 1966

Manley EB: The organic structure of enamel. Br Dent J 84: 132, 1948

Meckel AH: The formation and properties of organic films on teeth. Arch Oral Biol 10: 585, 1965

Meckel AH, Griebstein WJ, Neal BJ: Structure of mature human dental enamel as observed by electron microscopy. Arch Oral Biol 10: 775, 1965

Mellberg JR, Nicholson CR: In-vitro fluoride uptake by erupted and unerupted tooth enamel. J Dent Res 47: 176, 1968

Miller WA, Massler M: Permeability and staining of active and arrested lesions in dentin. Br Dent J 112: 187, 1962

Sarnat H, Massler M: Microstructure of active and arrested dentinal caries. J Dent Res 44: 1389, 1965

Sognnaes RF: The organic elements of the enamel IV: the gross morphology and histologic relationship of the lamellae to the organic framework of the enamel. J Dent Res 29: 260, 1950

Takuma S, Sunohara H, Sekiguchi K, Egawa I: Electron microscopy of carious lesions in human dentin. Bull Tokyo Dent Coll 8: 143, 1967

Travis DF: Comparative ultrastructure and organization of inorganic crystals and organic matrices of mineralized tissues. In Biology of the Mouth. Washington DC, American Association for the Advancement of Science 1968, p 237

Weatherall JA, Robinson C, Halsworth AS: Variations in the chemical composition of human enamel. J Dent Res 53: 180, 1974

Wei SHY: Remineralization of enamel and dentin—a review. J Dent Child 4th quarter, 444, 1967

Yoshida S, Massler M: Pulpal reactions to dentinal caries. NY J Dent 34: 215, 1964

10 Clinical Cariology

CARL A. OSTROM

Introduction
Enamel Caries
   Biological Mechanisms
   Enamel Sieve Concept
      Development of the Enamel Lesion
Dentin Caries
   Structural Features of Dentin
   Fluid Flow in Dentin
   The Dentin Caries Lesion
      The Infected Zone
      The Affected Zone
      The Hypermineralized Zone

Zone Differentiation Within the Lesion
Internal Mineralization
External Mineralization
Fate of the Microbial Infection
Clinical Management of Dental Caries Lesions
   Pit and Fissure Lesions
   Cervical Lesions
   Interproximal Lesions
Summary
Glossary
Suggested Readings

INTRODUCTION

Although impressive new knowledge has been developed during recent decades, there remains much to be learned concerning the biological mechanisms that are involved in dental caries. The disease is a multifactorial one, so that the areas needing further exploration range from the physics and chemistry of mineralized tissues through biological processes of adaptation and maturation to factors affecting the personal habits of the host. Nevertheless there is a sufficiently established body of knowledge from current research and clinical experience to permit the practicing dentist to treat the subject with logic and confidence.

This chapter has as its objectives the following: to describe the features that are involved in the development of caries lesions; to reach an understanding of the responses of the dental tissues to caries lesions; and to provide methods for applying this knowledge to clinical control of the disease. Thus the ultimate goal is to present a logical basis for conservative clinical management of caries lesions in teeth.

Dental caries may be defined as a process of enamel or dentin dissolution that is caused by microbial action at the tooth surface and is mediated by physicochemical flow of water dissolved ions (see Chaps. 4, 13, and 19). When the plaque-mineral equilibrium is in its demineralization phase, enamel (or dentin as the case may be) mineral ions are leached toward the plaque. By physiologic reversal of the equilibrium to a remineralization episode, ions that remain in or that may be carried back into the lesion are deposited in the form of mineral salts which are less soluble than the original and render the enamel or dentin more resistant to subsequent demineralizing attacks (see Chap. 19). If the sum of the remineralization effects becomes equal to or greater than the sum of the attack episodes, the remaining caries lesion will contain altered tooth substance and remnants of other materials, but the caries process will have been arrested and the lesion will not progress. The enamel or dentin can then be considered to have adapted itself to its cariogenic environment. Thus, detectable enamel caries lesions that have clinically intact surfaces may be arrested and often become highly resistant to subsequent caries attack. Such adaptation of the enamel at the sites of caries initiation may be enhanced if the cariogenic attack is minimized by adequate reduction of dietary sugar intake frequency, or if meticulous daily removal of plaque is practiced. Adaptation of the enamel may also occur in the presence of plaque and moderate dietary sugar frequency if fluoride ion is provided. Similarly in dentin, in selected circumstances, the lesion does not progress, and the remaining bacteria slowly die off after the enamel surface has been sealed by a restoration or a sealant that will serve as a barrier between the caries attack and the susceptible tissue. Extending further, after the enamel cover has been removed or lost, dentin caries may be arrested spontaneously by exposure to saliva. This process may be augmented by fluoride therapy to reduce the dentin's solubility, or by elimination of dietary sugars to the extent necessary to reduce the caries attack to a level that will be less than the host's remineralizing capability. Independent of the described surface mechanisms, the dentin is capable of additional responses that are mediated from the pulp.

To describe the biologic processes applicable to clinical cariology, it is necessary to describe briefly certain elements of anatomy, biochemistry, crystallography, and pathology. The concepts presented in the present chapter are based on published research. The reader is enjoined constantly to keep in mind the fact that physiologic and pathologic processes in living tissues may vary in successive patients, with the result that various authorities hold different opinions concerning the applicability of certain findings to clinical practice. For more detail, texts on each subject covered here are available. The Suggested Reading list provided at the end of this chapter contains several recent comprehensive reviews and selected articles that provide additional supportive material.

ENAMEL CARIES

Biological Mechanisms

It has been well established that microbial activity is responsible for dental caries. There are at least three theories on the processes of cariogenic disease. The acidogenic theory is most widely accepted today (see Chap. 8). There can be no doubt that acid demineralization is essential to the process. Experimental caries produced *in vitro* with acidic buffers results in lesions that are indistinguishable from natural caries both histologically and in their ability to remineralize. Thus, caries occurs on enamel surface areas where the plaque may stagnate and the microbial flora finds a suitable environment for multiplication, colonization, and the metabolism of carbohydrates to form organic acids.

Dental enamel may be described as a three component system that consists of a mineral phase which comprises about 96 per cent of enamel by weight, an organic phase that plays an essential role in its original calcification and remains present in the finished tissue, and a water phase. The mineral phase consists almost entirely of hydroxyapatite crystallites (see Chap. 7) which are located in the enamel prisms where they are aligned in a repetitive structural pattern and contained in insoluble protein (keratin). The mineral phase is also present in the interprismatic areas where small hydroxyapatite crystallites are contained in a matrix of soluble protein. Soluble protein is also present in the prism cores and cross striations, the Striae of Retzius, lamellae, and cracks, all of which also contain imbedded hydroxyapatite crystallites. At the surface of normal enamel there is a prism free layer of hydroxyapatite crystallites which is about 25 μm. thick.

The water phase comprises a variable 2 to 4 per cent of enamel, by weight. It is present as water—bound to proteins in the organic phase. In the mineral phase there are three forms of water - the hydration shell that is bound to each crystallite, the tumbling water caged within each crystallite structure, and free water. The free water permits the transportation of ions through the enamel, as evidenced by the globules of free water that may be seen on the enamel surface of a freshly extracted tooth after its cleaned and dried surface is viewed under oil immersion.

The mineral phase of enamel is almost pure hydroxyapatite, but it contains variable quantities of other substances. At least 41 elements of the periodic table have been detected in sound enamel, 35 of which having been detected in quantifiable concentration. It is known, for instance, that small ions may fit into the hydroxyapatite crystallite by ionic substitution in the crystal structure. Thus, fluoride may fit into the crystallite replacing a hydroxyl ion, and creating a crystallite of fluorapatite that is less soluble than hydroxyapatite. Larger ions such as citrate must be located outside of the crystallites (see Chap. 7).

Other such ions present in higher concentration in the deeper portions or in uniform concentration throughout the enamel are considered to have been incorporated during tooth development. Octacalcium phosphate crystals are usually present throughout the enamel and are more concentrated in the deeper portions. Since ameloblast activity is reduced as the enamel nears completion, the lower concentration of octacalcium phosphate in the more superficial areas of enamel is consistent with the interpretation that it is a residue of ameloblast activity. Similarly, since magnesium participates in cell enzyme activity and carbonate is a product of cell metabolism, these moieties are higher in concentration in deep areas of enamel where ameloblast metabolism is more active than in the superficial areas. The concentrations of other trace elements throughout the depths of enamel have been shown to relate to their presence in the soils and water supplies of geographic areas, and to foods grown on such soils. In the enamel, these appear to be of nutritional origin, mediated systemically by the tissue fluid during amelogenesis.

After tooth eruption the saliva and plaque provide sources for various substances that may be adsorbed to the surface or may be imbibed by the superficial portions of sound enamel. As a result, the composition of superficial enamel changes rapidly during the first few months after tooth eruption. Thereafter, as enamel matures, the enamel composition continues to change more slowly as influenced by the pressure gradients in saliva and plaque, and in the enamel itself. As a result of such maturation, dicalcium phosphate and β-tricalcium phosphate are usually higher in concentration near the enamel surface and people who reside in a community with less than 1.0 ppm fluoride in its drinking water have low enamel fluoride concentration at the time of tooth eruption and acquire increasing concentrations of fluoride in the superficial enamel for up to 50 years.

Caries occurs when hydrogen ions from the plaque diffuse into the enamel where they cause changes in the mineral composition. When the caries attack is terminated by a rise in plaque pH, as described in the Stephan Curve (see Glossary), the saliva and plaque provide remineralizing activities. Within the caries lesion, calcium and phosphate ions derived from altered hydroxyapatite remain as residue in the lesion during a remineralization phase, and reprecipitate in a variety of complex salts of calcium and phosphate. If fluoride ions have been imbibed from the plaque, complex calcium-fluoride-phosphate salts will precipitate in the caries lesion. Since such salts are less soluble than hydroxyapatite, the resultant microscopic caries lesion will be less susceptible to subsequent caries attacks. After repeated cycles of demineralization and remineralization with fluoride present, increasing concentrations of fluoride salts accumulate, and the lesion becomes increasingly resistant to subsequent caries attacks.

The significance of trace elements, ions, and salts in dental enamel lies in the fact that enamel is not a pure substance and that other components influence the resultant enamel caries susceptibility. During the preeruptive period other trace elements may be acquired by ameloblast cell metabolism or by the host's nutrition. Still others are acquired posteruptively by adsorption to the enamel surface from dietary sources in a process termed *enamel maturation*. Some trace elements such as selenium, magnesium, and cadmium have been associated with increased caries susceptibility, while others such as fluoride, molybdenum, vanadium, and strontium appear to make the enamel more resistant to caries attack. While a variety of such influences have been demonstrated in research, only the fluoride ion is of practical therapeutic effectiveness for reducing dental caries in humans. It may be deposited in the tooth structure by incorporation during development, posteruptive imbibition, and remineralization. Figure 10-1 displays the potential fluoride distribution that might result in a molar of a young adult who had resided

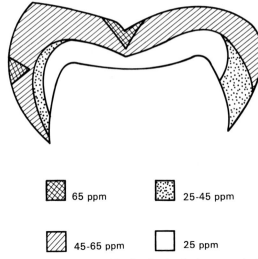

| 65 ppm | 25-45 ppm |
| 45-65 ppm | 25 ppm |

Fig. 10-1. Typical fluoride distribution in the enamel of a tooth that acquired the ion by three routes—incorporation during original development, posteruptive imbibition by sound enamel, and incorporation during remineralization of minimal caries lesions. (Modified from Weatherell JA: Br Med Bull 31: 115–119, 1975)

in a community with a low water fluoride level, and who had received no topical fluoride treatments. In such a case the fluoride levels displayed might have been of dietary origin. However, that same specimen might contain over 2,000 ppm fluoride on the surface and in the caries lesions if the person had lived in a community with a high fluoride level, or had received topical fluoride treatments (see chapter 20).

Enamel Sieve Concept

Enamel imbibition of hydrogen ions from the plaque causes dissolution of hydroxyapatite crystallites to their ionic components. In response to the increased pressure gradient, calcium and phosphate ions diffuse toward the plaque, leaving behind microspaces in the enamel mineral. After the acid attack has been terminated by depletion of the fermentable sugar in the plaque and by action of buffers in the plaque, a remineralization episode occurs within the enamel lesion that is subjacent to that plaque. The residue of calcium and phosphate ions in the microspaces, together with other ions that diffuse from the plaque back into the enamel lesion, tend to be precipitated in a variety of complex salt crystals. In a succession of demineralization-re-

mineralization cycles, if the sum of the demineralization episodes is greater than that of the remineralization episodes, there is a continuing loss of calcium and phosphate, and increasing porosity of the enamel until it physically collapses to form a cavity.

Development of the Enamel Lesion

To analyse the nature of enamel caries it is necessary first to define the lesion. The dentist finds it easy to recognize a frank open cavity. Clinical identification of the carious pit or fissure lesion is accomplished by tactile sense with an explorer. The dentist recognizes "white spots" on buccal and lingual smooth surfaces, and identifies similar early enamel lesions on the interproximal surfaces as a cone shaped radiolucency on X-ray film. Pit and fissure lesions occur because developmental faults retain plaque. As a result, such caries lesions usually are considered irreversible. However, as long as their surfaces are intact, smooth surface lesions can be arrested and remineralized. To understand this, one must remember that even the minimal enamel lesion may be months or years old. Therefore, it is essential to understand the stages of enamel caries that occur even before they can be seen *in vivo*, at stages earlier than the clinically visible "white spot" or the minimal radiolucency on X-ray film.

Microscopic examination of radiographs and of thin sections of ground enamel are effective methods for studying early stages of the enamel caries lesion. Use of polarized light and sections that have imbibed substances of different molecular sizes give information on the sizes and distribution of the micropores. Based on such studies, Darling described the enamel caries lesion as occurring in a series of six stages. Additionally, he demonstrated four zones that are developed in the progressing lesion (See Fig. 10-2). Using such parameters as pore size, pore per cent of volume, pore distribution, and changes in composition, the differential features associated with the six successive stages can be described. The key features of these stages are listed as follows and will be discussed in the following paragraphs.

Stage 1. Translucent zone is present.
    2. Dark zone appears.
    3. Body of lesion appears.
    4. White spot lesion appears, subsur-

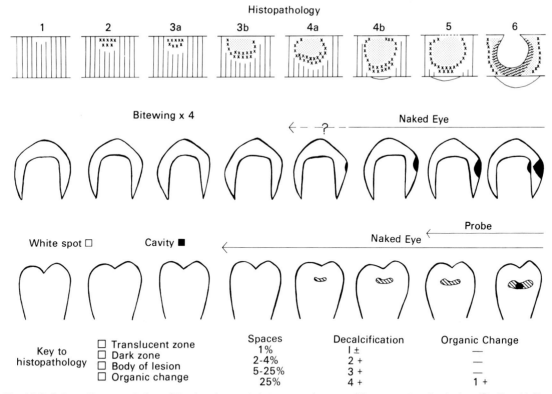

Fig. 10-2. Schematic presentation of the developmental stages and zones of the enamel caries lesion. (Darling AI: Br Dent J 107: 287–296, 1959)

face organic change is first detectable and dentin is invaded.
5. Intact surface becomes chalky.
6. Cavitation occurs.

To gain an appreciation of the complex processes of caries formation it should immediately be pointed out that stage 6 is the earliest lesion that can be seen as a frank clinical cavity. Furthermore, Stage 4 is the earliest seen on clinical radiographs or as white spot lesions. Stages earlier than 4 can be seen only in microscopic examination of thin slices of extracted teeth. In this system, penetration of the dentoenamel junction occurs late in Stage 4. In contrast, histologic study of demineralized teeth has shown that white spot lesions (Stage 4) usually relate to an inflammatory pulp response. Therefore the ionic exchange that eventually results in clinically detectable demineralization of the enamel apparently can precede the demineralization to the extent that it also penetrates the dentin and elicits a reaction in the pulp. Although not established, it is logical to interpret this to mean

that the ionic changes can penetrate the tubules to the pulp without detectable demineralization of the dentin matrix.

Subsurface Demineralization. At Stage 1 in a ground section soaked in quinolin, the minimal subsurface lesion appears translucent. However, the same section viewed under polarized light shows that the translucent zone contains spaces or micropores that make up about 1 per cent of the zone's volume. These spaces vary from small to moderately large in size. The micropores appear along the Striae of Retzius and are seen in relation to the striae at the points of entry through the visually intact surface layer. Since the Striae of Retzius are of high organic content, it has been speculated but not established that the striae act to impede the progress of acid demineralization, with the result that the demineralizing activity spreads laterally at each stria.

Stage 2 is closely similar to, but more advanced than Stage 1. A section that has imbibed quinolin and is viewed under transmitted light shows a dark central zone preceded by the translucent zone. At this stage, the dark zone's volume contains 2 to 4 per cent micropores that are similar to those of the translucent zone, and are mixed in size from small to moderately large. It seems that as the lesion progresses, the translucent zone moves deeper into the enamel and the newly created dark zone represents a further development of the former translucent zone. The continuing demineralization of the dark zone is demonstrated by the larger number of similar sized micropores as compared to the advancing translucent zone.

At Stage 3 transmitted light viewing of quinolin treated sections reveals three zones. The translucent zone has progressed deeper and is still at the advancing front. The dark zone generally is wider than it was at Stage 2, but remains the same in position, pore volume, and pore size. The newly visible body of the lesion is immediately subsurface, in the area formerly occupied by the translucent and dark zones. Different areas of this body of the lesion show various sized micropores that make up 10 to 25 per cent of its volume, indicating that 75 to 90 per cent of the enamel mineral is still intact.

A Stage 3 lesion is not visible on a clinical radiograph and only the body of the lesion is sufficiently porous to be seen on a microradiograph. In studying both dry and water soaked specimens, as well as after imbibition of media with refractive indexes of 1.41 and 1.47, Silverstone diagrammed the pore distribution of Stage 3 lesions. Figure 10-3 gives a summary of the changes seen in the caries lesion at Stage 3.

A Stage 4 lesion of enamel may be described simply as an advance from Stage 3. The surface layer is still intact and microradiographs

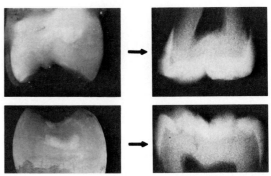

Fig. 10-4. Examples of Stage 4 caries lesions of enamel at the proximal subcontact area of two molars that had been extracted from mature adults. The photographs (at left) display the clinically intact mesial surfaces that have the characteristic semilunar "white spots" that are smooth and vitreous. The radiographs (at right) are buccolingual views of the same teeth. The radiolucency in the maxillary molar (arrow) presents distinct evidence of subsurface demineralization associated with the white spot lesion. The mandibular molar shows no radiolucency associated with its white spot lesion. Thus a Stage 4 caries lesion of enamel may or may not be detectable by radiographs. These illustrations are magnified 3.3×.

still show involvement of the Striae of Retzius. It is not until the latter part of Stage 4 that the dentoenamel junction is penetrated. This is the earliest stage of caries that can be detected as a white spot on visible smooth surfaces or in radiographs of interproximal surfaces (see Fig 10-4).

At Stage 5 the superficial enamel becomes chalky and can be scratched with an explorer. At Stage 6 the surface collapses. Although changes in the organic composition have been quantitated at Stage 6, and have been qualitatively detected as early as Stage 4, it is probable that future advances in research technology will make it possible to study such changes at even earlier stages.

Surface Layer Retention. Striking features of the processes involved in development of the caries lesion are the retention of the surface layer until Stage 6, and the appearance of pulpal inflammatory response simultaneous with or shortly after the lesion has penetrated the dentoenamel junction. Thus acid demineralization at the advancing front of the lesion appears to be the primary caries mechanism in enamel. Once this demineralizing attack reaches the dentin, it penetrates the dentinal tubules very rapidly. Current consensus holds that the intact enamel surface layer survives so late into the lesion development because of

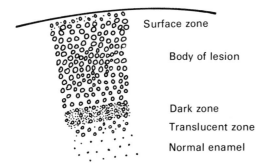

Surface zone

Body of lesion

Dark zone

Translucent zone

Normal enamel

Fig. 10-3. Diagrammatic representation of micropores in a Stage 3 enamel caries lesion. (Silvertone LM: Oral Science Rev 3: 100–160, 1973)

its changing compositon. The surface layer is usually about 25 μm. thick. Although its mineral content is usually about 10 per cent less than that of adjacent sound enamel, its fluoride content is higher than that of normal enamel. This layer lies between the plaque, from which the demineralizing acid enters the enamel, and the subsurface lesion, from which minerals are leached during each acid attack. Subsequently, the plaque provides minerals that pass through the surface layer into the body of the lesion during the intermittent remineralizing phases. Between these alternating actions, and supported by plaque mediated minerals from the saliva, a variety of CaP and CaFP salts precipitate. Thus the end result is that the surface layer of the early enamel caries lesion contains a mineral content that is similar in *quantity* but different in *specific nature*, as compared to normal intact enamel.

The question that remains is how the plaque-mediated acid attack penetrates the surface to demineralize the deeper zones. *In vitro* studies with extracted teeth have shown that strong acids will dissolve the surface enamel, while mild acidic buffers produce subsurface demineralized zones which are closely comparable to the earliest stages of clinical caries as described by Darling. Therefore, the mechanism appears to depend in part on the intensity of the acid attack. It has been proposed that the initial leaching out of the soluble proteins creates the micropores, which subsequently permit the sieve—like flow of water borne hydrogen ions. Alternatively, it has been shown that sound enamel is permeable to water and small ions. Therefore, it may very well be that the overall process can be explained as a simple water borne diffusion of hydrogen ions.

Remineralization. In enamel samples that have been partially demineralized, exposure to saliva alone will remineralize the enamel. Other minerals play roles also. Probably most important to clinical practice of dentistry is the influence of the fluoride ion on remineralization. Not only does fluoride ion accelerate remineralization, it also results in almost complete rehardening of previously softened enamel. Furthermore, the complex salts that it forms within the lesion render the remineralized site more resistant to future acidogenic attacks than was the original enamel. A more in-depth description of remineralization is presented in Chapter 19.

DENTIN CARIES

Structural Features of Dentin

Dentin is a unique tissue that is admirably suited to its functions providing the physical body of the tooth, as well as physiologic support to the related tissues. In embryologic origin and physiologic activities, the dentin and pulp are parts of the same tissue.

The dentin matrix consists of an organic phase and a mineral phase. Although it forms the bulk and contour of the dentin, the organic phase contributes only about 20 per cent of the weight of the matrix. Of this organic phase, about 90 per cent is a dense network of insoluble collagen fibers and the remainder consists of soluble proteins (see Chap. 6). The mineral phase of the matrix consists of hydroxyapatite crystallites that are contained in the soluble protein in considerably less systematic orientation than those of enamel. The soluble protein permits rapid passage of hydrogen ions. The crystallites being smaller than those of enamel offer more surface area and therefore are more rapidly dissolved under acid attack. Those two structural features permit caries to progress much more rapidly through the dentin matrix than through enamel.

The matrix contains dentinal tubules that number 70,000 to 90,000 per mm.^{2} at the outer surface, and range from about 3 μm. in diameter at the outer end to about 5 μm. at their pulpal terminus. With age, the tubules become progressively smaller in diameter through deposition of peritubular mineral. The tubules normally are occupied by odontoblastic processes while the odontoblast cell bodies remain in the pulp (see Chap. 9).

Fluid Flow in Dentin

It has been estimated that about 25 per cent of normal dentin volume is occupied by fluid. The tubular structure permits flow of fluids, ions, and molecules. The fluoride content of dentin may continue to increase for many years after tooth eruption (see Chap. 20) and this is mediated by tissue fluid flow through the tubules of normal dentin. As described earlier in this chapter, pulp reaction has been observed internal to the tubules that are subjacent to a late Stage 4 enamel caries lesion.

This is interpreted as an effect of the rapid penetration of the dentin tubules by hydrogen ions. In otherwise sound teeth, the tissue fluid pressure within the pulp has been measured at about 30 mm. Hg. This indicates that the pressure should cause a continuous outward flow of tubule contents wherever dentin surface is exposed and the tubules are patent. Flow through the tubules in either direction can be influenced by osmotic pressure; hypotonic solutions at the dentin surface cause water to flow toward the pulp, while hypertonic solutions cause fluid to flow outward. However, exposure of the peripheral ends of the tubules to pain producing stimuli, (e.g., $CaCl_2$ or sugar solution cause an outward flow at a rate greater than that predicted on the basis of osmotic and pulpal fluid pressure alone. The permeability of dentin tubules is also influenced by the size, shape, and charge of the particles in a solution in addition to the properties of the tubules that act as diffusion channels. Passage of molecules from the pulp to the dentin surface was demonstrated in extracted teeth when niacin added to the pulp chamber supported growth of niacin dependent bacteria at the outer surface of freshly cut dentin tubules where they were provided with a niacin free media. Alternatively, passage of molecules from the dentin surface to the pulp was demonstrated in experimental animals with atraumatically cut cavities to the dentin. In this experiment, botulinus toxin that was placed in the cavity penetrated the dentin and reached the systemic circulation to produce classical botulinus paresis in the animal. Thus the tubules comprise the circulatory system of normal viable dentin and permit rapid passage of fluid, ions, and molecules.

The Dentin Caries Lesion

Dentin caries is a process of matrix alteration that occurs as a result of microbial metabolism. Although the tubules become altered, their participation appears to be passive. The carious lesion in dentin appears to result from acid demineralization of the matrix, followed by proteolytic degradation of its organic phase. The dentin caries lesion contains three recognizable zones.

The Infected Zone

The *infected zone* is the superficial area that comprises the body of the carious infection. Comparable to fully mature plaque, this zone contains about 10^8 viable microbial cells per gram. It consists almost entirely of a mixture of bacteria with a predominance of proteolytic cells and a low concentration of about 0.1 per cent aciduric cells. Clinically, this material is a soft, yellow mass of cheesy texture.

The Affected Zone

In gradual transition from the infected zone, the *affected zone* appears deeper in the dentin. This is an area of partially demineralized dentin which retains much of its tubular structure, albeit the tubular arrangement becomes distorted. The extent of tubule distortion is great in the superficial area and progressively approaches a minimum of tubule distortion at the front of the affected zone. This zone contains about 10^5 viable microbial cells per gram, less than 0.1 per cent as many as the infected zone. This concentration can be misleading because the transition is gradual, so that at the front of the affected zone there are virtually no viable bacterial cells at all. Within this zone, with its microbial content one thousandth that of the infected zone, there is a marked increase in the proportion of bacteria that are aciduric and a corresponding decrease in the proportion that are proteolytic. This observation is compatible with the interpretation that acid demineralization plays a predominant role in the affected zone, while proteolytic activity (collagen degradation) is more active in the infected zone. Clinically, the affected zone becomes progressively more dark brown and leathery in texture. Massler considers the affected dentin as an area of partial demineralization but otherwise morphologically intact dentin. He holds that the infectious challenge of caries is in the infected zone and that the few remaining viable cells that may be recovered from the affected zone are considered as "contaminents" that cannot survive after the infected zone has been removed and the remaining affected zone has been sealed off from contact with the cariogenic plaque. To distinguish between these two zones is important to preventively oriented, conservative dental practice. Indirect pulp capping is a technic that is frequently used when a carious lesion is so close to exposure of the vital pulp that a mechanical or accidental exposure appears imminent. Selection of this form of therapy is based on the principle that the caries process will be arrested after the infected zone has been removed and the sealed-in affected zone is allowed to remain in situ long enough for reaction dentin to form on the pulpal wall subjacent to the associated tubules.

The Hypermineralized Zone

Consisting of increased mineral content, the *hypermineralized zone* is found at the active front of the advancing carious lesion in dentin. Its thickness varies with the intensity and chronicity of the caries attack. This zone is narrow in cases of acute caries, but is considerably wider subjacent to the front of chronic, more slowly progressing caries. Specific to dentin caries, its developmental mechanism is unknown. It is considered probable that this zone occurs as a result of the precipitation of mineral salts at that site during each reversal of the demineralization-remineralization equilibrium. Thus the formative mechanism of the hypermineralized zone of dentin caries apparently depends on microbial metabolism within the infected body of the lesion, and parallels the remineralization of the surface layer of enamel caries.

Zone Differentiation Within the Lesion

A variety of stains have shown that the infected zone may be heavily colored, the stain becomes progressively weaker in the depths of the affected zone, and the hypermineralized zone is essentially impermeable to stains. The progressive loss of stainability illustrates the gradual change in composition between the zones. However, clinical application of stains to identify the zones is of negligible usefulness because the color and texture of unstained zones are more definitive. Hardness changes in dentin have also been correlated with microscopic recognition of the zones. In chronic, slowly progressing lesions, the zones are distinct and relatively broad. In acute, rapidly progressing dentin caries, the zones become more difficult to demonstrate by hardness changes, suggesting that the caries progress is too rapid for definitive zones to be developed. However, the typical dark brown color is always present in the deeper parts of the affected zone. Therefore, both color and texture are the essential criteria for clinical differentiation between the zones.

Internal Mineralization

While the hypermineralized zone is specific to dentin caries, other forms of mineralization that occur in response to a variety of stimuli, including caries, also are of interest. The dentist's understanding of these mechanisms is useful in management of dentin caries.

Reaction dentin is an irregular form of secondary dentin that is deposited on the pulpal wall when a challenge to the pulp exceeds that which would stimulate secondary dentin formation. When the challenge has been sufficient to cause death and disruption of the odontoblast layer, atubular reaction dentin may be deposited on the dentin-pulp wall subjacent to those tubules which transmit the irritant to the pulp. With subsequent regeneration of the odontoblast layer, irregular tubular dentin and ultimately secondary dentin are deposited internal to the atubular dentin.

Sclerotic dentin or "blind tract dentin" formation is a process in which the affected tubules are slowly filled by mineralization. This is routinely observed when both ends of a group of tubules have been occluded. It may also be observed subjacent to arrested dentin caries. While sclerosis makes the dentin less permeable, it does not completely seal the tubules. Thus the formation of sclerotic dentin appears to be a self protective mechanism of the dental pulp.

Although therapeutic remineralization of carious dentin remains in limited use in dental practice, there is clear evidence that it can be made to occur. When the affected zone of carious dentin is covered with a calcium hydroxide lining and the cavity is sealed by a restoration, subsequent analysis will reveal an increased phosphate content, indicating that mineralization has occurred. Since only calcium ion was applied, it is clear that the increased phosphate content was provided from an *in vivo* source. This explains the clinical usefulness of a calcium hydroxide lining on the dentin surface during the restoration of teeth that have carious lesions with deep involvement of the dentin.

External Mineralization

Under appropriate conditions, the outer surface of dentin that had previously been demineralized by caries can be remineralized. When the overlying enamel is removed to the extent that the exposed carious dentin surface is maintained free of plaque by self cleansing, exposure to saliva alone usually will be followed by arrestment of the caries and remineralization of the exposed dentin surface. Such surfaces become stained dark brown, vitreous, and fluoride rich. This process may occur spontaneously as occasionally observed in adults in whom the undermining dentin caries had progressed laterally to the extent that the enamel walls had collapsed, leaving the carious dentin surface exposed to saliva and self cleansing.

Numerous studies have shown that partially demineralized dentin surfaces can be remineralized by calcifying solutions. Calcium, fluoride and several heavy metals have each been shown to remineralize carious dentin *in vivo*. Of these, a ten per cent stannous fluoride solution has been shown to remineralize the dentin most effectively. Electron dense crystals have formed within the dentin matrix, and crystalline salts of tin have been detected. These findings are compatible with the clinical evidence that topical application of stannous fluoride is effective in arrestment of clinical caries lesions that involve the dentin.

Fate of the Microbial Infection

The microbial mass that is responsible for dentin caries depends on the plaque and the oral milieu for the nutrition that will permit both continuing multiplication and further caries activity. The numbers of surviving bacteria will be sharply reduced, however, when sealed by an amalgam restoration placed in a cavity with clinically recognizable carious dentin of the affected zone. A small number of viable cells may still be recovered after as long as two years. During that time the caries process is stationary. After all clinical signs of carious dentin have been removed and the cavity has been sealed, viable acidogenic streptococci and lactobacilli also may be recovered upon reopening the cavity after as long as two years. This indicates that clinical judgment is not a reliable criterion for complete removal of the cariogenic flora. Even more pertinent is the knowledge gained from recent research wherein placement of a sealant in the fissures over otherwise undistrubed moderately deep dentin lesions demonstrated that there was about a 95 per cent reduction in numbers of viable cells during the first two weeks and a continuing reduction to less than 0.05 per cent of the origi-

nal number of bacteria after two years. Most importantly there was no detectable dentin caries lesion increase. Thus the bacteria of the infected zone of dentin caries also are dependent upon oral nutrition sources for continuing significant rates of survival, multiplication, and cariogenesis. In contrast, the small number of viable bacterial cells which may be recovered after as long as two years suggests that these cells may receive nutrients from the tissue fluids via the pulp, and possibly from degradation products of remaining dead bacterial cells in amounts sufficient to support a highly limited number of viable bacterial cells. Whether this limited nutrition will support survival of the infection much more than two years remains to be determined. Although an increase of the dentin caries lesions could not be detected after two years, this does not preclude the possibility that measurable caries advance might occur over many years. For this reason, sound dental practice makes logical the complete removal of all clinically detectable carious dentin before placement of permanent restorations. At the same time, the described reduction in bacterial count and two year absence of caries progress also makes logical the indirect pulp capping technic in which the affected zone is sealed in for a relatively short period of weeks during which deposition of protective reaction dentin is allowed to occur.

CLINICAL MANAGEMENT OF DENTAL CARIES LESIONS

Application of cariology knowledge to clinical treatment of caries lesions requires professional discretion concerning the location of the lesion and the site's potential for arrestment and remineralization. Since caries normally invades the dentin before the enamel surface collapses, it is logical to consider the clinical management of both dentin and enamel caries in the same context.

Pit and Fissure Lesions

The pit or fissure lesion by definition is not in a self cleansing area, and caries occurs because the physical dimensions permit retention of plaque. Clinical studies have shown that sealants or amalgam restorations that are placed in the presence of remaining caries in pits or fissures tend to be followed by arrestment of the process and slow dying off of the remaining bacteria over as much as two years. Thus the caries process is interrupted by placement of a barrier between the early caries lesion and the cariogenic plaque. A widely held scientific attitude advocates the application of sealants to all pits and fissures of children's teeth, with the exception of sites that have advanced dentin caries which is detectable by its leathery texture to an explorer or by the color of enamel that is undermined by dentin caries. For the latter, a restoration is normally indicated.

Cervical Lesions

A second area of concern is the frequently observed white spot lesion at buccal or lingual cervical areas, principally on the posterior teeth of young patients. From clinical experience the dentist usually learns that many such lesions do not progress to cavitation. Historically, it has been recognized that these lesions usually appear near the gingival crest during the first few years after tooth eruption and do not progress after the gingival crest had been relocated apically as the patient matures. This conversion of the site to a self cleansing area is the mechanism that halts the caries process. The observations of Backer-Dirks strongly support the interpretation that such clinical caries lesions usually will not progress to cavitation and may remineralize without therapeutic intervention. He examined 90 children annually from age 8 to 15 years. As illustrated in Figure 10-5, of 72 such lesions on the maxillary first molars, 9 progressed to cavitation, 26 remained as white spots, and 37 reverted to clinically normal appearing enamel. Thus 63 lesions were arrested, with 26 clinically unchanged and 37 apparently remineralized to the extent that they disappeared at some time during the seven year observation period. For these reasons operative restoration of cervical lesions seems to be contraindicated until the process has advanced to Stage 6 and the enamel surface has collapsed.

Interproximal Lesions

On freshly extracted, clinically sound teeth that have been washed and air dried, the proximal subcontact area often shows either a

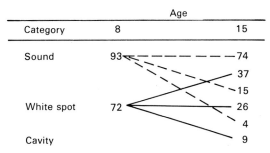

Fig. 10-5. Fate of sound and of white spot carious enamel at buccal and lingual cervical surfaces of maxillary first molars. (Modified from Backer-Dirks O: J Dent Res 45: 503–511, 1966)

brown or an opaque white spot. Each represents an earlier caries lesion that had progressed approximately to Stage 4. The opaque white spot consists of enamel that was partially demineralized before the tooth was extracted. It may have been an active caries lesion or it may have been arrested and remineralized to some degree. The brown spot represents a former white spot in which the caries process has been reversed for a longer period of time. It has been remineralized to some degree, and the color is imparted by organic material imbibed from the plaque. A brown spot usually contains a higher content of both fluoride and organic material than a white spot, and analysis of the subsurface material will demonstrate the presence of a variety of complex calcium-fluoride-phosphate salts that have precipitated in the lesion during remineralization episodes.

Spontaneous arrestment of such interproximal lesions detectable only by X-ray has been reported. Shiller and Scola observed such lesions in 115 men aged 18 to 23 years who were in the untreated control group of a clinical trial. These investigators reported that 60 per cent of the lesions either were already arrested before the study or they were arrested during the study.

If clinically sound teeth from a variety of subjects (e.g., those extracted for periodontal reasons) are cleaned, dried and examined, a significant number of proximal subcontact areas will reveal white and brown spots. If the latter teeth are aligned in a manner similar to their intra arch relationships, simulated clinical radiographs of most of the white and some of the brown spots will present the typical cone shaped radiolucency that is diagnostic of caries. However, an appreciable number of such white and brown spots will not be detectable in clinical radiographs, indicating that remineralization had progressed to the extent that the arrested lesion and adjacent sound enamel were of such similar radiodensity that they were indistinguishable from one another. This indicates that incorporation of organic material is not essential to remineralization in white spot lesions. The relative infrequency of brown spot cervical lesions, compared to the disappearance of white spot lesions observed by Backer-Dirks, supports this interpretation. The highly important application of this knowledge is that the proximal caries lesion which may be diagnosed by radiograph but which does not present clinical cavitation, may be a candidate for arrestment. In fact, it may be remineralized and become even more resistant to future caries attack than the adjacent sound enamel. Published studies have shown that such lesions have made no progress for as long as 17 years. Still unanswered is the question of at what stage surgical intervention and restoration of a carious proximal surface is justified. Current consensus holds that (with the exception of special cases such as those with rampant caries) radiographic evidence of dentin involvement should be the criterion. Conservative dentists who have confidence in their preventive dentistry delivery system may hold to the attitude that a proximal smooth surface caries lesion which is detectable only in radiographs should be recorded as a candidate for arrestment until consecutive semiannual examinations reveal recognizable increase in the depth of the lesion's dentin penetration.

SUMMARY

The biology of dental caries involves loss of tooth mineral in accord with the physicochemical laws. Acids that are generated in the superficial microbial infection penetrate the enamel and dentin where they solubilize tooth minerals during each demineralization phase of the equilibrium that normally exists at the interface between the active microbial mass and the tooth surface.

Diffusion of the dissolved mineral ions toward the microbial plaque results in increasing porosity of the enamel at that carious site until the surface collapses to form a cavity. Alternatively, prior to the surface collapse, each time that the equilibrium shifts to a remineralization phase the dissolved ions diffuse back into the porous enamel lesion where they may be reprecipitated in the form of complex salts that are less soluble than the original sound tooth mineral. When this reversal of ion flow and precipitation of less soluble salts has occurred to the extent that the site has become insoluble relative to the usual caries attack, the lesion will be arrested.

After the enamel surface has collapsed, the cariogenic microflora reach the dentin. Dentin caries appears to be primarily a process of acid demineralization of the matrix followed by proteolytic degradation of the organic phase of the dentin matrix. Three zones are developed in carious dentin. The superficial infected zone consists almost entirely of bacterial cells and may be recognized as an amorphous yellow mass of cheesy texture. The affected zone is deeper in the dentin lesion. It is a partially demineralized area that retains its tubular structure although in distorted arrangement. This zone may be identified clinically by its leathery texture and brown color. In the affected zone the tubular morphology and bacterial content change progressively until, at the zone's front, the dentin morphology appears normal and the viable bacterial cells become almost nonexistent. Deep to the affected zone, the hypermineralized zone is found at the surface of morphologically intact dentin. Related to dentin caries, both internal and external forms of mineralization may occur. While not impermeable, these mineralizations act to impede the progress and to protect the pulp from the caries process. Their degree and rate of formation appear to be related to the chronicity or acuteness of the caries attack.

The described processes which retard caries progress can occur spontaneously in some subjects. With an understanding of the principles described in this chapter, their occurrence may be enhanced therapeutically. For the practice of sound dental medicine, it is essential that our patients receive the benefits of these advances in dental science.

GLOSSARY

Acidogenic. "Acid Generating." Term applied to microorganisms that are capable of generating a high hydrogen ion concentration in the environment.

Aciduric. "Acid Enduring." Term applied to microorganisms that, although they may prefer a neutral environment, are capable of enduring acidities as low as pH 4.0 without undue damage.

Adsorbed. To attach atoms, ions, or molecules to the surface of a substance by means of unsatisfied valence bonds.

Affected zone. The area of a carious dentin lesion that is subjacent to the infected zone. It is a leathery, brown mass of partially demineralized dentin that contains distorted tubules and an average of about 10^5 microbial cells per gram, about one-thousandth that of the infected zone. The concentration becomes progressively lower and the proportion that are acidogenic becomes progressively greater as the front of the affected zone is approached, so that microbial cells are almost absent at the front of the affected zone.

Atubular dentin. Reaction dentin formed with no tubules. This is the first variety to be formed after an injury or irritation that was so severe as to cause death of the odontoblasts associated with the site.

Bound water. Water caged within the hydroxyapatite structure but freely tumbling within the crystallite. Removable at 900–1300 C, with irreversible changes to the hydroxyapatite.

Demineralization. A loss or decrease of the mineral constituents of a tissue. In dental caries, demineralization results in loss or decrease of the calcium and phosphate ions from hydroxyapatite.

Enamel sieve. The concept that the free water of dental enamel is capable of transporting ions through the apparently solid enamel as if it were a sieve.

Free water. Loosely held water of dental enamel that is easily removed by dehydration at 100 C without irreversible changes in the enamel.

Hydration shell. A layer of tightly bound water that envelops the apatite crystal and provides a medium for ionic exchange within the crystal. This term is also sometimes used in reference to the first layer of water molecules surrounding an ion in aqueous solution. In demineralization of hydroxyapatite, water forms a hydration shell surrounding each dissolved Ca and PO_4 ion. In remineralization, crystallization occurs when Ca and PO_4 precipitate, converting the waters of their hydration shells to free water.

Hydroxyapatite. A mineral structure, $Ca_{10}(PO_4)_6(OH)_2$, which the crystal lattice of bones and teeth closely resembles.

Hypermineralized Zone. Subjacent to the affected zone of a dentin caries lesion, the hypermineralized zone is a relatively narrow zone that contains a higher mineral concentration than normal dentin.

Imbibition. "To drink in." The absorption of fluid or dissolved ions by a solid body such as enamel, without resultant significant change in the body.

Infected zone. The superficial zone of a dentin caries lesion. The infected zone consists of a soft, cheesy yellow mass containing about 10^8 microbial cells per gram, that are predominantly proteolytic forms, together with degraded dentin material components.

Irregular dentin. A variety of reaction dentin that may be formed when some odontoblasts survive the causal injury, or may be deposited internal to atubular dentin after odontoblast cells have been regenerated at the site.

Microspace. Synonymous with micropore. A space of microscopic dimension. In enamel caries, demineralization of a limited number of hydroxyapatite crystallites and diffusion of the resultant ions to another location leaves microspaces in the formerly solid enamel.

Polarized light. A change effected in a ray of light passing through certain media, whereby the transverse vibrations occur in one plane only instead of in all planes as occurs in the ordinary light ray.

Primary dentin. The original dentin that forms the main body of the tooth and is laid down prior to tooth eruption.

Quinoline. C_9H_7N; a volatile nitrogenous, colorless, odorless liquid distilled from coal tar. Quinolin has a characteristic refractive index that so differs from the refractive index of enamel that, after quinolin has been imbibed by a microscopic enamel caries lesion and the specimen is viewed under polarized light, the quinolin displays the micropores size and location.

Reaction dentin. (Reparative Dentin). Dentin deposited locally on the pulpal wall as a response to any irritant, (i.e., caries, medications, or operative procedures). The type of reaction dentin formed depends on the severity of the causal irritant and the resultant speed with which the reaction dentin is formed.

Refraction, refringence. The deflection of a ray of light when it passes from one medium into another of different density.

Refractive index. The relative velocity of light in a medium compared to its velocity in air. The ratio of the sine of the angle of incidence to the sine of the angle of refraction when light passes obliquely in a medium.

Remineralization. The deposition of mineral salts in an area or tissue from which mineral previously had been removed. In enamel and dentin, this new mineral consists primarily of calcium and phosphate, but it may include other substances, such as organic material, when remineralization occurs.

Sclerotic dentin. Blind tract dentin. A zone of calcified dentinal tubules that may have been caused by a variety of stimuli. The resultant sclerotic dentin is harder, more dense and less permeable than normal dentin. Sclerosed dentin usually forms when both ends of the tubules are obtunded, (i.e., by atubular dentin at the pulpal end and a restoration at the peripheral end).

Secondary dentin. The dentin which continues to be formed posteruptively, throughout life. It may be differentiated from primary dentin by a change in the course, regularity, and numbers of tubules. With time after the pulp has recovered from an injury, secondary dentin may form internal to reaction dentin.

Stephan curve. The classical graphic correlation between hydrogen ion concentration in dental plaque and time after exposure to sugar. The plaque pH falls rapidly early in microbial metabolism of the sugar and rises over a period of time as the acid concentration is reduced by salivary flow, neutralized by plaque buffers, ammonia, and amine production, and further metabolism of strong acids to weak acids.

Striae of retzius. A series of widely spaced bands that reflect intermittent changes in the overall calcification pattern of enamel. The resultant striae make circumferential arcs that progress occlusally or incisally from the dentoenamel junction to the outer enamel surface where they end in grooves that parallel the cementoenamel junction and are known as the perikymata.

Tumbling water. Synonymous with bound water. Molecular water bound to the hydroxyapatite surface and capable of transfering its bond from one site to another.

SUGGESTED READINGS

Backer-Dirks O: Posteruptive changes in dental enamel. J Dent Res 45: 503–511, 1966

Bergman G: Microscopic demonstration of liquid flow through human dental enamel. Arch Oral Biol 8: 233–234, 1963

Brännström M, Lind PO: Pulpal response to early dental caries. J Dent Res 44: 1045–1050, 1965

Curzon MEJ, Losee FL: Dental caries and trace element composition of whole human enamel: Eastern United States. J Am Dent Assoc 94: 1146–1150, 1977

Darling AI: The pathology and prevention of caries. Br Dent J 107: 287–296, 1959

Darling AI: Ultrastructure of enamel in relation to mineralization, demineralization and remineralization as revealed by microradiography, polarised light and plane microscopy. Int Dent J 17: 684–692, 1967

Darling AI, Mortimer KV, Poole DFG, Ollis WD: Molecular sieve behaviour of normal and carious human dental enamel. Arch Oral Biol 5: 251–273, 1961

Eidelman E, Finn SB, Koulourides T: Remineralization of carious dentin treated with calcium hydroxide. J Dent Child 32: 218–225, 1965

Fehr FR von der: Maturation and remineralization of enamel. In Hardwick JL, Held RR, König KG (eds): Advances in Fluorine Research and Dental Caries Prevention. London, Pergamon Press, 1964, pp 83–98

Fusayama T, Okuse K, Hosoda H: Relationship between hardness, discoloration, and microbial invasion in carious dentin. J Dent Res 45: 1033–1046, 1966

Handelman SL, Washburn F, Wopperer P: Two year report of sealant effect on bacteria in dental caries. J Am Dent Assoc 93: 967–970, 1976

Johansen E: The nature of the carious lesion. Dental Clinics of North America. St. Louis, CV Mosby, 305–320, 1962

Koulourides T: Experimental changes of enamel mineral density, In Harris RS (ed): Art and Science of Dental Caries Research. New York, Academic Press, 1968

Koulourides T, Feagin F, Pigman W: Remineralization of dental enamel by saliva in-vitro. Ann NY Acad Sci 131: 751–757, 1965

Levine RS: Distribution of fluoride in active and arrested carious lesions in dentin. J Dent Res 51: 1025–1029, 1972

Little MF, Casciani FS: The nature of water in sound human enamel. Arch Oral Biol 11: 565–571, 1966

Losee FL, Ludwig TG: Trace elements and caries. J Dent Res 49: 1229–1235, 1970

MacGregor AB: The extent and distribution of acid in carious dentine. Proc Roy Soc Med 55: 1063–1070, 1962

Massler M: Preventive endodontics: vital pulp therapy. In Dental Clinics of North America. St. Louis, CV Mosby, 1967, pp 663–673

Mercer VH, Muhler JC: The clinical demonstration of caries arrestment following topical stannous fluoride treatments. J Dent Child 32: 65–72, 1965

Moore DL: Preventive operative dentistry. In Bernier JL, Muhler JC (eds): Improving Dental Practice Through Preventive Measures. St. Louis, CV Mosby, 1975

Sarnat H, Massler M: Microstructure of active and arrested dentinal caries. J Dent Res 44: 1389–1401, 1965

Scott DB, Simmelink JW, Nygaard V: Structural aspects of dental caries. J Dent Res 53 (2): 165–178, 1974

Shiller WR, Scola FP: Two year observations of enamel caries on posterior interproximal surfaces. US Navy Med News Letter 48: 19–21, 1966

Silverstone LM: Structure of carious enamel, including the early lesion. Oral Sc Rev 3: 100–160, 1973

Silverstone LM: Remineralization phenomena. Caries Res [Suppl] 11 (1): 59–84, 1977

Stanley HR, White CL, McCray L: The rate of tertiary (reparative) dentine formation in the human tooth. Oral Surg 21: 180–189, 1966

Weatherell JA: Composition of dental enamel. Br Med Bull 31: 115–119, 1975

Wei SHY, Kaqueler JC, Massler M: Remineralization of carious dentin. J Dent Res 47: 381–391, 1968

PART THREE

The Agents:

MICROBIOLOGIC INTERACTIONS WITH ORAL TISSUE

11 Composition and Ecology of the Oral Flora

ROBERT MORHART

ROBERT FITZGERALD

Introduction
Composition of the Oral Microbiota
    Problems in Determining the Composition of Oral Microbial Ecosystems
    Sample Collection
    Transport and Dispersion Methods
    Isolation and Cultural Procedures
    Identification of Isolates
    Method of Expressing Results
Primary Oral Ecosystems
    Tongue

    Coronal Plaque
    Crevicular Microbiota
    Saliva
Microbial Succession of the Oral Flora
    Acquisition of the Oral Flora
    The Development of an Ecosystem: Coronal Plaque
Summary
Glossary
Suggested Readings

INTRODUCTION

Microorganisms have been known to be ubiquitous to the oral cavity of man since their direct observation by van Leeuwenhoek, the pioneer microscopist in the 17th century. About the turn of the last century, the work of W. D. Miller, G. V. Black, and J. L. Williams led to the concept that dental caries was the result of the localized activity of the bacteria that coated the teeth, and the term "gelatinous microbic plaque" was coined to describe this entity. However, it was as recent as the mid 1950's when it was demonstrated that certain plaque forming oral streptococci could produce dental caries in experimental animals and in the mid 1960's when it was experimen-

tally proven that a direct correlation existed between the amount of dental plaque and marginal gingivitis in humans.

The seminal work in the period between the mid 1950's and 1960's which led to the discovery that certain microorganisms, notably *Streptococcus mutans*, could cause dental caries opened a new era in oral microbiology. These studies demonstrated once and for all that dental caries is a microbial disease, and that the microbiota inhabiting the oral cavity of man is composed of a variety of distinct microbial ecosystems. Prior to this time the oral microbiota was viewed to be homogeneously distributed, a belief that led many investigators to mistakenly seek for caries producing organisms in readily obtained saliva samples. Yet it is ironic that the eventual discovery of specific cariogenic organisms, a longstanding research goal, did not really simplify our understanding of dental caries but instead made more evident the complexity of this disease.

The multifactorial nature of dental caries (see Chap. 8) can be viewed in several ways. When viewed from the ecologic standpoint, as we do in this book, it is apparent that the incidence and severity of dental diseases are determined by a dynamic relationship between three factors: the microbial agent of the disease, the defensive capability of the host, and the environmental conditions which may affect each of the first two factors. In such a relationship it is possible for agent and host factors to be modulated by environmental variables to such an extent that disease may or may not result. Microbial ecologic concepts can then be used to view the microbial agents of disease as well as the dynamic nature of the oral microflora in general. The main concern of this and the following two chapters is to show how host and environmental factors serve as ecologic determinants for the implantation, establishment, distribution, growth, metabolism, and transmissibility of organisms within the oral microbiota in the normal state and when dental caries is present.

This chapter presents information on the predominant members of specific oral ecosystems at various points in man's life cycle. Chapter 12 introduces certain microbial eco-

logic concepts and considers general factors that are necessary for the growth of oral microorganisms, specific characteristics of microorganisms that allow for their implantation and propagation within certain habitats, and factors that control and modulate the growth rates and metabolic properties of microorganisms within these habitats. Chapter 13 considers the cariogenic organisms from both a microbial ecologic and a general ecologic perspective.

It is the goal of the present chapter to develop the concept that microbial flora of the mouth is composed of a variety of distinct microbial ecosystems at different sites, often with subsystems existing within the same site. An understanding of this principle is essential to the understanding of dental caries and to the appreciation of the advances made in oral microbiology in recent years.

COMPOSITION OF THE ORAL MICROBIOTA

The oral microbiota is composed of a number of distinct microbial ecosystems. In turn, each of the ecosystems is formed by a variety of bacterial types that favor certain habitats within the mouth. A habitat is a natural environment where organisms can grow. The major habitats of the oral microbiota include

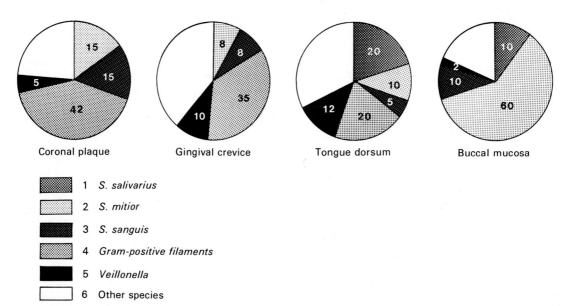

Fig. 11-1. Approximate proportional distribution of the predominant cultivable flora of four oral habitats.

the teeth, mucous membranes, saliva, tongue, and gingival crevice. The microbial populations that comprise these ecosystems differ in both qualitative and quantitative aspects. Quantitative studies have shown that the largest biomass of bacteria exists on the surfaces of the teeth and on the dorsum of the tongue. Microorganisms make up more than 90 per cent of the mass of coronal plaque according to optical and electron micrographs of plaque sections, and number between 10^{11} and 10^{12} organisms per gram wet weight. Epithelial cells scraped from the dorsal surface of the tongue average well over 100 adherent bacteria per cell, whereas epithelial cells removed from the cheek and palatal surfaces harbor only 5 to 25 bacteria per cell. Figure 11-1 shows a graphic representation of the approximate proportional distribution of selected bacterial types found within four oral habitats. Streptococci and gram positive filamentous organisms comprise major segments of the flora present in most sites. It can be seen, however, that each of these ecosystems contains its own characteristic collection of bacterial species. For example, *Streptococcus mitis* is the predominant species colonizing the buccal mucosa, S. *salivarius* preferentially colonizes the dorsal surface of the tongue, and S. *sanguis* preferentially colonizes the teeth. In addition to these broad differences in distribution, other representatives of the more than 40 species so far identified that make up the oral microbiota also seem to preferentially colonize one or more of the oral habitats. Furthermore, not only are there both qualitative and quantitative variations between different sites within the same mouth, and at different times within the same site, but also variations commonly occur between the same habitat in different individuals.

Problems in Determining the Composition of Oral Microbial Ecosystems

The significance of the complexity and variability of the oral microbiota has only recently been appreciated. This slow development can be attributed largely to the extreme difficulties in obtaining accurate quantitation of the mixed microbial populations of the mouth. While advances in anaerobic techniques and the development of selective media have been significant aids to the understanding of the oral microflora, there are still no universally applicable methods for isolation and enumeration of the full complement of dental plaque microorganisms. Depending on the study objectives and the available resources, investigators are often forced to make various compromises in their final choice of procedures. Some of the technologic problem areas encountered in determining the composition of oral microbial ecosystems include the following: sample collection, sample preservation and dispersion, isolation and cultural procedures, identification of isolates, and methods of expressing results. It is worth our while to briefly consider some of these factors.

Sample Collection

The realization that saliva might not be a suitable site for the search for the agent factor of dental caries led to direct sampling of the affected tooth surfaces. One technique was to pool plaque collected from a number of teeth. While this approach had the advantage of obtaining the quantities of materials required for accurate weighing and for biochemical studies, it had the serious disadvantages of lacking precision and obscuring between-site variations which could be relevant to understanding caries activity. Methods are required that allow for more precise assessment of specific areas such as buccal and lingual smooth surfaces, pits, fissures. Generally dental explorers or similar instruments are used for sample collection at these sites. For the more inaccessible approximal surfaces, plaque specimens can be collected with dental floss or extra fine explorers. For studies in which optical and/or electron micrographs of plaque sections are needed along with cultural studies, investigators have restored to a variety of artifical intraoral devices for the collection of intact plaques at desired sites. When properly applied, this approach is especially valuable since the organization and spatial relationships of bacteria in plaque are preserved, and ultrastructural assessments can be made about the physiologic state of the organisms, the characteristics of the intercellular matrix, and the interrelationships between various species.

Techniques have also been developed for the collection of samples at various levels within the gingival crevice free of contaminants from the surrounding area. Depending on the objectives of the investigator, the choice of an appropriate sampling procedure is of fundamental importance to the validity of any study of the composition of the oral microflora.

Preservation and Dispersion Methods

Early quantitative culturing procedures for plaque samples could only recover about 20 per cent of the microscopically visible organisms as viable colonies on plate counts. This was because some of the organisms were non-viable, some were killed during processing, others were unable to grow under the cultural conditions used, and still others occurred in masses that could not easily be dispersed for proper plating. Subsequent studies have shown that if plaque is collected and manipulated under systems of complete anaerobiosis, (e.g., sample collection under nitrogen gas, preservation in reduced transport media, and the use of roll tube techniques or an anaerobic chamber) the recoveries of bacteria are tripled.

Quantitative examination of plaque based on viable bacterial counts necessitates the use of serial dilution procedures. This approach presents certain technical problems since the plaque mass must be disrupted to release individual cells that presumably will then grow as individual colonies when plated on suitable growth media. Unfortunately, because of the sticky, cohesive nature of plaque, completely single cell dispersions are almost impossible to obtain in practice. This problem is further complicated by the varying susceptibility of different species both to the physical forces that are employed to disperse plaque and to the presence of oxygen. In practice, ultrasonic devices, vortex mixers, shaking with glass beads or tissue homogenizers are most commonly used, either alone or in combination, in atmospheres that maintain reduced oxygen levels. The final choice of method can generally only be determined by trial and error in each specific case. Usually it comes down to a compromise between maximum preservation of viability and satisfactory dispersion of cells.

Isolation and Culture Procedures

The uneven distribution of widely dissimilar organisms within plaque presents problems in processing of samples. Procedures such as the streaking of plaque directly on agar media, or the direct inoculation of broth select out only the fastest growing organisms for the specific media employed and thus give no indication, or at best a biased indication, of the total number or types of bacteria present in a sample. To meet this objection it is preferable to use a range of different media and cultural conditions. Commonly, a combination of nonselective and selective media are used, some for aerobic and others for anaerobic incubation of aliquots of each sampling. Selective media may be especially helpful for the isolation of strains that are present in low concentrations. Selective media are also frequently used to isolate and/or quantitate selected bacterial species when the total viable count is not needed. Over the years a number of selective media have been described for isolation of various oral bacteria.

Identification of Isolates

Only after an organism has been isolated and established to be a pure culture can it be subjected to final identification procedures. Although taxonomic problems still exist within several broad groups of commonly isolated oral microorganisms, including the numerous gram stain, colonial morphology and growth identify most plaque isolates to the genus level by a relatively small number of criteria. These would include cell morphology and motility, gram stain, colonial morphology and growth in different atmospheres and the application of a limited number of biochemical tests, (e.g., hydrogen peroxide decomposition, nitrate reduction, indole production, H_2S production, the oxidase reaction and the fermentation of a number of sugars). Identification to the species level is possible for many strains, but this may require further biochemical testing, as well as fermentation end product analyses, serological tests, and cell wall composition studies.

Methods of Expressing Results

Having taken appropriate steps to get an accurate estimation of the numbers and kinds of organisms present in a series of samples, it is important to find a meaningful expression for these results. The following methods are among the most generally used:

1. Frequency of occurrence, that is, the number of instances in which various organisms are present (or absent) in a population, subject, tooth or site on a tooth, without reference to the actual numbers present.
2. Number of organisms of various types per unit weight (or volume) of a sample, expressed on a wet or dry weight basis and either as a proportion of total viable count or total microscopic count.
3. Modifications of (2) in which the absolute weight of the sample is replaced by some analytically determinable parameter which is related to it, such as the protein, nitrogen, or deoxyribonucleic acid content of the sample.
4. Procedures in which the numbers of specific organisms are expressed as proportions of the total cultivable flora of a sample, or as proportions of a predominant group of microorganisms (e.g., the per cent of *S. mutans* in the total streptococci cultivable on a medium selective for this group of bacteria).

Each of these methods has some inherent advantages and associated errors. Most errors have their source in the problems already enumerated in the sections on sample processing, adequacy of culture procedures, and identification of microorganisms. The advantages of one procedure over another will depend on the balance between the convenience with which it can be carried out and the reliability of the information it yields in the context of the study objectives. For example, in a study intended to determine numbers of plaque organisms at various sites it would be of no value to reduce the data to numbers of bacteria per milligram of plaque since a given weight of plaque, regardless of source, will nearly always contain a constant number of organisms (approximately 10^{12} per gram wet weight). In the case cited, therefore, the correct way to express the data would be as the total number of organisms per site since this would reflect differences in the amounts of plaque which accumulated at the different sites.

Primary Oral Ecosystems

The major oral ecosystems include the tongue, the tooth crown, the gingival crevice,

and saliva. Table 11-1 lists the types and distribution of organisms that predominate in the various sites of the mouth. The main purpose of this Table is to illustrate the point that certain genera and/or species have a primary habitat, whereas others are distributed throughout the oral cavity. It should be borne in mind however, that we are dealing with dynamic ecosystems and marked variability can exist in the microbial composition within these sites, so much so, that the microflora at a particular site or even within the same site in the same individual may differ at different sampling times. These differences can involve alterations not only in numbers of organisms but qualitative changes in types as well. Heterogeneity of the oral microbiota is thus the normal state of affairs.

The data presented in the following sections are at best only an estimate of the types and counts of bacterial species present at the various sites since bacteriologic censuses can only describe the situation at the moment the sample was collected. While it is also beyond the scope of this chapter to give detailed information concerning the microbiologic and biochemical characteristics of the various bacterial species referred to in the following sections, the reader is encouraged to read any one of the several texts referred to in the Suggested Readings for more complete coverage.

Tongue

The predominant cultivable organisms (approximately 50%) found on the dorsum of the tongue are gram positive cocci. Collectively, the viridans group of *Streptococcus* species constitutes the majority of this group. *S. salivarius* accounts for over 50 per cent of the viridans streptococci, followed by *S. mitior* (approximately 30%) which is also found in large numbers on other oral mucous membranes, and *S. sanguis* (approximately 20%) making up the bulk of the remaining streptococci. *S. salivarius* is a fairly well defined species which characteristically produces large quantities of extracellular levans (polyfructans) when grown in the presence of sucrose (see Chap. 14). The *S. sanguis* group is in the process of being subdivided on serological grounds. *S. sanguis* was formerly called *Streptococcus S.B.E.* because of its association with subacute bacterial endocarditis. It characteristically produces extracellular polyglucans causing

TABLE 11-1. APPROXIMATE DISTRIBUTION OF THE CULTIVABLE BACTERIA IN VARIOUS ORAL HABITATS

Group	Coronal Plaque	Gingival Crevice	Tongue Dorsum	Buccal Mucosa	Saliva
1. Gram-positive cocci	40%	35%	50%	80%	55%
Streptococcus mutans	R	V	V	—	T
S. mitior	R	R	R	R	T
S. sanguis	R	R	R	R	T
S. salivarius	V	—	R	R	T
S. milleri	R	R	V	V	T
Staphylococcus	R	R	R	—	T
Micrococcus	V	V	R	—	T
Enterococcus	—	V	—	—	T
Peptostreptococcus	R	R	R	—	T
2. Gram-negative cocci	10%	10%	20%	2%	17%
Neisseria	R	V	R	—	T
Veillonella	R	R	R	V	T
3. Gram-positive rods	40%	30%	20%	<0.1%	16%
Actinomyces species	R	R	R	—	T
Nocardia species	R	V	V	—	T
Rothia species	R	V	V	—	T
Bacterionema species	R	V	V	—	T
Lactobacillus species	V	—	V	—	T
4. Gram-negative rods	9%	20%	10%	<0.1%	7%
Bacteroides oralis	R	R	R	V	T
Bacteroides melaninogenicus	V	R	—	—	T
Vibrio sputorum	V	R	—	V	T
Spirillum sputigenum	V	R	V	—	T
Fusobacterium species	R	R	V	—	T
Haemophilus species	R	—	—	—	T
5. Spirochetes	1%	1–3%	<0.1%	<0.1%	—
Treponema microdentium	V	R	—	—	T
Treponema denticola	V	R	—	—	T
Borrelia vincentii	V	R	—	—	T

R = Resident to site, T = Transient to site, V = Variable to site, — = Present in low numbers or absent from site.

broth cultures to gel when growing in the presence of sucrose. The S. *mitior* group is the least well characterized of the viridans streptococci. Organisms that cannot be placed with certainty into other streptococcal species usually end up by default in the S. *mitior* group. It is, therefore, not uncommon to find some strains in this group which possess one or more of the properties of the other species. For example, some S. *mitior* stains can form extracellular polyglucans. After the streptococci, the most numerous groups are the gram negative cocci, mainly *Veillonella* (approximately 20%) and the gram positive rods (approximately 20%). Gram-negative rods account for 10 per cent of the cultivable flora of the tongue.

Coronal Plaque

In ecologic terms, dental plaque is a community of organisms living together and existing with their abiotic constituents on the various surface areas of the tooth. Operationally, plaque may be described as the adherent microbial deposit on the tooth surface. This distinguishes it from food and cellular debris that may collect loosely around the teeth (see Chap. 5). A further distinction should be made between plaque deposits on the coronal portion of the teeth and those found in the region of the gingival crevice. Hereafter, the former will be referred to as coronal plaque and the latter as crevicular or gingival crevice microbiota. Each type of plaque may exist as a separate entity, or they may merge into each other, especially when oral hygiene is neglected.

In coronal plaque the gram positive cocci (approximately 40%) and the gram positive rods (approximately 40%) make up the predominant flora. S. *mitior*, S. *sanguis*, and S. *milleri* make up the major portion of the gram positive cocci, whereas gram positive rods usually consist mainly of actinomycetes and diphtheroids. Gram negative cocci (approximately 10%), mainly *Veillonella* and *Neisseria* species, and gram negative rods (*Bacteroides* and *Fusobacterium*) may also represent a significant part of the flora in mature plaque. In regions of active caries S. *mutans* and *Lactobacillus* may be present in large numbers, whereas in cemental lesions *Actinomyces* may predominate.

The flora of the pits and fissures has been difficult to quantitate because of sampling problems. However, the virtual absence of gram negative rods and spirochetes, as well as an apparent difference in the proportional distributions of streptococcal species, suggest that pit and fissure plaque should be viewed as a separate dental plaque ecosystem. Direct microscopic counts of fissure plaque suspensions have shown cocci to constitute 70 to 90 per cent of the organisms, the remaining part being gram positive rods. Viable counts showed that S. *sanguis* is commonly the most prevalent streptococcal species observed. S. *salivarius* has also been observed frequently, and the mean percentage of S. *mutans* has been reported to range from between 10 to 40 per cent of the total streptococcal count. The gram negative cocci consist mainly of Veillonella species. The gram positive rods, when present, are usually lactobacilli.

The composition of plaque at various sites on the same tooth surface has been studied by only a few investigators. From the limited number of reports available, however, it is clear that wide variations exist in the relative proportions of some bacteria isolated from closely adjacent sites on the same tooth. Such findings, as shown in Table 11-2, substantiate the concept derived from microscopic examination of sections that plaque contains numerous communities of different organisms in the form of microcolonies.

Crevicular Microbiota

The compostion of the gingival crevice microflora has been the subject of a large number of investigations which have sampled the gingival crevice in a healthy state, as well as in various disease states, (i.e., gingivitis, periodontitis, periodontosis, and rapid onset destructive periodontitis). The microbiota of the gingival crevice exists in two distinct locations and in two distinct forms. The first of these, the adherent plaque deposits at or below the height of the gingiva, also differs qualitatively and quantitatively in composition from plaque on the coronal surfaces. In addition to the adherent microbial deposits on the tooth surface, the second type of plaque seen in the gingival crevice is what has been called "free floating plaque." In reality this "plaque" is composed of an unattached mass of motile organisms and loosely packed gram negative organisms residing between the outer portion of the adherent plaque and the crevicular epithelium. Depending upon the gingival health of an individual, the microbial content of the gingival crevices may range from virtually none to a gram or more, with a thickness of 100 to 300 cells when many teeth are affected due to poor oral hygiene.

In gingival health the gram positive cocci (approximately 35%), consisting of S. *sanguis*, S. *mitior*, S. *milleri* and enterococci, compose one of the major groups of adherent plaque at the gingival margin, followed by the gram positive rods (approximately 30%), with *Actinomyces* species predominating. The gram negative flora (approximately 20%) consists

TABLE 11-2.   VARIATIONS OF CULTIVABLE PLAQUE FLORA ON 3 SITES OF THE SAME TOOTH

| Subject | Site | Percentage of Total Viable Count of | | | | |
		Streptococci	Actinomyces	Bacteroides	Fusobacterium	Veillonella
1	A	11.4	0.04	8.5	0.85	11.4
	B	65.5	5.7	9.0	11.4	0
	C	0.4	0.56	0.08	0.26	73.0
	Mean	25.7	2.1	5.9	4.2	28.1
2	A	8.6	85.3	0.65	0	1.7
	B	71.5	18.7	8.0	0.93	0
	C	14.3	56.6	0	0	16.6
	Mean	31.2	53.5	2.9	0.3	6.1
3	A	30.0	14.0	2.0	0	23.0
	B	65.0	7.0	25.0	3.0	14.0
	C	64.0	25.0	0	0.5	10.0
	Mean	53.0	15.3	9.0	1.2	15.6
Mean for all sites		36.6	23.6	5.9	1.9	16.6

Site A, contact area; Site B, gingival crevice below contact; Site C, buccal surface
(Hardie JM and Bowden GH: The normal microbial flora of the mouth. In Skinner FA and Carr JG (eds.): The Normal Microbial Flora of Man. P. 58. New York, Academic Press, 1974)

mainly of *Bacteroides*, *Fusobacterium*, and *Vibrio* species. Spirochetes may make up one to three per cent of the crevicular flora. Early gingivitis is associated with an increase in the number of gram positive organisms as reflected by an increase in proportions of the members of the genus *Actinomyces*. In longstanding gingivitis, however, approximately 25 per cent of the microflora may be gram negative cells which appear to be located in the free floating microbial community. Species of *Fusobacterium*, *Campylobacter*, *Veillonella*, as well as spirochetes and protozoa contribute to this increase.

A gram negative fusiform shaped rod which exhibits a gliding motion on agar surfaces has been reported to be the predominant organism found in typical periodontosis lesions. A new genus *Capnocytophaga* has been proposed for this organism. In addition, other gram negative anaerobic bacteroides-like organisms have been found in periodontosis lesions. Several types of gram negative organisms have also been found to be associated with rapid onset destructive periodontitis. These include an unnamed genus of anaerobic vibrios, "corroding" *Bacteroides*, *Eikenella corrodens*, *Fusobacterium nucleatum* and a newly described group of fusiform shaped, "gelatin loving" *Bacteroides*.

Saliva

It is debatable whether saliva has an indigenous flora of its own. The proportions of streptococci, *Veillonella*, and other species in saliva are very similar to their proportions on the tongue and mucosa. Saliva is free of bacteria if it is collected directly from the ducts of the various glands. It is constantly being removed and replenished. It does not provide an especially good growth medium for many of the organisms present, and there is rapid reestablishment of the microorganisms in saliva following use of mouth rinses. All these factors tend to support the concept that the microflora of the saliva is derived from other oral tissues.

MICROBIAL SUCCESSION OF THE ORAL FLORA

The process leading up to the final microbial assemblage of mature plaque, or the "climax community," is called *microbial succession*. For the most part, the general ecologic concepts concerning the oral flora presented in this section and in the following chapter have been adapted from Martin Alexander's now classic text, *Microbial Ecology* (see Suggested Readings). Succession is the replacement of one type of community by another in response to modifications in the environment affecting the habitat. Microbial succession is a dynamic process that often involves a sequence of continuous replacements of the microbial communities located in a particular place. Two kinds of succession, allogenic and autogenic, have been described. *Allogenic succession* is the replacement of one type of community by another because the habitat has been altered by nonmicrobial factors, (i.e., by alterations in local environmental conditions induced by abiotic agencies or by modifications in the host). Birth is the first in the myriad of environmental events which influence the microbial succession within the oral cavity. Other alterations can result from growth and maturation of the host, eruption and loss of teeth, insertion of dental restorations and appliances, changes in dietary habits, oral hygiene procedures, hard and soft tissue oral pathoses, certain hormonal changes, various systemic diseases, certain systemic and local drugs and antimicrobial agents.

In contrast, an *autogenic succession* is brought about because the resident community alters the environment to such a degree that it is replaced by other species more suited to the modified habitat. Thus, the pioneers create an environment which is either more suitable for the proliferation of secondary feeders or which results in a habitat that becomes increasingly unfavorable to themselves (i.e., by the removal of nutrients or by the formation of acids or other autoinhibitory products). Figure 11-2 illustrates an example of autogenic succession occurring during the development of coronal plaque. During the first 8 hours *S. sanguis* and *Actinomyces viscosus* act as codominants in the developing community with *S. mitior* contributing in the early hours. But by the two day mark, *S. sanguis* has proliferated to the point where it represents 70 per cent of the total viable flora and *S. mitior* has fallen out. By the eighth day, however, a climax community has more or less been established with the addition of another dominant population, namely, *Actinomyces naeslundii*.

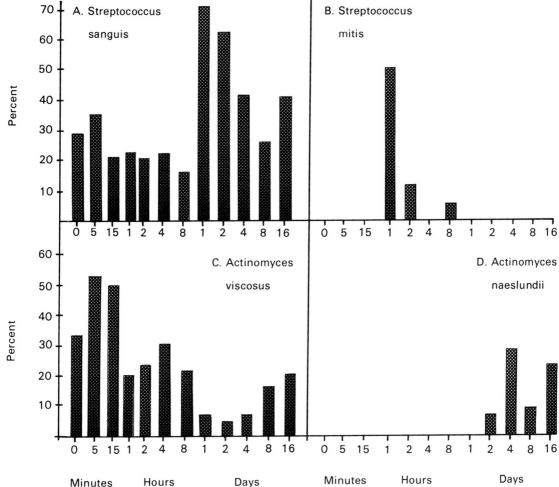

Fig. 11-2. Autogenic succession during development of coronal plaque on a buccal tooth surface. Data are expressed as percent distribution of total viable count. Strains of *S. sanguis* (A) and *A. viscosus* (C) are present at each stage of coronal plaque development. *S. mitis* (B) contribute to early coronal plaque development whereas *A. naeslundii* (D) acts as a secondary invader in later stages of coronal plaque formation. (Socransky SS, Manganiello AD, Propas D, et al. Bacteriological studies of developing supragingival dental plaque. J Periodontal Res 12: 90–106, 1977)

Acquisition of the Oral Flora

Pioneer colonization of the oral cavity of a neonate begins within hours after birth. In predentate infants streptococcal species, mainly, the *S. salivarius* and *S. mitior* groups, account for up to 70 per cent of the cultivable oral bacteria. Presumably the early pioneer species are transmitted to the neonate from the parents or attendants. Commonly, species of *Staphylococcus*, *Veillonella* and *Neisseria* are also detected within the first year. *Actinomyces*, *Lactobacillus*, *Nocardia* and *Fusobacterium* species are less frequently detected, while *Bacteroides*, *Leptotrichia*, *Candida*, and coliforms are sporadically found. Obligately anaerobic species, when present, occur in low numbers and probably then in only a close symbiotic relationship with oral aerobes.

The eruption of teeth introduces other habitats, namely, the smooth surfaces and the pits and fissures of teeth and also the gingival crevice area. At this stage the oral flora begins to take on the characteristics of the adult microflora. *S. sanguis* appears for the first time shortly after the eruption of the first teeth and, with the eruption of more teeth, *S. mutans* will make its first appearance. The development of 'anaerobic niches', as a result of reducing conditions created by the original inhabitants or by anatomical features such as gingival crevices, leads to a gradual shift in the plaque from an aerobic-facultative flora to a facultative-anaerobic flora in which organisms such as micrococci and *Neisseria* are replaced by *Veillonella* and *Actinomyces*. Interestingly, infants without teeth but with acrylic obturators, used, for example, to cover cleft palate defects, can harbor S. *sanguis* and S. *mutans* on those devices.

The Development of an Ecosystem: Coronal Plaque

The sequence of events leading to the formation of "mature" plaque, or climax community, has been studied by both cultural and microscopic techniques. Because of the technical complexity of carrying out sequential studies over extended time periods, most such investigations have been performed in adults and on easily accessible tooth surfaces which have been first denuded of plaque by a thorough prophylaxis. Figure 11-3 illustrates the typical shifts which occur in the microbial composition of developing coronal plaque on the labial surfaces of adult maxillary incisors over a 9-day period. One of the salient fea-

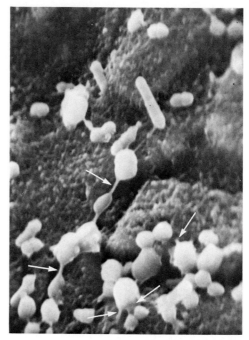

Fig. 11-4. One day plaque. A glue-like material extends between single organisms as threads or between pellicle and bacteria as threads or a coat (arrows). × 7,100 SEM microphotograph. (Lie T: Early dental plaque morphogenesis. J Periodontal Res 12: 77, 1977)

tures observed in this study was the progressive shift from mainly aerobic and facultative species in the earliest stages, to a situation where facultative and anerobic organisms became dominant. It should be borne in mind, however, that even under experimental conditions plaque development is not uniform and does not reach the same stage of development at the same time over the whole surface studied. (The ecologic raison d'être will be described in detail in the following chapter, and the biochemical characteristics of developing plaque are presented in Chap. 14.) Based on cultural studies and microscopic studies the dynamics of plaque formation can be considered to involve four characteristic stages: 1) formation of an acquired pellicle, 2) initiation of a pioneer community, 3) formation of an intermediate community, and 4) establishment of a climax community.

Stage 1. Following a prophylaxis, acellular, amorphous coating begins to form within minutes on the cleaned enamel surface. This coating is termed the *acquired pellicle*. It is formed mainly by the selective adsorption of

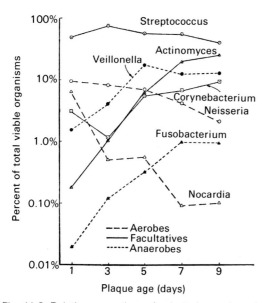

Fig. 11-3. Relative proportions of selected organisms in developing coronal plaque. (Ritz HL: Microbial population shifts in developing human dental plaque. Arch Oral Biol 12: 1561, 1967)

certain salivary glycoproteins to the enamel surface, and its properties determine to a large degree the types of microorganisms which will first attach to the tooth surface. For a detailed description of the acquired pellicle see Chapter 5.

Stage 2. The second stage of plaque formation, the initiation of a pioneer community, also begins within minutes following a pumice prophylaxis and consists of two phases: a colonization phase occupying the first 8 hours, and a rapid growth phase spanning from 8 hours to approximately 48 hours. The predominant cultivable organisms of the pioneer community are strains of *S. sanguis* and *A. viscosus.* Initially these organisms sorb onto the acquired pellicle in a weak or reversible state of attachment, but eventually a number of these organisms will become firmly attached and begin to proliferate. Scanning electron micrographs of early colonizers indicate that the attachment of cells to the pellicle and to each other is sometimes mediated by thread-like extensions from the surface of bacterial cell walls, while in other instances the extracellular extensions resemble a glue-like coat or intermedium (Fig. 11-4). Scattered epithelial cells, often colonized by bacteria, are also observed frequently in the early phases of plaque formation. At this phase of Stage 2 there are often discrepancies between the numbers and morphologic types of microbes reported from microscopic studies and results obtained from bacteriologic culture studies. One explanation suggested is that many of the weakly adherent organisms which show up in cultured plaque samples may be lost during the processing of samples for microscopic examination. The later phase of Stage 2 is characterized by rapid growth of organisms, leading first to the formation of a spreading monolayer and then to columnar palisades of seemingly similar organisms radiating perpendicularly from the tooth surface (Figs. 11-5, 11-6, 11-7, 11-8, 11-9). At the end of this stage, growth slows and the total number of organisms remains relatively constant thereafter.

Stage 3. The third stage, formation of an intermediate community, begins with the ingress and proliferation of secondary invaders. This stage is characterized by an increase in the complexity of the microbial composition of plaque, with *A. naeslundii,* *Veillonella* and *Peptostreptococcus* strains becoming more prominent. Early in this stage the plaque still exhibits well defined columnar arrangements

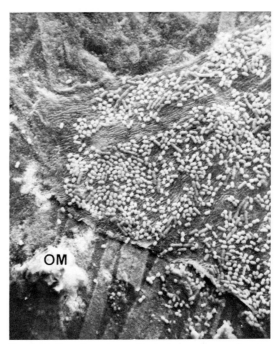

Fig. 11-5. Two day plaque. Bacteria, mostly cocci, colonizing a nonkeratinized epithelial cell while most of the surrounding splint surface is uncolonized. OM—Organic material. ×1,600 SEM microphotograph. (Lie T: Early dental plaque morphogenesis. J Periodontal Res 12: 79, 1977)

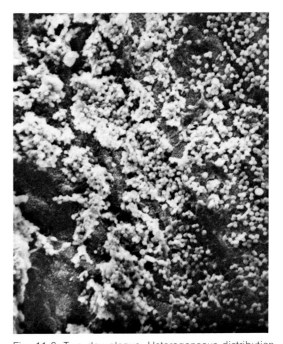

Fig. 11-6. Two day plaque. Heterogeneous distribution of bacterial growth. Areas of initial colonization interspersed with areas of more extensive plaque growth. ×2,000 SEM microphotograph. (Lie T: Early dental plaque morphogenesis. J Periodontal Res 12: 83, 1977)

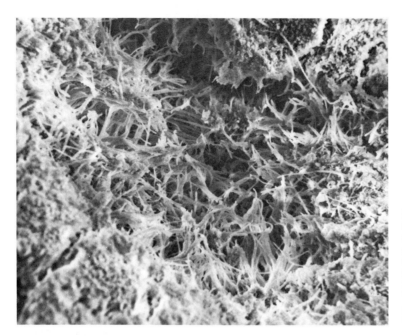

Fig. 11-7. Two day plaque. Bacterial thread-like forms totally dominate within deeper layers of plaque. Several organisms appear attached by one end, the other extending freely into the space. × 800 SEM microphotograph. (Lie T: Early dental plaque morphogenesis. J Periodontal Res 12: 85, 1977)

Fig. 11-8. Two day plaque. Some of the filaments are covered by cocci resembling "corncob" formation (CC) in an area demonstrating an increasing degree of structural complexity. × 4,000 SEM microphotograph. (Lie T: Early dental plaque morphogenesis. J Periodontal Res 12: 85, 1977)

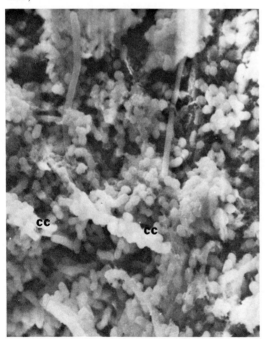

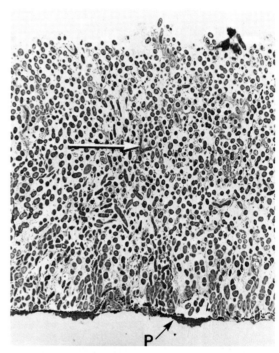

Fig. 11-9. One day plaque. The majority of bacteria are coccal shaped cells. Note the presence of isolated, elongated bacteria, including a branching filament (arrow) and of an electron dense pellicle (P) at the plaque-crown interface. × 3,800 TEM microphotograph. (Listgarten MA, Mayo HE, and Tremblay R: Development of dental plaque on epoxy resin crowns in man. J Periodontal Res 46: 14, 1975)

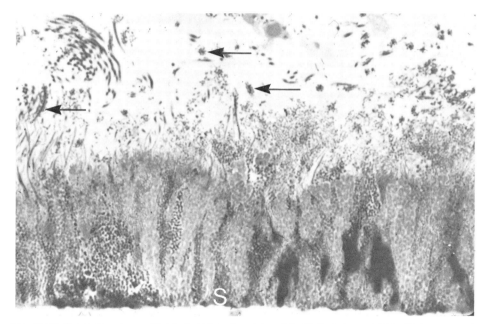

Fig. 11-10. Three day plaque. The bulk of the plaque consists of densely packed bacteria arranged into well-defined, columnar microcolonies extending from the crown surface (S). Some filamentous forms extend beyond the densely packed bacterial mass. They may be associated with cocci in "corn cob" formations (arrows). × 1,050 Light microphotograph. (Listgarten MA, Mayo HE, and Tremblay R: Development of dental plaque on epoxy resin crowns in man. J Periodontal Res 46: 16, 1975)

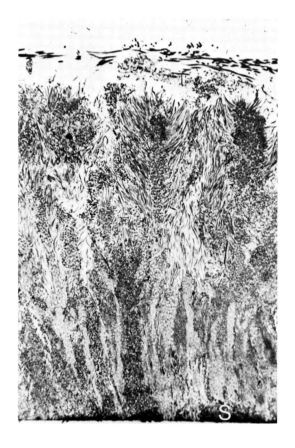

Fig. 11-11. One week plaque. Filamentous forms appear to invade and replace the coccal forms occupying the deeper layers. S, epon surface. × 860 Light microphotograph. (Listgarten MA, Mayo HE, and Tremblay R: Development of dental plaque on epoxy resin crowns in man. J Periodontal Res 46: 16, 1975)

(Fig. 11-9); later in this stage filamentous forms appear to invade the underlying bacterial mass, gradually replacing the coccal forms (Figs. 11-10, 11-11). Apparently, these secondary colonizers are able to adhere to other plaque organisms or matrix materials. In addition, the metabolic activity of this locally concentrated mass of organisms soon begins to exert selective effects on the plaque flora. One consequence is that aerobic species in the deeper layers are gradually replaced by facultative and anaerobic types of organisms as the oxidation reduction potential (Eh) drops. Furthermore, organisms which can withstand the acidic products associated with anaerobic metabolism, or which can use these acids (e.g., *Veillonella*) become more prominent.

Stage 4. Finally, a stage is reached where only a few new organisms are introduced, such as spirochetes located at the gingival margin (Fig. 11-12). The climax stage is

275

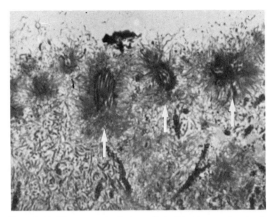

Fig. 11-12. Three week plaque. Spiral forms predominate along plaque surface facing gingival tissue. Note bacterial aggregations consisting of large, centrally located filaments, surrounded by a halo of thin, filamentous bacteria (arrows). × 1,750 Light microphotograph. (Listgarten MA, Mayo HE and Tremblay R: Development of dental plaque on epoxy resin crowns in man. J Periodontol Res 46: 20, 1975)

characterized by a fairly well balanced dynamic equilibrium. Although this equilibrium is always subject to some internal variations and fluctuations, it tends to retain its essential composition within limits, provided that no major environmental changes are superimposed.

SUMMARY

Distinct microbial ecosystems exist within the major habitats of the oral cavity, namely on the surfaces of the mucous membranes, tongue, teeth, and gingival crevice. The microbial populations inhabiting these various sites differ in both qualitative and quantitative respects with certain bacteria distributed throughout the oral cavity while others inhabit only specific sites within the oral cavity. The microbial succession within the oral cavity begins at birth with the establishment of certain pioneer species and culminates with the formation of climax communities. This dynamic process, however, continues in varying degrees throughout an individual's life cycle in response to alterations in local environmental conditions induced by the host or the resident microbial community.

GLOSSARY

Aerobic microorganisms. Bacteria capable of growing in the presence of free oxygen.

Allogenic succession. Replacement of one type of community by another because the habitat is altered by nonmicrobial factors. Alterations caused by changes in ecologically significant physical or chemical properties of the region induced by abiotic agencies or by modifications in the host within or upon which the microorganisms reside.

Anaerobic microorganisms. Bacteria capable of growing in the absence of free oxygen.

Autogenic succession. Replacement of one type of community by another because the resident population alters their surroundings in a manner such that they are replaced by species better suited to the modified habitat.

Climax community. The final microbial assemblage in a region. At this stage the species composition is maintained reasonably constant with the passage of time.

Colony. A macroscopically visible growth of microorganisms on a solid culture medium.

Community. The organisms inhabiting a given site.

Dental plaque. The assemblage of microbial species which are firmly adherent to the tooth surface embedded in organic and inorganic constituents derived from host and microbial sources; a microbial ecosystem on the tooth surface.

Ecosystem. The complex of organisms in a specified environment and the abiotic surroundings with which the organisms are associated. The ecosystem includes the assemblage of species and the organic and inorganic constituents characterizing the particular site.

Facultative microorganisms. Bacteria that are capable of growing under aerobic or anaerobic conditions.

Free-floating plaque. A population of loosely packed motile microorganisms residing within the gingival crevice between the outer portion of the adherent plaque and the crevicular epithelium.

Habitat. The location in nature where the organism actually grows, essentially its address.

Intermediate community. One or more series of communities formed by later arriving species which find the now modified environment of the pioneer community more suitable for their existence than for the pioneer species.

Koch's postulates. A statement of the kind of experimental evidence required to establish the etiologic relationship of a given microorganism to a given disease. The conditions included are (1) the microorganism must be observed in every case of the disease; (2) it must be isolated and grown in pure culture; (3) the pure culture must, when inoculated into a susceptible animal, reproduce the disease; and (4) the microorganism must be observed in, and recovered from, the experimentally diseased animal.

Mature plaque. The final assemblage of microorganisms on the tooth surface which will form between 7 and 12 days if dental plaque is left undisturbed. A climax community.

Microbiota. All of the microorganisms of a region; the combined flora of a region.

Niche. Refers to the role of the species in its habitat. Niche implies the function of the organism in a particular habitat, its occupation.

Oxidation-reduction potential (Eh). Tendency of a compound to give up electrons. Expressed by the electrical unit, the volt (V).

Pioneer community. A community formed by one or more pioneer species. The organisms first proliferating in a particular circumstance, in a region initially devoid of microbial life.

Plate count. A method used for quantitative analysis of viable microorganisms on solid medium, also called viable count.

Selective media. Media specially designed to isolate desired types of bacteria from natural environments such as saliva, dental plaque, or milk, in which many different kinds of organisms are present.

Serial dilution. Successive dilution of a specimen.

Strain. A pure culture of bacteria composed of the descendants of a single isolation.

Succession. The replacement of one type of community by another in response to modifications in the habitat.

SUGGESTED READINGS

Alexander M: Microbial Ecology. New York, John Wiley & Sons, 1971

Burnett GW, Scherp HW, Schuster GS, et al: Oral Microbiology and Infectious Disease, 4th ed. Baltimore, Williams & Wilkins, 1976

Gibbons RJ, van Houte J: On the formation of dental plaques. J Periodontol 44: 347–360, 1973

Hardie JM, Bowden GH: The normal microbial flora of the mouth. In Skinner FA, Can JG (eds): The Normal Microbial Flora of Man. New York, Academic Press, 1974, pp 47–83

Hardie JM, Bowden GH: The microbial flora of dental plaque: bacterial succession and isolation considerations. In Stiles HM, Loesche WJ, O'Brien TC (eds): Microbial Aspects of Dental Caries, Vol 1. Washington DC, Information Retrieval, 1976, pp 63–87

Lie T: Early dental plaque morphogenesis. J Periodont Res 12: 73–89, 1977

Listgarten MA, Mayo HE, Tremblay R: Development of dental plaque on epoxy resin crowns in man. J Periodontol 46: 10–26, 1975

Socransky SS, Manganiello AD: The oral microbiota of man from birth to senility. J Periodontol 42: 485–496, 1971

Socransky SS, Manganiello AD, Propas D, Oram V, van Houte J: Bacteriological studies of developing supragingival dental plaque. J Periodont Res 12: 90–126, 1977

van Houte J: Oral bacterial colonization: mechanisms and implications. In Stiles HM, Loesche WJ, O'Brien TC (eds): Microbial Aspects of Dental Caries, Vol 1. Washington DC, Information Retrieval, 1976, pp 3–31

12 Ecologic Determinants of the Oral Microbiota

ROBERT MORHART

RICHARD COWMAN

ROBERT FITZGERALD

Introduction
Physical Factors
Adherence Factors
  Salivary Aggregation
  Direct Interspecies Attachment
  Extracellular Polysaccharides
  Site Specific Receptors
  Physical Entrapment
Nutritional Factors
  Endogenous Nutrient Sources: General
      Considerations
    Carbohydrates
    Amino Acids
    Peptides
    Proteins
  Interbacterial Nutritional Relationships
  Exogenous Nutrient Sources
    Diet
    Exogenous Carbohydrates
    Exogenous Proteins and Fats
    Physical Consistency
Inhibitory Factors
  Salivary Inhibitors
    Lysozymes
    Thiocyanate Mediated Inhibitory Systems
    Lactoferrin
    Salivary Immunoglobulins
    Salivary Glycoproteins
    Leukocytes
  Intermicrobial Antagonisms
    Metabolic Factors
    Bacteriocins
  Mechanical Factors
Effects of Environmental Changes on
  Plaque Flora
Summary
Glossary
Suggested Readings

INTRODUCTION

The complex of organisms in a specified habitat and the abiotic surroundings with which the organisms are associated is known as an *ecosystem*. Each ecosystem has a collection of organisms and abiotic components unique to it and it alone. Microbial ecosystems are initially colonized with only a limited number of species because a habitat contains a certain set of conditions which selectively favors

278

them. In turn the metabolic activities of this initial population, or pioneer community, will alter the environment and influence the subsequent development and composition of the mature, or climax, community. This process, characterized by shifts in the species composition and in the relative abundance of the resident species of a community in response to modifications in the habitat, is called *microbial succession*. The ability of microorganisms to make use of the resources of their habitat is quite varied, but each must have an ecologic raison d'être.

As was seen in Chapter 11 the oral microbiota is composed of a number of distinct microbial ecosystems which exist within the various habitats of the oral cavity. Considered in this chapter are general factors that are necessary for the growth of oral microorganisms, specific characteristics of microorganisms that allow for their implantation and propagation within certain habitats, and factors that control and modulate the growth rates and metabolic properties of microorganisms within these habitats. These factors are referred to as ecologic determinants, and for the oral microbiota four sets of factors have been identified: physical, adherence, nutritional, and inhibitory. These factors may derive from the host, the external environment, or the microorganisms themselves. The complexities and dynamic state of the various ecosystems of the oral microbiota become more evident when one considers the large number of interactions and modulations that can take place both between and within these groups of factors. Because of this dependency, the absence of a species from a habitat may be ascribed to the lack of one or more ecologic determinants which it requires. In addition, the population size may be regulated by an essential factor whose concentration or rate of formation is too low to maintain maximum cell numbers. Conversely, the growth of an organism in an environment is of itself evidence that the essential factors are present, even though they may not be detectable because they are used as quickly as they are generated. It must be recognized, however, that no single factor is of itself a sole determinant of the oral microbial ecology. It is rather, as elsewhere in nature, the result of an enormously complex series of interactions of physical, biochemical and biologic factors that decides the ecology of each site individually.

The goals of this chapter are to show: 1) that

membership in a specific oral habitat is determined by interactions between physical, adherence, nutritional and inhibitory factors emanating from either endogenous or exogenous sources so that the resultant microenvironment is truly dynamic and subject to periodic fluctuation, 2) that organisms within these habitats—and this most certainly includes coronal plaque—can survive and grow even when endogenous factors are the only source for nutrition, 3) that diet composition will affect the composition and metabolism of coronal plaque, and 4) that a previously established oral microbiota may serve to protect the host by preventing the implantation and establishment of pathogenic organisms.

PHYSICAL FACTORS

Each microbial species grows, reproduces, and survives within a finite range of external conditions which define its tolerance range or ecologic amplitude for critical environmental factors. Thus, the key environmental factors must not only be present but must not exceed the tolerance limits of the population in order for individuals in a population to proliferate or merely survive when not growing. For the oral cavity habitats these abiotic factors include temperature, moisture, pH, and oxidation-reduction potential (Eh).

By comparison with the microbial ecology of the skin, the endogenous factors which are available to support the oral microflora make the oral cavity a virtual "Garden of Eden." On the skin, water is the primary rate-limiting factor for the growth of bacteria which normally have a water content of 80 per cent or more and depend on water for the exchange of nutrients, for metabolic reactions, and for removal of inhibitory waste products. In contrast, water is abundantly available throughout the oral cavity. In addition, the oral environment maintains a favorable temperature range for mesophilic (25 to 40°C) microorganisms and a pH range between 6.0 and 7.8, which is optimal for most of these organisms.

Most members of the oral microflora are facultatively anaerobic to anaerobic. Oxidation-reduction potentials have been shown to range from +60 to +310 mV for the tongue, saliva, and attached gingiva, to Eh levels as low as −200 mV for the coronal plaque and

−360 mV for the gingival crevice area. The attainment of anaerobic conditions is facilitated by the surface morphologies of oral structures (i.e., crypts of the tongue, gingival sulci, and fissures and approximal areas of the teeth) which limit the penetration of oxygen. However, a major contributory factor is the reducing capacity of the organisms themselves. In fact, organisms such as streptococci and *Neisseria* species are thought to play a vital role in early coronal plaque formation by creating local anaerobic conditions favorable to the subsequent establishment of more anaerobic organisms. Thus, wide local differences in Eh balances can be created by the combination of the reducing activities of certain resident organisms and anatomical features which limit the ingress of environmental oxygen.

Some oral microbes are known to have a narrower niche and can only become established when their particular needs are met. For example, the oral spirochetes require strongly anaerobic conditions. Thus a low Eh must be established by other organisms before the spirochetes can initiate growth.

ADHERENCE FACTORS

Gibbons and van Houte (see Suggested Readings) have clearly demonstrated that the preferential localization of some bacteria in different oral sites may depend on their ability to selectively adhere to a particular surface. The oral cavity is an "open" ecosystem; that is to say, it is subject to a continual flow of saliva and periodic influences of foods and drinks plus the microorganisms associated with them. Under these circumstances, in order for a given microbe to establish permanent residence in the oral cavity, it must be able to resist the various forces which tend to propel it through the mouth and into the gut. If an organism cannot come into contact with, and attach to, a favorable intraoral surface, it will soon be washed away by saliva. Adherence as an ecologic determinant plays an important role in the microbial successions within the various oral habitats, and the selective nature of bacterial attachments also helps to account for the microbial diversity observed between the various oral microfloras (Chap. 11).

For some bacteria adherence consists of two sequential steps. One is a reversible adsorption by which an organism is able to bind onto a specific receptor site on a surface; the other process allows for the organism to become irreversibly bound to that surface. Most probably different cellular mechanisms are involved in each step. While attachment mechanisms have been described for some microorganisms, the mode of attachment for a major portion of the oral microflora remains to be determined. Adherence mechanisms that are known include: the production of compatible receptor substances by the host and organism; the production of extracellular polymers by bacteria; interactions between bacterial surface coatings of different species; and nonadhesive retention via mechanical entrapment on various host surfaces.

Salivary Aggregation

Strains of *Streptococcus sanguis*, *Streptococcus mitior*, *Streptococcus mutans* serotype c and *Actinomyces* species have been shown to aggregate in the presence of whole saliva, parotid and/or submaxillary saliva. Some of these interactions seem to involve various high molecular weight salivary glycoproteins and divalent cations such as calcium. Different salivary glycoproteins have been found to act as separate agglutinins for S. *sanguis*, S. *mitior* and S. *mutans*, suggesting that a considerable degree of specificity is characteristic for all these interactions. Recent *in vitro* studies using purified salivary glycoproteins suggest that this specificity may depend on the composition and distribution of oligosaccharide side chains with specific binding characteristics along the protein backbone. Such reactions are reminiscent of those between certain plant proteins (lectins) and animal cells or glycoproteins, where agglutination or precipitation occurs due to interactions with specific sugar moieties. Experimentally, certain lectins have been shown to inhibit *in vitro* the saliva-induced aggregation of S. *mutans*. Although the mechanism is not known it could be due either to blocking the sugar moieties of salivary glycoproteins at sites which bind to bacteria or to the induction of conformational changes in the glycoproteins, with a resulting loss in aggregating activity. While it is tempting to speculate that their adsorption and attachment is aided by salivary constituents present on the tooth or on the outer cell surface, the exact process which

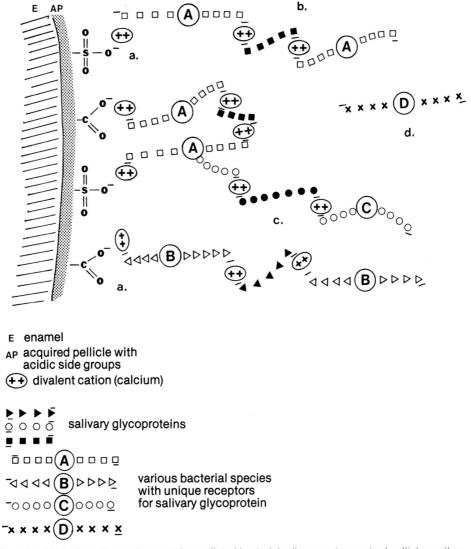

E enamel
AP acquired pellicle with
    acidic side groups
(++) divalent cation (calcium)

salivary glycoproteins

various bacterial species
with unique receptors
for salivary glycoprotein

Fig. 12-1. Model for salivary glycoprotein-mediated bacterial adherence to acquired pellicle or other microorganisms. **a.** Attachment of bacteria to the acquired pellicle by electrostatic interaction. A divalent cation bridge is formed between specific negatively charged receptors on the bacterial cell wall and negatively charged side groups of salivary glucoproteins previously adsorbed onto the tooth surface. **b.** and **c.** Attachment of similar or dissimilar species via divalent cation bridges formed between specific salivary glycoproteins and specific receptors on the bacterial cell wall. **d.** A bacterial species which lacks a proper attachment receptor.

brings about their firm attachment *in situ* is presently unknown.

Figure 12-1 shows three hypothetical adherence situations involving electrostatic interactions via calcium bridges, between salivary glycoproteins, and various oral bacteria that may be active in coronal plaque development. Situation *a* (Figure 12-1) depicts the initial attachment of certain organisms to the acquired pellicle. Situation *b* shows additional attachments taking place mediated by salivary glycoproteins between similar species, while situation *c* shows attachments mediated by a different glycoprotein between dissimilar species. Although bacterial adsorption may occur continuously during plaque formation, most of the increase in plaque mass is considered to be due to subsequent growth of attached microorganisms.

Figure 12-2 depicts a similar hypothetical

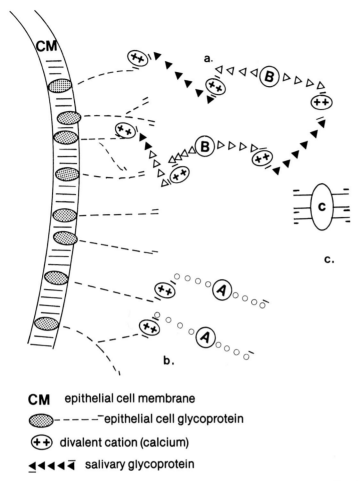

CM   epithelial cell membrane

⬭- - - - - epithelial cell glycoprotein

(+ +)   divalent cation (calcium)

◀◀◀◀◀   salivary glycoprotein

○○○○ (A) ○○○○
◁◁◁◁ (B) ▷▷▷▷
     ╟╢
     (C)
     ╢╟

**various bacterial species
with specific receptors**

Fig. 12-2. Model for bacterial adherence to epithelial cell. **a.** Indirect attachment of bacteria to epithelial cell surface or to similar species mediated by specific salivary glycoproteins and divalent cation bridges. **b.** Direct attachment of bacteria to specific glycoproteins on the epithelial cell membrane via divalent cation bridges. **c.** A bacterial species which lacks a proper attachment receptor.

adherence mechanism, this time involving the attachment of certain organisms to oral epithelial cells mediated by salivary glycoproteins (Fig. 12-2, situation *a*).

While saliva can facilitate the attachment of some bacteria, some salivary glycoproteins have been shown to specifically block the attachment of other types of microorganisms to oral surfaces (see section below).

Direct Interspecies Attachment

Bacterial attachment can also involve a direct interaction between the bacterial surface

coatings of dissimilar microbial species. These interactions appear to be highly specific and occur via cell surface receptors. For example, certain strains of *Actinomyces viscosus* will aggregate only with certain strains of *S. sanguis* or *Veillonella* species. Electron microscopic studies on mature coronal plaque have revealed that the so called "corn-cob" structures seem to be composed of filamentous bacteria coated with cocci. Figure 12-3 shows that thin surface fibrils of the cocci appear to be binding to the cell envelope of the filament. In addition, other structures such as the "bristle brush" or "bottle brush" formation seem to be composed of filamentous bacteria coated with perpendicularly attached shorter filaments (Fig. 12-4). This type of attachment also could account for the addition of different bacterial species that are seen during succeeding stages of plaque formation.

Extracellular Polysaccharides

The best known example of adhesion due to bacterial polysaccharides is provided by the cariogenic organism S. *mutans*. This organism has been found to synthesize high molecular weight dextrans and other insoluble glucans from sucrose (Chap. 14), and these polymers seem to be involved in the adherence of this organism to hard surfaces. Both *in vivo* and *in vitro* studies have shown that sucrose markedly fosters plaque formation by S. *mutans*, and that polyglucan hydrolases, specific glucan-degrading enzymes, are capable of inhibiting plaque formation. Although S. *mutans* will aggregate in the presence of dextran, it is thought that the main function of the glucan polymers is to act as an insoluble extracellular matrix which irreversibly binds these organisms together and to the tooth surface. Thus in humans while sucrose may not be indispensible for the initial colonization of S. *mutans*, it may be of special significance for the accumulation and prolonged retention of S. *mutans* on the tooth surface. A hypotheti-

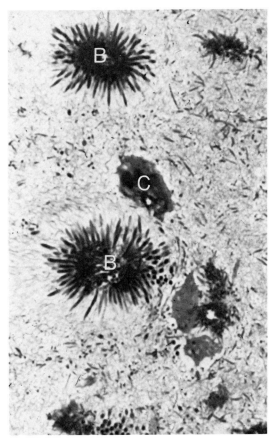

Fig. 12-4. The external surface of subgingival plaque consists of a flora with many spirochetes, bacterial formations (*B*) resembling "bristle brushes" (cross section) and occasional mammalian cells (*C*). (×1,400 Light microphotograph) (Listgarten MA, Mayo HE and Tremblay R: Development of dental plaque on epoxy resin crowns in man. J Periodontol 46: 20, 1975)

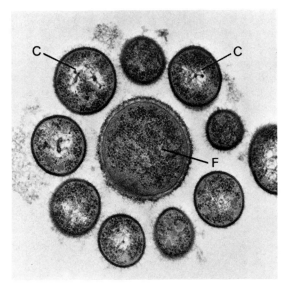

Fig. 12-3. Cross section of "corn cob". A coarse, fibrillar material attaches the cocci (C) to the central filament (F). ×22,500 TEM microphotograph. (Listgarten MA, Mayo HE and Tremblay R: Development of dental plaque on epoxy resin crowns in man. J Periodontol 46: 18, 1975)

cal model for the adherence of S. *mutans* mediated by polyglucans is shown in Figure 12-5. For intercellular adherence to be induced by sucrose the cell requires cell bound glucan, sucrose, and a cell bound glucan receptor (situation *a*). For adherence to be induced by preformed dextran the cell requires only the cell bound glucan receptor (situation *b*). Apparently, cell to surface adherence of S. *mutans* has only two requirements: first, that adherent glucans be formed by enzyme molecules which are in close proximity to the surface, either as components on a cell momentarily adsorbed to the tooth surface by some nonspecific mechanism or as cell free molecules which have adsorbed to the tooth surface; and second, that the cells specifically bind to these adherent dextrans via a cell surface dextran receptor (situation *c*).

Certain other types of bacteria also appear

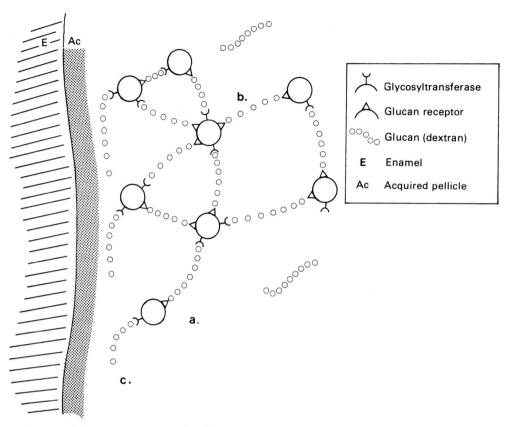

Fig. 12-5. Model for extracellular glucan (dextran)-mediated adherence of *S. mutans*. **a.** Intercellular adherence induced by glucan synthesized by glucosyltransferase on one cell and glucan receptor on cell wall of another. **b.** Intercellular adherence induced by performed glucans attaching to glucan receptors on different cells. **c.** Bacterial cell adherence to acquired pellicle mediated by glucans on the cell surface.

to adhere in plaque by synthesizing polymers. For example, strains of *A. viscosus* are known to produce a nonglucan polymer which enables them to form cohesive bacterial masses which adhere to solid surfaces. At least one cariogenic strain of *Streptococcus salivarius* is known which forms coronal and crevicular plaques due to elaboration of an adhesive extracellular polyfructan. Many other oral species can also synthesize extracellular glucans including strains of *S. sanguis, S. mitior, S. salivarius* and *Lactobacillus* species. These organisms, however, do not exhibit dextran induced aggregation apparently because they lack the appropriate cell receptors.

Site Specific Receptors

Electron microscopic studies have shown that *S. salivarius* and *S. mitior* each possesses a distinct, but morphologically different, fibril-

lar "fuzzy" surface coating. The attachment of these organisms to germ-free rat cheek cells seems to be mediated by their fuzzy coats, because treatment of these organisms with trypsin results in a loss of much of their fuzzy surface coat and impairs their adherence to oral epithelial cells (Fig. 12-2, situation *b*). As mentioned earlier (Chap. 11), *S. sanguis* and *Actinomyces* species primarily colonize the tooth surface, whereas *S. salivarius* primarily colonizes the tongue surface, and *S. mitior* can be found on a variety of oral surfaces.

Physical Entrapment

Finally, many oral microbes appear to be unable to adhere directly to epithelial, bacterial or salivary components, extracellular polymers, or tooth surfaces. Apparently these organisms are physically entrapped in the pits and fissures of the teeth, around dental appliances, in carious lesions in the gingival crevice, in periodontal pockets, and within the plaque matrix itself. Thus lactobacilli are found in open carious lesions and around orthodontic bands, whereas strains of spirochetes, vibrios, and *Bacteroides* species are predominantly found in the gingival crevice. Of course, the nature of the prevailing growth conditions will also determine the types of microorganisms that will survive in these areas.

NUTRITIONAL FACTORS

In common with all other forms of life, microbes require a supply of nutrients for the maintenance of life and for growth. Nutrients provide the organisms with the energy necessary to perform biosynthetic reactions as well as with the building blocks for the synthesis of

cellular components. The oral microflora can draw on a pool of nutrients that is at times overabundant and diverse but at other times is intermittent and limited in required substrates. The sources may be the host's tissues and secretions, the host's diet, and also microorganisms living in close proximity.

As seen in Table 12-1, oral microbes exhibit great diversity in nutrient requirements. Some organisms can use carbohydrates as an energy source, whereas others may prefer amino acids or organic acids. Nitrogen requirements can be satisfied by peptides, amino acids, or, in some cases, by ammonia. One or more water-soluble vitamins such as biotin, pantothenate, nicotinic acid, thiamine, riboflavin, pyridoxal, menadione or folic acid may be required for growth, depending on the species. Purines, pyrimidines, fatty acids, and more esoteric growth factors may enhance or even be essential for

TABLE 12-1. SOME CHARACTERISTICS OF THE ORAL MICROFLORA OF POTENTIAL ECOLOGICAL SIGNIFICANCE

Group	Relation to Oxygen	Energy Source*	Distinctive Characteristics**	
			Enzymes	Metabolic Products
1. Gram-positive cocci				
Streptococcus mutans	Facultative	CHO	Glucosyltransferase, fructosyltransferase	GLU, LEV, IPS
S. mitior	Facultative	CHO	Glucosyltransferase	GLU, IPS
S. sanguis	Facultative	CHO	Glucosyltransferase	GLU, IPS, NH$_3$, H$_2$O$_2$
S. salivarius	Facultative	CHO	Fructosyltransferase	LEV, IPS
S. milleri	Facultative	CHO		NH$_3$
Staphylococcus	Facultative	CHO, AA	Proteases, catalase, hyaluronidase	
Micrococcus	Aerobic	CHO	Catalase, urease	
Enterococcus	Facultative	CHO	Protease	NV acids
Peptostreptococcus	Anaerobic	CHO, NV acids	Protease	NV acids
2. Gram-negative cocci				
Neisseria	Facultative	CHO	Urease, oxidase	EPS, NV acids
Veillonella	Anaerobic	Lactate, NV acids	Peroxidase	H$_2$S, H, NV acids
3. Gram-positive rods				
Actinomyces species	Anaerobic	CHO		EPS, IPS, NV acids
Nocardia species	Aerobic	CHO		EPS, IPS, NV acids
Rothia species	Aerobic	CHO	Catalase	NV acids
Bacterionema species	Facultative	CHO		
Lactobacillus species	Facultative	CHO		EPS, IPS
4. Gram-negative rods				
Bacteroides oralis	Anaerobic	CHO	Proteases	
Bacteroides melaninogenicus	Anaerobic	CHO, AA	Proteases, collagenase	
Vibrio sputorum	Facultative	formate, H		H$_2$S
Spirillum sputigenum	Anaerobic	CHO		
Fusobacterium species	Anaerobic	AA, CHO	Proteases	NV acid, H$_2$S, indole
Haemophilus species	Facultative	CHO		
5. Spirochetes				
Treponema microdentium	Anaerobic	CHO		
Treponema denticola	Anaerobic	AA		
Borrelia vincentii	Anaerobic			

* CHO, Carbohydrate; AA, amino acids; NV acids, nonvolatile acids; H, hydrogen
** GLU, glucans; LEV, levans; IPS, intracellular polysaccharides; EPS, extracellular polysaccharides

the growth of the more fastidious organisms. Various minerals are required in trace or substrate amounts. Many organisms (including streptococci) require or are stimulated by carbon dioxide. This great nutritional diversity among oral microbes points out the role of nutrition as a major ecological determinant. Thus it is to be expected that the distribution of individual oral organisms would be greatly influenced by the availability of required nutrients in specific sites.

Not every essential nutrient is of ecological significance. A needed substance present at all times in concentrations sufficiently high to satisfy the demand of all indigenous and invading populations is of little ecological consequence. Chemical analysis of an environment prior to invasion tells more about the pioneers that cannot multiply than those that do. Organisms requiring substances not initially present are excluded, but many that should be able to grow, at least on the basis of their nutritional patterns, fail to become established for reasons not related to nutritional factors. Analysis of a habitat supporting a climax community likewise provides limited information on the nutrition of the indigenous forms. This is because nondemanding organisms can multiply where readily assimilable growth factors are available, ignoring the complex compounds all around, and conversely, a fastidious population may use the entire supply of a required growth factor leaving none for the analyst to find. For these reasons assessments of nutritional conditions *in vitro* frequently provide more useful information than chemical analyses of the ecosystem.

Endogenous Nutrient Sources: General Considerations

Endogenous nutrients are those produced in the oral cavity of the host. In this context, the host derived nutrients, being constantly present could potentially be of greater nutritional significance to the oral microflora than those of intermittent dietary origin. Sources of these nutrients include saliva, crevicular fluid, desquamated epithelial cells, and blood constituents. In comparison to saliva, only small amounts of crevicular fluid are normally secreted into the oral cavity, but its presence is indicated by the occurrence in whole saliva of albumin, a crevicular fluid protein constituent. This protein is not found in the separate

TABLE 12-2. RELATIVE AMOUNTS IN MG% OF GLUCOSE, FREE AMINO ACIDS, AND PROTEIN IN WHOLE SALIVA, PAROTID SALIVA, AND SUBMANDIBULAR SALIVA

| Nutrient | Secretion Examined | | |
	Whole	Parotid	Submandibular
Glucose	<1.0	<1.0	<1.0
Amino acids	3.4	1.5	1.1
Protein	100–300	250	150

glandular secretions. Moreover, crevicular fluid also is the apparent endogenous source of hemin, a specific requirement for *Bacteriodes melaninogenicus*, and of alpha-2-globulin required by *Treponema dentium*, both members of the gingival crevice microbiota.

Although the foregoing examples represent special cases, the occurrence of abundant plaque deposits on the teeth of patients fed solely by gastric tubes clearly attests to the significance of the endogenous nutrients as sources of growth substrates for the complex array of microorganisms which comprise the wider oral ecosystem. Since most of the oral microbial inhabitants need carbohydrates for energy and all require nitrogenous constituents for growth, there is intense competition between the various organisms to obtain their own specific growth needs from those available in the "endogenous" pool. The net result of this nutritionally mediated selective pressure is that only those organisms able to successfully obtain their growth needs will prosper as permanent members of the oral microbiota.

To provide a general perspective, Table 12-2 lists amounts of carbohydrate (as glucose), amino acids, and protein which have been reported to occur in whole mixed saliva and the separate parotid and submandibular gland secretions (see Chap. 3 for a more detailed review). The metabolic fate of each of these types of endogenous nutrients will now be considered.

Carbohydrates

Although the level of free glucose is understandably low in saliva, carbohydrate for energy can be derived endogenously from the salivary glycoproteins, a class of complex proteins containing oligosaccharide side chains. Many members of the oral microbiota, particularly the streptococci and micrococci, elaborate extracellular glycosidase or neuraminidase enzymes capable of dissociating the carbohydrates from the mixture of glycoproteins. The fact that only trace amounts of glycoprotein-associated carbohydrates are ever detectable in the proteins of the acquired pellicle or dental plaques indicates that these sources are rapidly attacked and utilized. Despite these different endogenous sources of carbohydrate however, soluble exogenous dietary carbohydrates are more probably the energy source most readily available to the oral ecosystem.

Amino Acids

Some strains of oral streptococci apparently can utilize inorganic ammonium salts as a sole nitrogen source for growth. However, most species of oral streptococci, lactobacilli, and a wide assortment of other organisms require organic nitrogenous compounds for growth. This requirement arises from the fact that these organisms are unable to synthesize all of the amino acids needed to manufacture cellular proteins. As might be expected, the oral microbiota varies considerably in its needs for amino acids; some types require only a few while other types have more complex requirements. The amino acids required by different strains of a single species and between species of a given genus may also vary considerably. For example, some strains of S. *mutans* require only two or three amino acids while other strains may require five or more. S. *mutans* and S. *sanguis* have relatively simple requirements compared to S. *mitior* or S. *salivarius* which may require seven to nine different amino acids.

As indicated in Table 12-2, whole saliva contains only low levels of free amino acids. Glycine, phenylalanine, leucine, and isoleucine generally appear to be the major amino acids present, whereas cysteine, histidine, and methionine are not found. Dental plaque also contains free amino acids, with glutamic acid, aspartic acid, glycine, alanine, and proline representing the major amino acids present. Cysteine, cystine, methionine, arginine, leucine, isoleucine, tyrosine, and phenylalanine are absent. Moreover, extensive amino acid decarboxylase activity appears to be present in plaque as indicated by the reported occurrence of putrescine from ornithine, cadaverine from lysine, gamma aminobutyric acid from glutamic acid, and histamine from histidine. These amine-producing enzymes function under acidic conditions and represent a competitive factor to those organisms requiring these types of amino acids.

Peptides

Knowledge of occurrence and role of salivary peptides as nitrogenous growth substrates for the oral flora was developed in an interesting manner. The concept that acids produced from the glycolytic fermentation of carbohydrate by the oral microbiota were important in the caries process created a focus of attention on the acidogenic potential of salivary microorganisms, many of which are also members of the plaque flora. The intrinsic glycolytic activity of saliva is associated with the sedimentable material, consisting of microorganisms, epithelial cells, and leucocytes. This fraction exhibits only half the activity that is demonstrable in whole saliva, but glycolytic activity can be restored fully by the addition of saliva supernatant, which has no activity alone. Although simple amino acids do enhance the glycolytic capability of salivary sediment, concentrations eight to ten times those normally occurring in saliva are required to equal the glycolytic activity seen in whole saliva. In studies on the nature of the stimulatory factor in saliva supernatant, certain peptides were found to be particularly effective. It is now thought that stimulation of glycolysis by salivary peptides probably occurs because, as readily assimilatable sources of essential amino acids for the salivary flora, they induce cellular anabolic (i.e., cell building) reactions which in turn require added energy production obtained through increased glycolytic activity.

Proteins

Saliva contains reasonable amounts of proteins (see Table 12-2) and approximately 30 to 40 per cent of the dry weight of plaque is protein, mainly of salivary and microbial origin. Both saliva and plaque contain numerous exopeptidases of microbial origin which cleave single amino acids from the ends of the protein macromolecules. Especially active are reactions causing the release of proline, alanine, methionine, leucine, lysine, and arginine. However, it should be recalled that these amino acids may also serve as substrates for amino acid decarboxylases under acid conditions, or amino acid deaminases under alkaline conditions. In addition, a number of oral microorganisms possess peptidase or proteolytic activities. They include the enterococci (found occasionally), diptheroids, bacteroids, lactobacilli and the oral streptococci. *B. melaninogenicus*, for example, possesses enzymes for collagen degradation. The end products of these enzymatic activities include peptides, via proteinases, and degradation of the peptides, by peptidases, to amino acids.

The supernate of centrifuged saliva, as the only source of nitrogen in a chemically defined medium, has been found to support the *in vitro* growth of *S. mutans, S. sanguis,* and to a lesser extent that of *S. mitior* and *S. salivarius.* As shown in Figure 12-6 for *S. mutans,* fractional ultrafiltration of mixed saliva into three fractions based on molecular weight ((a) nitrogenous constituents having molecular weights greater than 10,000 (proteins), (b) ni-

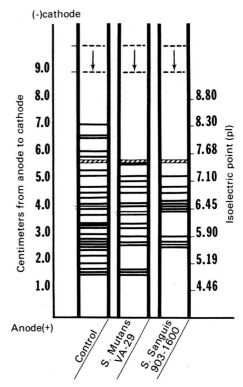

Fig. 12-7. Schematic representation of isoelectric-focusing protein patterns of saliva supernatant before and after growth by *S. mutans* VA-29 and *S. sanguis* 903-1600. Samples were applied at 9.0 cm, direction of migration as indicated by arrow toward anode. Cross-hatched zone represents location of β-amylase. Cowman RA, Fitzgerald RJ, Schaefer SJ: Role of salivary factors in the nitrogen metabolism of plaque-forming oral streptococci. Stiles HM, Loesche WJ O'Brien TC (eds.): Microbial aspects of dental caries: vol 2, p. 473. Washington D.C., Information Retrieval Inc., 473, 1976.

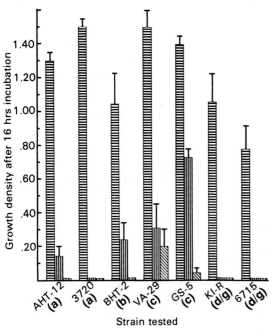

Fig. 12-6. Growth of different serotypes of *S. mutans* in basal medium containing different molecular weight fractions of saliva supernatant. **a.** Horizontal bars, nitrogenous constituents > 10,000 MW; **b.** Vertical bars, nitrogenous constituents between 1,000–10,000 MW; and **c.** Cross-hatched bars, nitrogenous constituents < 1,000 MW. (Cowman RA, Fitzgerald RJ, Perrella MM, Cornell AH: Human saliva as a nitrogen source for oral streptococci. Caries Res 11: 5, 1977)

trogenous constituents between 1,000–10,000 MW, and (c) nitrogenous constituents of less than 1,000 MW (free amino acids, small peptides)), clearly demonstrates that the greatest growth-promoting activity is associated with the protein subfraction. Thus *S. mutans* and *S. sanguis* apparently possessed the ability to meet all of their amino nitrogen needs by a direct attack on the salivary proteins. Electrophoretic studies indicated that upon incubation of mixed saliva with washed cells of *S. mutans* or *S. sanguis,* different salivary proteins were attacked by each of these species of oral streptococci. The apparent specificity in proteins susceptible to hydrolysis and utilization for growth is illustrated in Figure 12-7. On the basis of amino acid analyses, only small amounts of degradation products were found in the medium after growth, suggesting that these oral streptococci confine their attack on the proteins to the extent needed to obtain essential amino acids for growth. However, the organisms were also found to utilize considerable amounts of nonessential amino acids when available. While S. *mitior* and S. *salivarius* also hydrolysed salivary proteins, the appearance of considerable amounts of degradation products in the growth culture supernatants seems to indicate that they are less efficiently utilized by these streptococci. It has now been established that there are at least eight salivary proteins susceptible to attack by S. *mutans* that are seldom attacked by S. *sanguis*, S. *mitior* or S. *salivarius*. Conversely, these organisms may degrade proteins which are not affected by S. *mutans*.

Interbacterial Nutritional Relationships

Still another source of endogenous nutrients may derive from the ability of some microorganisms to utilize metabolic end products or surplus growth factors released by neighboring organisms. Some typical examples of potential oral significance are the ability of *Veillonella* species to use as an energy source lactate formed during glycolysis by streptococci, lactobacilli, and other organisms; the ability of various plaque organisms to degrade bacterial extracellular glucans or fructans and utilize the simple carbohydrates produced as energy sources; and the ability of S. *mutans* to obtain some of its vitamin requirements from S. *sanguis*. Similarly, when an organism hydrolyses a protein any unused amino acids or peptides that are liberated would be available to other organisms in the vicinity. Since the information on these processes has been derived in the main from *in vitro* studies or experiments in gnotobiotic animals involving pure cultures, it is difficult to estimate their significance in the complex ecologic situation in the human oral cavity. However, in view of the opportunistic nature of most microorganisms, it seems highly unlikely that they would ignore local sources of available nutrients, whenever present, in preference to making them *de novo*. Rather, it is reasonable

to believe that mutualistic interbacterial nutritional interactions are among the more powerful influences on the ecology of densely crowded microbial habitats such as dental plaque.

Exogenous Nutrient Sources

Diet

The consistency, form, and composition of the diet as well as the frequency of diet intake are important factors to be considered when attempting to understand the relationship between microbial utilization of foodstuffs and the bacterial composition of oral ecosystems. The action of the oral musculature and the washing and buffering effects of saliva contribute to limit the duration that foodstuffs are in contact with fixed oral ecosystems. The result is that foodstuffs are quickly cleared from the mouth and little food can be detected on the tooth surface a few minutes after eating. Except for special situations, food elimination is completed within a half hour. Furthermore, nutrients from foodstuffs rarely affect the gingival crevice microflora since the outward flow of crevicular fluids acts to prevent the penetration of saliva and ingesta into this habitat. With few exceptions, the most notable of which is the interrelationship between sucrose and certain streptococci in coronal plaque accumulation, there is little documentary evidence of direct linkages between specific dietary substances and the ecology of individual oral microorganisms.

Exogenous Carbohydrates

The influence of the sugar content of the diet on oral ecosystems has been studied more than any other factor. Numerically, a large preponderance of oral microorganisms preferentially utilize simple carbohydrates as their principal energy source. Most of them produce organic acids as end products of this process, so that in areas where acids can accumulate aciduric organisms will have an ecological advantage. As a corollary, those species which can utilize these acids will also be favored.

Since the availability of carbohydrates from

dietary sources occurs only intermittently, it is significant from an ecological standpoint that certain of the oral microorganisms have the capability to adapt to this situation. As seen in Table 12-1 some oral organisms possess enzyme systems by which they can convert excess sugar to storage materials for later use (Chap. 14). For example, S. *mutans*, S. *sanguis*, A. *viscosus* and some lactobacilli and diphtheroids can convert simple carbohydrates to intracellular amylopectin-like storage polymers. The first two organisms mentioned can also convert excess sucrose to extracellular soluble and insoluble polyglucans, whereas S. *mutans* and S. *salivarius* can also synthesize extracellular polyfructans from sucrose.

These functions can have important ecologic consequences. For example, during fasting periods the intracellular polysaccharides can be catabolized for energy by those organisms which are able to synthesize them. Certain plaque organisms may be able to hydrolyse extracellular polysaccharides for the same purpose. However, a major ecologic function of the extracellular polysaccharides, particularly the 1-3 branched glucans, seems to be their role in the structure of the coronal plaque matrix. While the stickiness of these substances aids in plaque adhesion, their gel-floc nature can selectively influence the concentration of nutrients and metabolic products within the plaque as well as serving to control the diffusion of external substances into plaque.

Frequent ingestion of foods containing readily soluble carbohydrates will affect the composition of the oral microbiota by promoting the growth of acidogenic and aciduric types of organisms and preventing the survival and growth of more acid-sensitive types. The consequences of frequent consumption of sucrose are particularly evident in coronal plaque where S. *mutans* and lactobacilli increase in numbers and S. *sanguis* decreases.

Exogenous Proteins and Fats

The specific effects of dietary proteins on the oral flora are largely unknown. The slow rate of dissolution and liberation of proteins from foodstuffs, coupled with short exposure time to the weak proteolytic enzyme activity in saliva, suggests that amino acids from dietary protein sources are not readily available to oral microorganisms. All that can be said at present is that some of the effects that have been observed following an increase in the protein content of diets, such as reductions of the acidogenic flora, seem to be mainly reflections of the replacement of carbohydrates by nonfermentable substances. In the case of fats the same explanation can be adduced, although it has also been suggested that fat-containing foodstuffs are less likely to adhere to the teeth and other tissues, and that fatty coatings on carbohydrates render them less soluble and hence less available to the oral flora.

Physical Consistency

The physical consistency of the diet will affect its retention in various sites in the oral cavity and thus may influence the microflora at those sites. Diet consistency and taste also have a selective influence on salivary gland function (Chap. 2). Liquid diets have been shown to cause a significant reduction in volume, amylase activity, and total protein content of the parotid gland secretion which also contains the principal salivary buffer, bicarbonate. Submaxillary saliva is not affected. Hard or fibrous foods have the opposite effects.

INHIBITORY FACTORS

Despite seemingly ideal conditions and the astronomic number of organisms inhabiting the various sites within the mouth, it seems clear that these organisms ordinarily do not grow and multiply rapidly *in vivo*. It has been estimated that oral microbes average only three to four divisions per day. While this is attributable in part to limitations in the amount of available nutrients, a number of inhibitory factors apparently are also important in determining microbial distribution and population size and in governing succession within the various oral habitats.

These inhibitors may arise from host tissues and secretions, from the resident microorganisms, or from oral hygiene practices. Host derived factors which prevent the establishment of transient organisms or hold the population size and activity in check are referred to as barriers. These include salivary antibacterial factors such as lysozyme, lactoperoxidase, lactoferrin, certain glycoproteins and glycolipids, and the immunoglobulin, secretory IgA. Other host-associated barriers to microbial colonization would include salivary flow, functional and other mouth movements, and natural sloughing of oral epithelial cells, all of which help to eliminate organisms from the mouth. Resident microorganisms may also regulate the community's composition by excreting metabolites deleterious to cohabitant or transient populations. In addition, dental habits, (i.e., toothbrushing, dental flossing and tongue brushing) will affect, at least temporarily, the ecologic balances at these sites.

Salivary Inhibitors

Considered here and also in Chapters 3 and 15 are some of the antibacterial factors contained in saliva. All of these factors are known to possess antibacterial effects against some species *in vitro*, however, the extent of their effectiveness *in vivo* is not known. It appears likely that their main action is directed against transient microorganisms and that they exert only a relatively weak selective influence on the indigenous oral microflora.

Lysozymes

Lysozymes are low molecular weight (14,000) basic proteins with isoelectric points approximating *p*H 11. They are enzymes which break down bacterial cell wall components by hydrolysing the 1-4 linkage between N-acetylglucosamine and N-acetylmuramic acid residues. Lysozymes are usually thought to exert their bactericidal effects by bacteriolysis, however, they are also known to kill susceptible bacteria without lysing them.

Lysozymes are widely distributed. They occur in body tissues, in body secretions (including the saliva), in gingival tissues, in the gingival crevice fluid as well as in leukocytes. They are active against strains of *Neisseria*, *Micrococcus*, *Sarcina*, *Klebsiella*, *Streptococcus*, *Staphylococcus* and *Mycobacteria*.

Thiocyanate Mediated Inhibitory Systems

Two anti-lactobacillus systems have been found to occur in saliva. The first of these involves lactoperoxidase acting in concert with hydrogen peroxide and thiocyanate. The enzyme has been purified from human parotid saliva. The reaction functions aerobically with sulfite and sulfate as end products. *In vitro* studies have shown this system is particularly effective against lactobacilli and streptococci, apparently by inhibiting hexokinase and other glycolytic enzymes. The second system also requires thiocyanate but does not require peroxidase. It functions under both aerobic and anaerobic conditions, but sulfite and sulfate do not appear as end products.

Lactoferrin

This iron binding protein was originally described in bovine milk. Lactoferrin is present in most external secretions including saliva. A similar iron binding protein, transferrin, is present in serum. Both of these proteins have a molecular weight of approximately 80,000 and bind two atoms of iron per molecule, however lactoferrin possesses a greater affinity for metals and retains this property under more acidic conditions. Apparently, lactoferrin achieves its *in vitro* bacteriostatic effect by depletion of iron in the environment to a concentration below that required for bacterial growth.

Salivary Immunoglobulins

The major immunoglobulin of saliva is secretory IgA (Chap. 15). The bulk of salivary IgA is synthesized in the salivary glands by plasma cells located around the intralobular ducts, and it appears in saliva as a dimer composed of two IgA molecules joined together by a secretory piece. Although secretory IgA is the major immunoglobulin of saliva, its concentration is lower than the IgA in serum. Saliva also contains small amounts of IgG, IgD, IgM and IgE which enter the oral cavity as components of the crevicular fluid.

Secretory IgA possesses viral neutralizing properties and can act as an antibody to bacterial antigens and probably food antigens. For example, secretory IgA is absorbed on oral microorganisms *in vivo* and will specifically agglutinate certain oral microbes *in vitro*. The effectiveness of salivary IgA as an intraoral defense mechanism is uncertain, although agglutinated organisms may be prevented from attaching to oral surfaces and thus be more effectively removed from the oral cavity.

Salivary Glycoproteins

Some salivary glycoproteins are known to bind specifically to certain bacteria and, as discussed previously, these glycoproteins may mediate the attachment of some organisms to various oral surfaces. On the other hand, salivary glycoproteins may also inhibit the attachment of other species to oral surfaces. It is theorized that salivary glycoproteins may prevent attachment by blocking receptor sites required for adherence that are located on the bacterium itself or on a host tissue surface.

Leukocytes

In whole saliva leucocytes will round up and take on morphologic characteristics that do not resemble leukocytes in blood. For this reason salivary leukocytes frequently are referred to as salivary corpuscles. Individuals with clinically healthy gingiva have few salivary leukocytes, while those with gingivitis may have up to 12 million leukocytes per milliliter of saliva. The gingival crevice is the principal portal of entry for leukocytes. While they are in the gingival crevice, leukocytes are known to ingest bacteria, and in this habitat they probably act as a host defense mechanism. Their antibacterial function in other oral habitats is uncertain.

Intermicrobial Antagonisms

Cooperative interactions among microorganisms have been already discussed as ecologic determinants. Less well understood, but of potentially equal importance, are the antagonistic effects which may exist between different organisms in the oral environment. Microbial communities supporting high densities of dissimilar populations are characterized by interactions detrimental to many of the inhabitants. Often prominent among these harmful interrelationships is *amensalism*, a form of symbiosis in which one population (or species) is adversely affected and the other unaffected. Studies *in vitro* have identified a variety of microbially produced agents which can inhibit other oral microorganisms. They include hydrogen peroxide, organic acids, free fatty acids, bacteriocins, and bacteriophages. One of the best known examples of this phenomenon is the inhibition of the diphtheria bacillus by oral streptococci. However, in spite of the abundance of evidence for antagonism between oral microorganisms *in vitro*, it is very difficult to determine the extent to which such antagonisms are operative *in situ*. Furthermore it has been a common experience of students of these phenomena to find that both members of an antagonistic pair *in vitro* may exist in apparent harmony *in vivo*. Incongruous as this may appear, it does not necessarily imply that bacterial antagonisms are of little consequence as determinants of oral microbial ecology. They could be operative at close range within the confines of a given microcosm where the inhibitor concentrations would be maximally effective against nearby susceptible organisms. The inhibitory effects need not be absolute, for even partially inhibitory interactions would still be meaningful in regulating the balance between competing organisms. It is also conceivable that some of the most potent antagonistic relationships within the oral cavity have thus far eluded detection simply because the victims were so effectively eliminated that no evidence of their existence remains.

Metabolic Factors

Common mechanisms of amensalism would include the production of organic acids, hydrogen peroxide, ammonia and hydrogen sulfide, as well as oxygen consumption. Suppressions based on these kinds of interactions are probably operative in oral microhabitats. Acid tolerant organisms such as S. *mutans* and *Lactobacillus* species, H_2O_2 producing organisms such as S. *sanguis*, organisms which maintain a low Eh and produce additional toxicants, H_2S and organic acids in particular, will all benefit by maintaining an environment that is unfavorable to other species. Organic acid toxicity is greatest at low *p*H. Growth inhibition, however, is not merely a direct acidity effect but is probably due also to the fact that these acids penetrate cell membranes only in the undissociated form, which increases with decreasing *p*H. Furthermore, only specific organic acids are functional, namely, acetic, butyric, propionic, and formic acids. Interestingly, these volatile fatty acids are found in fasting coronal plaque and are commonly produced by oral streptococci when growing under sugar limitation. This may very well be a mechanism for protecting against secondary invaders when the resident population is at a competitive disadvantage because its energy requirements are restricted.

Bacteriocins

Some microorganisms are noted for their capacity to form highly potent antimicrobial agents, the antibiotics and bacteriocins. The bacteriocins are of particular interest to the ecology of the oral microflora because numerous oral microbes are known to produce them and/or to be sensitive to them. Bacteriocins are a class of antibacterial agents composed of a chemically heterogeneous group of substances ranging from polypeptides or simple proteins to proteins complexed with carbohydrates and lipids. Their mode of action is unlike that of antibiotics in that they are irreversibly adsorbed on the outer wall of the cells of sensitive bacteria, and are bactericidal rather than bacteriostatic. Those produced by gram negative bacteria act only against strains of the same or closely related species while those from gram positive bacteria often have a wider spectrum of activity, even including species of other gram positive genera. Activity against gram negative organisms has yet to be demonstrated for bacteriocins produced by gram positive bacteria.

Strains of S. salivarius, S. mitior, S. sanguis, and S. mutans produce bacteriocins under in vitro conditions. The active substances produced by these strains differ with respect to chemical composition and activity spectrum. These bacteriocins show varying degrees of activity against strains of S. salivarius, S. sanguis, S. mitior, S. mutans, Streptococus faecalis, Streptococcus pyogenes, enterococci, Staphylococcus aureus, Staphylococcus epidermidis and A. vicosus but not against gram negative organisms. As a group, the c serotype strains of S. mutans are observed to produce bacteriocins more frequently than strains of others S. mutans serotypes. This is of ecologic interest because the c serotype of S. mutans is the most prevalent type found in human plaque (Chap. 13). Furthermore, bacteriocins produced by S. mutans are commonly active against strains of S. sanguis. This observation is also of ecologic interest

because it has been reported that as the number of S. mutans increases in plaque, there is a concomitant decrease in the number of S. sanguis present. Figure 12-8 shows the inhibitory effect of four c serotype strains of S. mutans against S. mutans strain FA-1R (serotype b) and S. sanguis strain 167.

Gram positive organisms which are not normally indigenous to the oral microflora also produce bacteriocins which are active against the oral streptococci. For example some strains of Staphlococcus aureus and Staphylococcus epidermidis produce bacteriocins which are active against strains of S. salivarius, S. sanguis and S. mutans. Figure 12-8 shows the inhibitory effect of a purified bacteriocin from Staphlococcus epidermidis strain 1580 against various strains of S. mutans and S. sanguis.

Compared to antibiotics, bacteriocins have a narrow activity spectrum and are highly effective in their lethal action. It has been suggested that purified (cell free) bacteriocins, having selective activity against S. mutans, may be ideally suited to specifically eliminate these cariogenic organisms from the oral cavity without drastically altering the normal oral microbial ecology. These agents could be applied topically to the teeth, similar to the manner in which topical antibiotics are applied to skin infections.

Mechanical Factors

The host is provided with a number of defense mechanisms which help to control the microbiota of mucosal surfaces of the mouth. Salivary flow, aided by muscle movement and chewing forces, provides a means for clearance of bacteria from these surfaces with final removal provided by swallowing. Epithelial cell desquamation also serves to limit bacterial accumulation, thus bacterial growth on individual epithelial cells is limited by the turnover rate of oral epithelial cells. Mucus secreted by the mucous tissues can form a mechanical barrier to the attachment of organisms to these surfaces.

Since coronal plaque is tenaciously adherent to the tooth surface, and since the tooth surface does not shed, the above host defense mechanisms are less effective in limiting the population density of coronal plaque. Thus, the need for tooth brushing and flossing.

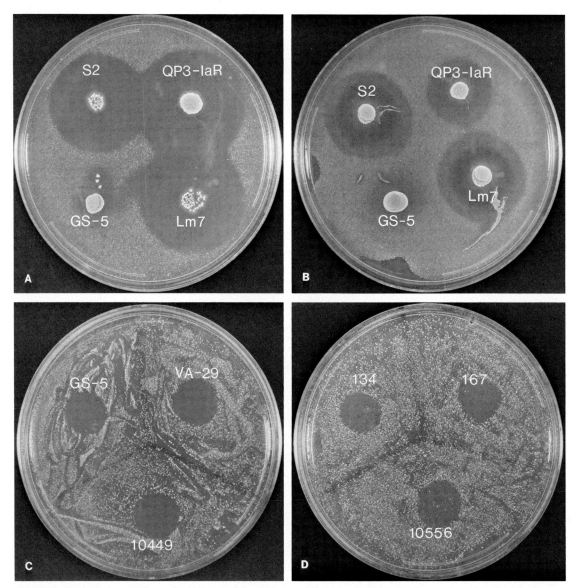

Fig. 12-8. Bacteriocin activity against strains of *S. mutans* and *S. sanguis*. Bacteriocins produced by four *S. mutans* strains active against *S. mutans* strain FA-1R **A.** and *S. sanguis* strain 167 **B.** Purified bacteriocin from *Staphylococcus epidermidis* 1580 active against three strains of *S. mutans* **C.** and three strains of *S. sanguis* **D.**

These measures for oral hygiene will temporarily remove accessible plaque from the tooth surface; however, the process of plaque development will immediately start once again. Succession stages will vary depending on how thoroughly each tooth area was cleaned, thus the cleanest areas will start with a relatively aerobic streptococcal flora while areas with plaque remnants will already be at a stage to support a more anaerobic flora.

EFFECTS OF ENVIRONMENTAL CHANGES ON PLAQUE FLORA

The interdependence of various environmental factors in regulating oral microbial ecology becomes evident when one or more factors is altered experimentally or as a result of some medical problem. When the teeth are removed *S. mutans*, *S. sanguis* and *Lactobacillus* populations decline rapidly in the oral cavity, only to return again when dentures are worn. Similar changes occur when diets which are restricted in carbohydrates are consumed. The effect of sucrose restriction on polyglucan forming streptococci such as *S. mutans* and *S. sanguis* has already been alluded to. In addition, mechanical factors, such as eating and tooth brushing, will also modify oral habitats. This is reflected in the range of values for bacterial populations found at different times of the day. For example, salivary bacterial counts are reported to decrease after a meal, gradually increase between meals, and to be the highest in the morning upon arising.

Radiation induced xerostomia is also known to have a profound effect on the oral microflora. It has been demonstrated that in coronal plaque, lactobacilli, staphylococci, candida, and *S. mutans* show progressive increases during radiation treatment that last for at least three months post-radiation. In contrast, *S. sanguis*, neisseria and fusobacteria decline in numbers (Chap. 13, Figs. 13-7, 13-8, 13-9) under these conditions. These changes cannot be attributed solely to the reduction in salivary flow. There were also concomitant changes in eating habits, especially during the weeks of radiation treatment when the bulk of the diet consisted of soft or liquid foods. Even when the dietary choices returned to pretreatment types of foods, the liquid intake remained elevated. These findings illustrate the problems encountered in attempts to isolate and examine separately the effects of individual factors on the microbiota *in vivo*. More often than not a change in one parameter leads to a series of changes in other parameters which can make it impossible to postulate a simple cause and effect relationship. Virtually all of the ecologic factors which have been described in this chapter can be implicated in some degree in the microbial changes which follow radiation induced xerostomia.

For example, the loss of the buffering and cleansing power of saliva, the resultant change in plaque-buffering capacity, the reduced oral clearance time for food and microorganisms, the changes in diet consistency and eating habits, and the loss of nutrient, metabolites and adherence factors normally provided by saliva, all affect existing members of the plaque microbiota to varying degrees. Once these changes occur, additional changes can be expected in Eh levels, inhibitory and stimulatory metabolic products, and microbial interactions which tend to evoke compensatory changes in the plaque microbiota.

SUMMARY

Consideration of endogenous and exogenous factors as overall determinants of oral microbial ecology leads to the conclusion that endogenous factors play a prominent role. The interactions between specific microorganisms and physical, adherence, nutritional, and inhibitory factors provided by the host selectively determine the kinds of microorganisms which will initially reside in the oral cavity and the habitats which they will colonize. The effects of exogenous factors on the ecology of the oral microbiota, nevertheless, are not inconsequential. The diet and oral hygiene habits may modulate such endogenous factors as the salivary secretions, bacterial clearance, and the local resistance of the gingival tissues to infections. The metabolism of dietary sucrose by oral microorganisms with the production of acids and intracellular and extracellular polysaccharides has a specific influence on the microbial composition, metabolic activities and mass of coronal plaque. In the final analysis it must be recognized that no single ecologic factor, whether it be exogenously or endogenously derived, is of itself a sole determinant of the oral microbial ecology.

GLOSSARY

Amensalism. A form of symbiosis in which one population (or species) is adversely affected and the other unaffected.

Bacteriocins. Protein-like substances produced by various species of bacteria which kill only strains of the same or closely related species.

Barrier. A physical, chemical, or biologic condition preventing the establishment of a species or holding the population size or activity in check.

Climax community. The final microbial assemblage in a region. At this stage the species composition is maintained reasonably constant with the passage of time.

Crevicular fluid. A serum-like fluid which enters the gingival sulcus after transversing the crevicular epithelium. When gingivitis is present the fluid resembles an inflammatory exudate.

Ecosystem. The complex of organisms in a specified environment and the abiotic surroundings with which the organisms are associated. The ecosystem includes the assemblage of species and the organic and inorganic constituents characterizing the particular site.

Fastidious organisms. Organisms that are difficult to isolate or cultivate on ordinary culture media because of a special physical or nutrient requirement.

Habitat. The location in nature where the organism actually grows, essentially its address.

Niche. Refers to the role of the species in its habitat. Niche implies the function of the organism in a particular habitat, its occupation.

Oxidation-reduction potential (Eh). Tendency of a compound to give up electrons. Expressed by the electrical unit, the volt (V).

Pioneer community. A community formed by one or more pioneer species. The organisms first proliferating in a particular circumstance, in a region initially devoid of microbial life.

Symbiosis. Denotes a reasonably long lasting relationship in which two or occasionally more different species live in immediate proximity and derive reciprocal benefits from their interaction.

Tolerance range. A definite range or level of environmental factors within which each species grows, reproduces, and survives.

Transient population. Those microorganisms which are only present sporadically in a habitat. They are unable to survive for any length of time with the resident floras.

SUGGESTED READINGS

Alexander M: Microbial Ecology. New York, John Wiley & Sons, 1971

Bibby BG: Influence of diet on the bacterial composition of plaques. In Stiles HM, Loesche WJ, O'Brien TC (eds): Microbial Aspects of Dental Caries, Vol II. Washington DC, Information Retrieval, 1976, pp 477–490

Brown LR, Dreizen S, Handler S: Effects of selected caries prevention regimens on microbial changes following irradiation-induced xerostomia in cancer patients. In Stiles HM, Loesche WJ, O'Brien TC (eds): Microbial Aspects of Dental Caries, Vol 1. Washington DC, Information Retrieval, 1976, pp 275–290

Burnett GW, Scherp HW, Schuster GS: Oral Microbiology and Infectious Disease, 4th ed. Baltimore, Williams & Wilkins, 1976

Geddes DAM, Jenkins GN: Intrinsic and extrinsic factors influencing the flora of the mouth. In Skinner FA, Carr JG (eds): The Normal Microbial Flora of Man. New York, Academic Press, 1974, pp 85–100

Gibbons RJ, van Houte J: Bacterial adherence in oral microbial ecology. Annu Rev Microbiol 29: 19–44, 1975

Hardie JM, Bowden GH: The normal microbial flora of the mouth. In Skinner FA, Carr JG (eds): The Normal Microbial Flora of Man. New York, Academic Press, 1974, pp 47–83

Newman HN, Poole DFG: Structural and ecological aspects of dental plaque. In Skinner FA, Carr JG (eds): The Normal Microbial Flora of Man. New York, Academic Press, 1974, pp 111–134

Olson GA, Guggenheim B, Small PA Jr: Antibody-mediated inhibition of dextran/sucrose-induced agglutination of *Streptococcus mutans*. Infect Immunol 9: 273–278, 1974

Reeves P: The bacteriocins. In Klunzeller A, Speinger GF, Wittman HG (eds): Molecular Biology, Biochemistry and Biophysics, Vol 11. New York, Springer-Verlag, 1972

Rölla G: Inhibition of adsorption-general considerations. In Stiles HM, Loesche WJ, O'Brien TC (eds): Microbial Aspects of Dental Caries, Vol II. Washington DC, Information Retrieval 1976, pp 309–324

van Houte J: Oral bacterial colonization: mechanisms and implications. In Stiles HM, Loesche WJ, O'Brien TC (eds): Microbial Aspects of Dental Caries, Vol 1. Washington DC, Information Retrieval, 1976, pp 3–31

13 Microbial Aspects of Dental Caries

ROBERT MORHART

ROBERT FITZGERALD

Introduction
The Natural History of Caries
Early Theories of Caries Etiology
Bacterial Specificity in the Initiation of Dental Caries
    Evidence from Animal Studies
    Types of Microorganisms Cariogenic in Animal Models
    Evidence from Human Studies
    Longitudinal Studies
Microflora of Deep Caries Lesions

Ecology and Virulence of Cariogenic Microorganisms
    Virulence
    Intrinsic Microbial Factors in Virulence
    Sucrose and Cariogenicity
    Host Defenses
    Caries as an Ecologic Consequence
Summary
Glossary
Suggested Readings

INTRODUCTION

Dental caries, as a microbial disease of childhood, causes loss of tooth substance mainly in the pits and fissures and on the interproximal surfaces of the crown. Dental caries occur less frequently on the buccal and lingual surfaces (see Chap. 8). Dental caries has no single cause but instead it is a disease in which environmental factors play a decisive role. The general ecologic triad for dental caries is discussed in Chapter 8 (see Fig. 13-1). Briefly, caries susceptibility can be modified by physiologic and dietary circumstances that may directly affect the tooth's morphology, composition, or maturation process. Additionally, these factors may affect the quantity and composition of saliva. Chapters 9, 10, and 19 view the relationships between agent and host factors in light of current theories on the odontolytic process of this disease. This chapter will examine the question of microbial specificity in cariogenicity and consider the profound effect that environmental factors have on the cariogenic potential of the oral microflora.

There are practical reasons for emphasizing the ecologic concept of disease at this point, the main one being the need to maintain a balanced perspective on the role that the microbial agents play in the ecologic triad of dental caries. In humans the incidence and progression of caries is governed by the natural interplay of these ecologic factors. In the experimental approach to this disease, however, considerations of expediency often result

297

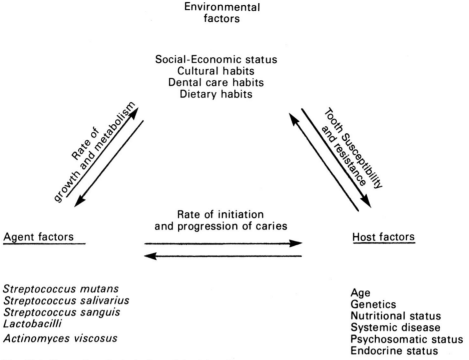

Fig. 13-1. General ecologic factors of dental caries.

in the use of study models that dispropor-tionately emphasize the factor under inves-tigation at the expense of the other contri-buting factors. For example in studies of the microbial agent factor, animal model test sys-tems are deliberately exaggerated in terms of the cariogenic challenge applied, (i.e., the size of the microbial inoculum and the su-crose content of the diet). By the same token clinical studies are frequently designed to em-ploy human populations in which the disease is rampant. While there is no longer any doubt that dental caries is an infectious micro-bial disease, realistically it can best be de-scribed as a disease of altered ecology. Thus, students and practitioners with interest in this disease will profit most by understanding this ecologic concept of caries, especially as it relates to contemporary caries preventive methods, and should not be sidetracked by controversy on the more limited questions such as the microbial specificity of this dis-ease.

The aims of this chapter are to identify the oral microorganisms that have been found to cause dental caries in animal model systems; to give evidence from clinical studies that bears upon the association of certain orga-

nisms with human caries; and to consider the ecologic determinants that may be governing these potentially cariogenic organisms.

THE NATURAL HISTORY OF CARIES

By present day standards caries occurred rela-tively infrequently in early man, a fact attrib-uted in part to the coarse types of diets con-sumed that tended to have a cleansing effect on the dentition, stimulate salivary flow, and resist impaction in the occlusal fissures of the teeth. Nevertheless, archeological and anthro-pological evidence shows that caries existed in all the ages of civilized man. The distribu-tion pattern of the lesions was considerably different than is observed at present. A series of studies by Moore and Corbett (see Suggested Readings) of the dentition of Britons of various periods from the Iron Age to the 19th Century showed that until about 1850 overall caries prevalence was quite low and that lesions in the region of the cementoenamel junction made up a major proportion of the caries experience. The data showed a gradual increase over the ages of all types of caries (Fig. 13-2). However after 1850, coinciding with the availability of cheap cane sugar, highly refined flour, and the industrialization of many British communities, much of the working class diet consisted of bread, jam, and highly sweetened tea. From that time there was an explosive increase in dental caries, primarily in the occlusal fissures and the approximal areas. The same high prevalence and pattern of carries distribution still exists today, not only in England but in all "civilized" populations. It should be noted that in England annual sugar consumption before 1850 was about 25 pounds per capita. After 1850 it rose to about 90 pounds, and at the present time it is over 100 pounds per capita in most European and American populations. It is also worthy of note that the predominantly root surface pattern of caries seen in ancient Britons has a close counterpart in present day primitive populations such as the New Guinea indigenes studied by Schamschula and his colleagues (see Suggested Readings).

Although the prevalence of caries was lower in olden days than in recent times it was still a problem which concerned the early healers. Without much of anything in the way of pre-ventive care, extraction was the main treatment as carious lesions often proceeded unchecked until the patient became agonizingly aware of their extension to the dental pulp. From the earliest records there is evidence that caries was generally associated with diet, especially rich and sweet foods. However, the manner in which the lesion began and progressed was unknown and many different explanations were advanced which were long on theory but short on factual information.

EARLY THEORIES OF CARIES ETIOLOGY

Most of the early theories of caries causation were examined critically in 1890 by the pioneer oral microbiologist W. D. Miller in his book *The Microorganisms of the Human Mouth* (see Suggested Readings). In general there were three main ideas concerning the origin of caries. The first was that it arose internally in the tooth as a result of an inflammation provoked by excessive or improper food consumption. Another theory held that minute worms in the mouth bored holes in

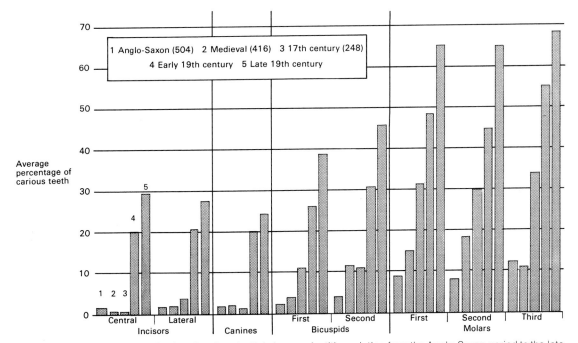

Fig. 13-2. Frequency and distribution of carious teeth in human dentitions dating from the Anglo-Saxon period to the late 19th Century in England. Number in parenthesis refers to the number of dentitions examined. (Moore WJ, Corbett ME: Distribution of dental caries in ancient British populations. Caries Res 9: 163–175, 1975)

the teeth. This was later changed to substitute microorganisms when their existence became known through the studies of van Leeuwenhoeck in the 17th Century. The third school of thought held that caries was variously due to acidic foods, putrefaction of retained food, or chemicals resulting from breakdown of foods in the the mouth. Miller rejected each of these explanations and formulated his chemicoparasitic theory of caries which held that caries was caused by the combined interaction of microorganisms with carbohydrate foods to produce tooth-destructive acids. Miller also rejected the concept that specific microorganisms could cause caries, holding instead that any and all of the acidogenic microorganisms in the mouth contributed to the process. Strangely, Miller ignored the significance of the dental plaque as an entity in his theory although he was well aware of the presence of microbes on the tooth surfaces and in carious lesions. In later years, following the description of the plaque by J. Leon Williams and G. V. Black the chemicoparasitic theory was amended to embrace the plaque as a component element of caries causation.

After the discoveries of Louis Pasteur, Robert Koch, and their followers that specific microorganisms caused specific diseases, there appeared claims by dental researchers that one or another organism was the specific cause of caries in humans. The earliest claims were based on histological evidence of the presence in carious lesions of certain organisms which were named on the basis of morphology alone. Other investigators isolated various organisms from caries lesions on the crude culture media available to them and claimed that they were the etiological agents. None of these investigators demonstrated that their candidate organisms actually could induce caries either in man or in laboratory animals.

Through the first half of the present century the two principal suspects were the streptococci and the lactobacilli; the former organisms because of their numerical predominance in plaque and their acid forming capability, and the lactobacilli because their numbers increased with increasing caries activity, and because of their acid-producing ability and their inherent ability to survive better than most organisms in environments of high acidity. Yet here too the evidence favoring these organisms as being cariogenic was entirely inferential, being based on epidemiologic studies rather than on an experimental demonstration of their ability to produce the disease.

During this period, however, investigators began to use animal models to study caries. Of the various animals used in caries research only the rat and the hamster and several primate species are now used with any regularity. The methodology, rationale, and details of the carious process in animals have been covered elsewhere in this book and also in the book *Animal Models in Dental Research* by Navia (see Suggested Readings).

BACTERIAL SPECIFICITY IN THE INITIATION OF DENTAL CARIES

Current concepts of the etiology of caries have been derived from both laboratory animal models and from clinical studies and epidemiological surveys in humans. Various animal models are used to directly assess the cariogenic potential of microorganisms whereas in the human situation clinical studies are used to indirectly determine the association of suspected organisms with the initiation and progression of caries. Chapter 23 deals with the general methodologies used in caries experimentation and Chapter 11 examines problems that are commonly encountered with cultural studies on dental plaque.

Evidence from Animal Studies

In 1946, shortly after penicillin became available, McClure and Hewitt (see Suggested Readings) demonstrated that it could inhibit experimentally induced caries in rats when administered in the diet and drinking water. This report had several major implications. First, it was an important concrete support for the concept that bacteria were involved in caries production. Secondly, because the antimicrobial spectrum of penicillin is limited mainly to gram positive bacteria, it narrowed the range of suspected cariogenic organisms to this group. Thirdly, it provided hope that caries in humans could be controlled by the use of specific antibiotics.

The next major advances in this field have been described by Navia (see Suggested Readings). In brief, Orland and his colleagues demonstrated that germfree (gnotobiotic) rats did not develop caries even when challenged with a diet which was caries conducive in rats with a normal oral microflora. When gnotobiotic rats were monoinfected with an enterococcus, caries was produced. Subsequently, investigators at the National Institute of Dental Research found that strains of an organism now known as *Streptococcus mutans* were highly cariogenic in gnotobiotic rats and in a special strain of hamsters which did not develop caries when challenged with high sucrose, cariogenic diets. Extension of these studies led to the conclusions that dental caries was transmissible from animal to animal, that specific strains of streptococci (i.e., *S. mutans* isolated from caries lesions in animals or man) were the most actively cariogenic of a number of bacterial strains tested, and that various agents such as fluorides or antibiotics could arrest active lesions or prevent new lesions in animal models.

By "labelling" specific strains of *S. mutans* through the induction of streptomycin resistance it was possible to show that these organisms formed coronal plaque, that they were present in caries lesions, and that the organisms and caries activity could be transmitted to caries inactive hamsters caged with infected animals, or infected with plaque or pure cultures of the "labelled" *S. mutans* isolated from caries lesions of infected animals. Essentially, these experiments fulfilled Koch's postulates that are required to establish the causative role of an organism in a disease process.

Koch's postulates require that an organism be isolated from a diseased site in pure culture, that it be used to infect a disease-free host animal, that it induce the typical lesions of the disease, and that it can be reisolated from the disease site in the test animal. The fact that an organism can be shown to fulfill these postulates does not mean that it can be considered the sole cause of a disease, however, since other organisms with the same capabilities may exist.

Types of Microorganisms Cariogenic in Animal Models

It is now known that a number of different organisms induce caries in appropriate test animals and some are selective for different areas of the dentition. Strains of *S. mutans* seem to be the most versatile of the cariogenic organisms, experiments in animals having shown

them to be capable of initiating caries in pits and fissures, on buccal and lingual smooth surfaces, in approximal areas, and even on root surfaces. *S. mutans* has also been shown to induce or enhance caries activity in every type of rodent or primate which is known to develop caries in the laboratory. Most of the other organisms listed as caries active in Table 13-1 have more restricted cariogenic potentials than *S. mutans* both in the type of host that will harbor them and their preferred site of attack on the dentition.

Various gram positive filamentous species are able to induce the breakdown of the periodontium and elicit root surface lesions in both the rat and hamster models. In contrast, some strains of *S. salivarius*, *S. sanguis*, *S. mitis*, enterococci, lactobacilli, and *Actinomyces* will produce fissure lesions only in the gnotobiotic rat (Table 13-1). It should be pointed out that most conventional laboratory strains of rats harbor a potentially cariogenic, indigenous microflora that in conjunction with a diet rich in sucrose will elicit varying amounts of fissure lesions. Figure 13-3 shows the variations in caries patterns occurring in two strains of rats in response to two different dietary and microbial challenges. It can be clearly seen that noninfected animals of either strain developed substantial amounts of sulcular lesions but little smooth surface caries. In contrast, animals superinfected with *S. mutans* developed increased amounts of smooth enamel lesions and only a slight increase in fissure lesions. The pattern of caries varied both with the strain of rat and the diet employed. The apparent cariogenicity of cer-

TABLE 13-1. TYPES OF DENTAL CARIES INITIATED BY VARIOUS BACTERIA IN THE GERM-FREE RAT

Smooth Enamel Lesions	Fissure Lesions	Root Surface Lesions
S. mutans*	S. mutans	S. mutans
	S. sanguis	
S. salivarius	S. salivarius	S. salivarius
	S. mitior	
	S. faecalis	
	A. viscosus	A. viscosus
	A. naeslundii	A. naeslundii
		Rothia species
	L. acidophilus	
	L. casei	

* All wild type strains of *S. mutans* exhibit some degree of cariogenicity, while only certain strains of other species may be active.

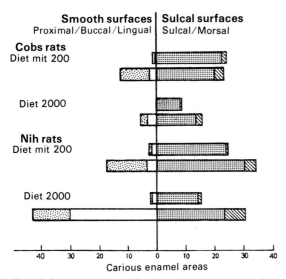

Fig. 13-3. A comparison of carious enamel areas on the smooth and sulcal surfaces for COBS and NIH rats fed either Diet MIT 200 or Diet 2000. The top bar in each set is for the non-infected control rats and the bottom bar for the *S. mutans* infected rats. (Laison RH: Rat caries model: interlaboratory standardization. In Stiles HM, Loesche, WJ, O'Brien TC (eds): Microbial Aspects of Dental Caries, vol. III. p. 757. Washington DC, Information Retrieval Inc., 1976.

tain strains of acidogenic organisms which produce only fissure caries in the gnotobiotic rat models (Table 13-1) is probably due to their ability to establish in the absence of competing organisms via physical entrapment within an already highly susceptible site and in the presence of fermentable carbohydrates to produce enough acid to decalcify the tooth in that area.

An important aspect of the use of conventional animals for testing the cariogenic potential of human plaque microorganisms is the requirement for these organisms to implant orally in the host animal in the presence of a complicated preexisting microbiota. The normal oral flora of most experimental animals, especially the rodents, is quite distinct from the human oral flora, undoubtedly as a reflection of the special oral ecologic and environmental conditions which exist in different species. While the gnotobiotic rat model by its nature is free from the restraints of a competitive microflora, conventional animals are not. Hence it is understandable that many more organisms have been shown to be cariogenic when assayed as monoinfectious in gnotobiotic rats than when they are used to superinfect conventional rats or conventional

hamsters. This poses a major problem in interpretation of experimental findings in terms of the potential importance of a specific organism in human caries causation. On one hand an organism which is demonstrably cariogenic in gnotobiotic rats may actually be insignificant in the causation of caries in the human due to an inability to achieve an effective cariogenic potential in the human plaque environment. Conversely, an organism which may be a major cariogenic agent in humans may not be able to achieve this potential in the ecologic environment of a foreign host (i.e., a conventional rat or hamster).

For these reasons and also because, as discussed in Chapter 23, so many other factors can influence the disease process, caution must be exercised in extrapolating the results of animal caries tests to the human situation. Nevertheless, the utilization of animal models for investigations into the etiology of caries has been a major technologic breakthrough in dental research and has provided both the impetus and the research tools for future advances in this field, particularly when the findings can be viewed in the light of clinical observations in humans.

Collectively, animal studies have demonstrated that in the presence of sucrose, S. mutans can initiate all three types of caries lesions recognised in humans, that gram-positive filamentous organisms initiate root surface lesions, and that a number of other oral streptococci and lactobacilli species can cause fissure lesions when fermentable carbohydrates are abundantly present. As an example of the above situations, Figure 13-4 shows the three types of caries lesions produced by three different oral bacteria in the rat model.

Evidence from Human Studies

Direct clinical demonstration of the causative association of specific bacterial agents with development of human caries is difficult both from practical, ethical, and methodological aspects. Therefore indirect approaches using epidemiologic methods have been employed. Since causation in the epidemiologic sense implies increased risk for the occurrence of disease, results from this type of study cannot be interpreted to define unequivocally the microbial etiology of dental caries. Three epidemiologic approaches have been used in caries studies:

1. Correlations between isolated organisms from pooled plaque or saliva samples and various degrees of caries activity.
2. Correlations between the presence of certain organisms obtained from dental plaque specimens removed from a caries active site and from a nearby normal site on the same surface of the tooth.
3. Longitudinal studies requiring periodic sampling of an initially caries free, but highly susceptible, tooth surface over an extended period of time in order to associate the presence and numbers of certain organisms with the development of dental caries which may occur at that particular site.

To date results from investigations using these approaches suggest that organisms similar to those which are known to cause caries in the animal models are also associated with human caries.

Following the discovery of the cariogenic potential of S. *mutans* in the animal models, intensive characterization studies of this species revealed that while S. *mutans* is phenotypically a fairly homogeneous species, it exhibits a great degree of antigenic and genetic heterogeneity. Presently, this species can be separated into five biotypes (Fig. 13-5). Epidemiologic studies of S. *mutans* prevalence in human populations indicate a worldwide distribution of this organism. Biotype I is most frequently found in human populations, followed by Biotypes IV and V respectively. Biotypes II and III are least often found in human populations.

Associations of increased numbers of S. *mutans* and/or lactobacilli, in saliva or pooled plaque samples collected from all teeth, have been made with an increased prevalence of dental caries in various population groups. While such associations have been useful in establishing general caries status on a group basis they do not establish a direct cause and

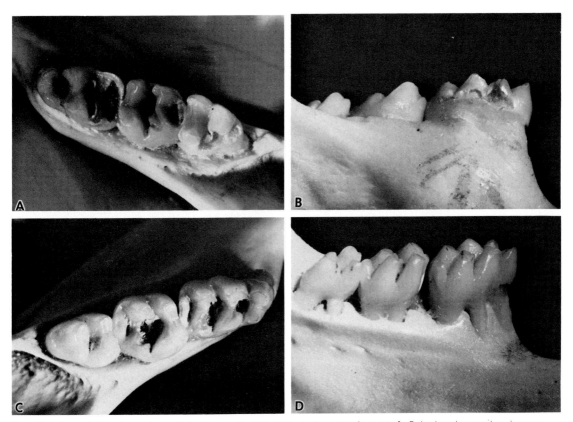

Fig. 13-4. Types of dental caries initiated by various bacteria in the germ-free rat. **A.** Sulcal and morsel caries produced by S. *mutans* **B.** Typical buccal caries on the first molar produced by S. *mutans* **C.** Sulcal caries produced by lactobacilli and **D.** Gingival and root surface caries on the mesial lingual root of the first molar produced by A. *viscosus.*

		Biochemical tests					
Biotypes	Serotypes	Mannitol	Sorbitol	Raffinose	Melibiose	NH³ from Arginine	Bacitracin 2u/ml+ Mannitol
I	c, eˣ, f	+	+	+	+ˣ	—	+
II	b	+	+	+	+	+	+
III	a	+	+	+	+	—	—
IV	d, g, SL-l	+	+ˣˣ	—	—	—	+
V	e	+	+	+	—	—	+

x = strains fermenting Melibiose   xx = some strains do not ferment Sorbitol

Fig. 13-5. A biochemical scheme for the separation of *S. mutans* into 5 biotypes. (Shklair IL and Keene HJ: Biochemical characterization and distribution of *Streptococcus mutans* in three diverse populations. (In Stiles HM, Loesche WJ, O'Brien TC (eds): Microbial Aspects of Dental Caries. vol II, 203. Washington D.C., Information Retrieval Inc., 1976)

effect relationship between these organisms and caries causation. In the first place the sampling methods are too crude to permit inferences about the nature of the microflora at the site of caries activity and secondly, the organisms present in the caries lesion at the sampling time may not be the types which originally intitated the disease process.

Pooled plaque samples from similar sites (i.e., pooled approximal and pooled occlusal samples) show statistically significant associations between levels of *S. mutans* and caries scores at those particular surfaces. However, caries has been found in subjects from whom detectable levels of *S. mutans* could not be recovered. When plaque sampling is confined to caries surfaces *S. mutans* is frequently but not invariably, found. However, under these circumstances the average proportions of *S. mutans* in the total anaerobic counts from carious sites is generally greater than from noncarious sites. Conversely, the proportions of *S. sanguis* are significantly greater on noncarious teeth. Not only have greater percentages of *S. mutans* been reported in cariogenic plaque but the conversion of sucrose into lactic acid and insoluble products (primarily intracellular polysaccharides and extracellular glucan) by these plaques is greater compared to similar amounts of noncarious plaque. Figure 13-6 shows the distribution of by-products of sucrose metabolism in cariogenic plaque and noncariogenic plaque. Approximately 40

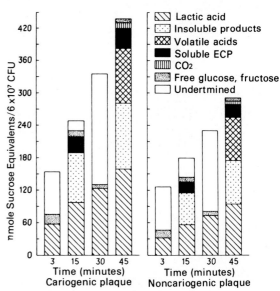

Fig. 13-6. Distribution of by-products of sucrose metabolism in cariogenic plaque and non-cariogenic plaque. The height of each bar represents the amount of sucrose consumed during the particular time interval. The height of each bar segment represents the proportion of the consumed sucrose recovered as the product indicated by the code on the figure. (Minah GE, Loesche WJ; Sucrose metabolism in resting cell suspensions of caries-associated and non-caries-associated dental plaque. Infect Immun 17: 51, 1977)

per cent more lactic acid is formed from sucrose by cariogenic plaque than by noncariogenic plaque. Although this type of metabolic study reveals clear differences between the plaque types, which coincide with the relative proportion and numbers of S. *mutans* in the plaques, this type of data is still not conclusive enough to prove that S. *mutans* was the caries-initiating agent.

Longitudinal Studies

A promising clinical approach to demonstrate the involvement of one or more bacterial species in the initiation of caries would be through longitudinal studies using periodic microbial sampling of initially caries-free surfaces at which carious lesions are most likely to occur. Results of the limited studies of this type to date indicate that high numbers of S. *mutans* in approximal plaque may be one situation under which a carious lesion can be produced. However, domination by S. *mutans* is not obligatory for the production of a lesion. These studies also indicate that in general after a lesion has been initiated, dramatic changes in the plaque over the lesion do not occur. Furthermore, an inverse relationship between S. *mutans* and S. *sanguis* is not usually noted in these studies.

A variation of this approach has been to ex-amine microbial changes following perturbations to the oral environment that result in patients becoming extremely susceptible to developing rampant caries. An example of this situation is radiation-induced xerostomia. In this situation a pronounced shift to a highly acidogenic plaque microflora occurs concomitantly with the saliva shutdown and the resulting radical changes in dietary habits and patterns of eating (see Chap. 12). Specifically, in coronal plaque S. *mutans*, lactobacilli, candida and catalase positive diphtheroids show progressive increases during radiation treatment that last for at least 9 months post-radiation (Fig. 13-7). In contrast, S. *sanguis*, neisseria and fusobacteria decline in numbers (Fig. 13-7). This shift is reminiscent, but on a more accelerated scale, of the microbial changes which frequently occur in response to high sucrose diets (see Chapter 12).

The microbial profile of the onset of rampant caries is also shown in Figures 13-8 and 13-9. An accelerated increase in plaque S. *mutans* which closely parallels the onset of rampant caries is seen in Figure 13-8, whereas the increase in *Lactobacillus* species appears to lag behind the increase in both the numbers of S. *mutans* and DMFS increments (Fig. 13-9). Thus, in the case of rampant caries in the xerostomia patients, it appears that S. *mutans* is responsible for caries initiation and that *Lactobacillus* species act as oppor-

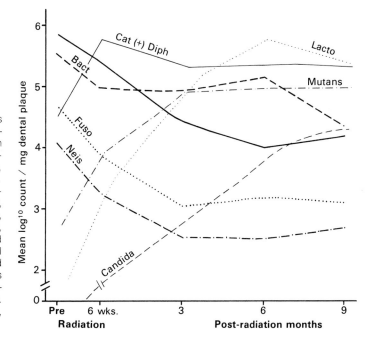

Fig. 13-7. Statistically significant changes in the cultivable plaque microflora following irradiation-induced xerostomia in 42 cancer patients. (NEIS, *Neisseria* species; BACT, *Bacteriodes* species; FUSO, *Fusobacterium* species; SANGUIS, S. *sanguis;* CAT (+) DIPH, catalase positive anaerobic diphtheroids; MUTANS, S. *mutans;* LACTO, *Lactobacillus* species, CANDIDA, *Candida* species.) (Brown LR, Dreizen S, Handler S: Effects of selected caries prevention regimens on microbial changes following irradiation-induced xerostomia in cancer patients. In Stiles HM, Loesche WJ, O'Brien TC (eds): Microbial Aspects of Dental Caries, vol I, p. 278. Washington DC, Information Retrieval Inc., 1976)

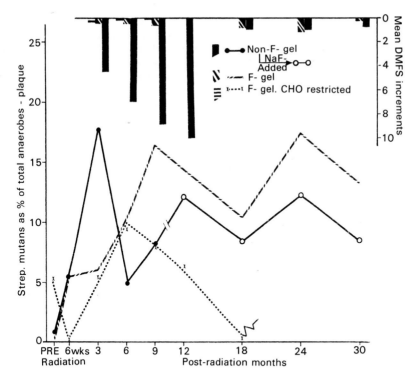

Fig. 13-8. Relationship between caries preventive regimens, changeover from non-fluoride to fluoride gel, plaque *S. mutans* and DMFS increments following irradiation-induced xerostomia. Brown LR, Dreizen S, Handler S: Effects of selected caries prevention regimens on microbial changes following irradiation-induced xerostomia in cancer patients. (In Stiles HM, Loesche WJ and O'Brien TC (eds): Microbial Aspects of Dental Caries. vol I. p. 286. Washington, D.C., Information Retrieval Inc., 1976)

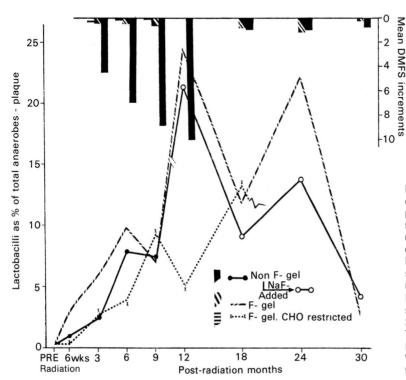

Fig. 13-9. Comparative effects of caries preventive regimens on plaque lactobacilli and successive mean 3-month DMFS increments following irradiation-induced xerostomia. Brown LR, Dreizen S, Handler S: Effects of selected caries prevention regimens on microbial changes following irradiation-induced xerostomia in cancer patients. (In Stiles HM, Loesche WJ, O'Brien TC (eds): Microbial Aspects of Dental Caries. vol I, p. 285. Washington D.C., Information Retrieval Inc., 1976)

tunist in caries progression. A striking finding of the study shown in Figures 13-8 and 13-9 was the impressive ability of one per cent sodium fluoride gel to prevent lesions in these patients when topically applied to the teeth daily. Since the fluoride only slowed the rate of increase of S. mutans, the fluoride effect may be more pronounced on the metabolism of the plaque microflora than in inhibiting bacterial growth. This effect, in addition to reducing enamel solubility and enhancing remineralization at the enamel surface, explains the impressive effectiveness of the daily topical application of fluoride in preventing caries despite the continuous presence of a highly cariogenic plaque microflora.

Few clinical studies have considered the microbial agent of root surface lesions. Those that have, have examined only the flora associated with active root surface lesions. S. mutans, S. sanguis and A. viscosus have been found in high numbers over the surface and in the deeper carious dentin of root caries lesions. In addition S. mutans, Staphylococcus epidermidis, Propionibacterium acnes, and an aerobic gram positive diptheroid with characteristics of the genus Arthrobacter have been isolated from the advancing front of root surface lesions.

In summary, evidence from human studies provides strong circumstantial evidence that S. mutans is associated with caries causation. The burning question that remains is whether S. mutans is the only organism involved. The available evidence from epidemiologic studies in humans suggests that this is not so in every case. It thus seems likely that, while S. mutans must be regarded as a major etiological factor in caries of humans, other acidogenic organisms may in some cases also be involved in the initiation and progression of caries.

MICROFLORA OF DEEP CARIES LESIONS

Compared to our understanding of coronal plaque, less is known about the microbiology of deep carious dentin. Even less is known about specific microorganisms, if any, which might be involved in the pathologic process at the advancing bacterial front of carious dentin. Further, it is not clear which biochemical properties function in the spread of bacteria in the dentin. Histologic studies of advanced caries lesions (Chap. 9) indicate that once a nidus of the penetrating caries becomes established at the dentinoenamel junction, microorganisms frequently spread along this junction and toward the pulp along the dentin tubules. It has been assumed that microbial products, such as organic acids and various enzymes which can be found ahead of the bacterial front line, might prepare the dentin for the microbial invasion. These microbial substances may originate from the bacteria in the deeper part of carious dentin or from the biochemical activities of all the bacteria in the whole caries lesion.

Microbiological examination of carious dentin indicates that it has a variable microflora which tends to be more aciduric than coronal plaque isolates. Species of Streptococcus and Actinomyces, Lactobacillus, and a large number of other unidentified gram positive rods are frequently isolated from carious dentin. However, large variations in the distribution of these organisms commonly are observed between carious dentin lesions. This suggests that once the caries process begins, a variety of ecologic factors affect the autogenic succession of organisms within a developing dentin lesion leading to the emergence of the species that will ultimately become dominant.

A comprehensive study which attempted to isolate and identify the cultivable bacterial flora of the advancing front of the carious dentin lesion from extracted teeth was carried out by Edwardsson (see Suggested Readings). Successive samples of dentin material were removed from the pulp chamber in the direction toward the lesion. The first positive culture was considered to represent the flora of the advancing bacterial front. A summary of the study results is presented in Table 13-2. Lactobacillus organisms were observed in approximately half of the teeth extracted and this genus accounted for the largest incidence of the genera observed. The next most populous group was the gram positive pleomorphic rods and filaments. The incidence of gram positive cocci was low which is in contrast to their ubiquitous presence in coronal plaque and to their role in coronal plaque development in initiation of the caries lesion.

Because of the complexity and broad variations for all the genera and species observed in carious dentin, no simple statement can be made concerning the floral composition of this tissue.

TABLE 13-2.   THE MEAN PERCENTAGE
             DISTRIBUTION OF THE PREDOMINANT
             CULTIVABLE ORGANISMS
             RECOVERED FROM THE ADVANCING
             BACTERIAL FRONT OF
             CARIOUS DENTIN*

Organisms	Mean†	Range
Gram positive anaerobic rods	44	0–100‡
Arachnia spp.	12	
Bifidobacterium spp.	9	
Eubacterium spp.	9	
Propionibacterium spp.	11	
Gram positive facultative anaerobic rods	38	0–100
Actinomyces spp.	5	
Lactobacillus spp.	33	
Gram positive anaerobic cocci	7	0–100
Streptococcus spp.	7	
Gram positive facultative anaerobic cocci	6	0–100
Streptococcus spp.	6	

* A total of 46 teeth were analyzed.
† Mean does not add to 100 per cent since percentages less than 1 are not included in this table.
‡ 100 per cent means that the organisms were observed in pure culture.
Edwardsson S: Bacteriological studies on deep areas of caries dentin. Odontol Revy 25: Suppl 32, pp. 100–103, 1974.

ECOLOGY AND VIRULENCE OF CARIOGENIC MICROORGANISMS

A unique aspect of caries is the degree of influence which ecologic factors exercise over the microbial agents involved. Moreover some of the same factors which facilitate the establishment of specific cariogenic organisms in the plaque microbiota also play a direct role in the pathogenesis of these organisms as far as caries is concerned. An understanding of this complex relationship is necessary to any consideration of the question of virulence in cariogenic organisms. This section will deal with the distinctive factors which govern the ecology of cariogenic organisms and which are also involved in their virulence.

Virulence

Virulence is generally defined as the ability of an organism to overcome the defense mechanisms of the host and to cause damage to host tissues. Such a definition implies that virulence is not an absolute entity since the resistance of the host and environmental factors necessarily enter into its assessment. In some instances virulence must also be defined in terms of the target tissue. For example, strains of *S. mutans, S. sanguis, S. mitior* and *S. faecalis* may cause endocarditis as well as dental caries. The complexity of caries as a disease process makes it far more difficult to explain what constitutes virulence in caries-associated organisms than in the case of organisms such as *Corynebacterium diphtheriae* or *Clostridium botulinum* where virulence can be directly related to the production of a specific destructive toxin.

A large number of laboratory investigations have been aimed at discovering the factors which determine virulence, or cariogenicity of oral microorganisms. Since S. *mutans* has been the most thoroughly studied of these organisms most of the discussion to follow is based on findings with this organism. However, within reasonable limits the basic concepts involved are applicable to other cariogenic organisms as well.

In the laboratory cariogenicity is usually assayed in animal model systems with the expressed or implied caveat that the extrapolation of findings to caries in humans must be done with caution. Furthermore, in the interests of scientific precision, most laboratory investigations have concentrated on single strains of microorganisms despite the fact that caries in humans invariably occurs in the presence of a very mixed microbiota. Thus, while it is possible to single out a characteristic which makes one bacterial strain more or less cariogenic than another in the laboratory there is no absolute assurance that the mechanism involved will be responsible for the same effect in humans.

With these reservations in mind a number of factors which are related to cariogenicity of oral microorganisms can be considered. As we shall see, there is no single characteristic that can be equated with virulence. Instead, an organism must possess a combination of characteristics to be potentially cariogenic. In addition, its ultimate virulence will depend as much or more on its response to environmental conditions at the tooth surface as it does on its intrinsic characteristics.

Intrinsic Microbial Factors in Virulence

The following characteristics have been found to be determinants of cariogenicity in S. *mutans.*

1. Acid-Producing Ability. Ultimately caries is initiated by acid demineralization of the surface enamel. Therefore acid production is an essential prerequisite for a cariogenic organism. In support of this concept it has been found that mutants of cariogenic parent strains of *S. mutans* which are impaired in their ability to produce lactic acid from sugars are also less cariogenic when tested in gnotobiotic rats.

2. Aciduric Potential. The continued production of acid by microorganisms can eventually result in their death due to the drop in *p*H below life sustaining levels. Thus while the most acidogenic organisms might be thought to be the most cariogenic this will not be the case unless they can survive the acid conditions which they cause. As will be shown later *S. mutans* is more tolerant of acid than most streptococci.

3. Formation and Utilization of Storage Polysaccharides. Most cariogenic organisms have the ability, when excess amounts of sugar are available, to convert a portion to intracellular storage polysaccharides (ISP). Later when exogenous carbohydrates are exhausted these organisms metabolize these reserves for energy requiring reactions with the production of lactic acid. This has the effect of prolonging the concentration of acid in the plaque and thereby prolonging the cariogenic challenge to the tooth. Laboratory studies have shown that mutant strains of *S. mutans* which lack this capability are less cariogenic in animals than their parent strains which produce abundant amounts of ISP although there are some naturally occurring strains of *S. mutans* which are still highly cariogenic in animals despite the inability to form large amounts of ISP. It is also of interest to note that while fluoride is an effective inhibitor of ISP synthesis it is relatively ineffective in preventing the formation of acid from ISP once it has been synthesized.

4. Formation of Insoluble Extracellular Glucans From Sucrose. The formation of insoluble extracellular adherent polysaccharides from sucrose is a common characteristic of *S. mutans* and cariogenic strains of *S. sanguis*, *S. mitior* and *S. salivarius*. These polysaccharides play an important role in the adherence and buildup of these organisms on the tooth, and they form a protective matrix for other organisms as well. They may also serve to concentrate for the plaque organisms required growth substances present in suboptimal concentrations in the saliva. Finally they may act

as a barrier to the diffusion of acids from the plaque and the ingress of salivary buffers, thus prolonging the concentration of acids in proximity to the tooth surface. The importance of these polysaccharides in plaque formation and cariogenicity of *S. mutans* has been demonstrated by the use of mutants of *S. mutans* which are deficient in their production. Such mutants are less able to colonize the smooth surfaces of the teeth of animals and hence produce less smooth surface caries. However their ability to cause caries in pits and fissures is generally unchanged, presumably due to the retentive and protected nature of the latter sites.

Sucrose and Cariogenicity

Since sucrose is by far the most commonly ingested sugar in humans, and its consumption has long been associated with caries, the reactions of the plaque microbiota to sucrose are of special interest in relation to cariogenicity. In an environment where sucrose is in abundance *S. mutans* enjoys a number of competitive advantages over other plaque organisms. Figure 13-10 shows that compared to other plaque species *S. mutans* produces more lactic acid and more insoluble extracellular glucans from sucrose, two factors in cariogenicity which have been discussed above. Furthermore, as shown in Figure 13-11, when growing in the form of concentrated masses (as colonies on agar) *S. mutans* forms acid from glucose, fructose, or sucrose more rapidly than *A. viscosus* or *S. mitior* and can maintain a low environmental *p*H without decreasing cell viability (i.e., it is more aciduric).

> /o impt.ce on smooth surfaces

Host Defenses

Besides the inherent characteristics of the microorganisms which have just been discussed in relation to cariogenicity it is necessary to take into account the second aspect of virulence, namely the host defences. From the standpoint of the host the major known defensive factors against caries are related to the saliva and the teeth themselves. A copious, well buffered salivary secretion may abort caries initiation by neutralizing acid and recalcifying demineralized or hypomineralized areas. Saliva may also contain specific inhibitory factors for oral microorganisms. Although it is not yet known how important

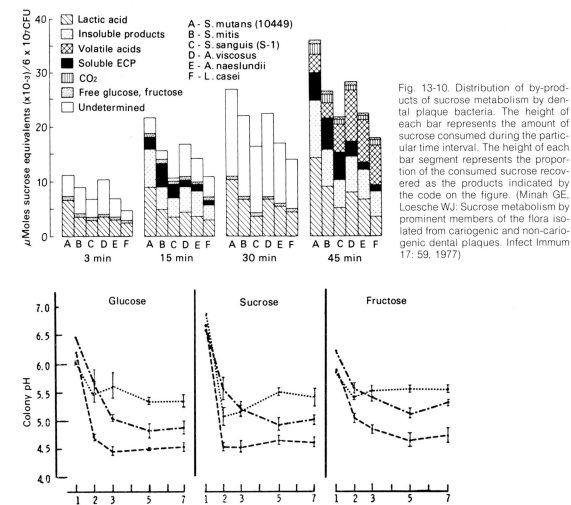

Fig. 13-10. Distribution of by-products of sucrose metabolism by dental plaque bacteria. The height of each bar represents the amount of sucrose consumed during the particular time interval. The height of each bar segment represents the proportion of the consumed sucrose recovered as the products indicated by the code on the figure. (Minah GE, Loesche WJ: Sucrose metabolism by prominent members of the flora isolated from cariogenic and non-cariogenic dental plaques. Infect Immun 17: 59, 1977)

Fig. 13-11. pH changes for colonies of *A. viscosus*, *Streptococcus mutans* and *Streptococcus mitis* grown on tryptic soy agar containing either glucose, sucrose, or fructose. Each value represents the mean of *pH* values obtained for 5 strains. Vertical bars represent the standard error of the mean. (Ellen RP and Onose H: pH measurements of *Actinomyces viscosus* colonies grown on media containing dietary carbohydrates. Arch Oral Biol 23: 106, 1978)

these latter factors are in humans, there is evidence from animal experiments that antibodies secreted in saliva, and possibly in the gingival fluid as well, may inhibit caries production by S. *mutans*. On the other hand, patients whose salivary flow has been abolished or seriously reduced as a result of disease or X-radiation quickly become susceptible to a rampant type of caries which affects all tooth surfaces.

The defensive factors associated with the teeth themselves are of two types. The first of

these is related to the anatomy of the tooth. Teeth with shallow molar cusps and fissures and nonretentive approximal contact points are less apt to develop decay in those areas than teeth in which bacteria and food remnants are provided with natural lodging sites. By far, the most effective tooth associated resistance factor to decay is the presence of fluoride in the enamel. Even the ordinarily overwhelming cariogenic challenge brought on by radiation-induced xerostomia can be effectively controlled by assiduous topical application of fluoride gels (Figs. 13-8, 13-9). Such treatments do not eliminate the infection and the rampant decay will resume shortly after the fluoride applications are discontinued, but this provides a dramatic illustration that in caries, as in many other infectious processes, the clinical outcome depends upon the balance between the virulence of the infectious agents and the defensive factors that can be mustered to protect the target tissue.

Caries as an Ecologic Consequence

Much of the information that we have discussed about caries causation has come from controlled laboratory investigations in which the experiments have been designed to limit the possible variables as far as possible. However in humans the plaque which overlays an incipient lesion is rarely a pure culture of a single organism and environmental conditions are rarely ever static. If we accept that acids produced by microbial metabolism of sugars are the prime factor in enamel demineralization then it makes little difference to the tooth whether the acid comes from S. mutans, from a *Lactobacillus*, from an *Actinomyces*, from another *Streptococcus*, or from all of them together. Once plaque is formed the key factors are whether the plaque microbiota is comprised of a mixture of organisms which produce enough acid to demineralize the enamel and whether enough of this acid gets to the tooth surface or is utilized by other organisms or neutralized by saliva. Of course, as we have seen, if the tooth surface is adequately fortified by fluoride its resistance to acids will be enhanced to the point where demineralization will either not occur or where remineralization will take place so rapidly that the caries process is effectively aborted at that site.

Only when considered from this ecologic point of view does it become possible to piece together a rational picture of the pathogenesis of caries initiation and to understand why car-

ies occurs on some tooth surfaces and not on others. Many of the same ecologic factors which govern the nature of the climax microbial community that we call dental plaque also govern the cariogenic potential of that plaque (Chap. 12). These include the mechanisms by which specific organisms adhere to the tooth, the acidogenic and aciduric capabilities of those organisms, their mutualistic and antagonistic metabolic interactions, and their special interactions with sucrose and saliva. S. mutans seems to be specially endowed with most of the attributes which are considered to relate to cariogenicity in a microorganism. There is every reason to regard its presence in plaque as a danger signal that conditions are favorable for caries initiation at that site. There is good evidence also that the risk of caries increases as the proportion of S. mutans in plaque increases. However we must not lose sight of the fact that under appropriate environmental conditions other organisms may cause caries and that the initial caries lesion as seen clinically is most probably the net result of the total ecosystem which comprises the plaque at that site.

SUMMARY

Only a limited number of microbial species apparently have the ability to produce dental caries, but even this ability is clearly governed by environmental factors which play a decisive role in the outcome of this disease. Environmental factors affect both the microbial composition of plaque and the behavior of the cariogenic plaque microorganisms. These factors affect the caries process by altering the ability of potentially cariogenic microorganisms to colonize on tooth surfaces. They emerge as a major determinant of the ecosystem at that site and allow/prevent these microorganisms to fully express their odontopathic capability.

GLOSSARY

Acidogenic microorganism. An organism which produces acid from fermentable carbohydrates.

Aciduric microorganism. An organism capable of survival in an acidic environment.

Biotype. Any one of a number of strains of a species of microorganisms that have differentiable physiologic characteristics.

Cariogenicity. Capacity of an organism to cause dental caries.

Cariogenic plaque. Dental plaque located within an active caries lesion.

Gnotobiotic. A word derived from the Greek "gnotos" and "biota" meaning known flora and fauna.

Monoinfection. Infection with a single kind of organism.

Superinfected. Infection of a conventional animal with a microorganism which is not a member of its normal microflora.

Transmissible. Capable of being transmitted from one individual or one species to another.

Virulence. Capacity of a microorganism to cause disease. Virulence of a microorganism is determined by its toxigenicity and/or invasiveness. Synonymous with pathogenicity.

Xerostomia. Dryness of the mouth from lack of normal secretion.

SUGGESTED READINGS

Brown LR, Dreizen S, Handler S: Effects of selected caries prevention regimens on microbial changes following irradiation-induced xerostomia in cancer patients. In Stiles HM, Loesche WJ, O'Brien TC (eds): Microbial Aspects of Dental Caries, Vol 1. Washington DC, Information Retrieval, 1976, pp 275–290

Burnett GW, et al: Oral Microbiology and Infectious Disease, 4th ed. Baltimore, Williams & Wilkins, 1976

Edwardsson S: Bacteriological studies on deep areas of carious dentine. Odontol Revy [Suppl] 25 (32): 7–143, 1974

Fitzgerald RJ: Dental caries research in gnotobiotic animals. Caries Res 2: 139–146, 1968

Gibbons RJ, van Houte J: Dental caries. Annu Rev Med 26: 121–136, 1975

McClure FJ, Hewitt WL: The relation of penicillin to induced rat dental caries and oral *L. acidophilus.* J Dent Res 25: 441–446, 1946

Miller WD: The Microorganisms of the Human Mouth. New York, S. Karger, 1973

Moore WJ, Corbett ME: Distribution of dental caries in ancient British Populations. Caries Res 9: 163–175, 1975

Navia JM: Animal Models in Dental Research. Tuscaloosa, University of Alabama Press, 1977

Schamschula RG, Keyes PH, Horrabrook RW: Root surface caries in Lufa, New Guinea. I. Clinical observations. J Am Dent Assoc 85: 603, 1972

Tanzer JM, Freedman ML, Woodiel FN, Eifert RL, Rinehimer LA: Association of *Streptococcus mutans* virulence with synthesis of intracellular polysaccharide. In Stiles HM, Loesche WJ, O'Brien TC (eds): Microbial Aspects of Dental Caries, Vol III. Washington DC, Information Retrieval, 1976, pp 597–616

14 Plaque Biochemistry

Introduction
Plaque Morphogenesis
Characteristics and Composition of Pellicle
and Dental Plaque
    Composition and Origin of Acquired Pel-
    licle
    Chemical Composition of Plaque
        Proteins in Plaque
        Inorganic Components of Plaque
        Carbohydrates in Plaque
        Microbial Plaque Components
Biochemical Activities of Plaque Bacteria
    Plaque Extracellular Activities
        Polysaccharide Formation

Adhesion, Agglutination, and Coloniza-
tion
Plaque Intracellular Activities
    Carbohydrate Metabolism in Plaque:
    Acid Production
    Amino Acid Metabolism: Ammonia,
    Amines
Factors that Modify Plaque Metabolism
    Dietary Carbohydrates and Dietary Pat-
    terns
    Fluoride
Conclusion
Glossary
Suggested Readings

INTRODUCTION

Dental plaque, the bacterial system found on tooth surfaces, is largely responsible for the development of specific oral diseases. Dental caries and periodontal diseases are examples of two major oral diseases which are influenced by the pathologic activity of dental plaque. Preventive programs designed to control and eradicate these oral diseases have made use of the understanding about the nature and biochemical properties of plaque obtained through research to interfere with those processes that determine plaque pathogenicity. Furthermore, dental disease preven-

tive programs are based on the recognition that bacterial disease processes are enhanced by increasing the virulence and numbers of etiologic agents, and retarded by improvements in host resistance. Therefore, broadly conceived programs should be designed not only to control plaque, a major etiologic agent, but also to enhance the resistance of oral tissues against disease agents. It follows then, that understanding the composition of dental plaque and those factors that determine its morphogenesis and biochemical activity is essential to the proper design and application of a disease preventive program in the dental office.

It is well known that the oral cavity has such propitious environmental conditions that large numbers of a variety of microorganisms

* Supported in part by NIH-NIDR Grant No. DE07020
and DE02670

313

grow and develop in the mouth in commensal or parasitic relationships with the host. Less recognized is the fact that the oral cavity is not a single microbial habitat, but a diversity of oral habitats characterized by specific microenvironmental conditions (see Chap. 12). Examples of such selected sites are the dorsum of the tongue, the gingival crevice, the palatal mucosal surface, and the smooth surfaces of teeth. As already discussed (see Chaps. 11 and 13), a specific microflora will develop in each of these sites depending on type of surface, local chemical and physical characteristics, effectiveness of oral hygiene procedures, degree of accessibility to oral fluids, and other ecologic factors. Dental plaque constitutes a tenaciously adhering film of bacteria and salivary components which attaches to tooth surfaces, one of the ecologic sites previously mentioned. There are a variety of dental environments because these tooth surfaces can be found in a variety of locations in the mouth (e.g., approximal, lingual, buccal, occlusal surfaces). Therefore, it is not surprising to find that the composition and bacterial activity in these microsystems differ depending on the tooth site where dental plaque is formed.

Dental plaque, therefore, represents a tenacious, bacterial structure formed on tooth surfaces which can not be washed off with water sprays, and which contains large numbers of closely packed microorganisms surrounded by extracellular materials of bacterial and salivary origin. Dental plaque has two major interphases, an internal one with enamel where cell free salivary components are found in an intervening cuticle or layer referred to as pellicle (see Chap. 5), and an external one in contact with the oral cavity called plaque-saliva interphase. Bacteria at this interphase have ready access to a variety of nutrients essential to bacterial growth. A third interphase could be defined as the plaque-gingiva interphase. Bacteria at this site receive nutritional input from gingival fluids, and their metabolic end products could affect the gingival tissues in close proximity. The accurate study of this complex and dynamic ecologic microcosm is made extremely difficult by large variations in bacterial composition due to differences in site, opportunism, time of colonization (plaque age), nutritional input, and other factors. Regardless of these complications it is fundamental to design and implement a sound and effective preventive program based on plaque control to ensure oral health.

PLAQUE MORPHOGENESIS

To understand the biochemistry of dental plaque and its implication for oral health, it is helpful to review briefly the developmental stages of plaque formation as well as its composition (see Chaps. 11 and 12). If a tooth were to be thoroughly cleaned and pumiced, thus exposing to the oral environment the bare enamel surface containing hydroxyapatite, it would be covered within an hour by an organic film, the *acquired pellicle* (see Chap. 5). The pellicle is primarily of salivary origin, and is formed by the selective adsorption to hydroxyapatite of specific glycoproteins from saliva. Adsorbed proteins are usually very acidic in nature. An example of these proteins is a sulphated glycoprotein which has been frequently identified in pellicle. As many as 13 specific immunologically categorized proteins have been detected in pellicle, including IgA, IgG, IgH, albumin, transferrin, and lactoferrin.

After 4 to 6 hours of enamel exposure to the oral environment, the accummulation of pellicle has increased and may reach 0.1 to 1 μm. in thickness. After 10 to 20 hours, the moist, warm conditions in the oral cavity, together with optimal pH and oxygen concentration, propitiate selective bacterial colonization at different sites on the tooth surface. Examination of the tooth surface with the scanning electron microscope (SEM) reveals globular structures (Fig. 14-1A) which eventually coalesce with each other as these bacterial colonies grow in size. A soft aggregate of salivary proteins and inorganic salts of salivary origin eventually covers these bacterial structures in one or 2 days. After 3 days of undisturbed growth and deposition of salivary components and bacterial debris, the plaque surface looses its globular or rough, undulating surface appearance, and it becomes smooth and devoid of shape. The plaque may continue to grow in thickness for some time, but after 6 to 9 days no further increase in plaque accumulation takes place, and it maintains the attained thickness if it continues to be undisturbed by oral hygiene procedures. Growth of this plaque material seems to start preferentially in cracks and fissures on the tooth surface. It is also initiated in other protected oral sites, such as those close to the gingival margin, and then it extends occlusally (incisally) to the rest of the tooth.

Elegant ultrastructural studies using light microscopy, replicas, and electron microscopic techniques have shed light on the complex structural features of plaque. Parallel filaments oriented at right angles to the enamel surface are seen frequently, surrounded by small coccal microorganisms (Fig. 14-1B) which seem to be firmly attached to the filament forms. Food debris, salivary constituents, and dead bacterial and epithelial cells provide a rich substrate which can be used by cells in the external layers of plaque to grow and accumulate in large numbers. Bacterial counts done on wet plaque samples indicate that it contains approximately 10^{11} to 10^{12} bacteria per gram of plaque. Bacteria in plaque, therefore, are closely packed together and this has great importance in determining the high metabolic output of such large numbers of cells within a small volume.

Several important considerations should be stressed in relation to plaque formation and development:

1. Bacteria in plaque are generally attached to an organic film of salivary origin, yet there may be sites on the enamel surface where they are found in direct apposition to enamel structures.
2. Initial colonization is random, but microecologic conditions favor growth of specific bacteria at selected sites within plaque (e.g., the areas close to the gingiva which are bathed by gingival fluids and which are less accessible to cleansing procedures, and the deeper layers in a thick section of plaque). Aerobic bacteria would develop best at external positions, while anaerobes would thrive best in deeper layers which are poor in oxygen.
3. The metabolism and nutritional activity of plaque bacteria are influenced by the availability of nutrients. Depending on diffussion characteristics of different molecules, availability of nutrients vary and bacterial metabolism is directed to cope with a deficiency of sugars, phosphates, or nitrogen depending on location within plaque.
4. The high density of plaque bacteria mentioned previously results in the formation and retention of different me-

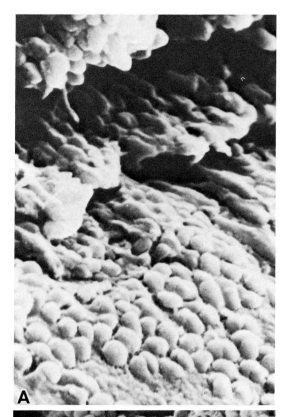

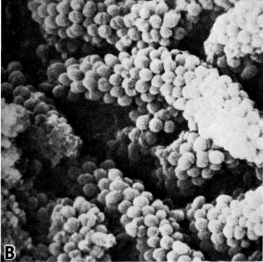

Fig. 14-1. Scanning electron microscope of bacterial structures in plaque globular structures on the enamel surface **A** Notice agglomeration in layers (×9,000); **B** coccal forms in plaque. (×13,000) (Courtesy of Dr. J. Shackleford)

tabolic end products in high concentrations at selected sites close to enamel or gingiva. These end products may affect the integrity and health of oral tissues.

5. Plaque is initiated and maintained by adhesive processes between cells, organic intermatrix, pellicle, and enamel (see Chap. 12) which are strong and which makes plaque tenacious, so that it is not easily dislodged by masticatory action. Elimination or control of plaque necessitates the use of some physical cleaning procedure. Prevention of its accumulation can be achieved by chemotherapeutic procedures against specific microorganisms known to be heavy plaque formers (see Chap. 18); interference with adhesion phenomena of cells (see Chap. 12); reduction of the amount and frequency of consumption of fermentable carbohydrates which are known to stimulate the formation of intercellular materials (see Chap. 16); and oral hygiene procedures such as brushing and flossing (see Chap. 22).

Evidently, plaque formed under the above described conditions is not a defined, stable structure. Plaque constitutes a dynamic and complex conglomerate of bacteria and organic matter plus inorganic materials. Plaque composition varies from person to person, from one site in the oral cavity to another, and even from one location on the tooth surface to another. It is unfortunate that plaque has received names such as *scum*, *slime* or *debris* because these terms do not describe the reality that plaque is a *living* structure containing organisms which have specific biochemical activities and metabolism, and whose enhanced pathogenic potential constitutes a threat to oral health by stimulating disease processes such as dental caries and periodontal disease. Proper understanding of the viable nature of plaque and the various interrelations it has with food and oral fluids (Fig. 14-2) should lead to procedures to control, inhibit, or remove plaque. The suggestion that teeth should be "cleaned", as if plaque were an inert deposit on the tooth surface, involves a gross oversimplification of the nature of plaque.

CHARACTERISTICS AND COMPOSITION OF PELLICLE AND DENTAL PLAQUE

The composition of acquired pellicle and dental plaque has been studied in detail (see Chaps. 5 and 11) with a view to identifying their origin, biochemical characteristics, and possible chemical changes related to their pathogenic properties. Pellicle has been one of the most difficult structures to study because of the complications associated with sampling the very thin layer of organic material (0.1 μm.) deposited on enamel surfaces.

Composition and Origin of Acquired Pellicle

Methods have been developed by dental scientists to study the composition of pellicles produced under various experimental conditions. By way of review, results of their experiments indicate that both *in vivo* and also *in situ* pellicles collected on enamel slabs have identical amino acid and carbohydrate composition. This work suggests that all constituents found in short-term pellicles are pri-

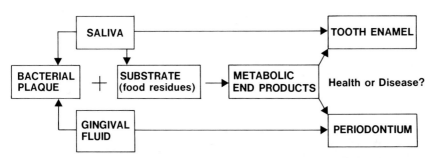

Fig. 14-2. Schematic diagram describing the relationship between bacterial plaque, the food residues used as substrate and the oral fluids. The end products from bacterial metabolism affect oral tissues, such as enamel and the periodontium, determining the development of disease or the maintenance of health.

marily originated from saliva, and that the process seems to be a highly selective one where bacteria or their breakdown products appear not to be essential.

Interestingly, glucose has been found in approximately equal concentrations to galactose in both *in vivo* and *in vitro* pellicle. Fucose, mannose, and sialic acid also have been demonstrated by paper chromatography; glucosamine and galactosamine are also found on the amino acid chromatograms of all pellicle samples collected. When pellicle formed from submandibular saliva was compared to pellicle formed from parotid saliva, the carbohydrate components were found to be remarkably similar, thus suggesting that similar glycoproteins, present in both salivas, were selectively deposited as initial pellicle on enamel slabs. Studies on the amino acid composition of pellicles formed *in situ* from submandibular, parotid, and mixed saliva have reinforced the concept of specific adsorption of selected proteins, as there were major differences in protein composition between the pellicle formed and the saliva from which it was formed. In general, the proteins adsorbed on enamel are acidic sulphated glycoproteins from sublingual and submandibular salivary glands.

Many aspects of the physiochemical mechanism for the *in vivo* formation of pellicle remain unexplained, however, some are now understood. It has been documented that the composition of experimental pellicle formed on plastic films or glass is quite different from that formed on etched enamel slabs. It is also known that hydroxyapatite selectively binds different proteins depending on the negatively or positively charged groups on the molecule. Based on this it is assumed that the physicochemical status of the enamel will determine a specific surface energy for different sites on enamel that can determine the binding or repulsion of specific salivary proteins. It remains to be elucidated which factors modify the electrochemical property of enamel, the type of proteins adsorbed under different conditions, and finally, what is most important, which proteins provide a protective effect and which ones (if any) enhance the demineralization reactions on the tooth surface. Understanding these factors, and others, such as the role of fluoride in pellicle formation, will bring about improvements in the implementation of clinical procedures to prevent enamel demineralization and influence the selection of bacteria which adhere to acquired pellicle.

Chemical Composition of Plaque

The composition of plaque has been investigated with a view to characterize it chemically, and also to attempt to identify relationships between plaque composition and virulence. While sampling of plaque is easier than pellicle collection, major problems have arisen from attempts to correlate plaque composition with tooth site, age, time after food consumption, and other factors known now to affect plaque chemistry. Because plaque is essentially a dense agglomeration of cells with some intercellular material, its water content resembles that of bacteria and fluctuates between 70 and 80 per cent. Recent studies have pointed out that there are two main compartments in dental plaque: an aqueous phase, also refered to as "plaque saliva" or plaque fluid, which contains extracellular components, and a cellular phase. The *extracellular phase* contains a fluid which is in direct contact with the underlying enamel and is responsible for the chemical interactions taking place at this interphase. The *aqueous phase* can be physically separated from total plaque and represents approximately 10 to 25 per cent of plaque by weight. Analysis of this fluid in comparison to mixed saliva and gingival fluid is given in Table 14-1.

All components except pH and aF^- (fluoride activity) were reported to be at higher concentrations in plaque fluid than in either saliva or gingival fluid (sodium excepted). The major free amino acids in plaque fluid were reported to be glutamate, aspartate, and alanine. Ammonia was also found. The presence of NH_3 as ammonium compounds and the absence of basic amino acids suggests that metabolism leading to NH_3 release is continuously going on.

Proteins in Plaque

The major component of the cellular or solid phase of plaque is protein which may vary in concentrations from 30 to 50 per cent of dry weight. Several specific proteins have been detected in plaque such as IgA and IgG. Only trace amounts of IgM have been found. Other salivary proteins and plasma-type proteins include secretory component, albumin, lysozyme, amylase, and the C_3 component of complement which is also found in gingival crevice fluid. Therefore, both salivary secre-

TABLE 14-1. COMPOSITION OF PLAQUE FLUID COMPARED WITH MIXED SALIVA-AND GINGIVAL FLUID*

	Saliva	Concentration (mmol/L) Plaque Fluid	Gingival Fluid†
	Mean (range)	Mean ± S.D. (n)	Mean ± S.D.
Sodium	13 (6.5–26)	35.1 ± 9.0 (7)	88.8 ± 31.8
Potassium	20.5 (13.6–32)	61.5 ± 13.5 (21)	17.4 ± 9.0
Calcium	1.45 (0.55–2.85)	6.5 ± 2.1 (16)	4.9 ± 1.8
Magnesium	0.41 (0.29–0.53)	3.7 ± 1.1 (17)	0.4 ± 0.3
Inorganic phosphate	5.4 (2.0–23)	14.2 ± 3.1 (43)	1.3 ± 0.9
Carbohydrate (glucose)	0.06 (0.03–17)	13.9 ± 2.3 (7)	1.6 ± 0.7‡
pH	6.5 (4.5–8.5)	6.54 ± 0.26 (5)	8.2 ± 0.14§
Protein (g%)	0.28 (0.18–0.42)	1.49 ± 0.06 (7)	6.83 ± 1.26**
aF⁻	2 (1–5)	2.0 + 0.7 (11)	

* Calculated from Jenkins GN: *The Physiology of the Mouth.* 3 ed. Oxford, Blackwell Scientific Publications, 1966.
† Calculated from Kaslick RS, Chasens AL, Mandel ID, *et al.:* J. Periodontol 41: 93, 1970, and J. Dent. Res 52: 180, 1973.
‡ Calculated from Kjellman. Swensk. Tandlark Tidska 63: 11, 1970.
§ Smith LB, Golub LB and Duperon DF. Results in subjects with full permanent dentition. J. Dent. Chi. 41: 128, 1974.
** From Bang J and Cimasoni G: Data derived from 20 patients with periodontal disease. J. Dent. Res. 50: 1683, 1971.
(From Tatevossian, Gould CT: Arch Oral Biol 21: 319–323, 1976)

TABLE 14-2. QUANTITATION OF PLAQUE COMPONENTS: COMPARISON WITH WHOLE SALIVA AND GINGIVAL CREVICE FLUID

Preparation	n	Dry Weight (mg)	Protein	μg/ml IgA	IgG	HSA	Ratio IgA/IgG	IgA/HSA
Plaque 1	18	145.7	13,590	217.7	63.0	171.0	3.5	1.3
Plaque 2	30	117.4	11,270	300.6	248.0	164.0	1.2	1.8
Plaque 3	60	390.0	41,700	239.0	344.6	441.2	0.7	0.5
Plaque 4	130	300.0	24,900	361.0	455.0	ND	0.8	ND
Whole saliva (unstimulated)				194.0*	14.4*	12.5†	13.5	15.5
				152.0‡	6.0‡	13.0‡	25.3	11.7
Gingival crevice fluid				1,568§	14,631§	ND	0.1	ND
				1,100**	3,510§	ND	0.3	ND

(Key: ND, not determined; n, number of individuals from whom plaque was sampled)
* Values calculated from the data of Brandtzaeg P: Clin. Exp. Immunol. 8: 69, 1971
† Values calculated from the data of Oppenheim FG: Helv Acta Odontol. Scand 14: 10, 1970
‡ Determined in Taubman's laboratory from whole saliva of three persons.
§ Values calculated from the data of Holmberg K and Killander: J. Periodontal Res 6: 1, 1971
** Values calculated from the data of Shillitoe EJ and Lehner TG: Arch Oral Biol 17: 241, 1972
(From Taubman MA and Smith DJ: J Dent Res 55: C153–62, 1976)

tion and gingival crevice fluid seem to contribute to dental plaque protein components which vary in concentrations as shown in Table 14-2. Studies of amino acid composition indicate that tyrosine, phenylalanine, threonine, methionine, valine, and proline are commonly found in plaque in concentrations which seem to be fairly constant compared to other plaque components. Lipids are also found in plaque in small concentrations ranging from 10 to 15 per cent dry weight. Larger concentrations of lipids are found in the acellular than in the cellular fraction. More studies are needed to identify the nature of these lipids, probably of bacterial origin, and to understand their role in the metabolic activity of plaque and its virulence.

Inorganic Components of Plaque

The inorganic and the carbohydrate components of plaque are the ones which seem to vary the most, probably because they are influenced by a large number of factors. Approximately 5 to 10 per cent of dry weight of plaque is contributed by inorganic materials in which calcium, phosphorus, and potassium seem to predominate. Magnesium, sodium and a wide variety of trace elements such as zinc, copper, lead, iron, lithium, strontium, and fluoride are also found in plaque. Variations in calcium, phosphorus, and fluoride concentrations are important because they are probably related to enamel dissolution and remineralization processes (see Chap. 19).

Still, other elements such as strontium and lithium may play important roles in determining the caries pathogenicity of plaque. Concentrations of calcium and phosphate within plaque seem to be dependent on factors such as plaque location on the tooth surface, age of the host, ability of the host to form calculus, length of time the plaque remains undisturbed, and carbohydrate intake and its pattern of consumption by the host.

Trace elements in plaque vary depending on the mineral content of water and foods consumed by the individual and the composition of the underlying enamel. Fluoride, for example, is found in plaque of subjects consuming water and foods containing fluoride and may fluctuate from 5 to 50 ppm. Several epidemiologic studies in Columbia and in Papua, New Guinea have included measurements of trace element concentrations in dental plaque from subjects belonging to populations with different caries experience in an effort to detect meaningful correlations. While no clear pattern has yet emerged, certain elements such as lithium, strontium, and boron appear to be elements in plaque inversely associated with low caries activity.

Fluoride (see Chap. 20) continues to be the most important and effective cariostatic trace element and, therefore, a number of studies have attemped to define its metabolism in plaque. Its main source is probably water, foods, and saliva, with only a minimal amount coming from enamel. The chemistry of fluoride in plaque is not completely clear. It is assumed that when plaque pH is close to neutral, fluoride is loosely bound to the intercellar material, and that a large proportion is bound to calcium, so that little or no ionized fluoride is found in plaque. This might help explain why even though substantial amounts of fluoride have been reported in plaque, bacteria in plaque continue to grow and metabolize without seemingly being affected by the bacteriostatic and antienzymatic properties of fluoride ions. Further research is needed to understand the role of fluoride and other trace elements in plaque formation and caries.

Carbohydrates in Plaque

The other plaque component which is subject to wide variations in concentration and composition is carbohydrate. Plaque contains a large amount of carbohydrate (approximately

10 to 20 per cent by volume) in the form of polysaccharides synthesized by bacteria and accumulated extracellularly. Hydrolysis of the carbohydrate fraction of plaque yields large quantities of glucose, as well as some other sugars such as fructose, mannose, galactose, maltose, rhamnose, glucosamine, and others. The carbohydrate composition is largely determined by the type of bacteria in plaque, types of dietary substrates they metabolize, and the time elapsed since the last dietary intake.

Extracellularly the major polysaccharide isolated from plaque is a glucan, a polymer of glucose whose predominant linkages are $\alpha(1 \rightarrow 6)$ and a high proportion of $\alpha(1 \rightarrow 3)$ linkages. Detailed studies of large plaque samples indicate that the so called insoluble glucans are highly crosslinked polysaccharides with appreciable amounts of $\alpha(1 \rightarrow 3)$ linkages. The highly crosslinked polymer of glucose synthesized from sucrose by glucosyl transferases from *Streptococcus mutans* is named "mutan", a term coined for polysaccharide found in plaque (Fig. 14-3). Specific glycosyl transferases are used by different *S. mutans* strains to synthesize mutans which vary considerably in types and degree of crosslinkages.

Fructose is the major component of another polysaccharide found in plaque, commonly known as fructan or levan (Fig. 14-4). One of the important differences between the water soluble fructan and mutan is that fruc-

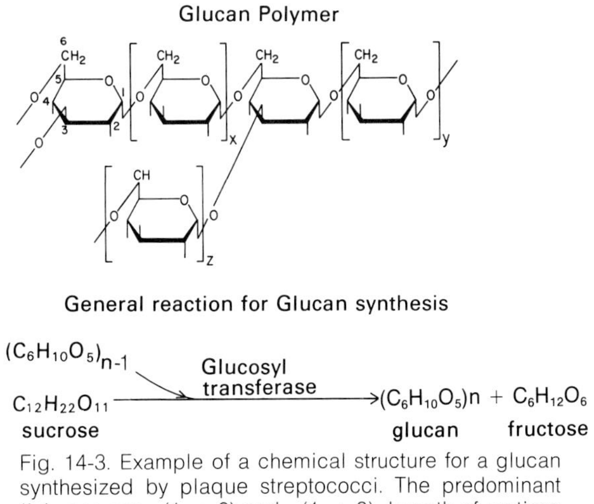

Fig. 14-3. Example of a chemical structure for a glucan synthesized by plaque streptococci. The predominant linkages are $\alpha(1 \rightarrow 6)$ and $\alpha(1 \rightarrow 3)$. Length of portions of the polymer (x, y, z) and the degree of crosslinkages varies depending on strain of *S. mutans* producing the glucan. The reaction describes the activity of glucosyltransferase utilizing sucrose as specific substrate for glucan synthesis.

Levan polymer

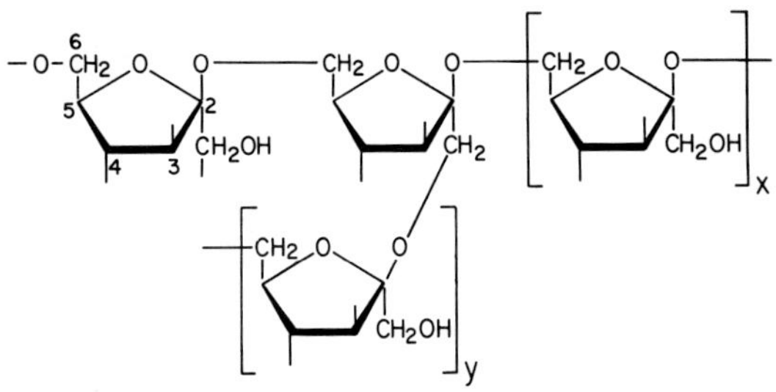

Fig. 14-4. Example of a chemical structure for a levan polymer synthesized by fructosyl transferase from plaque streptococci. Length of portions of the polymer (x and y) vary depending on streptococci producing the fructan.

tan can be degraded by bacterial plaque while mutan is highly resistant to hydrolytic enzymatic action. Therefore, levan frequently disappears from plaque after it has been synthesized, thus constituting a reservoir of fermentable sugars for the oral flora. Analysis of plaque which has not been exposed to sucrose for some time usually shows little fructan, while under these conditions large quantities of the more insoluble glucan or mutan can still be detected.

It should be understood that even though glucans and fructans are the most abundant extracellular products obtained when sucrose is metabolized by streptococci, other extracellular polysaccharides (some of these heteroglycans) may also be present in plaque. These polysaccharides can be produced from other sugars available in the diet and may even be produced in the absence of dietary carbohydrates. Since sugars are also present in the cell wall of the different bacteria, they also contribute to the carbohydrate pool found in plaque.

One other polysaccharide found in plaque is the polymer formed intracellularly by bacteria such as streptococci, leptothrichiae, and diphtheroids, among others. The intracellular polysaccharide (IP) resembles starch or glycogen and is made up of glucose units linked together by $\alpha(1 \rightarrow 4)$ bonds. As the polysaccharides are strongly iodophylic, the presence of IP can be detected microscopically by staining the cells with iodine.

The biologic significance of polysaccharides in plaque has been the subject of numerous studies. Briefly some of the most important points are:

1. sucrose is the specific substrate for the glycotransferase enzymes to form either glucan or levan;

2. polysaccharide formation represents a mechanism to store energy within and around cells which is available at times when there is a metabolic need for such energy rich molecules;
3. polysaccharide synthesis also represents a metabolic pathway that enables bacterial cells to handle large concentrations of carbohydrate without having to use the glycolytic or oxidative pathways;
4. extracellular polysaccharides (ECP) are important in adhesion processes between cells, and between cells and other tooth structures such as pellicle and hydroxyapatite;
5. ECP act as a diffusion barrier that protects the cells from major osmotic effects resulting from high concentrations of ions, and at the same time interfere with diffusion of nutrients and metabolic end products in or out of the plaque.

All of these factors have an important bearing on the determination of the pathogenicity of plaque and deserve careful consideration by oral health professionals.

Microbial Plaque Components

Enamel represents the only structure in the oral cavity that has no turnover rate in the manner seen in epithelial surfaces. It is also a surface of apatitic material (see Chap. 7) covered with proteinaceous material of salivary origin (pellicle). This surface is ideally suited for the attachment of specific bacteria which are ecologically fitted to that particular oral site (see Chap. 12). For these reasons, soon after the pellicle is formed on the enamel surface it becomes covered with aggregates of bacteria which, if not disturbed, reach bacterial concentrations of approximately 10^{11} bacteria per 100 mg. wet weight of plaque. Microscopic studies have revealed that while most bacteria in plaque adhere to pellicle, there are denuded areas where bacteria are observed in close apposition with enamel without an obligatory pellicle interphase. Saliva seems to play an important role in determining plaque composition not only through pellicle formation, but also by stimulating agglutination of specific bacteria through what has been refered to as salivary lectins (see Chap. 3).

It is important to realize that teeth offer a variety of surfaces, some of which are smooth and others which constitute retentive areas, such as pits and fissures where bacteria can be held independent of any of the adhesion phenomena previously described. In these latter sites, food debris can be physically held and packed into deep crevices where the trophic environment is different from that of smooth surfaces. Major organisms colonizing these pits and fissures include, among others, *S. salivarius*, *S. sanguis*, *S. mitis* and *S. mutans*. Of these bacteria, *S. sanguis* is primarily seen on smooth surfaces, followed by *S. mutans* which may reach a high proportion of the total streptococci if allowed to grow undisturbed. The ability of *S. mutans* serotypes to adhere to surfaces depends to a large extent on the presence of glycosyl transferases on its cell membranes and the extracellular polymers (glucan or fructan) it produces. Treatment of these cells with trypsin or antibodies to the transferases is known to interfere with cell ability to adhere to a variety of experimental surfaces.

Other bacteria also colonize various sites on the tooth surface. One such example is the filamentous bacteria, often seen in close apposition with streptococci. As the plaque is allowed to remain on the tooth surface undisturbed, lactobacilli and *Actinomyces* also become abundant. During early stages in the formation of plaque the environment on smooth surfaces is essentially aerobic, and the first organisms that attach to these sites are either aerobic or facultative anaerobes. It is therefore not suprising that oxygen-tolerant streptococci represent approximately 60 per cent of the total bacteria isolated from newly formed plaque. After a few days of growth, other organisms such as *Fusobacterium*, *Actinomyces* and *Veillonella* become abundant.

Data from longitudinal studies have demonstrated a pattern in the sequence of colonization of different bacteria with increasing age. The first bacteria to be detected in a baby soon after birth is *S. salivarius* followed by *S. sanguis* which is detected soon after eruption of the first teeth. *S. mutans* is commonly isolated from children who have developed caries, and lactobacilli is detected especially in children who have had some filled teeth.

As *S. mutans* is one of the major cariogenic species, a large number of studies have been conducted to understand its nature and biochemical activities in plaque. Distinguishing characteristics of *S. mutans* are that it ferments mannitol, sorbitol, raffinose, and inulin, but does not produce ammonia from arginine. *S. mutans* has been classified into 7 serotypes: a, b, c, d, e, f, g. The serological groupings, together with the subspecies and some of their characteristics are listed in Table 14-3. All subspecies have been isolated from carious lesions, however, serotype c seems to predominate.

Lactobacilli are mostly found in the oral cavity when the diet is rich in fermentable carbohydrate and when there are active carious lesions. Generally, they are present in low numbers in plaque, and tend to be found in saliva and in deep carious lesions. Lactobacilli attach poorly to enamel surfaces, are fastidious in their nutritional requirements, and produce acid. They are, therefore, usually found in retentive tooth areas, such as pits and fissures, or at carious sites where they are considered to be secondary invaders rather than primary etiologic agents.

Interactions between various bacteria in plaque are extremely important and in many situations determine the biochemical effect of plaque on enamel. For many years it has been recognized that dental plaques are heterogenous. As previously stated (see Chap. 11) bacterial evaluation of dental plaque from different individuals indicates that in mature plaques (the climax community) filamentous bacteria appear to predominate, while in other types of plaque coccal forms are abundant, and in yet another type of plaque combinations of these two resembling a "corncob" may frequently be found. Random colonization, ecologic factors, and specific interactions between bacteria determine plaque composition (see Chap. 12). *L. casei*, *S. faecalis* and *S. salivarius* in paired mixed plaque assay cultures with *S. mutans* caused notable inhibition of plaque formation by *S. mutans*. *C. albicans*, however, was observed to enhance plaque formation when added to cultures of *S. mutans*. Yeast forms have been isolated in large numbers from plaque and saliva of individuals with active caries, and may yet play an important secondary role in the establishment of pathogenic bacteria in plaque.

Another interesting metabolic interaction is the one described for Veillonella. These bacteria seem to utilize the metabolic end products of glucose fermentation produced by *S. mutans*. Veillonela also has the ability to adhere to *A. viscosus* to form mixed plaque aggregates.

Inhibitory or negative interactions have been reported between *S. sanguis*, one of the

TABLE 14-3. SUBSPECIES OF *STREPTOCOCCUS MUTANS*, THEIR CHARACTERISTICS AND BASIC DIFFERENCES. (COYKENDALL 1974, BRATTHALL AND KOHLER 1976, COYKENDALL AND LIZOTTE 1978)

Subspecies	Genetic Group	Serotype	Example of Strain	DNA Base Content (G & C, mol %) From TM-	From C_sCl	Wall Carbo-hydrate	Biotypes	Electrophoretic Modify Man P Dehydrogenase	Differential Biochemical Tests
S. *mutans* subsp. *Mutans*	I	c	NCTC10449; JC 2	37.1–37.9	36.9–37.5		1	1	No NH_3 from arginine Resists bacitracin Ferments raffinose Slow glycolysis of fructose when grown on glucose
	I	e	LM7; B2	No data	36.6–36.9	{glucose rhamnose	1	No Data	
	I	f	OMZ 175	No data	No data		1	No data	Some strains Lancefield E
S. *mutans* subsp. *Rattus*	II	b	Fa-1;	42.2–43.2	40.8–41.8	{galactose rhamnose	2	2	Produces ammonia from arginine
S. *mutans* subsp. *Sobrinus*	III	d	B 13; OMZ 176	No data	44.7	{glucose	3	4	Fail to ferment raffinose
	III	g	OMZ 65; K1R	45.2	45.3	galactose	3	4	
	III	—	SL-1	45.1	44.9	rhamnose	3	4	
S. *mutans* subsp. *Cricetus*	IV	a	AHT; E49	42.7–43.7	41.3–41.8	{glucose galactose rhamnose	1	3	Does not grow in air. Sensitive to bacitracin

(From Coykendall AL: J Gen Microbiol, 83: 327–338, 1974; Bratthall D, Kohler B: J Dent Res, 55: C15–C21, and Coykendall AL, Lizotte PA: Arch Oral Biol, 23: 427–428, 1978)

most effective colonizers of the tooth surface, and strains of S. *mutans*, S. *salivarius*, and some species of Corynebacterium. The mechanism of inhibition might be related to either some form of toxic substance produced or to a lack of some essential nutritional factor preferentially utilized by S. *sanguis*. Other types of negative interaction may be related to pH optima for growth and maintenance of the bacteria. For example, S. *mutans* is considerably more aciduric than S. *sanguis*, which could explain the disappearance of the latter and the increased numbers of the former in actively metabolizing plaque where the pH may be as low as 4.0. These types of chemical and metabolic interactions, as well as cell-cell relations (e.g., between A. *naeslundii* and *Streptococcus sanguis* and *Streptococcus mitis*), contribute to the determination of the bacterial composition of the different types of human dental plaque.

Recently some other bacterial interactions mediated by bacteriocins have received a great deal of attention. Streptococci are known to produce bacteriocins which have an antagonistic effect on other bacteria such as *Actinomyces viscosus*. However, it is not known whether such effects clearly demonstrated in *in vitro* studies, play a role in regulating the oral microflora within plaque. For a more detailed description of this phenomena the reader is directed to Chapter 12.

BIOCHEMICAL ACTIVITIES OF PLAQUE BACTERIA

Plaque Extracellular Activities

From a biochemical viewpoint the most important reactions taking place in dental plaque are those related to the metabolic utilization of substrate provided by the food-saliva mixture coming in contact with plaque bacteria. Enzyme systems from bacteria, and also from saliva, act on the various molecules in the oral environment to facilitate the implantation, growth, and maintenance of oral bacteria. For this reason, the type of foods and their frequency of intake are of utmost importance in determining the nature of the plaque formed, as well as its pathogenic potential in terms of caries and periodontal disease.

When food is masticated a certain amount of debris will be retained on mucosal and tongue surfaces, as well as on tooth surfaces, particularly at interproximal areas. Saliva contains α-amylase which acts randomly on starch molecules. The $\alpha(1 \rightarrow 4)$ D-glucosidic linkages of starch are split by this enzyme and the hydrolysis products are a mixture of maltose, glucose, dextrins, small glucose polymers (9-10 units) which are also held together by $\alpha(1 \rightarrow 4)$, and some $\alpha(1 \rightarrow 6)$ D-glucosidic bonds. This effect of salivary amylase has minor importance from the standpoint of food digestion, as the high acid concentration in the stomach inhibits the activity of this enzyme. However, in terms of oral health it should not be underestimated. Studies on retention and clearance rates for different starch-containing foods might bring further insight into the role of starch in plaque metabolism. Starches, because of their high molecular weight, are probably unable to diffuse into plaque, but their breakdown products may easily contribute readily fermentable substrate at a later time after mastication of food. These oral effects of salivary amylase can be even more pronounced in a laboratory animal, such as the rat, which is known to have high concentrations of amylase in its saliva and which is also characterized by its thorough masticatory habits. Saliva also contains enzyme systems such as the oxidoreductases or dehydrogenases which could convert, in the presence of NAD, some of the polyols, (i.e., sorbitol) into fructose which could in turn be further metabolized by plaque bacteria.

These enzymatic reactions have not been extensively evaluated relative to their contribution to plaque metabolism and need to be considered in future research. However, the metabolism of monosaccharides and disaccharides has been studied in greater detail.

Polysaccharide Formation

Sucrose is of special importance in plaque metabolism because streptococci, which are the major components of mature plaque, have extracellular homopolysaccharide synthesizing enzymes, the glycosyl transferases. These enzymes specifically use sucrose as substrate to form high molecular weight polymers. These extracellular enzymes are not only of importance because of their synthesizing abilities, but also because they represent binding mechanisms which cause cell aggregation and clumping (see Chap. 12). The two main groups of homopolysaccharide synthesizing enzymes are the glucosyl transferases and the fructosyl transferases.

The glucosyl transferases (EC2.4.1.5) are a group of extracellular enzymes found in bacteria such as S. sanguis and S. mutans which specifically use sucrose to form a glucose polymer and liberate the fructose moiety (Fig. 14-3). The reaction does not seem to require a metal cofactor or coenzymes and is not affected by fluoride ions. The enzyme has a broad pH optimum (between 5.0 and 7.0) and produces a variety of glucose polymers which have different bonding patterns. Some of the polymers formed are soluble and with predominant $\alpha(1 \rightarrow 6)$ linkages, while others constitute more of an insoluble fraction and contain other bonds (i.e., $\alpha (1 \rightarrow 3)$) in various proportions. Thus, there is a great deal of bond heterogenicity among this type of polymer formed by glucosyl transferases.

The other major extracellular polysaccharide formed by plaque bacteria is a homopolymer of fructose known as levan or fructan (Fig. 14-4). This is a D-fructofuranose polymer which shows a predominance of $\beta(2 \rightarrow 6)$ linkages. These high molecular weight polymers (approximately 20×10^6 daltons) are fairly soluble, easily degraded and are formed by the enzyme, fructosyl transferase found in bacteria such as S. salivarius, A. viscosus and some strains of S. mutans. Since these bacteria are also capable of degrading this polymer, it is difficult to determine the true output of fructan by plaque bacteria. The specific substrate for fructosyl transferases is sucrose, from which fructose is used to enlarge the fructofuranose polymer liberating a molecule of glucose in the process.

Even though glucan and fructan are the major extracellular polysaccharides formed in plaque from sucrose, they should not be considered as the only polymers in plaque, or that other sugars might not be used by other enzyme systems to produce different polysaccharides. Data have been reported which indicates that plaque polysaccharides can be formed in the absence of dietary sucrose and even in the complete absence of dietary carbohydrates. Whether these other polymers have an important role in disease processes remains yet to be determined.

Adhesion, Agglutination and Colonization

Characteristically, the enzyme activity of glycosyl transferases in streptococci is found associated with bacterial cell surfaces. The glucosyl transferases have a particularly strong tendency to associate with their products, the glucans. When cells are grown in a rich media containing some sucrose, 80 per cent or more of the glucosyl transferase is found associated with cells, and a small proportion is released into the culture media. Sucrose is quickly and completely converted to glucans which remain closely attached to the cells and increases the ability of cells to agglutinate and form clumps. Both glucans and fructans participate in this process, but glucans, being more insoluble and far less degradable than fructans, are considered to be more critical to cell adhesion and plaque formation. Addition of only a few molecules of high molecular weight, soluble dextran per bacterial cell results in rapid bacterial aggregation. The polymer, which binds to receptor sites of cell surfaces, causes multiple S. mutans cells to bind to the same polymer molecule. The model thus proposed to explain the adhesion and agglutination phenomena as a basis for plaque formation involves the presence of glucosyl transferase, the formation of receptor sites on the cell surface, the production of insoluble glucan polymers, and binding of the polymer to receptor sites on several cells to form a conglomerate. While this may not be the only possible mechanism of adhesion used by bacterial plaque cells, it is undoubtedly an important mechanism.

Recent studies directed towards the understanding of the molecular mechanism by which agglutination occurs have suggested that the spatial arrangement of HOC(3)H and 0(1) groups in dextran is important, but that the polymer receptor site responsible for agglutination is not identical with the dextran reactive site of glycosyl transferase. Other carbohydrates in addition to dextran, such as maltose, may serve as glucosyl acceptors and influence enzyme reactions, and yet, maltose has been found to be unable to block dextran mediated agglutination. These data also support the concept that glucosyl transferase and surface dextran receptors are different structures. The binding reaction and subsequent cell agglutination requires Ca^{++} or Mg^{++}, although specifically the exact reaction which requires these cofactors is not known.

These bacterial reactions, together with the different aggregating factors which exist in saliva, and which are responsible for the interaction between one or several of the different bacteria in the oral cavity are some of the factors that contribute to cell adhesion and plaque formation.

Extracellular polysaccharides (ECP) have important roles other than facilitating cell adherence to the tooth surface. They provide a source of available carbohydrates to be used by cells as they are hydrolyzed. ECP play an important role in diffusion processes taking place in plaque. They also may function to trap and concentrate trace elements and minerals. Extracellular polysaccharide formation is undoubtedly a major factor responsible for the odontopathogenic properties of plaque, and as such it needs to be understood clearly to help develop sound plaque control programs.

Plaque Intracellular Activities

Carbohydrate Metabolism in Plaque: Acid Production

Once dental plaque is formed on the tooth surface, bacteria continue to metabolize the available substrates to fulfill energy requirements and to produce structural components for maintenance and reproduction. Dietary carbohydrates are major sources of energy for bacterial cells in plaque and contribute the essential substrate to form the extracellular polysaccharides used as storage material. They are also instrumental in the colonization process. Disaccharides, such as sucrose, which enter the cell can be hydrolized by a β-D-fructofuranoside fructohydrolase (invertase: EC 3.2.1.26) to its monosaccharide components, glucose and fructose. This enzyme has been identified as an intracellular enzyme that can be induced by sucrose in S. *sanguis*, but has been found to be constitutive in S. *mutans*. An amylomaltase which can hydrolyze maltose also has been found in S. *mutans*. The latter is important as it could be a metabolic step in the utilization of starch breakdown products such as maltose and maltodextrins.

Carbohydrates from dietary residues remaining in the mouth and those released from salivary glycoproteins by plaque bacteria can be readily utilized to obtain the necessary energy for cells. Starches can be degraded to maltose and dextrins which ultimately yield glucose. In addition glycosyl transferases, in forming glucans or fructans, yield molecules of fructose or glucose as by-products of the polymer synthesizing activity. Plaque bacteria preferentially utilize these monosaccharides

through fermentative pathways (**glycolysis**) due to the anaerobic environment in which most of them exist. The major end product of such fermentation processes is lactic acid, although other organic acid end products such as acetic, propionic and formic acid can be formed. Fermentation of carbohydrates by plaque yields lactic acid in concentrations around 50 per cent of the total acid concentration. However, it is not uncommon in many plaque samples to find that acetic and formic acids represent the major acids present. The production of formic acid as opposed to lactic acid is an important variable considering the greater strength of formic acid. Large amounts of formic acid can be expected to be produced in the deeper layers of plaque next to enamel where a carbon-limited environment may be predominant.

The acid produced by the fermentation of monosaccharides brings about an increase in acidity of plaque. Following exposure to a 0.1 per cent glucose solution, the pH of human plaque may decrease by one unit within 5 minutes and will not return to the original value for 20 to 30 minutes. Higher concentrations of sugar (10%) will further lower the pH to values below 5.0 and proportionally increase the time necessary to return to original pH values. Stephan first described this behavior of plaque, and also reported that plaques on the labial surfaces of maxillary and mandibular teeth differed in pH minima obtained by these procedures. Relating this phenomena to caries activity on these tooth surfaces, and taking into consideration the physicochemical characteristics of enamel, he postulated the existence of a critical pH (4.5–5.5) below which enamel would demineralize and loose its integrity. Other investigators have extended these studies and made significant contributions to the understanding of the acid-base reactions of plaque and their significance to demineralization and remineralization processes on the tooth surface.

Glycolysis is probably the major pathway used to generate the necessary ATP to fulfill energy needs and synthesis reactions of plaque cells. Glucose and fructose enter this metabolic pathway directly through formation of glucose-6-phosphate and fructose-6-phosphate by hexokinases. Polyol sugars, such as sorbitol and mannitol, can also be fermented through this glycolytic pathway. Studies have been reported in which S. *mutans* cells adapted to grow on mannitol or sorbitol showed the presence of induced mannitol-1-

phosphate dehydrogenase and sorbitol-6-phosphate dehydrogenase which allows the conversion of these polyols to fructose-6-phosphate which then can enter the glycolytic pathway. S. *mutans* has as a specific biochemical characteristic the ability to ferment mannitol and sorbitol. When grown in the presence of these substrates, the concentrations and activity of these dehydrogenases are increased. It is possible that fermentation of sorbitol (which in the case of S. *mutans* adapted cells is marked by production of high levels of alcohol dehydrogenase and a shift away from the homolactic fermentation) might not represent an important contribution to acid plaque production. However, the ability to utilize and ferment polyols, such as sorbitol, which are widely used in some types of confectionary products, might contribute to the metabolism of S. *mutans*, thus providing a nutritional advantage in the colonization process and in their subsequent metabolic activities within plaque.

Xylitol differs from sorbitol and mannitol in that it is not metabolized by streptococci, especially *Streptococcus mutans*, and therefore, from the standpoint of plaque biochemistry, it cannot contribute to lowering of the pH. Human studies suggest that this polyol can be administered without danger of accommodation or adaptation of plaque streptococci. Some questions which arise relative to this polyol and other sugars proposed to substitute for dietary sugars are whether the other numerous bacteria in dental plaque and the oral cavity at large are capable of metabolizing the polyol; what, if any, will be the bacterial interactions (synergisms or antagonisms) stimulated by the continuous presence of this new substrate in the oral cavity; what will be the net oral health effect obtained by partial substitution in view of the ubiquitousness of other sugars; and what will be the cost, safety, and organoleptic acceptability of snack foods manufactured with such sugar substitutes?

Aside from the fermentation of various monosaccharides and polyols, plaque bacteria have other important metabolic pathways which utilize sugars present in the plaque environment. Several plaque microorganisms, such as S. *sanguis*, use phosphoenol pyruvate (PEP) and bicarbonate from saliva to form oxaloacetate via phosphoenol pyruvate carboxylase, and others, such as A. *viscosus* and A. *naeslundii*, use pyruvate and bicarbonate to form oxaloacetate via pyruvate carboxylase.

Thus, glycolysis not only produces ATP for energy reactions, but also provides important intermediate compounds such as oxaloacetate which can be converted to aspartic acid thus contributing to protein and nucleic acid metabolism and cell wall synthesis.

One other pathway of importance in the metabolism of carbohydrates by plaque bacteria is the formation of intracellular polysaccharide. Several strains of S. *mutans*, L. *casei*, S. *mitis* and others, have been shown to synthesize intracellular iodophilic polysaccharides of the amylopectin type from carbohydrates such as sucrose, maltose, or glucose. These polymers have been considered to have a role in storing energy reserves which can be utilized when there is a scarcity of carbon and energy sources. It has been suggested that a phosphoglucomutase intracellularly incorporates glucose-6-phosphate into the polymer containing glucose molecules linked with $\alpha(1 \rightarrow 4)$ bonds. Fluoride seems to inhibit the formation of intracellular polysaccharide at low pH, but the exact step at which the inhibition takes place is not clearly known. Even though a consistent direct relationship between ability to synthesize the intracellular polysaccharide and caries virulence is not always observed, this biochemical property of plaque bacteria is of metabolic importance as it allows bacteria to sustain their biochemical activity even in the absence of dietary carbohydrates.

Amino Acid Metabolism: Ammonia, Amines

Metabolism of carbohydrates by plaque bacteria usually results in acid production and determines a rapid and sustained decrease in plaque pH. However, in careful studies of the Stephan effect it has been noted that changes in plaque pH occur in both directions. A pH decrease occurs after a carbohydrate meal or a glucose rinse, while a pH increase occurs either slowly, mediated by the combined effects of salivary components and plaque, or quickly if plaque is subjected to a rinse with 1 per cent urea. The pH also increases, although slowly, under the influence of the buffering effect of saliva. Thus, plaque pH at any given time is the net effect of acid and base production by bacterial metabolism. Saliva, aside from its washing effects and its buffering capacity due to the presence of bicarbonate, contains urea which can be metabolized by plaque bacteria to liberate ammonia and to neutralize acids produced in fermentation of carbohydrates. Dietary carbohydrates are periodically available in large quantities provided by a meal or a snack, while urea in saliva is available at all times and in low concentration. Thus, plaque *p*H decreases rapidly after food intake. Longer periods of time are necessary to reestablish original *p*H levels. Fasting plaque has been repeatedly reported to have a high *p*H which has been mainly attributed to salivary urea breakdown. Regions of the dentition that have poor access to saliva and favor retention of carbohydrates have a low plaque *p*H, while areas exposed to saliva have higher *p*H values. Maxillary plaque *p*H is lower than plaque *p*H on the mandibular dentition. The lingual plaque *p*H is also usually higher than the corresponding plaque on the buccal side. These effects have been used as evidence to support the role of saliva in increasing plaque *p*H due to its urea content.

Dietary residues, saliva, and contents from dead cells in plaque also provide a number of proteins and amino acids that can be metabolized and therefore affect plaque *p*H. Deamination reactions yield strong keto acids which lower the *p*H. However, decarboxylation produces amines which tend to increase plaque *p*H. In addition, a small peptide (containing arginine) in saliva referred to as the "*p*H-rise factor" (*sialin*) has been described as inhibiting plaque *p*H fall at low glucose concentrations by enhancing its uptake and stimulating amino acid synthesis.

These fluctuations in plaque *p*H as a result of the interplay of carbohydrate metabolism and salivary effects are important to dental health because they influence the mineralization and remineralization process at the enamel-plaque interphase. Accumulation of protons and chelating organic anions stimulate the removal of calcium and phosphorus from enamel when the *p*H falls below a critical value of around 5.5 to 4.5 (see Chap. 19). Conversely, increases in plaque *p*H above 7.0 tend to precipitate Ca and P in plaque, resulting in the formation of brushite or apatitic precipitates. These minerals become more abundant and stable with time, especially when plaque *p*H increases at special sites such as the lingual surfaces of mandibular teeth. Precipitation of calcium and phosphorus in plaque can be a strict physicochemical phenomena influenced by various ions such as magnesium and fluoride, or the result of biological process taking place intracellularly in

organisms such as *B. matruchotii* and others which have been shown to be part of calculogenesis on the enamel surface.

Factors that Modify Plaque Metabolism

Dietary Carbohydrates and Dietary Patterns

Dietary carbohydrates are by far the most important factors affecting the chemical composition of plaque, the type of bacteria found in plaque, and the metabolic activity of bacteria found in plaque. Amount and frequency of carbohydrate intake determines to a large extent the mineral composition of plaque and the amount and type of extracellular polysaccharide present. While fermentable sugars are readily metabolized and diffuse easily through superficial layers of plaque, they do not necessarily reach the bacteria located at deeper layers of plaque. Therefore, these cells are not necessarily exposed to a carbon rich environment, and as a result their metabolism must necessarily adapt to this condition.

Starches are not directly available to plaque bacteria, but it should be noted that dietary carbohydrates influence plaque metabolism, not only as they come in contact with the tooth surface where plaque accummulates during mastication, but also later when they remain in the mouth as food debris. Starches can then be hydrolyzed by salivary amylases which break them down to readily fermentable sugar molecules. Food snacks which combine starch and sugars may be far more dangerous to oral health than commonly considered. The residence time of foods in the oral cavity, as suggested by many dental scientists, is important because it not only extends the availability of sugars in foods, but also generates new fermentable substrates from those previously considered inert substances. Starch fermentation is not only aided by salivary action, but also by the metabolic activity of specific bacteria which are present in the oral cavity of humans and which have powerful hydrolyzing enzymes to degrade such starch residues.

Dietary manipulations have long been known to control dental caries and plaque formation. It has been impossible to ascertain a carbohydrate intake that would be associated with the absence of virulent, cariogenic streptococci. Extreme dietary behaviors are clearly defined and predictable in terms of consequences to oral health. For example, those who meticulously avoid all types of sugar-containing foods, such as individuals afflicted with hereditary fructose intolerance, have low caries experience, while those who are exposed frequently to sugars such as infants fed sugared drinks in nursing bottles or sugar cane cutters who frequently consume sucrose generally have poor oral health. The definition of in-between dietary behavior which might be safe and hold caries incidence at a minimum is difficult. Considering the bacterial composition of plaque and the mechanism of action of many of the reactions that take place within plaque, it is sound to avoid the frequent consumption of sugar-containing snacks between meals. In view of the large differences that exist in dietary patterns and foods consumed in the U.S. this is the best general recommendation that can be offered. Dentists and dental hygienists involved in nutritional counselling to control plaque and prevent oral disease can offer more specific advice by taking nutritional histories and dietary evaluations and then correlating these with plaque indexes and overall clinical impressions. Gradual limitation of carbohydrate intake and frequency of intake will indicate which specific dietary regime will yield acceptable oral health conditions in combination, of course, with oral hygiene practices and fluoride therapy.

Several dietary manipulations have been proposed to reduce the caries potential of caries promoting foods. One has been the substitution of monosaccharides, such as glucose and fructose, for sucrose. Obviously, in the light of previous discussions in this chapter these substitutions are not effective. The use of polyols such as sorbitol has been recommended and implemented in the U.S. In spite of their inability to lower plaque pH and their lack of cariogenicity when tested in monkeys, the impact on human oral health of long term use of sorbitol in a dietary regime where other sugars are frequently consumed, remains to be clearly determined. Of further interest is xylitol, the most metabolically inert sugar alcohol for cariogenic streptococci. It is being considered as a potential candidate for future use in the manufacture of selected in-between-meal snacks (see Chap. 16).

Recently, there has been great interest in developing new noncaloric sweeteners similar to saccharin and cyclamates which are known not to be metabolized by plaque, and which are used in very small concentrations in food. Many different types of compounds are presently being tested, such as the dihydrochalcones, as well as taste modifiers (miraculin) which do not provide a sweet taste but modify the perception of acid taste to make it appear sweet. Other efforts involve the use of synthetic sweeteners coupled to large molecules which are not intestinally absorbed, yet provide a sweet taste as they come in contact with the mouth. Development of a synthetic sweetener with acceptable organoleptic properties and a high degree of safety is critical for certain confectionary products which are characteristically sweet, high in flavor, and intended for frequent use throughout the day. These products, traditionally made with sucrose and pressed into tablet shapes, would benefit from such technological developments as these substitutions would reduce their challenge to oral health.

Lastly, there are other modifications proposed to reduce the caries promoting properties of foods through food fortification with anticaries agents such as different phosphates and fluorides. Phosphates have been extremely effective in experiments using laboratory rats, but some of the clinical studies have provided conflicting results. Sodium trimetaphosphate, a cyclic phosphate, has been found effective in rodent experiments as well as in a clinical study recently reported. Further studies are necessary to identify optimal concentrations of such a cariostatic agent without disturbing the organoleptic properties of the fortified food or excessively increasing the phosphorus intake of a population which already seems to have large amounts of phosphates in its diets.

Fluoride

Fluoride, although discussed elsewhere (see Chap. 20), deserves special attention to emphasize its cariostatic effectiveness relative to plaque biochemistry. Unquestionably, fluoride administered at optimal concentrations in the drinking water has been the single, most effective caries preventive measure implemented around the world. Various proposed mechanisms to explain the cariostatic effect of fluoride have been extensively evaluated and studied. The mechanism relating the effects of fluoride to enamel surface structure and composition has received a great deal of attention. Research in this area has demonstrated that fluoride can increase the resistance of enamel to acid demineralization. However, fluoride has other possible effects which have not received enough attention. The modifications of surface charge and the chemicophysical properties of surface enamel treated with fluoride may alter the composition (in terms of proteins and calcium) and also may alter the amount of pellicle deposited on the tooth surfaces. These changes may in turn modify the adherence of bacteria and influence the colonization pattern on the tooth. Not enough information is available on the nature of such possible effects of fluoride on pellicle formation and initiation of plaque morphogenesis.

Fluoride may also exert its cariostatic action through its inhibitory effect on enolase, an important enzyme in the glycolytic pathway, that could then decrease the concentration of phoshoenol-pyruvate within the bacterial cell and affect its energy and biosynthetic pathways. It is difficult to explain the reason why fluoride, which seems to accummulate in fairly large concentrations in plaque, does not seemingly affect plaque bacteria which continue to grow and reproduce. The reason, as indicated previously may be that most of the fluoride in plaque is bound to calcium and therefore it is not present in ionic form. Another reason to be considered is that plaque has a heterogenous bacterial composition where some organisms may be affected by residual fluoride ions and others are not. Understanding of the biochemical characteristics of virulent versus nonvirulent cariogenic bacteria relative to fluoride levels in plaque would contribute to the understanding of such fluoride effects and lead to the identifica-tion of the best delivery system to be used in a preventive program based on fluoride administration.

CONCLUSION

Plaque is a tenacious, acquired structure formed on enamel surfaces and comprised of bacteria, their metabolic products, and salivary components. The enamel is to the tooth what the skin is to the body. Both are ectodermal in origin, and serve as limiting protective barriers between the homeostatically controlled internal environment and the variable external millieu. Like the skin, enamel has a characteristic bacterial flora that may include pathogens. Depending on the ecologic factors and the trophic environment, specific pathogens may develop a health disruptive activity which can be accentuated by the activity of other scavenger microorganisms as the lesion progresses. Thus, the integrity of enamel is disrupted and bacterial penetration progresses into deeper tissues through the initially opened sites of invasion.

Understanding the biochemical factors which determine the formation and virulence of plaque, as well as those factors that contribute to the strengthening of the enamel surface, will aid in the identification and development of methods to prevent plaque dependent diseases such as dental caries. Prevention procedures to be devised and implemented in the future will have to be based on clear understanding of the biochemistry and microbiology of plaque to obtain a maximum degree of effectiveness without disrupting the balanced ecosystem necessary to maintain oral health.

GLOSSARY

Acquired pellicle. An organic film on tooth enamel surfaces formed by selective adsorption to apatitic surfaces of specific glycoproteins of salivary origin.

Adhesion. A mechanism through which cells become attached tenaciously to other cells or to surfaces. Adhesion is considered important in the process of bacterial colonization.

Agglutination. Bacterial cells under the influence of specific molecules or cell mechanisms adhere together to form clumps and therefore exhibit agglutination behavior.

Bacteriocins. Antibacterial compounds produced by some streptococci against specific bacteria that may inhibit attachment or growth of the organism in the immediacy of the bacteriocinogenic streptococci.

Clearance time. The time required for particles from a given food to be completely removed from the oral cavity after mastication and swallowing.

Constitutive enzymes. Enzymes that are always found to be present in a given cell in nearly constant concentration.

Dental plaque. A tenacious structure formed on tooth surfaces which contains large numbers of closely packed microorganisms surrounded by salivary components and extracellular materials of bacterial origin.

Extracellular polysaccharide. Polymers produced extracellularly by plaque bacteria using sucrose or some other sugar as a substrate. Examples of extracellular polysaccharides (ECP) are glucans and fructans.

Fructan (Levan). A homopolymer formed by fructosyl transferase acting on sucrose as a substrate. This polymer is made of fructose units linked together by $\beta(2 \rightarrow 6)$ linkages.

Fructosyl transferase. The enzyme which is active in fructan synthesis.

Glucan (Dextran). A homopolymer made of glucose units linked together by $\alpha(1 \rightarrow 6)$ linkages and produced in plaque by the action of bacterial glucosyl transferase on sucrose.

Glucosyl transferase. The enzyme which is active in glucan synthesis.

Glycans (polysaccharide). A polymer consisting of recurring monosaccharide units with differing chain length and degree of branching.

Glycolysis. The biochemical pathway used by bacterial and mammalian cells to ferment (anaerobically) a glucose molecule to obtain 2 ATP molecules. It usually yields lactic acid as an end product.

Heteroglycans (heteropolysaccharide). A glycan which contains two or more different monomeric units joined together with different type linkages (i.e., glycosaminoglycans).

Homoglycans (homopolysaccharide). A glycan containing only one type of monomeric unit (i.e., dextran, starch).

Intracellular polysaccharide (IP). A polymer formed inside some bacterial cells found in plaque. This homopolymer resembles plant starch and glycogen and can be used by cells when there is no external supply of molecules capable of providing energy.

Lactoferrin. A compound of salivary origin capable of strongly chelating iron, therefore, interfering with bacterial colonization and growth.

Mutan. A glucan type polymer characterized by the high degree of crosslinking of the $\alpha(1 \rightarrow 3)$ type, which makes the molecule extremely insoluble and undegradable.

Plaque saliva. The fluid found in plaque and representing one of its chemical compartments. It has a characteristic chemical composition which differs from that of the cellular fraction of plaque.

Retention time. The time that food particles remain in the oral cavity after the food has been masticated and swallowed.

Serotypes. Classification of bacteria is done attending to different criteria such as biochemical characteristics and growth patterns. They can also be classified according to their serological response into specific serotypes (a, b, c, etc.) which are useful to identify a subgroup within a specific strain of bacteria.

Stephan's (Curve) response. Stephan noted that after ingestion of a food containing sugars, or after rinsing with sugar-containing solutions, plaque pH would decrease. After a certain period of time, plaque pH would start to increase until it returned to its original value. A plot of these pH changes occurring in plaque during these events is referred to as Stephan's curve.

Surface receptors. Specific proteins on the surface of bacterial cells which mediate recognition of specific molecules outside the cells. Streptococci have such surface receptors which are involved in the adhesion phenomena taking place between cells and extracellular polysaccharides such as glucans.

SUGGESTED READINGS

Ashley FP, Wilson RF: The relationship between dietary sugar experience and the quantity and biochemical composition of dental plaque in man. Arch Oral Biol 22: 409–414, 1977

Birkeland JM, Charlton G: Effect of pH on the fluoride ion activity of plaque. Caries Res 10: 72–80, 1976

Bjorn H, Carlsson J: Observations on a dental plaque morphogenesis. Odontol Revy 15: 23–28, 1964

Bowen WH: Nature of plaque. In Melcher AH, Zarb GA (eds): Preventive Dentistry: Nature, Pathogenicity and Clinical Control of Plaque. Munksgaard, Oral Science Reviews, 1975, pp 3–21

Bowen WH, Velez H, Aguila M, Velazquez H, Sierra LI, Gillespie G: The microbiology and biochemistry of plaque, saliva and drinking water from two communities with contrasting levels of caries in Columbia, SA. J Dent Res 56: C32–39, 1977

Bratthall D, Kohler B: S. mutans serotypes: some aspects of their identification, distribution, antigenic shifts and relationship to caries. J Dent Res 55: C15–C21, 1976

Brown AT: The role of dietary carbohydrates in plaque formation and oral disease. In Present Knowledge in Nutrition. Washington DC, Nutrition Foundation Series, 1976

Brown AT, Christian CP: Characterization of a novel nicotinamide adenine dinucleotide-dependent alcohol dehydrogenase from a strain of S. mutans. Arch Oral Biol 19: 397–406, 1974

Brown AT, Patterson CE: Ethanol production and alcohol dehydrogenase activity in S. mutans. Arch Oral Biol 18: 127–131, 1973

Carlsson J, Grahnen H, Jonsson G: Lactobacilli and streptococci in the mouth of children. Caries Res 9: 333–339, 1975

Cole JA: A biochemical approach to the control of dental caries. Biochem Soc Trans 5: 1232–1239, 1977

Coykendall AL, Lizotte PA: Streptococcus mutans isolates identified by biochemical tests and DNA base contents. Arch Oral Biol 23: 427–428, 1978

Edgar WM: The role of saliva in the control of pH changes in human dental plaque. Caries Res 10: 241–254, 1976

Ellen RP, Balcerzak-Raczkowski IB: Interbacterial aggregation of A naeslundii and dental plaque streptococci. J Periodontal Res 12: 11–20, 1977

Ericson T, Sandham J, Magnusson I: Sedimentation

method for studies of adsorption of microorganisms onto apatite surfaces in vitro. Caries Res 9: 325–332, 1975

Facklam RR: Physiological differentiation of viridans streptococci. J Clin Microbiol 5: 184–201, 1977

Gibbons RJ, van Houte J: Dental caries. Annu Rev Med 26: 121–136, 1975

Hay DI, Gibbons RJ, Spinell DM: Characteristics of some high molecular weight constituents with bacterial aggregating activity from whole saliva and dental plaque. Caries Res 5: 111–123, 1971

Holmberg K, Hollander HO: Interference between gram-positive microorganisms in dental plaque. J Dent Res 51: 588–595, 1972

Hotz P, Guggenheim B, Schmid R: Carbohydrates in pooled dental plaque. Caries Res 6: 103–121, 1972

Imfeld TH, Hirsch RS, Muhlemann HR: Telemetric recordings of interdental plaque pH during different meal patterns. Br Dent J 144: 40–45, 1978

Kashket S, Donaldson CG: Saliva-induced aggregation of oral streptococci. J Bacteriol 112: 1127–1133, 1972

Kelstrup J, Funder-Nielsen TD: Adhesion of dextran to Streptococcus mutans. J Gen Microbiol 81: 485–489, 1974

Kelstrup J, Theilade J, Paulsen S, Möller IJ: Bacteriological, electron microscopical and biochemical studies on dento-gingival plaque of Moroccan children from an area with low caries prevalence. Caries Res 8: 61—83, 1974

Kleinberg I: Formation and accumulation of acid on the tooth surface. J Dent Res 49: 1300–1316, 1970

Kleinberg I: The acid-base metabolism of the dental plaque and its effects at the saliva-dentogingival interphase. In Dental Plaque and its Relation to Oral Diseases. Center for Research in Oral Biology, Seattle, University of Washington, 1972

Knuuttila MLE, Makinen KK: Effect of xylitol on the growth and metabolism of S. mutans. Caries Res 9: 177–189, 1975

Kraus FW, Mestecky J: Salivary proteins and the development of dental plaque. J Dent Res 55: C149–C152, 1976

Krembel J, Frank RM, Deluzarche A: Fractionation of human dental plaques. Arch Oral Biol 14: 563–565, 1969

Levine M, Beeley JA, Beeley JG: Comparative biochemical studies on the composition of saline extracts of human dental plaque, saliva and serum. Arch Oral Biol 21: 741–747, 1976

Levine RS: The action of fluoride in caries prevention: a review of current concepts. Br Dent J 140: 9–14, 1976

Mayhall CW: Amino acid composition of experimental salivary pellicles. J Periodontal 48: 78–91, 1977

Mayhall CW, Butler WT: The carbohydrate composition of experimental salivary pellicles. J Oral Pathol 5: 358–370, 1976.

McCabe MM, Smith EE, Cowan RA: Invertase activity in S. mutans and S. sanguis. Arch Oral Biol 18: 525–531, 1973

Mikx FHM, van der Hoeven JS: Symbiosis of Streptococcus mutans and Veillonella alcalescens in mixed continous cultures. Arch Oral Biol 20: 407–410, 1975

Mikx FHM, van der Hoeven JS, Plasschaert AJM, Konig KG: effect of Actinomyces viscosus on the establishment and symbiosis of Streptococcus mutans and Streptococcus sanguis in SPF rats on different sucrose diets. Caries Res 9: 1–20, 1975

Miller CH: Degradation of sucrose by whole cells and plaque of Actinomyces naeslundii. Infect Immunol 10: 1280–1291, 1974

Miller CH, Kleinman JL: Effect of microbial interactions on in vitro plaque formation by S. mutans. J Dent Res 53: 427–434, 1974

Minah GE, Loesche WJ: Sucrose metabolism in resting-cell suspensions of caries associated and non-caries-associated dental plaque. Infect Immunol 17: 43–54, 1977

Minah GE, Loesche WJ: Sucrose metabolism by prominent members of the flora isolated from cariogenic and non-cariogenic dental plaques. Infect Immunol 17: 55–61, 1977

Mukasa H, Slade HD: Mechanism of adherence of Streptococcus mutans to smooth surfaces. Infect Immunol 9: 419–429, 1974

Navia JM: Fortification of sugars. In Handbook Series in Nutrition and Food. W. Palm Beach, CRC Press, 1980

Newbrun E: Cariology. Baltimore, Williams & Wilkins, 1978

Newbrun E, Frostell G: Sugar restriction and substitution for caries prevention. Caries Res 12: 65–73, 1978

Parker RB, Creamer HR: Contribution of plaque polysaccharides to growth of cariogenic microorganisms. Arch Oral Biol 16: 855–862, 1971

Poole EFG, Newman HN: Dental plaque and oral health. Nature 234: 329–331, 1971

Ritz HL: Microbial population shifts in developing human dental plaque. Arch Oral Biol 12: 1561–1568, 1967

Robinovitch MR, Sreebny LM: Dental Plaque and its Relation to Oral Diseases. Center for Research in Oral Biology, Seattle, University of Washington, 1972

Saxton CA: Scanning electron microscope study of the formation of dental plaque. Caries Res 7: 102–119, 1973

Schachtele CF, Loken AE, Knudson DJ: Preferential utilization of the glucosyl moiety of sucrose by a cariogenic strain of S. mutans. Infect Immunol 5: 531–536, 1972

Schanschula RG, Agus H, Bunzel M, Adkins BL, Barnes DE: The concentrations of selected major and trace minerals in human dental plaque. Arch Oral Biol 22: 321–325, 1977

Stephan RM: Intra-oral hydrogen ion concentrations associated with dental caries activity. J Dent Res 23: 257–266, 1944

Tannenbaum PJ, Posner AS, Mandel I: Formation of calcium phosphates in saliva and dental plaque. J Dent Res 55: 997–1000, 1976

Tatevossian A, Gould CT: Methods for sampling and analysis of the aqueous phase of human dental plaque. Arch Oral Biol 21: 313–317, 1976

Tatevossian A, Gould CT: The composition of the aqueous phase in human dental plaque. Arch Oral Biol 21: 319–323, 1976

Taubman MA, Smith DJ: Immune components in dental plaque. J Dent Res 55: C153–C162, 1976

Van Houte J, Gibbons RJ, Banghart SB: Adherence as a determinant of the presence of Streptococcus salivarius and Streptococcus sanguis on the tooth surface. Arch Oral Biol 15: 1025–1034, 1970

Weerkamp A, Bongaerts-Larik L, Vogels GD: Bacteriocins as factors in the in vitro interaction between oral streptococci in plaque. Infect Immunol 16: 773–780, 1977

15 Immunologic Aspects of Dental Caries

ROBERT J. GENCO

Introduction
General Immunologic Principles of Importance in Understanding Caries Vaccine Experiments
  Demonstration of Local vs. Systemic Systems of Immunity
  Demonstration of Heterogeneity of Immunoglobins
  Immunoglobulins and Antibodies in Secretions
  The Demonstration of T- and B-Lymphocytes and Their Subclasses
  Role of Gut-Associated Lymphoid Tissues Such as Peyer's Patches in Immunity
Immunology of Dental Caries

Significance of Research on Vaccines in the Prevention of Dental Caries
Rationale for Directing a Vaccine Against Streptococcus mutans
Caries Vaccine Studies in Animals
  Immunization of Rodents
  Immunization of Primates
Human Studies of Caries Immunity
  Role of Secretory IgA in Immunity to Dental Caries
  Possible Side Effects of a Caries Vaccine
Summary
Glossary
Suggested Readings

INTRODUCTION

Although evidence of dental caries, an ancient disease, is found in the remains of one-million-year-old Rhodesian man, relatively little caries existed even as late as 1200 A.D. Since then, the incidence and prevalence of this disease has increased so that today it is the most common chronic bacterial disease of man. Through the ages, many theories about the etiology of dental caries were advanced, including ideas that caries was initiated by tooth worms or screw-shaped organisms which bore holes in the teeth. But it wasn't until 1890 that W. D. Miller proposed that dental caries represents a chemical-parasitic process consisting of two distinctly marked stages, decalcification or softening of the enamel and dentin, and dissolution of the softened residue. Miller proposed that the initial decalcification of the tooth was caused by bacteria, which through their fermentation of carbohydrates, produced lactic and other acids capable of destroying enamel. In the 80 years since it was proposed, substantial clinical and laboratory evidence has supported Miller's hypothesis about the role of bacteria

332

in dental caries (see Chaps. 8-14). Since specific organisms were shown to cause dental caries, it was reasonable to attempt to vaccinate to protect against the disease. This chapter will describe the immunologic aspects of dental caries with an emphasis on those studies dealing with caries vaccination.

GENERAL IMMUNOLOGIC PRINCIPLES OF IMPORTANCE IN UNDERSTANDING CARIES VACCINE EXPERIMENTS

Knowledge in the field of immunology has advanced rapidly in the last two decades and several major concepts have developed from this information which have led to the basis for experiments with caries vaccines. These basic concepts and major findings are summarized below.

Demonstration of Local vs. Systemic Systems of Immunity

Early researchers found that immunity was not always related to serum antibodies but was often related to coproantibodies, (i.e., antibodies found in feces of infected or immunized animals). In studies of this phenomena with guinea pigs it was found that animals inoculated by feeding with *Cholera vibrio* organisms developed antibodies in the feces which appeared earlier and disappeared faster than antibodies in the serum. In addition, they found that irradiation of the guinea pigs eliminated or reduced the serum immune response leaving the fecal antibody response intact. They proposed that there was an immune system providing antibodies in intestinal secretions which was separate from that providing antibodies in serum. Similar observations were made in studies of respiratory tract antibodies, antibodies in milk and antibodies in saliva, demonstrating a dissociation or lack of correlation between antibodies in these secretions and antibodies found in serum. Hence, the concept of a discrete, local, or mucosal immune system separate from the systemic or serum immune system was developed. The molecular basis of this difference was to be determined.

Demonstration of Heterogeneity of Immunoglobulins

Many investigators working in the 1940's and 1950's described the existence of antibody activity in a heterogeneous family of serum glycoproteins. These are now known as *immunoglobulins* and they differ in carbohydrate content, molecular weight, and electrophoretic mobility and antigenicity; although they all show the property of specific binding to antigens. There are now five major immunoglobulin classes: IgG, IgM, IgA, IgD and IgE, and several subclasses. The immunoglobulins are all composed of a basic 7S unit or monomer with a molecular weight of 150-160,000. This basic unit has four polypeptide chains: a pair of heavy chains of 60,000-80,000 molecular weight, and a pair of light chains of 22,000 molecular weight. The light chains, of which there are several types, are shared by all immunoglobulins. However, each immunoglobulin class differs in heavy chain composition (see Fig. 15-1). There are specific heavy chain types which are unique to each immunoglobulin class and subclass. Some immunoglobulins, such as IgM and IgA, exist in plasma as polymers of the basic 7S unit, IgM as a pentamer of about 900,000 molecular weight, and IgA as a trimer or dimer. The other immunoglobulins exist basically as the four chain or monomeric 7S unit. Immunoglobulin concentrations of each class vary widely in plasma from approximately 12mg/ml for IgG to nanogram quantities for IgE. They also differ markedly in biologic activity with IgE responsible for reagenic or allergic-type reactions, and IgM and IgG able to fix complement and hence, participate in complement mediated reactions. IgD along with a form of IgM appear to be major surface immunoglobulins on lymphocytes and may be involved in development and triggering of lymphocytes.

Immunoglobulins and Antibodies in Secretions

IgA is found as the predominant immunoglobulin class in secretions. Workers in the early 1960's described IgA in secretions and also ascribed the properties of the secretory immune system to IgA antibodies. They

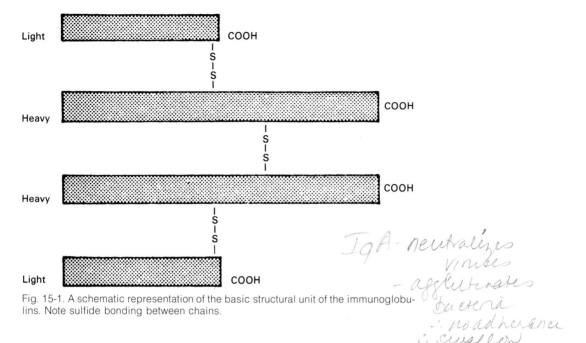

Fig. 15-1. A schematic representation of the basic structural unit of the immunoglobulins. Note sulfide bonding between chains.

[Handwritten margin note:] IgA- neutralizes viruses — agglutinates bacteria ∴ no adherence ∴ swallow

found that the IgA in secretions was different from serum IgA in several respects. For example, the IgA in secretions, termed secretory IgA (sIgA), not only has heavy and light polypeptide chains arranged into the same 4 chain monomeric units as other immunoglobulins, but it also possesses secretory component, a glycoprotein of 60–70,000 molecular weight, and a joining chain or J-chain of about 15,000 molecular weight. Hence, sIgA is comprised of 4 different polypeptide chains. The entire molecule is about 360,000 molecular weight and is comprised of 2 monomeric or 7S units, each comprised of 2 heavy and 2 light chains, 1 secretory component and 1 J-chain. It has been shown that sIgA is the major immunoglobulin in secretions such as saliva, tears, milk, genital-urinary secretions, gastrointestinal secretions and bronchial secretions.

Production of antibodies of the IgA class occurs independently of production of IgG and IgM antibodies of the serum. Several investigators have demonstrated that either local immunization or feeding of antigen can induce antibodies of the IgA class in secretions. The biologic function of secretory IgA has received considerable attention, and it is clear that this antibody can effectively neutralize viruses providing a first line of defense against viral infections which begin at mucosal surfaces. In a similar manner it has been proposed that IgA antibodies protect against bacterial infections of mucosal surfaces and their associated structures, such as teeth, by

inhibiting adherence and thereby preventing colonization by organisms which otherwise infect these surfaces. Secretory IgA antibodies are thought to agglutinate these organisms in the secretion (such as saliva), thus preventing their adherence to the mucosal surface or to the tooth suface, and facilitating their disposal by swallowing. This concept of IgA-mediated antibacterial immunity has received considerable support from investigators in dental caries research as well as those studying enteric or mucosal infections in which attachment or colonization of the mucosal surfaces is an important first step in pathogenesis.

The Demonstration of T- and B-Lymphocytes and Their Subclasses

The demonstration of two types of lymphocytes by Good and his colleagues was an important conceptual advance in immunobiology. T-cells are lymphocytes which mature under the influence of the thymus and are responsible for delayed hypersensitivity or cell-mediated immune reactions. These are mediated by lymphokines or by direct lymphocyte cytotoxic effects on target cells. B-cells, on the other hand, are lymphocytes which often are stimulated to develop into plasma cells which produce immunoglobulins. B-cells also can produce lymphokines. However, it appears that under most circumstances their main importance may be to become plasma cells which produce antibodies.

There are several cell interactions of importance in immune reactions. For example, macrophages interact with T- and B-cells in several ways, such as by processing and presenting antigens to the lymphocytes in the process of sensitization or antigenic stimulation. There are also T-cell-B-cell interactions of importance in the stimulation of immune responses. Subpopulations of T-cells can act as helper cells in B-cell stimulation and another subpopulation of T-cells, called T-suppressor cells, reduce the response of B-cells to antigen.

Role of Gut-Associated Lymphoid Tissues Such as Peyer's Patches in Immunity

Another major conceptual advance in understanding stimulation of the sIgA system comes from studies of T-helper or T-suppressor cells and their role in IgA antibody production. It is felt that Peyer's Patches contain T-cells which, when stimulated by antigen by direct injection or by feeding, will develop into helper and suppressor cells. These cells effect the differentiation and production of antibodies by plasma cells derived from antigen-stimulated B-cells. It appears that antigens which are ingested stimulate the production of T-helper cells which specifically aid in the differentiation and production of IgA antibodies. At the same time a population of T-suppressor cells is induced which specifically inhibits or suppresses the differentiation of B-cells which would otherwise produce IgG and IgM antibodies. These observations may explain why antigens administered by feeding stimulate the formation of B-cells which are aided by T-helper cells to produce sIgA antibodies. At the same time the gut antigens stimulate suppressor T-cells which inhibit the production of serum IgG or IgM antibodies. The immune response to fed antigens has been observed to result in induction of sIgA antibodies in secretions, and at the same time suppression of serum antibodies.

IMMUNOLOGY OF DENTAL CARIES

Thus far, the single most effective contribution to the prevention of dental caries has been the introduction of fluoride into many public water systems in the United States and in other countries (see Chap. 20). Since fluoridation was begun, a 55 to 60 per cent reduction has been noted in the number of decayed, missing, or filled permanent teeth of children continuously exposed to water-borne fluorides from birth. However, because fluoridation of the water supply is a subject to political decisions by local governments, and because it is often difficult to implement in rural areas, approximately half of the general public in the United States is not reached by this program. Therefore, current research has concentrated on other avenues of prevention such as alteration of the diet by reducing the intake of sucrose or other refined carbohydrates (see Chapters 16 and 17). Another focus of current research is the reduction of the bacterial flora on the tooth, especially the cariogenic flora such as *Streptococcus mutans* and possibly *Actinomyces viscosus* (see Chap. 18).

A number of methods are presently under evaluation to decrease the bacterial assault on the tooth surface. Among these are the mechanical removal of adherent organisms (see Chap. 22); chemotherapeutic procedures such as systemic or topical antimicrobials (see Chap. 18); the implantation of noncariogenic bacteria in the oral cavity with the capacity to antagonize or replace cariogenic organisms (see Chap. 18); and the production of vaccines against cariogenic bacteria.

The use of florides, dietary control, mechanical removal, and antimicrobial approaches to caries prevention will be discussed in other chapters. In this chapter we will concentrate on the possibility of vaccination as a method of preventing dental caries.

Significance of Research on Vaccines in the Prevention of Dental Caries

Active immunization against dental caries is an attractive potential public health measure. Considering that it would cost approximately $10 billion annually to repair the damage caused by caries in the United States alone, the cost of immunization, combined with current effective preventive measures such as fluoridation, would be small by comparison. Voluntary immunization would be particularly attractive if an oral means for antibody stimulation could be found. Aside from its public health value, research in immunization against dental caries offers the possibility of revealing basic phenomena regarding immune responses to infections in general.

Rationale for Directing a Vaccine Against *Streptococcus mutans*

Among the many oral organisms tested in the gnotobiotic, sucrose-fed rodent, it appears that *S. mutans* has a marked capacity for causing dental caries. Although other organisms such as lactobacilli, *Streptococcus faecalis* and *Streptococcus sanguis* have caused caries in animal models, these bacteria take much more time to develop caries lesions, and the lesions are less extensive than those caused by *S. mutans*. Animal studies demonstrate that *S. mutans* is markedly more virulent than other species of Streptococci commonly found in dental plaque. In addition, evidence obtained from human studies establishes a strong statistical relation between *S. mutans* and coronal caries. Hence, it is reasonable to propose that interference with *S. mutans* by vaccination will markedly reduce human coronal caries. Coronal caries would be a reasonable target for vaccination because it is more common in children and young adults than either cervical or root surface caries.

Caries Vaccine Studies in Animals

Immunization of Rodents

Early attempts to immunize rats against dental caries met with varied results. Conclusions were difficult to interpret because very often diets were uncontrolled, methods of scoring caries (see Chapter 23) were not fully described, and a number of mildly cariogenic organisms were used for immunization. Therefore, we will concentrate on more recent experiments, most of which demonstrate that caries in rodents can be reduced to some extent by immunization procedures.

In 1976 Smith and Taubman reported on a series of vaccine experiments with several groups of gnotobiotic as well as conventional rats. The animals were vaccinated in the region of the salivary glands using *S. mutans* in complete Freund's adjuvant, a mixture which enhances immunity. The animals were then infected with the same organisms 10 to 22 days after completion of the immunization schedule and the experiment continued for as long

as 180 days. Salivary, as well as serum-agglutinating antibodies, were detected in the immunized rats, and the salivary antibodies were mainly of the IgA class. In several experiments the mean caries scores were significantly lower in the experimental animals than in the controls. They also found that immunized rats had greater protection against smooth surface caries than against pit and fissure caries.

Other investigators reported on gnotobiotic rats injected subcutaneously near the submandibular region with a suspension of *S. mutans*. They recovered fewer *S. mutans* from the vaccinated animals and observed lower caries scores. It has been shown more recently that rat dams immunized with *S. mutans* will passively transfer immunity to *S. mutans*-induced caries to their pups. It is unclear whether this immunity is derived from the serum antibodies or from the milk antibodies. In either case, it appears that the immunity is antibody-mediated.

More recent studies have reported that feeding *S. mutans* to gnotobiotic rats from weaning to 90 days induced both salivary and milk IgA antibodies in the presence of barely detectable serum antibodies. These animals were also protected against caries induced by the same strain of *S. mutans* used to immunize. These results show that IgA antibodies in saliva can exert protective effects; however, the possible protective role of cellular and intestinal immunity (coproantibody) cannot be ruled out by these same studies.

Taken as a whole, the immunization experiments performed in the rat caries model system suggest a correlation between the presence of salivary antibody to *S. mutans* and a reduction of caries caused by *S. mutans*. Immunization which induces primarily IgA antibody in saliva appears adequate to confer protection against caries. This suggests that IgA antibody is the important antibody in protection against smooth surface dental caries. However, in the absence of salivary IgA antibody, IgG antibody, such as that observed in the passive transfer experiments, may also be effective.

Immunization of Primates

Recent studies in primates have shown that *Macaca fascicularis* (also called *Macaca irus*) monkeys can be useful models for the study of human dental caries. These monkeys rarely have S. *mutans* as a constituent of their normal flora and they have a dentition and immune system which closely resembles that of humans. They are essentially caries-free in the wild, and when infected with S. *mutans* and fed a cariogenic diet, develop caries which resemble the human disease in most important aspects. It has been found that M. *fascicularis* have little or no detectable serum or salivary antibody to S. *mutans* prior to immunization, simplifying control conditions used in immunologic studies. In several experiments it was possible to induce salivary IgA antibodies and reduce the S. *mutans* infection of the teeth of the immunized animals. In a pilot experiment three M. *fascicularis* monkeys were immunized intravenously with live, cariogenic S. *mutans* isolated from humans. Following immunization, the three immune and three non-immune monkeys were infected with the immunizing strain of S. *mutans*. The immunized group showed a significantly lower incidence of caries than the unimmunized control group. In more recent experiments, broken cells of S. *mutans* or preparations of S. *mutans* containing glucosyltransferase of varying degrees of purity were used to immunize the monkeys. In the animals immunized with broken cells, substantial reduction in dental caries was achieved and maintained up to 5 years.

It has also been reported that Rhesus monkeys were partially protected from spontaneous dental caries by extensive subcutaneous immunization with S. *mutans* cells. In a series of immunization experiments with S. *fascicularis* monkeys, it was shown that intraductal parotid immunization is more effective than parenteral immunization for producing salivary IgA antibodies to S. *mutans*. Animals that had relatively high titers of salivary antibodies of the IgA class were protected from oral infection by S. *mutans* in the later studies.

Human Studies of Caries Immunity

Many attempts have been made to correlate serum or salivary antibacterial activity with dental caries experience in man. These studies present difficulties for several reasons. One of the major problems is that dental caries is a chronic process and the appearance of a caries lesion is simply the clinical manifestation of what may have been occurring for months or years. At the time of sampling the lesion may have been restored, or the caries process arrested. It would not be surprising to find antibodies to cariogenic organisms in human serum and saliva since these organisms are constantly being introduced into the bloodstream through the gingival crevice during chewing. They are also being swallowed, and it is likely that antibody production is also stimulated by the intestinal route.

A number of studies have examined levels of human serum and salivary antibodies to cariogenic streptococci. Several investigators have found that levels of agglutinating antibodies directed to the cell walls of cariogenic streptococci were higher in serum from caries-free subjects than in serum from caries-rampant subjects. More recently it has been reported that serum and salivary antibody levels to four serotypes of S. *mutans* existed in subjects ranging from 18 to 25 years of age. It was concluded that dental caries is an infectious disease, and that antibodies may contribute to caries immunity in man. Antibodies in saliva to glucosyltransferase derived from S. *mutans* (serotype d) in groups of patients with low or high caries experience has also been studied. The data supports the concept that caries is an infectious disease in which antibody levels alter or are altered by the state of infection. More definitive data relating human serum and salivary antibody levels to caries may come from studies in which several well characterized, purified antigens specific to S. *mutans* are utilized.

Role of Secretory IgA in Immunity to Dental Caries

Whole human saliva contains many immunologic factors including antibodies of the IgG, IgA, and IgM classes, as well as complement components. It is well established that there are leucocytes in saliva which are probably derived from the gingiva via the gingival fluid. However, since secretory IgA (sIgA) is the predominant immunoglobulin in whole human saliva, antibodies of this immunoglobulin class are the most likely to afford protection against cariogenic organisms.

The secretory IgA system is of considerable importance as a potentially useful protective system against caries. It has been shown to be effective in rodent immunization experiments. Also, selective stimulation of this system might preclude possible adverse immunopathologic reactions resulting from stimulation of high levels of serum antibodies, immediate hypersensitivity, or cellular immunity. Selective stimulation of a secretory IgA response by S. mutans without a significant rise in serum antibodies is possible. It has been accomplished by feeding S. mutans in the gnotobiotic rat and by retrograde ductal inoculation of S. mutans cells into the parotid gland in monkeys. Mestecky and coworkers were able to stimulate human secretory antibodies by feeding S. mutans over a 2 week period. These antibodies were mainly of the sIgA class in saliva and tears, but serum antibodies were not detected. This experiment demonstrates the potential to selectively stimulate the secretory immune system while not stimulating or possibly even suppressing serum antibody production.

Although it is not definitively known that salivary IgA antibodies play a decisive role in caries immunity, they most likely do; and emphasis should be given to studies of their inducement and function in caries vaccine experiments. Antibodies derived from the gingival crevice may also contribute to caries immunity but their appearance in saliva is likely to be highly dependent upon inflammation of the gingiva. Immunization routes and schedules, and forms of antigen for the stimulation of optimal and persistent protective immunity to dental caries will depend upon a better understanding of the secretory immune system.

Possible Side Effects of a Caries Vaccine

Possible side effects of a potential vaccine involve, for the most part, toxicity of the vaccine and potential immunopathology, including that which may result from cross-reactivity with mammalian tissues by antibodies to the bacterial vaccine. On the basis of previous experiences with bacterial cell vaccines, injection with whole cells of Gram-positive organisms may give rise to local tissue destruction. However, use of purified antigens may eliminate this reaction.

It has been proposed that there are antigens present in strains of S. mutans which share antigenic determinants with human heart muscle. Several groups of investigators have not been able to confirm this and others have found no deleterious side effects as the result of extensive immunization of primates with S. mutans vaccines. One interesting study shows that high titered anti-S. mutans, rabbit antisera, stain heart muscle at a low dilution (e.g., 1/10). However, careful studies show that serum from these rabbits obtained prior to immunization (i.e., normal rabbit sera) also react with heart tissue in the same manner. These results suggest that naturally occurring material(s) in rabbit serum react with mammalian heart tissues and that this is likely not related to S. mutans. It has been further shown that there are at least 3 components in extracts of S. mutans and of Lancefield Group A (type 6) streptococci which bind to heart tissues directly. Further studies are necessary to evaluate the significance of these components which bind to mammalian tissues. It is clear, however, that if a caries vaccine were purified so as not to contain these components, any potential immunopathologic problem brought about by these binding substances would be circumvented. Certainly, any human vaccine will have to be carefully screened for the presence of hazardous side effects.

SUMMARY

Dental caries vaccine research has provided evidence which suggests that it may be feasible to develop a caries vaccine for humans. Major findings which lead to this optimism are: S. mutans is a major cariogenic organism; there is direct evidence of efficacy of S. mutans vaccination in rat, hamster and monkey models of S. mutans-induced dental caries; it is possible to selectively induce sIgA antibodies in secretions such as saliva; these antibodies likely inhibit the adherence and subsequent colonization of the teeth by S. mutans; and experiments in man have shown that feeding of S. mutans cells can induce a secretory IgA response in saliva and other secretions and at the same time not induce a serum response.

The potential hazards, however, still remain. The potential for toxicity of either fed antigen or parenterally administered antigens is real. Direct toxicity could be caused by the peptidoglycans and other cell components. The evidence of cross-reactive antigens of S. mutans and mammalian heart or muscle tissue is controversial. However, there is evidence for components of S. mutans which will bind directly to heart muscle. The immunopathologic consequences of such components are not known, however, purification of vaccines so as to not contain these substances may well eliminate these as potential problems.

It is clear that we have among our methods for reducing dental caries several very powerful tools including fluoride (particularly fluoridation of water supplies), careful monitoring of diet with reduction of refined carbohydrates, and mechanical plaque control. However, there may be populations for which these measures cannot be instituted properly and in such populations dental caries may occur at a very high rate. It is these target populations which may be helped by a caries vaccine. As caries is not usually a life-threatening

disease the risks of vaccine will have to be weighed against the protective effects. It is likely that only highly purified vaccines, administered to selectively stimulate only protective immune responses, will be acceptable in man.

Much has been learned recently about the secretory immune system and its potential for antibacterial protection, especially about the unique features associated with antibacterial protection against diseases of mucosal surfaces and their related structures such as teeth. Concepts derived from these studies, such as selective adherence and antibacterial activity directed at reducing this adherence, have given us considerable insight into protective immunity not only for dental caries but also for other infections of mucosal surfaces.

GLOSSARY

Agglutinating antibodies. Immunoglobulins which will cause aggregation of bacteria by specific interaction of the Fab portion of the immunoglobulins.

B cell. B lymphocyte. Derived from bone marrow. This cell lineage gives rise to antibody-producing cells.

Cellular immunity. Heightened activity to a foreign material, called an antigen, which is dependent upon cells for its manifestations. The major cells involved in cellular immunity are lymphocytes which are aided by macrophages.

Complement. A system of glycoproteins which interact with the immune system and potentiate many reactions such as phagocytosis and bactericidal activity. In the process of activation of the complement system, active fragments are released with marked biologic activity. One of these (C5a) functions as a chemotactic agent for neutrophils and monocytes, and others act as an anaphylactic agent which leads to release of heparin and histamine from mast cells.

Conventional animal. An animal whose flora has not been altered, but has come about by natural means through contact with other animals and with the environment.

Coproantibody. Immunoglobulins with specific reactivity to antigens (i.e., antibodies) which are found in feces.

Delayed hypersensitivity. A state characterized by skin test reactions which occur maximally at 24–48 hours and exhibit edema, induration, and necrosis at the site of intradermal or subcutaneous injection of the antigen. The major cells leading to the reaction are lymphocytes and macrophages, and much of the inflammation seen is likely due to either direct effects of the lymphocytes (T-cells) and activated macrophages, or effects of the

soluble substances produced by these cells called lymphokines.

Freund's adjuvant. A mixture of mineral oil and emulsifying agents, sometimes containing dried killed tubercule bacillus, which potentiates immunologic responses to injected antigens sometimes as much as 1000-fold.

Gnotobiotic. Animals that have been raised in germ-controlled or germ-free surroundings.

Glucosyltransferase. An enzyme which catalizes the split of sucrose into its component monosaccharides, fructose, and glucose. It then polymerizes the glucose units into glucans. This enzyme is produced by S. mutans and other oral organisms.

Humoral immunity. Heightened state of reactivity to a foreign antigen which is mediated by humoral factors, namely antibodies of one or another immunoglobulin class.

Hypersensitivity. Increased state of reactivity to a foreign substance or antigen.

IgA, IgM, IgG, IgD, IgE. These refer to a family of glycoproteins, or immunoglobulins, in which antibody activity is found.

Immediate hypersensitivity. A state characterized by a skin test reaction which occurs within minutes, and is seen as a wheal resulting from intradermal injection of the eliciting antigen or allergen. The antibody responsible for the reaction (IgE) can fix to mast cells or basophils. Subsequent reaction with the allergen causes the release of mediators such as histamine from these mast cells or basophils.

Immunity. Local or mucosal immunity is a heightened reactivity to a challenge with antigens or foreign substances which was initially induced by prior sensitization with these substances. Local secretory or mucosal immunity is expressed on surfaces which are covered with external secretions such as surfaces of the gastrointestinal tract, genital-urinary tract, oral cavity, and the eye and is likely mediated by secretory IgA antibodies. This is contrasted with systemic immunity which is mediated by antibodies and immunoreactive cells found in the vascular system and extravascular fluids.

Lymphokin. A soluble protein mediator produced by stimulated T lymphocytes. A number of these mediators have been described.

Passive transfer. Immune status passed from a donor to a recipient via serum or blood which contains antibodies or sensitized cells.

Peyer's Patches. Aggregates of lymphatic tissue in the gut associated with immunologic activity.

Reagenic. Relating to antibodies in the blood associated with allergic reactions.

Secretory component. A glycoprotein with a molecular weight of 60-70,000 daltons found in secretory immunoglobulin.

T-cell. Thymus-derived cell. Acts as a helper cell in antibody production or as effector cell in certain immunologic responses.

SUGGESTED READINGS

Bowen WH, Cohen B, Colman G: Immunization against dental caries. Br Dent J 139: 45, 1975

Burrows WE, Elliott ME, Havens I: Studies on immunity to Asiatic cholera. IV. The excretion of coproantibody in experimental enteric cholera in the guinea pig. J Infect Dis 81: 261, 1947

Emmings FG, Evans RT, Genco RJ: Antibody response in parotid fluid in serum of irus monkeys (*Macaca fascicularis*) after local immunization with *Streptococcus mutans*. Infect Immunol 12: 281, 1975

Evans RT, Emmings FG, Genco RJ: Prevention of *Streptococcus mutans* infection of tooth surfaces by salivary antibody in irus monkeys. Infect Immunol 12: 293, 1975

Fitzgerald RJ: The microbial etiology of plaque in relationship to dental caries (abstr). In Stiles HM, Loesche WJ, O'Brien TC (eds): Microbiology [Suppl] 3: 849, 1976 Washington, D.C., Information Retrieval Inc. 1976

Fitzgerald RJ, Jordan HV: Polysaccharide producing bacteria in caries. In Art and Science of Dental Research. New York Academic Press, 1968, pp 79–86

Genco RJ, Evans RT: Specificity of antibodies to *Streptococcus mutans* and their significance in inhibition of adherence to smooth surfaces. In Mestecky J, Lawton AR III (eds): The Immunoglobulin A System. New York, Plenum Press, 1974

Good RA: Disorders of the immune system. In Good RA, Fisher DW (eds): Immunobiology. Stanford, Sinauer Associates, 1971 p 3

Gustafsson DE, Quensel CE, Lanke LS, Lundquist C,

Grahnen H, Bonow BE, Krasse B: The Vipeholm dental caries study. The effect of different levels of carbohydrate intake on caries activity on 436 individuals observed for 5 years. Acta Odontol Scand 11: 232, 1964

Jordan HV: Cariogenic flora: establishment, localization and transmission. J Dent Res 55: C10, 1976

Keyes PH: Research in dental caries. J Am Dent Assoc 76: 1357, 1968

Krasse B: Approaches to prevention (abstr). In Stiles HM, Loesche WJ, O'Brien TC (eds): Microbial Aspects of Dental Caries. Microbiology [Suppl] 3: 867, 1976 Washington, D.C., Information Retrieval Inc, 1976

Lehner T, Challacombe S, Caldwell J: An immunological investigation into the prevention of caries in deciduous teeth of rhesus monkeys. Arch Oral Biol 20: 305, 1975

Mestecky J, McGhee JR, Arnold RR, Michalek SM, Prince SJ, Babb JL: Selective induction of an immune response in human external secretions by ingestion of bacterial antigen. J Clin Invest 61: 731, 1978

Miller WD: Microorganisms of the Human Mouth. Philadelphia, SS White Dental Manufacturing Co, 1890

Montagu MFA: An Introduction to Physical Anthropology, 2nd ed. Springfield, IL, CC Thomas, 1951, p 159

Smith, DJ, Taubman MA: Immunization experiments using rodent caries model. J Dent Res 55: C193, 1976

Stinson MW, Nisengard RJ, Bergey EJ: Binding of Streptococcal cell components to muscle tissue (abstr). American Society for Microbiology, D80, 1979

Tomasi TB Jr, Tan EM, Solomon A, Prendergast RA: Characteristics of an immune system common to certain external secretions. J Exp Med 121: 101, 1965

PART FOUR

The Environment:

CARIES PREVENTION

16 Nutrition in Dental Caries

MICHAEL C. ALFANO

Developmental Aspects of Nutrition and Dental Caries
  "Critical Periods" during Organogenesis
  Tooth Development
  Tooth Alignment
  Salivary Gland Development
  Immunocompetence
Post-Eruptive Effects of Nutrition on the Caries Process
  Enamel Maturation
  Oral Fluids
  Dietary Substrates for Bacterial Plaque
Epidemiologic Relationships
  General Trends
  The Exceptions
Clinical Dietary Trials
  Vipeholm
  Hopewood House
  Turku Sugar Studies
Prospects for Nutritional Modification of Dental Caries
  Optimal Host Resistance
  The Fortification, Processing and Organoleptic Properties of Foods and Sugar Substitutes
  Modification of Diet Composition and Food Intake Patterns
  The Challenge
Summary
Glossary
Suggested Readings

Virtually every oral health care professional and most laymen readily recognize the importance of diet in the etiology of dental caries. Indeed, the classical interlocking ring diagram, which is used to illustrate the factors involved in the dental caries process, indicates that one of the fundamentally important variables is substrate or diet (Fig. 16-1). However, diet and nutrition are so intimately related with dental caries that this classical diagram underestimates the importance of this factor in the overall process. For example, although the substrate component of Figure 16-1 accounts for one-fourth of the variables, it is critically involved in each of the other three factors, including selection and metabolism of microorganisms, development and maintenance of the teeth and host defenses, and the time frame during which the substrate is present and tooth destruction occurs.

The significance of diet and nutrition in dental caries can be underscored from several additional viewpoints. Food affects the oral cavity twice—once locally, during mastication, and again systemically after the nutrients in the food are digested and absorbed. Diet also affects the teeth during pre-eruption and post-eruption, two distinct developmental phases. Finally, one frequently overlooked fact is that nutrients in the diet, such as zinc and sucrose, may affect taste perception which in turn will modify dietary preference

343

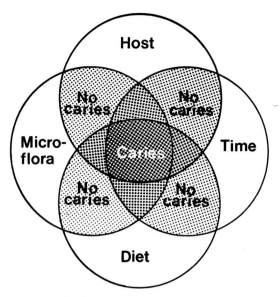

Fig. 16-1. The four circles diagrammatically represent the parameters involved in the caries process. All four factors must be acting concurrently (overlapping of the circles) for caries to occur.

and food intake patterns. Thus, diet and nutrition, via a series of complex interrelationships, are important in the developmental, pathophysiologic, and behavioral aspects of dental caries. The purpose of this chapter is to define the complex interactions of diet, nutrition, and caries. In addition, the potential for dietary control of dental caries is evaluated. Based on this evaluation, challenges are issued not only to the dentist and patient, but to the educational, industrial, and research grant systems as well.

DEVELOPMENTAL ASPECTS OF NUTRITION AND DENTAL CARIES

"Critical Periods" during Organogenesis

Every organ system develops in a sequence by which periods of slow growth are interrupted one or more times by spurts of rapid expansion in cell number and size. These rapid growth spurts or "critical periods" in development usually occur in three phases: a hyperplastic phase in which growth is accomplished primarily by an increase in cell number, an intermediate phase in which hy-

perplastic and hypertrophic growth occur simultaneously, and a final hypertrophic phase in which growth is primarily mediated by an increase in cell size. These three phases may be determined biochemically as illustrated in Figure 16-2. The hyperplastic phase is marked by an increase in DNA, the intermediate phase parallels an increase in RNA, and the hypertrophic phase is indicated by an increase in protein synthesis. Although this pattern of development is followed by each organ system, each system has its own unique timetable in which this pattern occurs. The brain may complete Phase I during week X, while the liver is not finished until week Y and the pancreas may not begin until week Z. Thus, although a variety of organs and systems may be developing simultaneously they develop in different phases, rates, and time sequences.

Oral tissues also follow differential growth patterns. For example, protein synthesis in the palate of the rabbit peaks at about day 18 of development, a time frame which is closely linked to palatal fusion in this species. However, protein synthesis in the rabbit tongue at day 18 or gestation is at a very low level (Fig. 16-3). Obviously, both tongue and palate are growing at day 18 but they are in different growth phases. These differential biochemical changes may be manifested morphologically as elevation of the palatal shelves from the vertical to a horizontal position and a relative drop in the position of the tongue.

The rapid growth spurts described above have been termed "critical periods" because they represent time frames during which environmental stress, such as malnutrition, may result in irreversible damage to the developing system. Although each system may grow differentially it cannot grow haphazardly, and the development of each system is regulated by both genetic and hormonal constraints. In the case of rabbit palate, for instance, the genetic and hormonal "green light" is on for protein synthesis at day 18. If an environmental stress, such as essential amino acid deficiency, is imposed at this time, the palatal shelves may not synthesize enough protein to elevate and fuse, and an irreversible defect, a cleft palate, will result. The timing is crucial because, even though the amino acids are supplied at day 19, the base of the skull will have expanded to the point where the shelves when elevated do not contact and cannot fuse.

The importance of differential growth, criti-

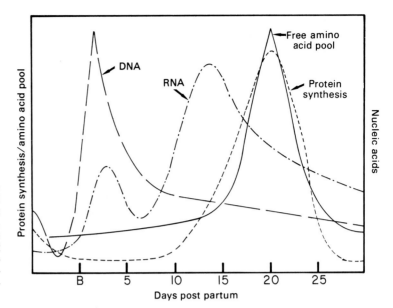

Fig. 16-2. An integrated, partially speculative schema of sequential changes in DNA, RNA and protein synthesis in developing organs. (From DePaola, DP, Kuftinec, MM: Nutrition in Growth and Development of Oral Tissues in Alfano, MC, De-Paola, DP (eds.) Symposium on Nutrition. Dent. Clin. N. Amer., 20, Philadelphia, W. B. Saunders, 1976.)

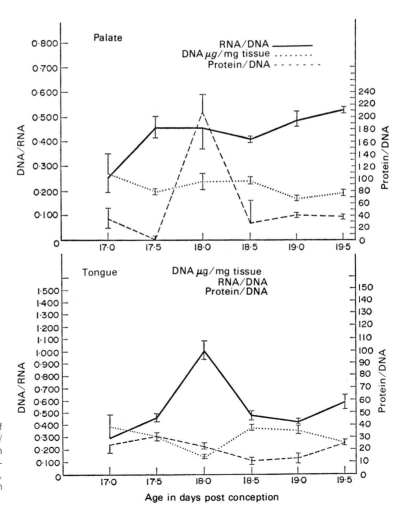

Fig. 16-3. Changes with time of DNA (μg./mg. tissue), RNA (RNA/DNA), and protein (protein/DNA) in the palate and tongue of the embryonic rabbit. (From DePaola, DP, Miller, SA, Drummond, JF: Arch Oral Biol 18: 1113–1119, 1973)

cal periods of development, and malnutrition in terms of development aspects of dental caries are outlined in the next four sections.

Tooth Development

Since teeth undergo rapid, well-defined critical periods of development, it is not surprising to note that numerous nutritional problems have been linked to alterations in the structure, size, composition, alignment, eruption, and caries suceptibility of teeth. For example, ascorbate deficiency will result in odontoblastic atrophy and porotic dentin formation in a developing tooth. In fact, the relationship between a reduction in ascorbic acid in the diet and the decrease in height of odontoblasts in the continuously erupting guinea-pig incisor is so close that this system was formerly used as a bioassay for quantitation of ascorbic acid activity. In addition, vitamin A deficiencies during development have been reported to result in ameloblastic atrophy, poor odontoblastic differentiation, enamel hypoplasia and pulp stones. A relatively common linear hypoplastic defect in the primary dentition of children from developing countries, the "Cauque" lesion, may be related to neonatal infection and low serum vitamin A levels in this population. These defects can contribute to extensive dental caries (Fig. 16-4).

The importance of dietary minerals in the development of a caries-resistant tooth is well known. Navia has classified the relationship between trace minerals and caries as illustrated in Table 16-1. It is important to note that these minerals may play a role not only in tooth development but also in the post-eruptive remineralization and bacterial colonization of the tooth surface. The present discussion will be confined to the pre-eruptive developmental effects.

Dietary fluorides can dramatically reduce the incidence of dental caries. Although it is known that the presence of fluoride ion during tooth development will result in the formation of enamel with reduced solubility and increased fluorapatite content, the mechanism of fluoride action may be considerably more complex than a simple alteration in the solubility product of the mineral phase of enamel. Several additional factors relative to fluoride cariostatic activity are discussed in Chapter 20.

The effects of the other trace minerals listed in Table 16-1 on tooth development and dental caries are not yet clearly defined and further research is required in this area. For example, although Mo, B, and Sr have been reported to be mildly cariosatic in epidemiologic studies, a recent animal study indicated that when these minerals were supplied during tooth development caries actually increased. Nevertheless, the macro-minerals, calcium and phosphorous, and the active metabolities of vitamin D associated with the absorption and metabolism of calcium and phosphorous, have been related to tooth development and caries.

Diets containing high-calcium-phosphorous ratios have been shown to increase the carbonate-phosphate ratio in the developing enamel of rodents. In addition, detrimental effects of vitamin D deficiency on tooth development have been repeatedly documented. These effects range from subtle alterations in calcification, such as the calciotraumatic line and Mellanby hypoplasia associated with a mild rachitic process, to excessive enamel hypoplasia associated with severe rickets. Moreover, clinical studies have suggested that an increased incidence and progression of dental caries is associated with a reduced vitamin D intake. The reader is cautioned, however, that vitamin D is quite toxic at high doses and its beneficial effect on dental caries can only be demonstrated in populations which are either deficient or marginally adequate in vitamin D nutriture. With the exception of overt calcium, phosphorous, or vitamin D deficiency during tooth development, calcium-phosphorous ratios and dietary phosphate levels *per se* are most important in dental caries from a post-eruptive viewpoint.

Although iron is generally considered to be a caries inert mineral (Table 16-1), recent studies by J. Sintes have suggested that a classical 56 per cent sucrose diet, routinely used to induce dental caries in the laboratory rat, is actually deficient in iron. Carefully monitored

TABLE 16-1.   RELATIONSHIP OF MINERAL ELEMENTS TO CARIES

Effect								
Cariostatic				F,	P			
Mildly Cariostatic	Mo,	V,	Cu,	Sr,	B,	Li,	Au	
Doubtful	Be,	Co,	Mn,	Sn,	Zn,	Br,	I	
Caries Inert			Ba,	Al,	Ni,	Fe,	Pd,	Ti
Caries Promoting			Se,	Mg,	Cd,	Pt,	Pb,	Si

From Navia JM: Int Dent J, 22: 431, 1972)

A

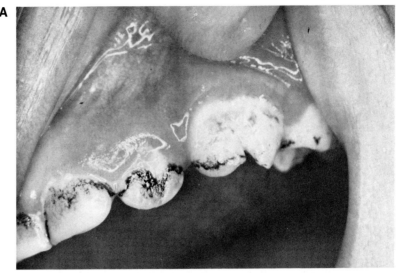

B

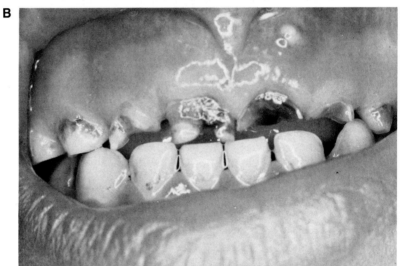

C

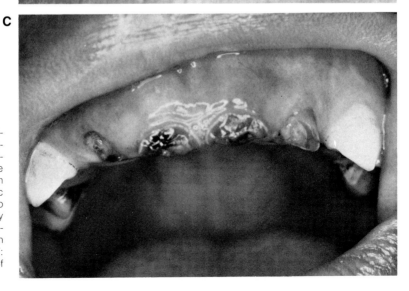

Fig. 16-4. **A.** Hypoplastic developmental defects (Cauque lesions) related to neonatal infection and malnutrition in the primary teeth of a Guatemalan child **B., C.** These hypoplastic defects predispose the child to rampant caries in the primary dentition (From Alfano, MC, Chasens, AI: Nutrition Education in the dental curriculum. Dialog. 7: 2–7, 1975, School of Dentistry of Fairleigh Dickinson University.)

rats, maintained solely on this diet, demonstrated poor growth, hair loss, anemia, skin lesions, and alterations in tooth color and saliva composition. Supplementation of the diet with iron not only reversed all of the above changes, but also markedly reduced the amount of dental caries. Considering the significant cariogenic challenge of a 56 per cent sucrose diet, it is indeed interesting to note the dramatic effect of iron supplementation on dental caries in animals maintained on this diet. This finding in conjunction with similar recent observations in zinc deficient animals underscores the complexity of nutrition in dental caries and the need for further study of the role of trace minerals in human caries.

Finally, several investigators, including Shaw, Navia, Menaker, Miller, and DiOrio have noted that protein deficient diets fed to experimental animals during tooth development result in smaller teeth, delayed eruption time, and increased caries susceptibility. However, the mineral composition of the teeth was not significantly altered. The increased caries experience in animals fed a protein deficient diet during tooth development cannot be explained based on alterations in tooth development alone. Therefore, these findings should also be related to possible adverse effects of protein deficiency on tooth alignment, salivary gland development, and immunocompetence.

Tooth Alignment

In view of the generalized emphasis on the genetic components of malocclusion and the small number of reports relating malnutrition to poor tooth alignment, any discussion of the effects of nutrition on tooth alignment must be largely speculative. Indeed, Shaw and Sweeney recently concluded that, "There has never been any thorough investigation to determine whether orthodontic problems may be related to nutritional deficiency during development." Nevertheless, since teeth differentiate early in development and undergo short critical periods, their ultimate, genetically determined size is established early in the developmental process. In contrast, the jaw bones develop during an extended period of time, undergo a prolonged critical period, and achieve their genetic size potential only after the teeth have developed. Therefore, if poor nutrition stunts jaw development after the teeth have differentiated, it is quite possible that Class I type malocclusions may result. That is, the jaws will not grow large enough to accommodate the teeth. Indeed, Tonge and McCance observed this effect when neonatal pigs were maintained on a calorie restricted diet for one year, and then rehabilitated for periods ranging up to two additional years.

Poor tooth alignment and crowding result not only in esthetic problems and masticatory insufficiency but also in increased caries and periodontal disease. Although improper nutrition participates in the caries process in many ways that are more dramatic than altered tooth alignment, this problem does affect human caries experience and is worthy of further study.

Salivary Gland Development

In an effort to delineate the mechanism by which neonatal protein deficiency in rats can decrease the subsequent resistance of the teeth to dental caries, Menaker and Navia studied the effects of early protein deficiency on salivary gland development and function. They noted that biochemical alterations in salivary gland composition and protein synthesis mediated by specific, but marginal, neonatal protein malnutrition were paralleled by functional changes in the salivary glands. For example, protein-limited rats secreted only one-fifth as much saliva and one-fourth the total protein of the control group. Considering the critical role of saliva in protecting the tooth from dental caries, it is probable that a significant portion of the increase in dental caries susceptibility caused by early protein deficiency is mediated by salivary dysfunction. Although the concentration of any of a dozen or more salivary components may be modified by neonatal protein deficiency, alterations in salivary volume, buffering capacity, and protein protective factors are the most likely choices for explaining the increased caries experience of the affected animals.

Recent studies by Alvares in primates confirm that protein malnutrition can alter the protein composition of the saliva. It will be interesting to determine whether the changes in protein composition are reflected in altered tooth-coating, pellicle forming glycoproteins (see Chap. 5), or in antibacterial proteins such as lactoperoxidase, lactoferrin, lysozyme, or secretory IgA (see Chap. 15). Irrespective of the mechanisms, the fact that neonatal protein deficiency can dramatically alter tooth resistance to dental caries in adult life is an exciting finding. It suggests that dentists should rethink their disdain for the "soft teeth" excuse offered by so many caries-prone individuals. The "soft teeth" excuse may actually be a reflection of poor salivary gland function and deminished remineralization capacity (see Chap. 19).

Immunocompetence

The fact that malnutrition can compromise host defense by numerous mechanisms has been documented in well over 1,000 reports and several texts. A particularly virulent or avirulent microbial species and a host with unusually high or low resistance may mask any effects of nutrition on host defense. However, nutritional status may be particularly important in the defense of a host with intermediate resistance from infection by a microbe of intermediate virulence. This relationship is diagrammed in Figure 16-5. In terms of dental caries, this diagram indicates that a highly resistant tooth would probably not decay when challenged by a typical cariogenic microflora and caries promoting diet. The reverse of this situation would also be true. Nevertheless, since individuals with highly resistant teeth are uncommon and since microorganisms have variable virulence

based on the particular strain, environment and so forth, it is probable that nutritional factors will influence the great majority of cases of dental caries in humans (Fig. 16-5).

It has been repeatedly demonstrated that malnutrition can decrease host resistance to infectious disease through altered cellular immunity, humoral immunity, and nonspecific immunity. Cellular immunity is not too important in the control of dental caries except as it interacts with the other two primary effector systems. However, humoral immunity, especially the secretion of salivary immunoglobulins, and non-specific immunity such as the secretion of lactoperoxidase, lysozyme and, lactoferrin, may be intimately involved in caries protection. Although malnutrition, most notably protein deficiency, has been shown to decrease the efficacy of each of these systems, the studies have usually been conducted on adult animals and salivary immune effectors have not been assayed.

Notwithstanding the problems listed above and the need for further studies, recent evidence suggests that malnutrition during critical periods of immunodevelopment can alter host resistance at a later time. In humans, for example, it is recognized that intrauterine growth retardation due to maternal malnutrition or placental insufficiency results in profound adverse effects on post-natal immunocompetence. In addition, significant impairment of antibody formation has been detected not only in the first generation of malnourished rats, but, incredibly, in the sec-

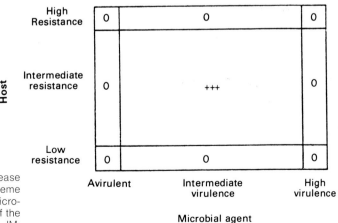

Fig. 16-5. Nutritional effects on disease processes will not be seen in extreme cases where the virulence of the microbial agent is high or the resistance of the host is extremely low. (From Navia, JM: Nutrition and Oral Disease in Caldwell, RC and Stallard RE (eds.) A Textbook of Preventive Dentistry, Philadelphia, W.B. Saunders, 1977.)

0: Area in which nutrition is ineffective in influencing disease process
+++ Area where nutrition will influence the prognosis of disease

ond generation as well. These facts in combination with the generalized decreased salivary protein synthesis mediated by developmental malnutrition, indicate that studies of the effects of developmental malnutrition on specific salivary immune effectors should be most interesting.

POST-ERUPTIVE EFFECTS OF NUTRITION ON THE CARIES PROCESS

Enamel Maturation

The minerals in the crystalline phase of enamel are in constant equilibrium with minerals from the saliva, tooth accumulated substances (primarily pellicle and plaque), gingival fluid, and possibly "enamel" fluid. This equilibrium results in constant de- and remineralization of the outer enamel layer particularly in newly erupted teeth. Radioisotope studies have demonstrated that recently erupted teeth can incorporate inorganic ions into the enamel surface at rates which are 10 or more times faster than teeth which have been in the oral cavity for prolonged periods. This observation is consistent with reports that newly erupted teeth have a propensity to take up dyes and are especially susceptible to caries formation in the presence of a cariogenic diet. The enamel "porosity" associated with recent tooth eruption reflects still another "critical period" in the development of a caries resistant tooth. A good diet, effective oral hygiene, and the presence of fluoride ion during this critical period along with the predominance of caries-resistant hydroxyapatite and flourapatite crystals will tend to promote remineralization of the enamel. In contrast, a particularly cariogenic diet in this time frame will promote development of a cariogenic microflora and hypomineralized enamel, and predispose the tooth to caries.

Although minerals from the enamel surface may exchange with minerals from a variety of environmental fluids and structures in the mouth, the preponderance of studies have evaluated mineral exchange at the interface of the tooth and saliva (see Chap. 19). In terms of nutritional effects on this exchange one must consider not only the local effect of food in the oral cavity discussed below, but also the

effect of diet on oral fluids, pellicle, and plaque which are discussed in subsequent sections.

The most familiar aspects of the local effects of food in the oral cavity relate to the so called "detergency" or "tooth-cleaning" properties of firm, fibrous foods. These foods are supposed to physically remove plaque from the teeth thereby decreasing the microbiologic insult and allowing for remineralization. Although this cleansing system functions well in certain animals, it has been repeatedly shown to be ineffective in humans. In fact, a recent study in our laboratories indicated that even vigorous chewing of gum containing abrasive calcium carbonate particles resulted in only a minimal amount of plaque removal during a ten minute test period. Thus the tooth cleansing benefits associated with the "apple-a-day" folklore appear to be overstated.

The chemical composition of food in the oral cavity is considerably more important in enamel remineralization than is its physical consistency. With the exception of fluorides (see Chap. 20), dietary phosphates have received the greatest attention for their cariostatic effects. A variety of organic and inorganic phosphate molecules have markedly reduced caries experience in experimental animals. Navia and co-workers have demonstrated that this cariostatic effect is mediated primarily by local rather than systemic factors, but the precise mechanism remains to be determined. Unfortunately, the use of dietary phosphate compounds in human caries trials, while encouraging, have been considerably less dramatic than observed in rodent models. This difference may merely be a reflection of the lower phosphate content of rat saliva relative to the human situation, or a manifestation of the fact that phosphates are already added in significant amounts to the human food supply for processing purposes.

The ratio of calcium to phosphorous in the adult diet has been related to caries experience in a series of about 200 dental patients. A Ca/P ratio of 0.55 was reportedly associated with little or no caries activity while ratios higher or lower than this figure were related to progressively higher levels of caries (Fig. 16-6). Although epidemiologic data tend to support this observation, large scale investigations are required to confirm the effect and determine the mechanism for Ca/P mediated alterations in caries experience.

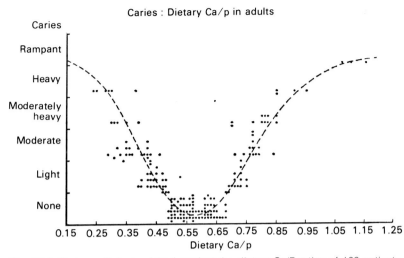

Fig. 16-6. Caries activity is plotted against the dietary Ca/P ratios of 183 patients. (From Stanton, G.: Diet and Dental Caries. N. Y. State Dent. J. 35: 399–407, 1969)

Oral Fluids

Saliva, gingival fluid and enamel fluid are three types of oral fluids which may modify the process of dental caries. Enamel fluid has been reported to form on the surface of a tooth from tissue fluids in the dental pulp. It has been postulated to serve as a systemic vehicle for nutritional modulation of dental caries. However, the very existence of this fluid "flow" is a controversial issue, and its composition is not defined; therefore, at this time no comment is warranted relative to its role in dental caries. In contrast, gingival fluid, arising from the crevice between the tooth and the free gingiva, is a well known entity, and its composition has been evaluated under numerous clinical conditions. Gingival fluid has a high content of urea and may serve as a caries protective factor in the gingival crevice region. Golub and Kleinberg have suggested that ureolytic microorganisms in the subgingival plaque may convert the urea to ammonia. This conversion would result in an elevation of pH and may partly explain the relative caries immunity in the subgingival area. Although recent studies have indicated that both vitamin E and folic acid can alter gingival fluid flow rates, no definite studies of the interaction of nutrition, gingival fluid, and dental caries have been reported.

Saliva is probably the most important host defense against dental caries. The flow rate, composition, and function of saliva have been altered by a variety of diet-related factors. For example:

1. Pre- and neonatal protein deficiency in rats results in a marked reduction in salivary flow rates and protein synthesis, and a subsequent increase in caries in adult rats.
2. The physical stimulation of chewing fibrous foods is generally considered to be an important factor in maintaining salivary secretory function.
3. Protein deficiency in adult monkeys has resulted in decreased levels of certain pellicle-like glycoprotein components in the saliva.
4. Salivary urea levels are directly related to dietary protein intake. High salivary urea levels may generate higher plaque pH's via the ammonia produced by ureolytic plaque microorganisms.

These observations, combined with the fact that saliva serves as the vehicle for facilitating taste sensation and dissolving cariostatic food ingredients, such as fluoride and phosphate, sets up an interesting cycle. That is, the nutritional status may affect the caries process either directly or by altering salivary function. Salivary function, in turn, may affect the caries process either directly or by altering taste perception, food intake, and nutritional status.

Dietary Substrates for Bacterial Plaque

The role of diet in supplying substrates, particularly sugars, for microbial growth, metabolism, and acid production is unequivocally important in the process of dental caries. However, this relationship is often discussed to the exclusion of all the other nutrition-related factors in dental caries. This unidirectional approach is misleading, and the emphasis for this chapter has been reoriented accordingly.

Dietary carbohydrates, particularly sugars, are the most important substrate for oral microbial metabolism. Brown has noted four aspects of dietary carbohydrate utilization by oral microorganisms which collectively contribute to their cariogenic potential. These four carbohydrate mediated microbial activities include the utilization of carbohydrates for glycolytic metabolism, and for the synthesis of adhesive bacterial extracellular polymers, intracellular storage polysaccharides, and extracellular storage polysaccharides.

The most direct role for carbohydrates in dental caries is their ability to serve as excellent fermentable energy sources for a variety of oral microbes. The production of lactic acid by glycolytic metabolism of oral carbohydrates is thought to be directly responsible for the initiation of the carious lesion (Fig. 16-7). Nevertheless, the synthesis of adhesive and storage polysaccharides is also critically important in the colonization of smooth tooth surfaces, the long term viability of the microflora, and perpetuation of the carious lesion.

The importance of sucrose in smooth surface caries is thought to be related to its role as a substrate in the synthesis of adhesive and storage extracellular polysaccharides, the glucans and levans (see Chap. 14). These polymers account for the "stickiness" required to initiate and maintain plaque formation on smooth tooth surfaces.

Biosynthesis of these polysaccharides occurs largely by the action of extracellular and membrane-bound enzymes with a high specificity for dietary sucrose. The enzymes,

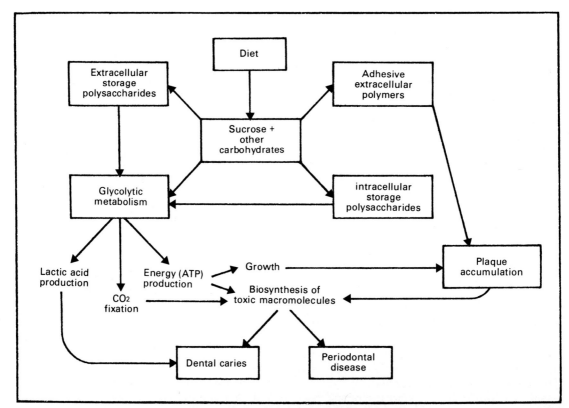

Fig. 16-7. Schematic representation of the role of dietary carbohydrates in oral disease. (From Brown, AI: The Role of Carbohydrates in Plaque Formation and Oral Disease. Nutr. Rev. 33: 353–361, 1975)

the glucosyl- and fructosyltransferases, have been isolated from *Streptococcus sanguis* and *Streptococcus mutans*, and have been characterized by Newbrun as follows:

1. They are highly specific for sucrose and will not utilize sugars such as fructose, glucose, maltose or lactose.
2. They have a broad pH optimum, 5.2-7.0, coinciding with the pH range prevailing in dental plaque.
3. In the presence of adequate nutrition the enzyme will be made by these organisms and sucrose is not a required inducer. Whenever sucrose is ingested, the organisms are ready to synthesize polysaccharides.
4. The equilibrium of the reaction shown below for glucan synthesis is far to the right.

$$nC_{12}H_{22}O_{11} \longrightarrow (C_6H_{10}O_5)n + nC_6H_{12}O_6$$
$$\text{(sucrose)} \qquad \text{(glucan)} \qquad \text{(fructose)}$$

Therefore, when sucrose is present in the plaque the glucosyltransferase enzymes will utilize it to form adhesive and storage polysaccharides as well as fructose. The fructose can be readily fermented by most plaque microorganisms to form organic acids.

In spite of the role of sucrose in plaque formation and caries, the reader is cautioned that a variety of other simple sugars can promote dental caries at rates which sometimes equal that of sucrose. Therefore, it is inappropriate to suggest that sucrose substitution by "natural" or "fruit" sugars will reduce the incidence of dental caries. Indeed, honey has been reported to produce dramatically more extensive occlusal caries when compared to sucrose in experimental animals. Moreover, even starch can support low levels of caries activity in both experimental animals and man.

Fats and proteins demonstrate an anti-caries effect. Fats may possibly decrease caries activity by altering surface properties of the enamel, by having a direct toxic effect on oral microbes, through interference with sugar solubilization, or simply by the replacement of dietary carbohydrates. The low to moderate cariogenic potential of milk chocolate relative to its sugar level has been attributed to its high fat content. However, this product also contains tannin derivatives from cocoa which demonstrate cariostatic activity. Proteins may function to reduce caries post-eruptively by a direct effect on plaque metabolism, replace-

ment of dietary carbohydrate, or by increasing salivary urea levels as previously discussed. In addition, dietary proteins are subjected to only weak proteolytic activity in the oral cavity. This factor, in combination with the short exposure time of proteins in the mouth, suggests that only small amounts of amino acids can be mobilized by plaque bacteria from dietary proteins.

Finally, two vitamins, thiamin and pyridoxine, have been specifically related to dental caries activity in animals. Thiamin has a caries promoting effect and pyridoxine seems to reduce dental caries. Although the precise mechanism for the caries influencing activity of these two vitamins has not been determined, they appear to function by local rather than systemic effects. These nutrients most probably affect the growth rates, metabolism, and microbial composition of the dental plaque by stimulating or inhibiting one or more microbial species in the plaque.

EPIDEMIOLOGIC RELATIONSHIPS

General Trends

In a recent review of the epidemiologic relationships between diet and dental caries, Russell noted that:

> The relationship between general nutrition and dental caries, worldwide, is inverse. In general those groups with the fewer nutritional deficiencies have the greater problems with dental caries.
> . . . no consistent relationship between nutritional states and dental caries could be developed in the series of international nutrition surveys conducted by the Interdepartmental Committee on Nutrition for National Development (ICNND) during the 1960's. On the other hand, there was a clear relationship between national usage of sugar in the diet and dental caries experience in the populations surveyed by ICNND teams.

Just as sugar, particularly sucrose, in the diet has been associated with increased caries, dietary fluorides have been related epidemiologically to reduced caries levels. In fact, the benefits of fluoride were first elucidated based on epidemiologic studies to relate the association between mottled enamel and reduced caries to various regions of the country.

The only well-defined epidemiologic relationships between nutrients in the diet and caries are for sugar and fluoride. Nevertheless, a number of other nutrients, especially trace minerals, have been related to caries experience. In this regard, the relative cariogenicity of the minerals listed in Table 16-1 were determined largely based on epidemiologic data. For example, the caries-promoting aspects of selenium were first determined epidemiologically and later confirmed in animal studies.

In spite of the usefulness of epidemiologic studies relating diet to caries, the reader is cautioned to consider certain problems in epidemiologic research particularly as it relates to diet. Some studies relate oral conditions to "per capita" intake of a number of foodstuffs. There is obviously a wide range of dietary intakes and usually storage spoilage and/or table waste which contribute to the per capita figure. Moreover, per capita data cannot be directly related to the individual with disease who may either be at the low or high end of the food intake scale. Another factor which is especially important in caries studies is the frequency at which a given nutrient is consumed. One hundred grams of sucrose consumed once a day would have a considerably different impact on the cariogenic microflora than the same dose given as twenty widely spaced five gram challenges. In this regard it is interesting to note that although the total amount of sucrose consumption has remained relatively constant in the United States on a per capita basis for more than 50 years (Table 16-2), some reports suggest that the prevalence of caries has increased. Although this increased prevalence has not been documented, if it does indeed exist it may be explained in many ways:

1. Although per capita levels of sucrose have remained constant, the distribution is such that individuals with high sucrose intakes are the ones with high caries levels.
2. There are better methods for detecting and reporting caries at the present time.
3. The genetic composition of the host and/or the virulence of the microflora has changed with time.
4. Caries promoting factors other than sucrose have been introduced into the diet.
5. Caries protective factors have been reduced or removed from the diet.
6. The relationship between sucrose and

dental caries is not as close as once was thought.
7. The form and frequency of sucrose consumption has changed in the last 50 years.

This last statement represents the most frequently cited reason for the apparent dichotomy. That is, although total refined sugar consumption has remained relatively constant in the last 50–60 years, the amount which is consumed in processed foods and beverages has increased from about 19 lbs. to more than 70 lbs. per person each year (Table 16-2). This suggests that although the total sugar challenge has remained constant, Americans are consuming more processed snack foods at greater frequencies. Nevertheless, it is important to note that each of the other six possible reasons cited may represent plausible explanations for any confirmed increase in caries incidence.

It is clear from the above example that the most useful type of epidemiologic data relating diet to caries is generated by investigations in which the food intake patterns and oral health status of the individuals in the study are directly and specifically related to one another. Even this approach will ignore the possible contributions of diet early in life (i.e., during tooth and salivary gland development) on the subsequent resistance of the host to caries. Therefore, dietary epidemiologic data must always be evaluated very carefully.

The Exceptions

It is important to note certain exceptions to the general epidemiologic observation that the dental caries experience of a population is directly and positively related to sugar consumption. First of all, dental caries does occur, sometimes at high levels, in populations that have never used sucrose or processed foodstuffs. Conversely, certain populations with high sucrose intakes may have low levels of caries. For example, the addition of sugar to the diet of Nauruan children has had little effect on their relatively low caries experience. It is also noteworthy that sucrose levels in the diet do not vary independent of other factors. In this regard, Kreitzman has noted that the high caries in Alaskan Eskimos from southern regions of the state, classically associated with increased sugar consumption via the trading post, may also result from an

TABLE 16-2. REFINED SUGAR—ESTIMATED PER CAPITA CONSUMPTION BY TYPE OF USE, SELECTED PERIODS 1909–13 TO 1971*

Type of Use	1909–1913 (Lb)	1925–1929 (Lb)	1935–1939 (Lb)	1947–1949 (Lb)	1957–1959 (Lb)	1965 (Lb)	1971 (Preliminary) (Lb)
In processed foods							
Cereal and bakery products	4.5	7.7	9.7	12.9	15.4	15.6	17.6
Confectionary products	6.5	8.0	8.2	9.8	9.6	10.4	11.0
Processed fruits and vegetables†	3.0	4.6	4.4	9.0	9.8	9.5	10.4
Dairy products	1.5	2.3	2.4	4.6	4.9	5.3	4.8
Other food products‡	0.3	0.7	1.2	1.5	1.7	2.5	2.6
Total food products	15.8	23.4	25.9	37.8	41.4	43.3	47.4
Beverages (largely in soft drinks)	3.5	5.0	5.2	10.6	12.6	16.9	22.8
Total processed food and beverages	19.3	28.4	31.1	48.4	54.0	60.2	70.2
Other food uses							
Eating and drinking places§	4.5	5.7	6.3	7.7	7.3	6.2	5.5
Household use‖	52.1	65.0	58.8	37.4	33.1	28.2	24.7
Institutional and other use**	0.5	0.9	0.9	1.3	1.0	1.4	1.1
Total	57.1	71.6	66.0	46.4	41.4	35.8	31.3
Total food use	76.4	100.0	97.1	94.8	95.4	96.0	101.5
Nonfood use***	0.3	0.4	0.4	0.4	0.7	0.6	0.9
Total consumption	76.7	100.4	97.5	95.2	96.1	96.6	102.4

* Prepared by Food Consumption Section, Economic Research Service, U.S. Department of Agriculture. (From Page, L and Friend, B: Level of use of sugars in the United States. In Sipple, HL and McNutt, KW (eds.): Sugars in Nutrition. New York, Academic Press, Inc., 1974, Ch. 7, with permission.)
† Canned, bottled, and frozen foods (processed fruit and vegetable products): jams, jellies, and preserves.
‡ Includes miscellaneous food uses such as meat curing, and syrup blending.
§ Includes hotels, motels, restaurants, cafeterias, and other eating and drinking establishments.
‖ Household use assumed synonymous with deliveries in consumer-sized packages (less than 50 lb).
** Largely for military use.
*** Includes use in pharmaceuticals, tobacco, and other nonfood use.

TABLE 16-3.   CALCIUM TO PHOSPHOROUS RATIOS
OF ALASKAN ESKIMO DIETS

Location	Ratio
South	
Hooper Bay	.79
Napaskiak	.99
Kewktok	2.35
Kasigluk	1.70
North	
Huslia	.53
Point Hope	.54
Shishmaref	.62

From: Kreitzman, SN. Nutrition in the Process of Dental
Caries. In Alfano, MC, DePaola, DP (eds.): *Symposium
on Nutrition,* Dent Clin N. Am *20:* 503, Philadelphia, WB
Saunders Co., 1976

alteration in the calcium to phosphorous
ratios in their diets (Table 16-3).

Another epidemiologic study which suggests that sucrose is not the only dietary variable important in dental caries was recently
completed by Alfano, Drummond and Guten-
tag. They studied a population in rural Guate-
mala and noted that the DMF experience of
females, 15 years and older, was significantly
greater than their male counterparts (Fig. 16-
8). This difference persisted throughout adulthood in spite of the fact that the males dem-

onstrated consistently poorer Oral Hygiene
Indices and consumed an average of three
times more sucrose than the females. This reversal of the more sucrose equals more caries
trend might be due to altered nutritional status of males vs. females during tooth, salivary
gland, and immunological development. It
might also simply reflect the nutrient drain on
the females in this population caused by frequent pregnancies and periods of lactation.
Regardless of the explanation, this example
serves, once again, to illustrate the care required in interpreting epidemiologic studies,
particularly those which deal with diet.

CLINICAL DIETARY TRIALS

The most clearly defined relationships between dietary sugar and dental caries have
been determined in a number of controlled
human clinical trials. These trials have provided the scientific basis for including dietary
modification programs in the comprehensive
practice of preventive dentistry (see Chap.
17). Accordingly a few of the more prominent
dietary trials are reviewed below.

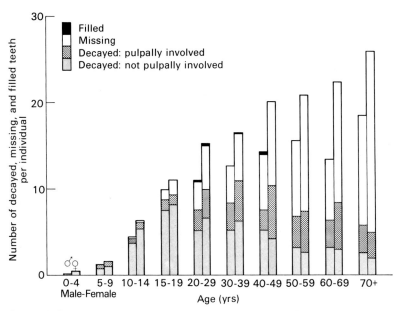

Fig. 16-8. The relative contribution of the number of decayed, missing, and filled
(DMF) teeth to the total DMF grouped by age and sex in a rural Guatemalan population. Note the increased caries experience in women relative to men even though
women had consistently better oral hygiene scores and consumed only one-third as
much sucrose as the men.

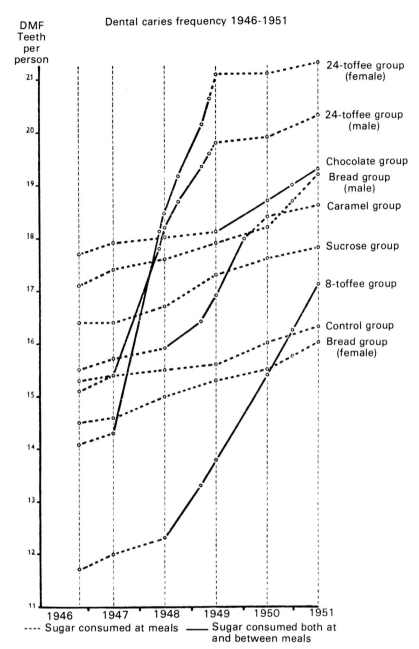

Fig. 16-9. Relation of carbohydrate intake to dental caries. (From Gustafsson, B., Quensel, C., Lanke, L., Lundquist, C., Grahnen, H., Bonow, B., Krasse, B.: The Vipeholm Dental Caries Study. Acta Odont. Scand. 11: 232–363, 1954.)

Vipeholm

The Vipeholm Dental Caries Study took place during a 5-year period in the late 1940's at a mental institution in Sweden. The more than 400 adult inmates in the institution were divided into 9 groups. The diets of these groups varied from a control group which received a basal diet containing essentially no sugar which was consumed only at mealtimes, to a group which received the basal diet supplemented with 24 toffees between meals each day. The results of this often quoted study are summarized in Figure 16-9. The data indicate quite clearly that frequent sugar intake can increase the rate of caries attack in individuals with poor oral hygiene. More importantly, however, this study revealed that the form and frequency with which sugar is consumed is of paramount importance. The sucrose group consumed as much as 5 times more sucrose at mealtimes than some of the candy groups consumed between meals during the day. However, the caries attack rate in the sucrose group was essentially no different than the control group. These data are particularly useful in the dietary management of patients with rampant caries. They suggest that if sweets are to be consumed, they should be eaten during rather than between meals.

Hopewood House

Institutionalized children at Hopewood House in Australia were raised on nutritionally adequate, vegetarian diets which were restricted in their content of sugar and other refined carbohydrates. In spite of the presence of low fluoride levels in the water and poor hygiene practices exercised by these children, they exhibited only 10 per cent of the caries prevalence which was seen in children of comparable age from the general population. It is particularly interesting to note that when the children grew older and ate a more conventional diet, the caries rate increased dramatically, paralleling that of the general population. Thus, refined carbohydrate restriction during childhood does not confer any long-lived immunity to dental caries. Apparently the virulence of the plaque microflora can readily adapt to metabolize the cariogenic substrates available.

Turku Sugar Studies

The most recent and pointedly exciting studies relating dietary factors to bacterial plaque and dental caries are the Turku Sugar Studies. These studies have been conducted in Turku, Finland, primarily by Scheinin and Mäkinen using 125 subjects with a mean age of 27.5 years. The subjects were divided into three groups and fed diets containing either sucrose, fructose, or the sugar alcohol, xylitol, as sweetening agents. The key to the success of the project is that the sweetening

agents were made available to the subjects in over 100 different processed products including candies, soft drinks, ketchup, pastries, crackers, chewing gum, and even cough syrup. The studies are also somewhat unique for the broad range of parameters studied such as caries increments, periodontal status, and general health status, as well as biochemical analysis of oral fluids, plaque, serum, and urine and microbiologic determinations.

The results of these studies can best be described as . . . . incredible! The xylitol diets reduced the incidence of dental caries by approximately 90 per cent, while the fructose diets reduced caries by 30 per cent relative to sucrose. Moreover, the xylitol diet prompted a significant number of caries reversals so that the net increment in decayed, missing, and filled tooth surfaces (DMFS-increment) for this group in two years was zero. This compares with DMFS-increments of 7.2 and 3.8 for the sucrose and fructose groups respectively. These results were further supported by a second study in which 100 subjects were given either sucrose of xylitol-containing gum to chew for a one-year period. This study indicated that although the DMFS-increment for the sucrose gum group increased by a factor of about 3.0 the xylitol gum group demonstrated a DMFS-increment which actually decreased by a factor of 1.0. Thus, xylitol might be not only cariostatic, but actually anticariogenic as claimed in one sensational newspaper report.

The remarkable potential benefits of xylitol outlined above may possibly be explained by a number of observations. Human dental plaque does not appear to have significant ability to bind xylitol nor do indigenous oral microorganisms metabolize this sugar-alcohol to any notable extent. Xylitol also increases the flow rate and calcium and phosphate concentrations of saliva which may promote increased buffering and remineralization of the tooth surface. Certainly this factor would help to explain the large numbers of caries reversals observed. Finally, xylitol can strongly stimulate the activity of the antimicrobial enzyme, lactoperoxidase, in saliva.

Notwithstanding the fact that the studies described above constitute one of the most comprehensive and far-reaching oral health research investigations in recent years, certain problems in the studies must be noted:
1. The mean age of the test subjects (27.5 years) was inordinately high for a caries

study, and constitutes an age range in which caries activity is normally low.

2. Subjects often selected which group they wanted to be in so that the subjects were not randomized.

3. Either by selecting their own groups or by means of slight taste differences in the foodstuffs the subject soon learned which group they were in; therefore, the study could not run on a double-blind basis.

4. Foodstuffs other than those in which the sugar composition was known were also consumed by the subjects during the study.

5. Differences in food intake patterns and frequencies were not clearly determined.

6. Caries scoring techniques were quite different than those used by other investigators.

7. Mild diarrhea and flatulence can accompany xylitol intake, although this side-effect does not appear to be intolerable.

In addition to these problems, serious questions have been raised about the potential carcinogenicity and other toxic effects of xylitol. Nevertheless, the potential benefits of xylitol warrant continued studies of its cariostatic effects and toxicity.

PROSPECTS FOR NUTRITIONAL MODIFICATION OF DENTAL CARIES

Optimal Host Resistance

Based on the discussions in the section entitled *Developmental Aspects of Nutrition and Dental Caries*, it is clear that nutritional inadequacies during development of the teeth, jaws, salivary glands, and immune system may substantially alter the resistance of the host to dental caries when the host matures. Although existing knowledge in this aspect of nutrition and oral health, particularly in terms of human studies, is scarce, the animal data which have been cited are exciting. Oral health researchers and clinicians as well should partly redirect their focus on dental caries. This focus should be broadened to include the very real possibility that nutritional stress, and perhaps other subtle environmental stresses during the development of the

craniofacial complex and immune systems may predispose the host to dental caries. The concept that a susceptible tooth is required for the initiation of a carious lesion should be expanded to include not only the size, shape, and composition of the tooth but also a variety of other host factors such as tooth alignment, salivary function, and immunocompetence. Moreover, the fact that dietary fluoride is only one of many nutrients during development which can affect the ultimate expression of dental caries should be emphasized.

The present basis of knowledge does not warrant statements that a certain child has more caries than another simply because of neonatal malnutrition. However, the data do suggest that clinicians should be concerned that pregnant women, infants, and young children consume nutritionally sound diets. In this regard, the traditional practice of supplementing the diets of needy school children with breakfast and lunch subsidies should be partially reoriented to include aid for the pregnant and lactating mother and preschooler. The new federal WIC (Women, Infants, and Children) programs may be most helpful in this matter.

Diet may also assist in maintaining oral tissues in an optimal state of caries resistance post-developmentally. The dietary variable with the greatest post-developmental impact on dental caries is the availability of refined carbohydrate. The form and frequency with which this carbohydrate is supplied to plaque microorganisms appears to be of greater importance than the total amount. Certainly a reduction in the frequency of refined carbohydrate intake, particularly sucrose, is usually accompanied by a reduction in dental caries. However, dietary sugars have been incorporated into a huge proportion of the processed food supply not because of an industrial plot to promote caries but because most consumers enjoy the taste and other properties it imparts to foods. The implications of this problem are discussed more fully in the following section, but it should suffice to indicate that the prospects that large segments of the population will reduce sugar intake simply by dietary discipline are remote. Therefore, alternatives should be examined.

A few questions concerning alternative dietary approaches which, combined with sugar substitutes or modified sugar consumption patterns, might have an impact on dental caries should be considered. First, the role of dietary phosphates and, perhaps more importantly, calcium to phosphorous ratios in dental caries should be further delineated. Is a dietary calcium/phosphorous ratio of 0.55 ideal in caries resistance as suggested by Stanton? What ratio or phosphate level promotes optimum remineralization? Any studies in this area must not fail to consider another recent suggestion that calcium/phosphorous ratios of greater than 1.0 promote optimal resistance to periodontal disease. Second, how does pyridoxine function to reduce caries? What microbial species are inhibited or enhanced? Can other vitamins alter the composition of bacterial plaque? Third, will higher salivary urea levels associated with high protein intake really affect caries activity in man? If so, is it economically and morally sound to increase dietary intake of a nutrient which is in worldwide short supply? Fourth, how does xylitol function to reduce dental caries? What is the relative importance of its sucrose replacement effect versus its stimulation of salivary calcium, phosphorous, lactoperoxidase, and flow rate? Pending clarification of the reported toxic effects of xylitol, it should continue to be studied as a model caries protective agent. In other words, one should not simply note that xylitol stimulates salivary calcium without asking how and whether other compounds might work better.

The Fortification, Processing and Organoleptic Properties of Foods and Sugar Substitutes

The food industry has come under increasing criticism for introducing high proportions of refined carbohydrates, particularly sucrose and more recently "glucose syrups" derived from corn products, into processed foods. Certainly the data in Table 16-2 indicate a dramatic increase in the consumption of sugar included in processed foods in the past 50 years. This factor, in conjunction with the high sugar content of many cereals, drinks, and snack products, and the sophisticated marketing programs which sell these items, support the food activist hypothesis that the food industry has "forced" sugar and possibly dental caries upon the masses. However, it is logical to assume that since the total amount of sucrose consumption has remained constant during the past 50 years, if industry had not added it to processed foods, sucrose would

probably be added in comparable levels at the table by the consumer. Moreover, as noted previously, the human preference for sweet taste is a primary factor in food selection. In fact, it has been argued that the preference for sweet is a fundamental drive which prevented primitive man from consuming toxic compounds. That is, most sweet tasting compounds are safe to eat. In contrast, bitter compounds such as the alkaloids not only taste unpleasant but are potentially life threatening. Moreover, the very fact that sugared products sell well, promotes a vicious cycle of more sugar equals more sales.

Sugar is not always added to products simply to obtain a sweet taste. It is added for a score of reasons including use as a preservative, flavor enhancer, and texturizing agent. These factors contribute to the overall organoleptic or sensory properties of a food; and, it is clear that the pleasant sensation associated with eating a good meal depends not only on the taste, but the smell, temperature, and texture of the food. Considering the multifaceted contributions of sugar to the overall pleasant organoleptic properties of foods, it is not surprising that this "gustatory godsend" permeates the food supply.

Perhaps it would be easier to fault the food industry for its sugar policy if it was ignoring the dental problems associated with frequent sugar intake. However, the industry has consistently searched for alternatives to the use of sugar (Table 16-4). The availability of "sugar-free" soft drinks and the so-called "sugarless" gums and mints are testimony to this effort. Nevertheless, there are a number of problems with these agents. Excessive intake of the sugar alcohols (sorbitol, mannitol, xylitol) used in gums and mints can cause gastrointestinal distress; therefore, the use of these agents cannot be expanded to include a large segment of processed food. Furthermore, saccharin, currently used in most sugar free and dietetic products, leaves a bitter aftertaste, and the Food and Drug Administration has declared that saccharin is a weak carcinogen. Therefore, new compounds are required and the search for caloric and noncaloric sweeteners is both continuous and difficult.

Industrial research programs and investigations at research institutions such as the Monell Center for the Chemical Senses are currently focusing on basic mechanisms of taste perception. An understanding of these mechanisms may make it possible to "engineer" safe

TABLE 16-4. RELATIVE SWEETNESS* OF SUGARS AND OTHER SUBSTANCES

Substance	Sweetness	Substance	Sweetness
Lactose	16	Cyclamate sodium	3,000–8,000
Raffinose	22	Ammoniated glycyrrhizin	5,000
Galactose	32	Naringin dihydrochalcone	
		Hesperidin dihydrochalcone	10,000
Rhamnose	32		
Maltose	32	L-Aspartyl L-phenylalanine methyl ester	10,000–20,000
Xylose	40	Dulcin	7,000–35,000
Sorbitol	54	Stevioside	30,000
Mannitol	57	Suosan	35,000
Glucose	74	Saccharin	20,000–70,000
Sucrose	100	Thaumatin	75,000
Xylitol	100	Neohesperidin dihydrochalcone	200,000
Glycerol	108	Monellin	300,000
Invert Sugar		1-N-Propoxy-2-amino-4-nitrobenzene	
glucose + fructose)	130	(ultrasuss)	400,000
Ethylene glycol	130		
Fructose	173		

* Sucrose is assigned a value of 100 for comparison. Sweet taste depends upon concentration of the sweetener, temperature, pH, type of medium used and sensitivity of the taster.
(Modified from Newbrun E, "The Role of Food Manufacturers in the Dietary Control of Caries" J Am Soc Prev Dent 4: 33–44, 1974)

compounds which either taste sweet themselves or modify the perception of other agents so that they taste sweet. Thus, the industrial research commitment to seek an alternative to sucrose is commendable. However, it is unfortunate that the marketing division, which maintains the ultimate corporate authority in new product development has generally been reluctant to embark on new food programs designed to foster dental health. Someday a company will market a cariostatic snack-food line with the same fervor as its traditional counterpart and be amazed to note that it sells.

Several compounds have been tested in an effort to fortify foods and decrease their cariogenic potential. The most notable example in this group are the organic and inorganic phosphates. These compounds have dramatic cariostatic activity in animals, but as already discussed their efficacy in human populations is variable. Certain factors extracted from cocoa beans have been reported to sharply reduce caries in hamsters. Indeed, one human trial indicated that individuals who consumed chocolate and skim milk powder for 5 days had significantly less plaque than after a similar period on a normal mixed diet. Moreover, the Vipeholm study also suggested that chocolate is less cariogenic than one might predict based on its sucrose content. Therefore, the caries protective potential of cocoa powder is worthy of further study. Finally, the dramatic results of the Turku Sugar Studies suggest

that xylitol may be an important caries protective agent not simply as a sucrose substitute but also as a food additive for its cariostatic activity *per se*. Once the Turku studies are confirmed using more conventional caries scoring methodology and if xylitol receives safety clearance, it is anticipated that there will be a marked increase in its utilization in processed foods.

Although the effects of food processing on the cariogenicity of foods is sometimes ignored, it has been shown to affect caries experience. The particle size of certain compounds, hydration state, physical consistency, and heat processing may each modify the cariogenicity of a food. These factors do not usually vary in a predictable fashion. For example, heat treatment of starch can either increase or decrease its ability to be fermented by *Streptococcus mutans* depending upon the temperature and duration of the heat treatment.

Modification of Diet Composition and Food Intake Patterns

Although a number of pre- and post-developmental nutritional factors in the host as well as food fortification programs have interesting potential in the control of dental caries, the practical application of these systems is several years away. Therefore, preventive oriented dental clinicians have resorted to traditional methods of dietary modification to effect improvements in the oral health of their patients. This modification program usually consists of substituting nutritious foods for their cariogenic counterparts, ensuring intake of a well-proportioned diet, and changing the frequency and time frame in which certain foods are consumed. The philosophy and methodology for this type of program is discussed extensively in the following chapter.

The Challenge

This chapter has underscored the unequivocal importance of diet and nutrition in the process of dental caries. In spite of the advances in this area the fact that nutrition plays a role in every phase of the caries process—host development and resistance, selection of a microflora, and substrate supply to that microflora—mandates that both research and applied programs in nutrition and oral health be accelerated.

At the level of the granting agencies such as the National Institute for Dental Research (NIDR), American Fund for Dental Health, foundations, and private philanthropies more funds should be allocated for basic nutrition research. The science of nutrition spans the entire spectrum of the NIDR scientific mission including craniofacial biology, periodontal disease, caries, and stomatology. In addition, advances in nutrition research using oral problems as models can almost definitely be applied to other biomedical situations. These advances should parallel the medical applications derived from the basic immunology, microbiology, and collagen research which was strongly supported by NIDR in the past. Thus, grant support for basic research in nutrition and oral health will pay dividends in many other health disciplines.

The corporate responsibility, including the various trade organizations, should be expanded to include funding for "mission oriented" research. Industry routinely uses universities in third party trials of new products in a specifically "targeted" research program. However, non-targeted industrial funding is in short supply most probably because corporate policy-makers want more immediate returns for their research dollars. Therefore, increased support for mission-oriented research programs funded by industry would serve a twofold purpose. First, university

based investigators working in a "mission-oriented" program would not be stifled by the immediate needs of a company for new product development. Second, by defining relatively narrow missions, corporate authorities could ensure that a high proportion of their investment was returned in areas relevant to long-range industrial goals.

Finally, the educational system should be reoriented toward preventive health care including nutrition at several levels. Every dental school should have a meaningful nutrition course, not simply a course on dietary counseling which focuses on *how* to modify diet rather than on *why* nutrition is important in oral health. NIDR has taken commendable steps to provide skilled manpower for these programs and, at the time of this writing, supports two programs to train dental research/educators in nutrition. From another point-of-view nutritionists and dietitians should be more thoroughly trained in oral health problems. They can then make viable contributions not only to preventive oriented health care teams in the dental office but also to large numbers of students in primary and secondary schools. Finally, an appropriate regulatory agency could require that a small portion of all corporate food advertising budgets should be channeled to an independent agency and used to support research in dental nutrition and to provide basic nutrition information to the masses via television, radio, and the press.

SUMMARY

Numerous aspects of the role of nutrition in the process of dental caries have been outlined. Nutritional inadequacy during development can alter the subsequent resistance of the host to dental caries by modifying tooth composition and alignment, salivary gland function, and immuno-competence. After eruption, diet is important in enamel maturation, salivary flow rate and composition, and the selection and metabolism of the oral microflora.

Epidemiologic studies and clinical trials have suggested a strong relationship between dental caries experience and sugar intake. However, this relationship does not seem to be linear and many factors other than the total amount of sugar consumed appear to modify the expression of dental caries. In this regard, the form and frequency of sugar intake is more important than the total amount eaten, and certain dietary variables such as fluoride, phosphates, and tannins can reduce the caries process. Based on this basic information, the prospects for dietary control of

dental decay were discussed. Moreover, specific challenges were issued to the research grant system, food industry research programs, the educational system, and the dental profession. If these challenges can be met, the public can expect some striking advances in oral preventive health care.

GLOSSARY

Calciotraumatic lime. A band of disturbed calcification in the dentin of young rats maintained on a rachitogenic diet.

Cauque lesion. A hypoplastic lesion of the enamel of the deciduous dentition. This lesion was named for the Guatemalan village of Santa Maria Cauque in which it was first identified. The lesion is thought to be related to neonatal malnutrition and infection.

Critical period. A time frame in the development of an organ or tissue during which environmental stress, such as infection or malnutrition, may result in irreversible damage to that organ.

Development. The manifestation of the combined effects of growth and differentiation; that is, an increase in cell number, size, and specialization.

Differentiation. A progressive increase in cellular specialization which can be demonstrated morphologically, biochemically and physiologically.

Enamel hypoplasia. A defect of enamel matrix formation which may be mediated by hereditary or environmental factors. Teeth with enamel hypoplasia are predisposed to dental caries.

Enamel fluid. A fluid thought to originate from the dental pulp by passage through the dentin and enamel. Neither the existence nor composition of this fluid has been definitely established.

Gingival fluid. A fluid, derived from gingival tissues, which flows from the orifice of the gingival crevice.

It contains electrolytes, proteins, urea, and other serum derived compounds but not in the same concentration as in serum.

Growth. The increase in cell number and/or cell size of an organism which is measurable either biochemically or anthropometrically.

Hyperplasia. An increase in cell numbers of a growing organ or tissue. This process can be biochemically estimated by measuring an increase in DNA per unit weight of tissue.

Hypertrophy. An increase in cell size of a growing organ or tissue. This process can be estimated biochemically by measuring an increase in protein per unit of DNA.

Mellanby hypoplasia. Microscopic defects in the enamel surface which may be caused by nutritional deficiency and are closely linked to increased caries susceptibility.

Organoleptic. The ability to stimulate any of the organs of sensation.

Sorbitol. A sugar alcohol of the hexitol group produced by catalytic hydrogenation of glucose. It occurs in the berries of many fruits and seaweeds and is often a component in the so-called "sugarless" gums and mints. It can be fermented by *Streptococcus mutans* but at rates which are usually lower than sucrose.

Xylitol. A five carbon sugar alcohol which can be commercially extracted from birch trees (birch sugar). It has not been shown to be fermented by *Streptoccus mutans* and demonstrates dramatic efficacy as a replacement for sucrose in caries control.

SUGGESTED READINGS

Alfano MC (ed): Changing Perspectives in Nutrition and Caries Research. New York, MEDCOM, Inc. 1979

Alfano MC: Effect of diet and malnutrition during development on resistance to oral disease. In Wei S (ed) National Symposium on Dental Nutrition, University of Iowa Press pp 23–35, 1979

Brown AT: Carbohydrate metabolism in caries-conducive oral Streptococci. In Sipple HL, McNutt KW (eds): Sugars in Nutrition. New York, Academic Press, 1974

Brown AT: The role of dietary carbohydrates in plaque formation and oral disease. Nutr Rev 33: 353–361, 1975

Carlos JP (ed): Prevention and Oral Health. Bethesda, National Institutes of Health, DHEW Pub No. (HIH) 74–707, 1974

Dawes C: Effects of diet on salivary secretion and composition. J Dent Res 49: 1263–1272, 1970

DePaola DP, Alfano MC: Triphasic nutritional analysis and dietary counseling. Dent Clin North Am 20: 613–634, 1976

DePaola DP, Alfano MC: Nutrition and oral health. Nutr Today 12: 6–32, 1977

DePaola DP, Kuftinec MM: Nutrition in growth and development of oral tissues. Dent Clin North Am 20: 441–460, 1976

Finn SB, Glass RB: Sugar and dental decay. World Rev Nutr Diet 22: 304–326, 1975

Golub LM, Kleinberg I: Gingival crevicular fluid: a new diagnostic acid in managing the periodontal patient. Oral Sci Rev 8: 49–62, 1976

Gustafsson B, Quensel CE, Lanke L, Lundquist C, Grahnen H, Gonow BE, Krasse B: The Vipeholm dental caries study: the effect of different levels of carbohydrate intake on caries activity in 436 individuals observed for five years. Acta Odontol Scand 11: 232–363, 1954

Harris R: Biology of the children of Hopewood House, Bowral, Australia. Observations on dental caries experience extending over five years (1957–1961). J Dent Res 42: 1387–1399, 1963

Hunt CE, Navia JM: Pre-eruptive effects of Mo, B, Sr and F on dental caries in the rat. Arch Oral Biol 20: 497–501, 1975

Kreitzman SN: Nutrition in the process of dental caries. Dent Clin North Am 20: 491–506, 1976

Menaker L, Navia JM: Effect of undernutrition during the perinatal period on caries development in the rat: II, III, IV. J Dent Res 52: 680–697, 1973

Menaker L, Navia JM: Effect of undernutrition during the perinatal period on caries development in the rat. V. Changes in whole saliva volume and protein content. J Dent Res 53: 592–597, 1974

Mäkinen KK: Sugars and the formation of dental plaque. In Sipple HL, McNutt KW (eds): Sugars in Nutrition. New York, Academic Press, 1974

Mäkinen KK: Dental aspects of consumption of xylitol and fructose diets. Int Dent J 26: 14–28, 1976

Navia JM, DiOrio LP, Menaker L, Miller S: Effect of undernutrition during the perinatal period on caries development in the rat. J Dent Res 49: 1091–1098, 1970

Navia JM: Prevention of dental caries: agents which increase tooth resistance to dental caries. Int Dent J 22: 427–440, 1972

Navia JM: Nutrition and oral disease. In Caldwell RC, Stallard RE (eds): A Textbook of Preventive Dentistry. Philadelphia, WB Saunders, 1977

Newbrun E: The role of food manufacturers in the dietary control of caries. J Am Soc Prev Dent 4: 33–44, 1974

Newbrun E: Etiology of dental caries. In Caldwell RC, Stallard RE (eds): A Textbook of Preventive Dentistry. Philadelphia, WB Saunders, 1977

Nizel AE: Nutrition and oral problems. World Rev Nutr Diet 16: 226–252, 1973

Nizel AE: Nutrition in Preventive Dentistry: Science and Practice. Philadelphia, WB Saunders, 1972

Russell AL: Carbohydrates as a causative factor in dental caries: epidemiological evidence. In Sipple HL, McNutt KW (eds): Sugars in Nutrition. New York, Academic Press, 1974

Scheinin A: Caries control through the use of sugar substitutes. Int Dent J 26: 4–13, 1976

Scheinin A, Makinen KK, Ylitalo K: Turku sugar studies. I. An intermediate report on the effect of sucrose, fructose and xylitol diets on the caries incidence in Man. Acta Odontol Scand 32: 383–412, 1974

Shaw JH, Sweeney EA: Nutrition in relation to dental medicine. In Goodhart RS, Shils ME (eds): Modern Nutrition in Health and Disease. Philadelphia, Lea & Febiger, 1973

Sweeney EA, Cabrera J, Urrutia J, Mata L: Factors associated with linear hypolasia of human deciduous incisors. J Dent Res 48: 1275–1279, 1969

Sweeteners: Issues and Uncertainties. Academy Forum, Washington DC, National Academy of Sciences, 1975

Tonge C, McCance R: Normal development of the jaws and teeth in pigs, and the delay and malocclusion produced by calorie deficiencies. J Anat 115: 1–22, 1973

17 Nutritional Analysis and Dietary Counseling

MICHAEL C. ALFANO

DOMINICK P. DePAOLA

LEWIS MENAKER

Nutritional Analysis
  Triphasic Nutritional Analysis
  Phase I: Medical and Social History, Clinical Exam, Qualitative Dietary Analysis
  Phase II: Semiquantitative Dietary Analysis, Laboratory Tests, Clinical Trials
  Phase III: Complex Tests of Metabolic Function
Dietary Counseling
  The "Caveat"

Behavioral Aspects of Food Intake
Nutrition Counseling Technique: A Team Approach
Integrating Nutrition into a Preventive Dentistry Program
Special Problems
Dietary Supplementation
Summary
Glossary
Suggested Readings

The oral health profession may take justifiable pride in the significant, often pioneering, role which it has played in the research, development, and delivery of preventive health care. The elucidation of the importance of fluorides in dental caries control, the untiring clinical educational and political efforts to deliver the benefits of fluoride to the public, and the continuing research on mechanisms of fluoride action constitute one of the most significant public health programs known to man. Nevertheless, many "preventive-oriented" dentists who conscientiously utilize fluorides, plaque control, hypertensive screening, and other effective preventive techniques are often incomplete in their approach

to preventive dentistry. In this regard, one of the most frequently neglected and improperly performed preventive services is dietary analysis and counseling. Although virtually all oral health professionals are aware of the role of diet in dental caries, many either ignore this important factor in oral disease or simply admonish the patient to "kick the sweet snack habit". This approach is at best naive and will probably lead to noncompliance with continuing decline in the oral health and possibly general health of the patient. The purpose of this chapter is to delineate an integrated system for the incorporation of nutritional analysis and dietary counseling into the clinical practice of preventive dentistry. The reader should review the fundamental aspects of nutrition in the process of dental caries discussed in the previous chapter in order to appreciate the rationale for the dietary analysis and counseling system presented in this chapter. The reader is also advised to examine the methods of Nizel, DiOrio, Pollack, Madsen, Clark and others which represent alternative approaches to dietary modification.

NUTRITIONAL ANALYSIS

The numerous social, ethnic, behavioral, and financial aspects of diet selection dictate that both haphazard, "How's your diet?", and unidirectional, "Cut-down on sweets", approaches to dietary management are doomed to failure. Moreover the complex interactions of nutrients in the development and maintenance of oral tissues indicate that no single nutrient can be singled out for an exclusive role in dental caries or periodontal disease. Thus the clinician must confront several problems if he is to succeed in improving the nutritional status and oral health of his patients. What nutrients are important in the disease process? What is the dietary intake of the patient? Why does the patient consume a particular diet? Do local or systemic factors complicate nutrient intake, absorption, utilization or storage? Can the food intake patterns of this individual be beneficially modified?

Each of the above questions can be answered by employing a systematic method for nutritional analysis which progresses in phases of increasing complexity as warranted by the needs of the patient. The triphasic method of nutritional analysis is particularly useful in clinical practice because, although all patients are screened, testing progresses only to the point at which a definitive nutritional analysis can be made. Patients are not subjected to complex tests of nutrient reserves and metabolic function unless warranted by data obtained in the initial phases of the program. The clinician can terminate the nutritional analysis after any phase provided that adequate information is available to insure a sound basis for diagnosis. Should the diagnosis indicate a nutritional problem the dentist can institute dietary modification and,

when indicated, refer the patient to an appropriately trained physician.

Triphasic Nutritional Analysis

Phase I: Medical and Social History, Clinical Exam, Qualitative Dietary Analysis

All dental patients should be screened for possible nutritional problems by means of a medical and social history, a comprehensive clinical examination and a qualitative dietary analysis. Although latent nutritional problems can rarely be diagnosed directly from a medical and social history, important indicators of potential nutritional problems may be uncovered. The patient may present with a history of such nutritionally related problems as chronic alcoholism, gastrointestinal resection, recent infection, celiac disease, or gastric ulcers. Moreover, physiologic processes such as pregnancy, lactation, and growth as well as other conditioning factors can markedly increase metabolic requirements and should be carefully evaluated for their impact on nutritional status (Table 17-1).

A good medical history is the critically important first step in the nutritional analysis of a patient. In this regard, the importance of systemic factors in the possible etiology of oral problems must be stressed to the patient, or in the case of children to their parents. Patients are often inclined to conceal systemic problems which they think are unrelated to caries and periodontal disease.

The clinician should also strive to develop a comprehensive social history of the patient. The social history is important in nutritional analysis because of the intimate associations between food habits and ethnic, religious, and socioeconomic factors. The data obtained in a social history is an absolute necessity if one is to be successful in modifying the dietary habits of an individual. This relationship will be discussed further in the section on dietary counseling.

In conducting the social history, the clinician should be careful to note the financial status of the patient or his parents. Can the individual afford to purchase the required foods? As the income of an individual decreases the relative expenses for food in his budget can increase dramatically; therefore, he must be counseled how to purchase high

TABLE 17-1. FACTORS IN THE MEDICAL HISTORY SUGGESTIVE OF NUTRITIONAL PROBLEMS

Factor	Example	Comments
Physiological stressors	Pregnancy, Lactation, Growth	Increased requirements for most nutrients but particularly folate, calcium, protein and iron
Food allergies and intolerance	Milk	Usually due to protein allergy or lactose intolerance, insure adequate protein and calcium intake.
	Celiac disease (non-tropical sprue)	Eliminate wheat and possibly milk products
Drug therapy	Contraceptive steroids	Increased requirements for: Folate, Ascorbic acid, B_6
	Anticonvulsants	Folate
	Cathartics	Impaired absorption of:
	Mineral oil	Fat soluble vitamins
	Magnesium salts	Calcium
Recent trauma or infection	Bone fractures, Oral surgical procedures, Measles	Trauma and infection may cause prolonged negative balances for a number of nutrients especially protein, ascorbate and zinc
Chronic diseases	Alcoholism	Probable multiple deficiencies particularly thiamin and folate
Gastrointestinal surgery	Gastrectomy	Intramuscular injections of B_{12} required
Non-specific symptomatology	Fatigue, Dizziness, Apathy, Glossodynia, Itchy skin	These factors are often considered to be psychological due to their vague nature; however, they should be evaluated for possible nutritional etiologies.
Parasitic infection	Hookworm	Increased iron requirements
Weight gain or loss	Dieting Systemic disease	Determine etiology of weight alterations, be suspicious of fad diets

quality, low cost foods. Asking the patient to describe a typical "daily routine" is a useful, indirect method for obtaining information about his social status. This method is also a useful supplement to a dietary history. For example, a child with a rampant caries problem may neglect to record all snacks during the day on a diet diary. However, when asked to describe a typical day he may indicate the following:

"Awake at . . . . juice and cookies for breakfast . . . . usually stop for cupcakes at the corner store on the way to school . . . . candy bar at morning recess . . . ."

Finally, in recording a social history, the clinician should note certain personality "keys." The elderly person living alone, food faddist, college student, alcoholic and others often have life styles which predispose to nutritional problems.

The dentist should routinely examine his patients for the clinical signs suggestive of nutritional inadequacy. As the patient walks into the examining room the dentist should note his height, weight, posture and gait. After the patient is seated in the dental chair, the following structures should be sequentially examined under good lighting: head, hair, eyes, nose, skin, neck, nails, lips, tongue, mucosa, gingiva, and teeth. These structures should be

studied for the problems listed in Table 17-2. It is interesting to note that the dentist has a particular advantage in detecting early clinical signs of malnutrition because many classic signs of nutritional deficiency occur in and around the oral cavity. It should be noted, however, that these tissues respond to stress in a limited number of ways, and that the changes noted are usually only suggestive of a nutritional problem. Therefore, problems noted in the clinical exam should be confirmed by medical, social, and dietary histories and, when appropriate, biochemical tests and clinical trials.

The dentist has more experience in evaluating the host response to chronic irritation than any other health professional. This experience provides the clinician with one final unique tool for detecting latent systemic problems - the "oral bioassay". As originally defined by Alfano, this assay is based on the subjective integration by the dentist of the amount of local irritants (plaque, calculus, overhanging restorations, etc.) present around the teeth with the degree of periodontal destruction present. Any exaggerated response of the local tissues which is inconsistent with the amount of local irritants present should greatly increase the clinician's suspicion of systemic involvement. Although this assay is nonspecific, variable, and based on

TABLE 17-2. COMPONENTS OF THE CLINICAL EXAM SUGGESTIVE OF NUTRITIONAL PROBLEMS

Component	Alteration	Possible Inadequacy*
Weight	Excessive or inadequate fat storage	Excessive or inadequate calorie intake
Head	Bossing	Vitamin D
Hair	Brittle, pluckable, sparse, depigmentation	Protein
Eyes	Xerophthalmia, photophobia, night blindness, Bitot spots, keratomalacia	Vitamin A
	Circumcorneal injection, canthal fissures	Riboflavin
Nose	Nasolabial seborrhea	Riboflavin
Skin	Edema	Protein
	Dyssebacea	Riboflavin
	Xerosis, follicular hyperkeratosis	Vitamin A
	Perifolliculitis, petechiae, purpura,	Ascorbate
	Pellagrous dermatitis	Niacin
Neck	Casal's necklace	Niacin
	Goiter	Iodine
Fingernails	Fragility, bands, lines	Protein
Lips	Angular cheilosis, angular scars	Riboflavin, B complex
	Pallor	Iron
Tongue	Pallor, magenta color, red color, papillary hypertrophy, papillary atrophy	Iron, B complex, particularly thiamin and riboflavin
	Fissuring	Vitamin A?
Oral Mucosa	Pallor	Iron, folate, B_{12}
	Red color	B complex
	Hyperkeratosis	Vitamin A
Gingiva	Red and spongy	Ascorbate
	Gingivitis	Multiple nutrient deficiencies
	Pallor	Iron, folate, B_{12}
Teeth	Caries	Fluoride, excessive sugar intake
	Linear Hypoplasia, melanodontia, malposition	Developmental nutrient deficiencies
Oral Bioassay	Excessive periodontal destruction relative to amount of local irritation	Multiple nutrient deficiencies

* It should be noted that the deficiencies listed are only suggested by the tissue alterations described. Confirmatory data must be obtained to determine the exact etiology of the tissue changes which may be due strictly to local factors as well as nutritional and other systemic problems.

considerably more "experience" than "science", it provides useful cues to the need for more definitive nutritional analysis.

Careful daily recording of food intake by the patient in the form of a diet diary can be converted into diet patterns and food groups which suggest nutritional problems to the dentist. This appears to be a straightforward, simple procedure and, indeed, this approach has been used to correct dietary imbalances successfully for many years. However, it suffers from several problems when applied to dental practice. First, the "Four Food Groups" method of dietary education has been overworked and, with the exception of children, may be too simplistic for today's sophisticated consumers. Second, there is great variability of nutrient composition within a given group. For example, a peach has 33 times more vitamin A than a pear but both are categorized in the fruit group. Finally, this analysis takes considerable time and when conducted by the dentist would be prohibitively costly for many patients. Therefore, it is recommended that this type of qualitative dietary analysis is most effective when conducted in conjunction with an appropriately trained auxiliary (e.g., nutritionist, dietitian, or specially trained dental hygienist). The interaction between the dentist, auxiliary, patient and physician will be discussed at length in the counseling section of this chapter.

Assuming that the oral health care team has the capability to interpret a diet diary in a qualitative manner, the additional factors of the diet diary being complete, honest, and recorded during an appropriate time frame must be considered. Many patients will not record certain "incriminating" items while others may either make up a false report to include several "good" foods or make an unusual effort to include these items in their menu.

Both approaches should be discouraged, and the patient must be informed that he is not being tested. He is receiving an important health service which is only valuable when accurate information is provided. In this regard the patient should be carefully instructed at the outset in recording the type, amount, and time of food consumption. Preprinted forms such as those developed by Nizel, Pollack, or DePaola or those which may be used by a local dental school are useful for this purpose. Diaries are usually recorded for 4 to 7 days including a weekend or holiday.

Should possible nutritional problems be detected based on the medical/social history, clinical exam, or qualitative dietary analysis, the evaluation should usually progress to Phase II. However, if enough information exists at the conclusion of Phase I to ensure a sound basis for therapy, the nutritional assessment can be terminated and appropriate dietary counseling instituted. For example, when the only problem is frequent sugar consumption by a caries-prone individual, dietary modifications can be implemented in conjunction with oral hygiene procedures at the end of Phase I.

Phase II: Semiquantitative Dietary Analysis, Laboratory Tests, Clinical Trials

When a nutritional problem is uncovered during Phase I analysis but this problem is not clearly defined, the analysis should progress to Phase II. For example, the medical history of a patient may reveal that he is easily fatigued and often tired, on clinical exam the tongue and mucous membranes are pale, and the qualitative dietary analysis indicates a lack of vegetables in the diet. These data are suggestive of nutritional anemia but the precise etiology remains unknown. Therefore more information is required. Depending upon the background of the dentist he may elect to refer the patient at this stage to an appropriately trained physician. However, most dentists should have the knowledge and confidence to proceed with the analysis, and most dental schools currently include the components of Phase II in their curriculum. These components include a semi-quantitative dietary analysis and a routine blood chemistry including a differential blood count, postprandial glucose determination, and possibly a glucose tolerance test.

The semi-quantitative approach to dietary analysis is comparable to the qualitative analysis of Phase I with the exception that the intake of individual nutrients is estimated more accurately. Several commercial computer-assisted dietary analysis services are available to facilitate the semi-quantitative listing of individual nutrients. Nevertheless, it is most important to note that these services are not all based on the same type of data input and, therefore, their relative usefulness is variable. Those services based on the "dietary intake frequency questionnaire", although relatively inexpensive, require that the patient indicate his food intake by selecting from a list of 50-60 predetermined foods in common use. This system suffers from the dual problem that the patient has to develop the listing entirely from "recall" and has limited opportunity to list the limitless range of ethnic, religious, or regional recipes consumed because of the restrictive questionnaire format. A superior method, in contrast, is the recording of a food diary as previously discussed which permits the patient to list each food consumed at the time it is actually eaten. The computer analyzed diet diary method is more costly because the information in the diary cannot simply be punched into the computer by a key punch operator but must be integrated first by a highly skilled nutritionist. Since "triphasic nutritional analysis" is a sequential but integrated method, the qualitative diet diary recorded in Phase I should be in a format which can be utilized without revision by the computer assisted dietary service. An example of the kind of information which a diet diary based computer analysis can provide is illustrated in Figure 17-1.

The medical laboratory provides important assistance in evaluating the health status of the patient, and the data provided may be used to rule out problems or focus on individual abnormalities. By means of automated techniques, a multiple test profile of the hematology and blood chemistry are available at low cost and are performed with reasonable accuracy. This profile typically includes such parameters as postprandial glucose, uric acid, alkaline phosphatose, serum proteins, blood urea nitrogen, calcium, phosphorous, hemoglobin, cholesterol, and triglycerides. In addition, a differential blood count in conjunction with hemoglobin, hermatocrit, mean corpuscular volume, and mean corpuscular hemoglobin determinations are useful in differen-

(*Text continues on p. 374*)

```
********************************************

                      NUTRAN

              DIET        ANALYSIS

     ********************************************

              DIET ANALYSIS OF..........
              PREPARED FOR DR. M. ALFANO 91175
                      PATIENT'S COPY


INSIDE YOUR PERSONAL NUTRAN REPORT
-----------------------------------
PAGE 2: QUICK REFERENCE SUMMARY OF NUTRIENT TOTALS
        AVERAGE AMOUNTS PER DAY AND THE PERCENT
        OF RECOMMENDED INTAKE FOR EACH.

PAGES 3-4: NUTRIENTS GROUPED BY METABOLIC FUNCTION.
           COMPARISON OF ACTUAL INTAKE WITH RECOMMENDED INTAKE.

PAGE 5: PROBLEM NUTRIENTS....THESE NUTRIENTS ARE LIKELY
        TO BE CONSUMED IN EXCESS.

PAGES 6-8: USING FOOD TO SUPPLY NUTRIENTS.....
           READY REFERENCE GUIDE TO FOODS RICH IN
           THE IMPORTANT NUTRIENTS NEEDED IN A HEALTHY
           DIET.  USE THIS HANDY GUIDE TO PLAN MENUS
           THAT WILL IMPROVE THE NUTRITIONAL VALUE OF
           THE DIET.
```

```
                                            PAGE TWO


THE RECOMMENDED VALUES LISTED BELOW ARE IN MOST CASES THOSE SUGGESTED BY THE NATIONAL RESEARCH COUNCIL (1973)
WHERE NO VALUES ARE SUGGESTED BY THE NRC, NUTRAN HAS SET RECOMMENDED VALUES BASED UPON THE BEST JUDGEMENTS OF OUR
CONSULTANTS AND THE CURRENT LITERATURE.  THE ACTUAL VALUES USED ARE PRESENTED IN THE SUBSEQUENT TABLE UNDER THE
HEADING....YOUR DIET SHOULD CONTAIN....

***NOTE....100% VALUES FOR FAT,SODIUM OR CHOLESTEROL SHOULD BE INTERPRETED AS A PRUDENT MAXIMUM INTAKE.****


                                              THIS SPACE FOR DOCTOR'S USE
                                              --------------------------
NUTRIENT          TOTAL    DAILY   PERCENT OF RECOMMENDED
                  4 DAYS  AVERAGE  AMOUNT PER DAY
========          =====   =======  ============================

CALORIES          8906.3  2226.6   106.0
CHO-GRAMS         1040.4   260.1    88.2
FAT-GRAMS          396.5    99.1   122.4 TOO HIGH
PROTEIN-GRAMS      264.5    66.1   143.8
SODIUM-MG         5976.9  1494.2    29.9 KEEP LOW
CALCIUM-MG        2392.9   598.2    74.8
PHOSPHORUS-MG     3604.7   901.2   112.6
THIAMINE-MCG      3988.2   997.0    90.6
NIACIN-MG           46.5    11.6    83.0
VIT.A-IU         15426.8  4106.7   102.7
MAGNESIUM-MG       443.8   110.9    37.0 TOO LOW
IRON-MG             39.3     9.8    54.6 TOO LOW
RIBOFLAVIN-MCG    5067.0  1266.8    90.5
VIT.C-MG           535.5   134.1   298.1
VIT.E-MG(IU)        46.1    11.5    96.1
VIT.B-12-MCG        16.6     4.1   138.3
FOLIC ACID-MCG     223.2    55.8    13.9 TOO LOW
FLUORIDE-MCG       574.1   143.5    14.4 TOO LOW
CHOLESTEROL-MG    1328.6   332.1    66.4 KEEP LOW


PERCENT CALORIES AS CARBOHYDRATE  48.1132

PERCENT CALORIES AS FAT  40.0269

PERCENT CALORIES AS PROTEIN  11.8598

THERE WERE   5  CUPS OF COFFEE CONSUMED DURING THE PERIOD
THERE WERE   0  CUPS OF TEA CONSUMED DURING THE PERIOD
THERE WERE  2.17  SERVINGS OF CARBONATED BEVERAGES CONSUMED
THERE WERE  1.5   SERVINGS OF ALCOHOLIC BEVERAGES, BEER OR WINE CONSUMED
```

Fig. 17-1. An example of the data output provided by a computer assisted dietary analysis service based upon a diet diary. (NUTRAN,™ PO Box 15464, Atlanta, Georgia)

```
                              PAGE THREE

           PROPER FUNCTIONING OF ALL SYSTEMS IS NECESSARY
           FOR A HEALTHY BODY.  CELLS AND TISSUES REQUIRE
           MANY NUTRIENTS WORKING TOGETHER AND AT THE SAME
           TIME TO PRODUCE OPTIMAL HEALTH.  FROM A STUDY
           OF BODY CHEMISTRY, SOME NUTRIENTS APPEAR TO BE
           MOST DIRECTLY ASSOCIATED WITH CERTAIN DISTINCT
           BODY FUNCTIONS.  THESE ARE GROUPED BELOW TO SUGGEST
           AREAS OF MAJOR IMPORTANCE FOR EACH NUTRIENT.  IT MUST
           BE REMEMBERED THAT ALL THE SYSTEMS ARE CONNECTED SO
           THAT PROBLEMS IN ONE AREA CAN LEAD TO MANY SECONDARY
           PROBLEMS.


WEIGHT PRODUCING FACTORS
-------------------------                  YOUR DIET CONTAINS              YOUR DIET SHOULD CONTAIN
                                           ------------------              ------------------------
CALORIES                                   2226 CALORIES                   2100   CALORIES
CARBOHYDRATE                               260  GRAMS                      100- 295   GRAMS
FAT                                        99   GRAMS                      LESS THAN 81 GRAMS

IF WEIGHT IS A PROBLEM, THE NUTRIENTS ABOVE SHOULD BE RESTRICTED

NUTRIENTS IMPORTANT IN ENERGY METABOLISM
----------------------------------------   YOUR DIET CONTAINS              YOUR DIET SHOULD CONTAIN
                                           ------------------              ------------------------
MAGNESIUM                                  110  MILLIGRAMS                 300 MILLIGRAMS
PHOSPHORUS                                 901  MILLIGRAMS                 800 MILLIGRAMS
IRON                                       9 MILLIGRAMS                    18  MILLIGRAMS
THIAMINE                                   997 MICROGRAMS                  1100   MICROGRAMS
RIBOFLAVIN                                 1266 MICROGRAMS                 1400   MICROGRAMS
NIACIN                                     11 MILLIGRAMS                   14  MILLIGRAMS
PROTEIN                                    66   GRAMS                      46  GRAMS

NUTRIENTS IMPORTANT FOR BLOOD BUILDING AND CLOTTING
---------------------------------------------------   YOUR DIET CONTAINS   YOUR DIET SHOULD CONTAIN
                                                      ------------------   ------------------------
IRON                                       9 MILLIGRAMS                    18  MILLIGRAMS
CALCIUM                                    598  MILLIGRAMS                 800 MILLIGRAMS
FOLIC ACID                                 55   MICROGRAMS                 400 MICROGRAMS
VITAMIN B-12                               4 MICROGRAMS                    3   MICROGRAMS
PROTEIN                                    66   GRAMS                      46  GRAMS



                              PAGE FOUR

NUTRIENTS IMPORTANT FOR TISSUE REPAIR AND HEALING
-------------------------------------------------   YOUR DIET CONTAINS     YOUR DIET SHOULD CONTAIN
                                                    ------------------     ------------------------
MAGNESIUM                                  110  MILLIGRAMS                 300 MILLIGRAMS
FOLIC ACID                                 55   MICROGRAMS                 400 MICROGRAMS
VITAMIN C                                  134  MILLIGRAMS                 45  MILLIGRAMS
PROTEIN                                    66   GRAMS                      46  GRAMS

NUTRIENTS IMPORTANT FOR MUSCLE DEVELOPMENT AND FUNCTION
-------------------------------------------------------   YOUR DIET CONTAINS   YOUR DIET SHOULD CONTAIN
                                                          ------------------   ------------------------
CALCIUM                                    598  MILLIGRAMS                 800 MILLIGRAMS
MAGNESIUM                                  110  MILLIGRAMS                 300 MILLIGRAMS
FOLIC ACID                                 55   MICROGRAMS                 400 MICROGRAMS
VITAMIN E                                  11   INTERNATIONAL UNITS        12  INTERNATIONAL UNITS
PROTEIN                                    66   GRAMS                      46  GRAMS

NUTRIENTS FOR BONES AND TEETH
-----------------------------              YOUR DIET CONTAINS              YOUR DIET SHOULD CONTAIN
                                           ------------------              ------------------------
CALCIUM                                    598  MILLIGRAMS                 800 MILLIGRAMS
PHOSPHORUS                                 901  MILLIGRAMS                 800 MILLIGRAMS
MAGNESIUM                                  110  MILLIGRAMS                 300 MILLIGRAMS
FLUORIDE                                   143  MICROGRAMS                 1000   MICROGRAMS
VITAMIN A                                  4106 INTERNATIONAL UNITS        4000   INTERNATIONAL UNITS
VITAMIN C                                  134  MILLIGRAMS                 45  MILLIGRAMS

NUTRIENTS THAT CAN INCREASE RESISTANCE TO INFECTION
---------------------------------------------------   YOUR DIET CONTAINS   YOUR DIET SHOULD CONTAIN
                                                      ------------------   ------------------------
VITAMIN A                                  4106 INTERNATIONAL UNITS        4000   INTERNATIONAL UNITS
VITAMIN C                                  134  MILLIGRAMS                 45  MILLIGRAMS
PROTEIN                                    66   GRAMS                      46  GRAMS
```

Fig. 17-1. (*Continued*)

PAGE FIVE

PROBLEM NUTRIENTS

WHEN CONSUMED IN EXCESS, THESE NUTRIENTS CAN
LEAD TO METABOLIC PROBLEMS AND ARE BELIEVED
BY MANY AUTHORITIES TO BE RISK FACTORS IN
VARIOUS DISEASES. IF YOUR INTAKE OF ANY OF
THE FOLLOWING NUTRIENTS IS EXCESSIVE IT WOULD
BE PRUDENT TO MAKE DIETARY ADJUSTMENTS.

	YOUR DIET CONTAINS	YOUR DIET SHOULD CONTAIN NO MORE THAN
CHOLESTEROL	332 MILLIGRAMS	500 MILLIGRAMS
FAT	99 GRAMS	81 GRAMS
SODIUM	1494 MILLIGRAMS	5000 MILLIGRAMS
CARBOHYDRATE	260 GRAMS	300 GRAMS
CALORIES	2226 CALORIES	2100 CALORIES

****

IF THIS ANALYSIS INDICATES THAT YOU ARE NOT EATING A BALANCED DIET, IT SHOULD BE AN INDICATION TO YOU THAT
ADDITIONAL NUTRIENTS ARE LIKELY TO BE MISSING FROM YOUR DIET AS WELL. WITHOUT THESE BODY COMPONENTS OBTAINED
FROM FOOD, THE BODY IS DEFENSELESS. THINK ABOUT YOUR NUTRIENT RESERVES IN THE SAME TERMS AS THE ELECTRICAL
CAPACITY IN YOUR HOME. THE SUPPLY MAY BE ADEQUATE UNTIL YOU ADD A STRESS SUCH AS A NEW TOASTER OR AIR CONDITIONER.
THERE ARE MANY TIMES IN OUR LIVES WHEN THE BODY RESERVES ARE STRESSED. BE SURE THAT YOUR BODY HAS THE NUTRIENT
RESERVES TO MEET THE CHALLENGE.

****

PAGE SIX

HOW TO USE FOOD AS A SOURCE OF NUTRIENTS

FROM FOOD COMES NUTRITION. NO PILL CAN MATCH NUTRITIOUS FOOD WITH REGARD TO HEALTH GIVING NUTRIENTS, SATISFACTION
AND GUSTATORY PLEASURE. LEARNING ABOUT THE NUTRIENTS IN THE FOODS YOU LIKE TO EAT CAN BE FUN, EDUCATIONAL,EASY
AND CAN PAY RICH DIVIDENDS IN RETURN. IT COULD BE THE DIFFERENCE BETWEEN LIFE AND DEATH.
   ON THIS SHEET, NUTRAN WILL TRY TO PRESENT A FEW OF THE BASIC FACTS ABOUT THE NUTRIENTS IN FOODS. IF YOU
DESIRE MORE INFORMATION CONSULT YOUR DOCTOR OR WRITE TO THE UNITED STATES DEPARTMENT OF AGRICULTURE, THE
AMERICAN MEDICAL ASSOCIATION OR THE AMERICAN DIETETICS ASSOCIATION. NUTRAN AS A MEDICAL SERVICE WILL AID YOUR PHYSICIAN
OR DENTIST WITH NUTRITION QUESTIONS. THESE PROFESSIONAL PEOPLE KNOW YOUR MEDICAL AND DENTAL HISTORY AND ARE BEST
EQUIPPED TO ADVISE YOU ON NUTRITION QUESTIONS. IT IS QUESTIONABLE JUDGEMENT TO TRUST YOUR HEALTH TO GUESSWORK.

** **

CALORIES:

   THE CALORIES IN FOOD COME FROM CARBOHYDRATE, FAT AND PROTEIN. EACH GRAM OF CARBOHYDRATE CONTRIBUTES 4 CALORIES, EACH
GRAM OF FAT CONTRIBUTES 9 CALORIES AND EACH GRAM OF PROTEIN CONTRIBUTES 4 CALORIES. SOME FOODS ARE HIGH IN CALORIES
BUT CONTRIBUTE LITTLE ELSE TO THE NUTRIENT NEEDS. THERE IS NOTHING SINFULL ABOUT THESE FOODS, BUT REMEMBER**ELECTRICITY
ALONE CAN DO LITTLE, FOOD ENERGY ALONE IS WORTHLESS ALSO.**

VITAMINS:

   IN THE COMPLEX CHEMISTRY OF THE BODY, THE VITAMINS CONTRIBUTE TO THE SECOND BY SECOND, HOUR BY HOUR CHEMICAL
ACTIVITY BY WHICH THE BODY CHANGES THE DINNER YOU ATE INTO BLOOD, BONES, MUSCLE AND SOUL WHICH IS YOU. WITHOUT
VITAMINS THERE IS NO LIFE, WITH A DEFICIENCY OF VITAMINS THERE IS NO HEALTH. THE SAME CAN BE SAID, OF COURSE, OF
EVERY OTHER NUTRIENT AS WELL. MINERALS, PROTEIN, FAT, WATER AS WELL AS THE VITAMINS MUST WORK TOGETHER TO SUSTAIN
LIFE AND HEALTH. A VITAMIN PILL IS NOT AN INSURANCE POLICY, VITAMINS SPRAYED ON BREAKFAST CEREALS WILL NOT COVER FOR
A POOR DIET. MOST PILLS DO NOT PROVIDE ALL THE NEEDED VITAMINS IN PROPER AMOUNTS. THE LIST BELOW WILL HELP YOU
SELECT THE FOODS THAT CONTAIN THE RICHEST AMOUNTS OF THE VITAMINS THAT YOUR NUTRAN ANALYSIS INDICATES ARE LOW IN
YOUR DAILY DIET.

VITAMIN C:

   THE BEST FOOD SOURCES OF VITAMIN C ARE FRUIT JUICES AND VEGETABLES. ASPARAGUS,BROCCOLI, BRUSSEL SPROUTS,
RAW CABBAGE, CANTALOUPE, GREEN PEPPER, STRAWBERRIES,TOMATOES, IN ADDITION TO THE JUICES OF THE ORANGE, GRAPEFRUIT AND
LEMON OFFER A GOOD SELECTION OF DELIGHTFUL FOODS TO PROVIDE VITAMIN C.

VITAMIN B-1 (THIAMINE)

ONE OF THE RICHEST SOURCES OF THIAMINE IS PORK. OTHER GOOD SOURCES ARE PEAS AND OTHER LEGUMES, WHOLE GRAIN
CEREALS, ENRICHED OR WHOLE WHEAT BREAD, AND FOR THOSE THAT ENJOY THE ESOTERIC... WHEAT GERM AND DRIED BREWERS
YEAST. THIS IS A NUTRIENT FOUND IN MOST ENRICHED CEREALS AND FLOURS AND IN JUST ABOUT ALL NUTRIENT SUPPLEMENTS.

VITAMIN B-2 (RIBOFLAVIN)

   RIBOFLAVIN IS PRESENT IN MANY FOODS. MILK IS A GOOD SOURCE, LIVER AND KIDNEY ARE EXCELLENT SOURCES, ALMONDS,
WHEAT GERM, BROCCOLI AND ASPARAGUS ALL PROVIDE RIBOFLAVIN IN THE DIET. THIS NUTRIENT IS ALSO FOUND IN MANY ENRICHED
CEREALS AND FLOURS.

NIACIN

   THE RICHEST SOURCES OF NIACIN ARE LIVER, POULTRY, BEEF, PEANUT BUTTER AND LEGUMES. ENRICHMENT OF CEREALS AND
FLOURS ADDS MUCH OF THE NIACIN THAT WAS LOST IN THE MILLING PROCESSES BACK INTO THESE PRODUCTS.

Fig. 17-1. (*Continued*)

FOLIC ACID

THIS IS PERHAPS ONE OF THE MOST DIFFICULT VITAMINS TO OBTAIN IN ADEQUATE AMOUNTS. THE BEST SOURCES ARE LIVER, MUSHROOMS, AND DARK GREEN VEGETABLES; SUCH AS ASPARAGUS, BROCCOLI, LIMA BEANS,SPINACH AND COLLARDS. FRUITS SUCH AS CANTALOUPE AND FRESH ORANGE JUICE ALSO CONTRIBUTE SOME FOLIC ACID.
THIS NUTRIENT IS RARELY FOUND IN SUPPLEMENTS AND IS NOT GENERALLY ADDED TO CEREAL AND ENRICHED PRODUCTS.

VITAMIN B-12

THIS VITAMIN IS FOUND ONLY IN FOODS OF ANIMAL ORIGIN. THE BEST SOURCE IS LIVER, ALTHOUGH BEEF, OYSTER, EGG, FISH AND DAIRY PRODUCTS CONTRIBUTE VITAMIN B-12

VITAMIN A

THIS NUTRIENT IS FOUND IN LARGE AMOUNTS IN LIVER, IN EGG YOLK, MARGARINE AND BUTTER. MOST DAIRY PRODUCTS ALSO SUPPLY VITAMIN A. CAROTENE, A PRECURSER OF VITAMIN A IS FOUND IN MANY VEGETABLES AND WILL EASILY SATISFY THE NEED FOR VITAMIN A. GOOD VEGETABLE SOURCES ARE SPINACH, CARROTS, BROCCOLI,KALE, ASPARAGUS,APRICOTS,WATERMELON AND PEACHES.

VITAMIN E

VITAMIN E IS FOUND IN VEGETABLE OILS. WHEAT GERM OIL, CORN OIL, COTTONSEED OIL, AND SOYBEAN OIL. SAFFLOWER OIL HAS CONSIDERABLY LESS. MAYONNAISE AND MARGARINES WHICH ARE MADE FROM THESE OILS ARE ALSO GOOD FOOD SOURCES OF VITAMIN E.

MINERALS

LESS WELL KNOWN THAN THE VITAMINS, BUT NO LESS IMPORTANT ARE THE MINERALS. THESE NUTRIENTS MUST BE PRESENT IN THE DIET OR ILL HEALTH AND DISEASE CAN RESULT AS READILY AS WHEN VITAMINS ARE DEFICIENT. SOME MINERALS ARE REQUIRED IN VERY SMALL AMOUNTS AND ARE KNOWN AS THE TRACE MINERALS, OTHERS SUCH AS CALCIUM, MAGNESIUM, IRON AND PHOSPHORUS ARE NEEDED IN LARGER QUANTITIES. IT IS CRITICAL THAT THE TRACE MINERALS BE PRESENT IN JUST THE RIGHT AMOUNTS, NOT TOO LITTLE AND ESPECIALLY IMPORTANT, NOT TOO MUCH. AS WITH THE OTHER NUTRIENTS, FOOD IS THE MOST DEPENDABLE SOURCE OF MINERALS.

CALCIUM

ONLY A FEW FOODS CONTAIN SIGNIFICANT AMOUNTS OF CALCIUM. DAIRY PRODUCTS SUCH AS MILK AND CHEESE ARE EXCELLENT SOURCES. THE NEXT BEST SOURCES OF CALCIUM ARE THE GREEN VEGETABLES, SUCH AS BROCCOLI, TURNIP GREENS, KALE, AND COLLARDS. THE CALCIUM IS MORE READILY AVAILABLE FROM THESE VEGETABLES AFTER COOKING.

PHOSPHORUS

GENERALLY, FOODS THAT ARE GOOD SOURCES OF PROTEIN ARE ALSO GOOD SOURCES OF PHOSPHORUS. CHEESE, BEEF, PORK, FISH, EGGS, WHOLE WHEAT BREAD AND PEANUTS ARE AMONG THE BETTER SOURCES.

SODIUM

SODIUM IS A MINERAL THAT FREQUENTLY IS EXCESSIVE IN AMERICAN DIETS AND NEEDS TO BE RESTRICTED. IN THE RARE CASE OF SODIUM DEFICIENCY, TABLE SALT WILL PROVIDE A LARGE DOSE OF SODIUM. WHEN SODIUM RESTRICTION IS DESIRED, IT IS IMPORTANT TO AVOID FOODS THAT HAVE BEEN CURED IN BRINE (SALT), SUCH AS HAM OR OLIVES. OTHER FOODS HIGH IN SODIUM THAT COULD BE AVOIDED IF RESTRICTION IS IMPORTANT INCLUDE GRAHAM CRACKERS, CHEDDAR CHEESE, CORNFLAKES, PROCESSED CHEESE AND SARDINES. REMEMBER ALSO THAT THE FLAVOR ENHANCER, MONO SODIUM GLUTAMATE (MSG,ACCENT) IS RICH IN SODIUM AND COULD BE AVOIDED.

MAGNESIUM

SOME OF THE RICHEST SOURCES OF MAGNESIUM APPEAR TO BE COCOA, WHOLE GRAINS, NUTS, AND SOYBEANS. GOOD SOURCES ALSO INCLUDE CLAMS, CORNMEAL, SPINACH, OYSTERS, CRAB, FRESH PEAS AND LIVER. DAIRY PRODUCTS AND FRUITS AND MOST VEGETABLES APPARENTLY CONTRIBUTE LITTLE MAGNESIUM.

IRON

LIVER IS A VERY RICH SOURCE OF IRON. GREEN VEGETABLES SUCH AS SPINACH,AND BROCCOLI ARE FAIR SOURCES. MEATS AND DRIED FRUITS SUCH AS APRICOTS AND RAISINS ALSO CONTRIBUTE IRON. COOKING IN IRON POTS CAN INCREASE THE IRON CONSUMPTION CONSIDERABLY, AS CAN DRINKING WATER COMING THROUGH IRON PIPES. OYSTERS, CLAMS AND COCOA ARE ALSO GOOD IRON SOURCES.

FLUORIDE

THOSE PEOPLE LIVING IN AREAS THAT HAVE ADDED FLUORIDE TO THE DRINKING WATER CAN BE ASSURED THAT THE FLUORIDE IN THE WATER WILL SATISFY THEIR NEEDS. OTHER SOURCES IN THE DIET ARE TEA AND COFFEE, SOYBEANS, SHELLFISH, AND OTHER SALT WATER FISH.

THE MAJOR NUTRIENTS....CARBOHYDRATE, FAT, AND PROTEIN

THIS IS THE STUFF OF WHICH WE ARE MADE. PROTEIN, THE SUBSTANCE THAT APPEARS TO FORM MUCH OF THE FUNCTIONAL ACTIVITY OF THE BODY, THE MATERIAL THAT MAKES UP MOST OF THE MUSCLE TISSUE, THE ANTIBODIES TO PROTECT US AGAINST DISEASE, THE HEMOGLOBIN THAT TRANSPORTS BLOOD TO ALL THE TISSUES,,,AND ON AND ON, IS ALL MADE OF PROTEIN. PROTEIN IS THE NUTRIENT THAT MUST BE CONSUMED MOST RELIGIOUSLY. IT IS ALSO THE MOST EXPENSIVE OF ALL THE NUTRIENTS. MOST FOODS CONTAIN SOME PROTEIN, HOWEVER, NOT ALL PROTEIN IS EQUALLY USEFUL TO THE BODY. THE MOST USEFUL PROTEIN COMES FROM EGGS, DAIRY PRODUCTS AND MEATS (INCLUDING FISH, CHICKEN, PORK, BEEF, LAMB ETC.) THE PROTEIN IN VEGETABLES IS MUCH LESS USEFUL AND CONSIDERABLE CARE MUST BE TAKEN IN BLENDING VEGETABLES IF THEY FORM THE MAJORITY OF THE PROTEIN INTAKE. IN SUCH A CASE IT IS ESSENTIAL TO DISCUSS THE FOOD CHOICES WITH A PROFESSIONAL WITH AN ADVANCED UNDERSTANDING OF NUTRITION.

FAT IS GENERALLY CONSIDERED TO BE PRESENT IN EXCESS IN MOST AMERICAN DIETS AND HAS BEEN SUGGESTED TO BE A RISK FACTOR IN HEART DISEASE WHEN CONSUMED IN EXCESS. MOST PEOPLE DO NOT REALIZE THAT SOME FAT MUST BE IN THE DIET, HOWEVER. IT APPEARS THAT THE MOST HEALTHY SOURCES OF FAT COME FROM THE UNSATURATED FATS IN VEGETABLE OILS. INCLUDING SOME CORN OIL OR SIMILAR VEGETABLE OIL WILL READILY PROVIDE SUFFICIENT DIETARY FAT. IT IS GENERALLY SUGGESTED THAT THE INTAKE OF SATURATED FATS (THAT FOUND IN BUTTER, MEATS AND BACON FOR EXAMPLE) SHOULD BE KEPT TO A MINIMUM CONSISTENT WITH ADEQUATE INTAKE OF HIGH QUALITY PROTEIN.

CARBOHYDRATE IS THE CLASS OF NUTRIENTS COMPRISED OF THE SUGARS AND STARCHES IN THE DIET. TABLE SUGAR, SOFT DRINKS, CANDY, AS WELL AS BREADS, POTATOES, CORN, AND CAKES PROVIDE LARGE AMOUNTS OF CARBOHYDRATE IN THE DIET. PROBLEMS CAN OCCUR IF CARBOHYDRATE IS TOO LOW ALTHOUGH THE USUAL SITUATION IS JUST THE OPPOSITE. MANY OF THE HIGH CARBOHYDRATE FOODS (SOME OF WHICH ARE LISTED ABOVE) CONTAIN LITTLE ELSE OF NUTRITIONAL IMPORTANCE. AS THEY ARE FILLING, THE TOTAL NUTRITION IS OFTEN POOR.

CHOLESTEROL

MANY AUTHORITIES CONSIDER DIETARY CHOLESTEROL TO BE AN IMPORTANT RISK FACTOR IN HEART DISEASE. IF YOUR DIET CONTAINS MUCH TOO MUCH CHOLESTEROL IT MAY BE NECESSARY TO HAVE A PHYSICIAN DETERMINE YOUR BLOOD CHOLESTEROL LEVELS AND RESTRICT THE INTAKE OF HIGH CHOLESTEROL FOODS SUCH AS EGGS, SHELLFISH, FATTY MEATS AND SOME DAIRY PRODUCTS. AS THIS QUESTION HAS NOT BEEN COMPLETELY RESOLVED, IT IS A GOOD IDEA TO CONSULT A PHYSICIAN BEFORE EMBARKING ON MAJOR DIETARY CHANGES THAT COULD LEAD TO OTHER SERIOUS DEFICIENCIES.

tiating normocytic, microcytic and macrocytic anemias. This data is useful in determining whether the anemia is mediated by iron, folate, B_{12}, or protein problems, or other factors such as chronic hemorrhage. Considering the widespread prevalence of anemia, these data narrow the diagnosis considerably and provide an effective basis for therapy.

Intelligent dietary modification and, if necessary, supplementation may usually be insti-

tuted at this time based on the semi-quantitative dietary analysis and routine laboratory tests described above. The clinician should note that clinical trials are a useful diagnostic adjunct during this Phase of analysis. In these trials patients are given prescriptions for the deficient nutrients. Correction of the problem by supplementation is acceptable proof of the diagnosis. In addition many dentists, suspicious of the role of diabetes and hypoglycemia

TABLE 17-3. SPECIAL LABORATORY TESTS OF VALUE IN NUTRITIONAL ASSESSMENT‡

Nutrient and Units	Age of Subject (years)	Criteria of Status		
		Deficient	Marginal	Acceptable
*Serum Ascorbic Acid (mg/100 ml)	All Ages	Up to 0.1	0.1–0.19	0.2+
*Plasma vitamin A (µg/100 ml)	All ages	Up to 10	10–19	20+
*Plasma Carotene (µg/100 ml)	All ages	Up to 20	20–39	40+
	Pregnant	—	40–79	80+
†Serum Folacin (ng/ml)	All ages	Up to 2.0	2.1–5.9	6.0+
**Serum vitamin B_{12} (pg/ml)	All ages	Up to 100	—	100+
*Thiamine in Urine (µg/g creatinine)	1–3	Up to 120	120–175	175+
	4–5	Up to 85	85–120	120+
	6–9	Up to 70	70–180	180+
	10–15	Up to 55	55–150	150+
	16+	Up to 27	27–65	65+
	Pregnant	Up to 21	21–49	50+
‡Riboflavin in Urine (µg/g creatinine)	1–3	Up to 150	150–499	500+
	4–5	Up to 100	100–299	300+
	6–9	Up to 85	85–269	270+
	10–16	Up to 70	70–199	200+
	16+	Up to 27	27–79	80+
	Pregnant	Up to 30	30–89	90+
**RBC Transketolase-TPP-effect (ratio)	All ages	25+	15–25	Up to 15
†RBC Glutathione Reductase-FAD effect (ratio)	All ages	1.2+	—	Up to 1.2
†Tryptophan Load (mg Xanthurenic acid excreted)	Adults (Dose: 100 mg/kg body weight)	25+ (6 hrs.) 75+ (24 hrs.)	— —	Up to 25 Up to 75
**Urinary Pyridoxine (µg/g creatinine)	1–3	Up to 90	—	90+
	1–6	Up to 80	—	80+
	7–9	Up to 60	—	60+
	10–12	Up to 40	—	40+
	13–15	Up to 30	—	30+
	16+	Up to 20	—	20+
*Urinary N'Methyl nicotinamide (mg/g creatinine)	All ages	Up to 0.2	0.2–5.59	0.6+
	Pregnant	Up to 0.8	0.8–2.49	2.5+
**Urinary Pantothenic Acid (µg)	All ages	Up to 200	—	200+
**Plasma vitamin E	All ages	Up to 0.2	0.2–0.6	0.6+

* Adapted from the Ten State Nutrition Survey.
† Criteria may vary with different methodology.
  Derived from Table of Current Guidelines for Criteria of Nutritional Status for Laboratory Evaluation in: Nutritional Assessment in Health Programs. Am. J. Public Health (Supp.) 63: 34, 1973, G Christakis, Editor.
  Also see: Sauberlich HE, Dowdy RP and Skala JH. Laboratory Tests for the Assessment of Nutritional Status in: Critical Reviews in Clinical Laboratory Science 4: 215–340, 1973.
‡ Butterworth CE, Blackburn GL, Nutrition Today 10: 18, 1975.

TRIPHASIC NUTRITIONAL ANALYSIS
SUMMARY DATA

	NO	YES	AMT/DAY	BRAND
COFFEE	____	____	____	_____
SMOKE	____	____	____	_____
MINTS	____	____	____	_____
GUM	____	____	____	_____
TEA	____	____	____	_____
VITAMINS	____	____	____	_____
	____	____		_____
	____	____		_____

NAME _____

ADDRESS _____

CHART NO. _____ OCCUPATION _____

AGE ____ SEX ____ HEIGHT _____ WEIGHT _____

PHASE I ANALYSIS

MEDICAL HISTORY

STRESS FACTORS ____	TRAUMA ____	
ALLERGIES ____	INFECTION ____	
DRUGS ____	G.I. SURGERY ____	
WEIGHT CHANGE ____	SYMPTOMS ____	

PROBLEMS: _____
_____
_____
_____

CLINICAL EXAM

HEAD ____	SKIN ____	TONGUE ____
HAIR ____	NECK ____	MUCOSA ____
EYES ____	NAILS ____	GINGIVA ____
NOSE ____	LIPS ____	TEETH ____

PROBLEMS: _____
_____
_____

ORAL BIOASSAY _____

SOCIAL HISTORY

	LOW	MED	HIGH
SOCIOECONOMIC STATUS	____	____	____
GENERAL HEALTH IQ	____	____	____
DENTAL HEALTH IQ	____	____	____
ETHNIC BACKGROUND	_____		
PERSONALITY TYPE	_____		
DAILY ROUTINE SUMMARY	_____		

_____
_____

DIAGNOSIS: _____

QUALITATIVE DIETARY ANALYSIS

FOOD GROUP	ADEQUATE		DEFICIENT		
	Norm.	Excess	Slight	Moderate	Severe
MILK PROD.	____	____	____	____	____
PROTEINS	____	____	____	____	____
FRUITS	____	____	____	____	____
VEGETABLES	____	____	____	____	____
CEREALS	____	____	____	____	____
FATS	____	____	____	____	____

DAILY SNACK FREQUENCY _____

DAILY SUGAR EXPOSURES:

(with meals)_____ (between meals) _____

PHASE II ANALYSIS

SEMI-QUANTITATIVE DIET ANALYSIS

PROBLEM NUTRIENTS: _____ % RDA

_____	_____
_____	_____
_____	_____
_____	_____
_____	_____

AUTOMATED BLOOD ANALYSIS

PROBLEMS: _____
_____
_____
_____

GLUCOSE TOLERANCE TEST

HOURS	0	½	1	2	3	4	5
mg/100 ml							

CLINICAL TRIALS

NUTRIENT	DOSE	DATES	EFFECT
_____	_____	_____	_____
_____	_____	_____	_____
_____	_____	_____	_____

DIAGNOSIS: _____

PHASE III ANALYSIS

ADDITIONAL LABORATORY TESTS INDICATED:

BLOOD:

PLASMA VITAMIN A	_____	
PLASMA CAROTENE	_____	
SERUM FOLACIN	_____	
SERUM IRON	_____	
TRANSFERRIN SATURATION	_____	
RBC GLUTATHIONE RED.	_____	

SERUM ASCORBATE	_____	
WBC ASCORBATE	_____	
RBC TRANSKETOLASE	_____	
PLASMA VITAMIN E	_____	
SERUM B$_{12}$	_____	
PLASMA CERULOPLASMIN	_____	

URINE:

RIBOFLAVIN	_____
THIAMIN	_____
PYRIDOXINE	_____
PANTOTHENIC ACID	_____
N. MET. NICOTINAMIDE	_____
FIGLU EXCRETION	_____
TRYPTOPHAN LOAD	_____
CREATININE	_____

MISCELLANEOUS TESTS:

BMR	_____	
THYROID FUNCTION	_____	
FECAL FAT	_____	
IMMUNE FUNCTION	_____	

PROTHROMBIN TIME	_____
BLEEDING TIME	_____
_____	_____
_____	_____

PATIENT REFERRED TO: _____

Copyright© M. C. Alfano, D. P. DePaola, 1977

Fig. 17-2. Tabular form used to summarize data gathered during Triphasic Nutritional Analysis.

in oral disease and concerned about these factors in the medical management of their patients, currently include a glucose tolerance test in their analysis. Moreover, this test is mandatory when abnormalities are detected in either postprandial or fasting blood glucose levels.

Phase III: Complex Tests of Metabolic Function

In the infrequent event that the nutritional diagnosis remains incomplete or clouded at the conclusion of Phase II, the analysis should progress to the final phase. This phase of the analysis is typically reserved for complex nutritional and metabolic problems, and should always be conducted by an appropriately trained physician. Comprehensive nutritional biochemical assays of blood, urine and tissues such as those illustrated in Table 17-3, as well as tests of metabolic and endocrine function are included in the Phase III analysis.

The results of Tri-phasic Nutritional Analysis should be tabulated on a summary sheet such as that illustrated in Figure 17-2. This summary serves as a data base during the dietary counseling phase of therapy and also as a reference point to which future nutritional analyses may be compared.

NUTRITION COUNSELING

The "Caveat"

The composition, form, and intake frequency of the diet is unequivocally important in the etiology of dental caries. Data from human clinical trails, animal research, and epidemiologic studies all indicate that the diet, particularly in terms of its refined carbohydrate content, is a critically important variable in the dental caries process. Therefore, the clinical rationale for attempting to modify the diet of caries prone individuals and thereby improve their oral health status rests on a strong scientific base. Nevertheless, the clinician should beware of a number of "caveats" associated with the process of dietary counseling.

First, virtually all of the dietary intervention and nutritional counseling studies related to oral health have been conducted on institutionalized populations. It is much easier to ensure compliance and monitor progress in these populations than in groups of free living, private dental patients. There is a glaring need for research studies to confirm the efficacy of diet modification in the typical non-institutionalized dental patient. Second, to ensure that the patient appreciates the relationship between nutrition and oral health, it is imperative that the dental team be knowledgable in nutrition and dedicated to the importance of diet modification in preventive dentistry. Any effort less than this commitment will certainly result in failure. Finally, the dental practitioner must recognize the appropriate scope for dietary therapy in his practice.

The comprehensive Triphasic Nutritional Analysis program outlined previously indicates that the authors deny neither the ability nor obligation of the dentist in diagnosing nutritional disorders. Indeed, the poor nutritional training received by the majority of practicing physicians and the fact that the patient presenting to a medical office usually considers himself to be systemically ill mandates an increasingly important role for the dentist in nutritional diagnosis and therapy. The dentist has an obligation to diagnose or refer for diagnosis all suspected nutritional problems and to treat those dietary problems which affect oral tissues but are not complicated by additional medical or systemic factors. The dentist, and unfortunately many physicians, should not supervise the dietary management of patients with such problems as diabetes, ulcers, hyperlipidemia, sprue, hypertension and so forth. In this regard, the authors are particularly concerned about the lecture circuit entrepreneurs who advise dentists to "balance body chemistry" or "manipulate trace mineral intake" to correct problems ranging from dental caries to sexual impotency. For example, mineral absorption is usually competitive and one mineral cannot usually be administered without affecting the absorption and metabolism of several others. Moreover, certain trace minerals have dramatic psychotropic effects. Most of these entrepreneurs consider themselves as pioneers and martyrs to the establishment politics of the scientific community; and, in fact, some of their recommended therapies may eventually prove to be correct. Nevertheless, their recommendations are often based only on subjective evaluations and case histories and are rarely published in reviewed journals. The moral commitment to the patient and the medicolegal situation warrant that only clearly established scientific principles be applied in clinical practice unless the patient is specifically advised of the experimental nature of a procedure and its possible consequences.

Behavioral Aspects of Food Intake

The dietary pattern of an individual is complex in origin and depends upon such variables as physiologic preferences, emotional state, religion, socioeconomic status, education, region, family customs, and cultural background. Obviously, food habits do not develop in a vacuum but are an integral part of an individual's total personality. Therefore, any attempt to modify food intake patterns which ignores the complexity of the problem cannot succeed. Thus, once the diagnosis of a nutritional problem is firm, the social history of the individual as discussed previously serves to set the stage for the direction which should be taken during dietary counseling. To illustrate this point, an elderly woman living alone may suffer from nutritional deficiencies because she has lost the behavioral stimulus for eating associated with mealtime family social interchange. She may also have limited financial resources. Therefore, during counseling she should be advised to share meals with friends, neighbors, and relatives whenever possible, and she should be instructed as to which foods within a group are most economical to purchase. This advice, though simple, will have much greater impact on her nutritional status than will a handful of preprinted "diets for senior citizens."

A comprehensive discussion of the ethnic, religious, and other behavioral factors associated with food intake is beyond the scope of this chapter. The reader is referred to the works of Nizel, Robinson, Williams and Anderson for further information. However, other aspects of behavioral modification of food intake for the dental patient should be briefly considered.

During diet counseling the role of food in the etiology of dental plaque, caries, and periodontal disease should be intimately linked together. For example, the patient must understand why the frequency of sugar intake is more important in dental caries than the total amount consumed if he is expected to comply with a recommendation to reduce the daily number of sugar exposures. Once the patient is convinced that diet is one of a few variables which he may modify to control dental caries, his level of compliance may improve considerably.

Finally the clinician should consider the fundamental principles of behavioral modification when offering dietary counseling services to his patients. In applying these principles to the counseling situation, Witteman has noted that:

Counseling normally involves two willing participants who meet to consider a problem, question or situation posed by one of the individuals.
Counseling is a face-to-face situation.

Counseling takes place in privacy.
Counseling demands a friendly, free atmosphere.
Counseling requires that the "counselor" have special skills and abilities acquired through prescribed professional training which equip him to participate in the counseling interview.

Dietary counseling, similar to most tools of preventive dentistry, requires modification of entrenched behavioral patterns by the patient. Unlike most traditional surgical and restorative oral health services success does not depend solely on the diagnostic acumen, artistic skills, and technical abilities of the dentist. The patient must cooperate . . . . the dentist must communicate. Only those dentists with patience, sincerity, and appropriate training and interest in nutrition can succeed in dietary counseling or, for that matter, preventive dentistry in general.

Nutrition Counseling Technique: A Team Approach

Once the nutritional analysis has been completed, the problems uncovered as well as suggestions to correct those problems should be explained to the patient in an understandable manner. Handing the patient a preprinted diet with the simple instruction to "follow this closely" is comparable to handing a European visitor an English phonics book with the simple instruction to "discontinue your accent". Obviously, dietary modification must be personalized and new diet patterns must be specifically developed for each individual. In view of the longstanding behavioral implications of food intake discussed in the previous section, it is clear that suggested dietary changes must be gradual.

An excellent step-by-step approach to dietary counseling has been developed by Nizel. This nondirective, personalized approach to dietary counseling is particularly useful since the patient learns not only what particular foods he eats but also when, where, and why he eats them, why he should change his diet, and how he can change his diet. The key to the success of this program is that the patient is permitted to develop his own diet based on what he has learned about nutrition and oral health and his own personal preferences. This system is based on the classic "four food groups" model and is simple, particularly for counseling caries-prone children. In the presence of the parent, the child is instructed as to which foods comprise each of the four groups and how many servings he should have from each group daily. The child can then determine those groups in which he is deficient and what foods he would like to add to his diet to improve nutritional balance. The form, amount, frequency, and time of consumption of sugar containing preparations is intimately linked to this counseling system as described later.

Although the four food groups serve as a useful tool in counseling children, the adolescent and adult population has become increasingly sophisticated and nutritionally oriented in recent years. Therefore, the four food groups approach is usually too simplistic for individuals in this older age category, and alternative methods for patient counseling must be employed. Food intake deficiencies may be converted to specific nutrient requirements either directly by a computerized dietary service or by the use of guides which have been developed by the Nutrition Section of the Office of International Research, National Institutes of Health. In addition, food exchange lists such as those developed by committees of the American Dietetic Association, the American Diabetes Association, and the Mayo Clinic are useful in meal and snack planning for more sophisticated patients. The exact system which is used (e.g., four or six food groups, computerized analysis, food guides, or exchange lists) is probably not as important as the manner in which it is applied. Each system must be personalized to the dietary needs, lifestyle and intellectual sophistication of the patient involved. The systems for nutritional analysis and dietary counseling which are best utilized in a given dental office will depend upon the physical facilities, patient population, and the interest and nutritional skills of the oral health care team.

The time involved in nutritional analysis and dietary counseling as well as the complexity of some of the nutritional problems which arise indicate that these services can be offered to the patient in the most efficient, effective, and economical manner by use of the team approach. The professional interaction which is required to achieve success is usually coordinated by the dentist and is diagrammed in Figure 17-3. In this interaction the great import provided by the involvement of the dentist or physician in nutritional services must be balanced by the economy and skills provided by specially trained auxiliaries. In other terms, should the dentist play no role in nutritional management, the patient would interpret this service as being relatively unimportant; conversely, if the dentist or physician

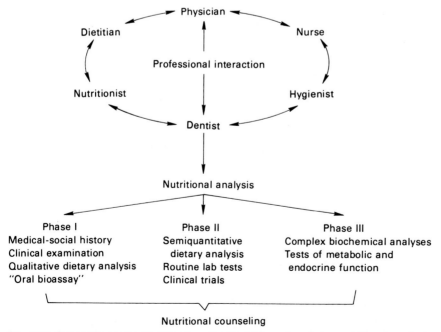

Fig. 17-3. Schematic representation of professional interaction during nutritional analysis and counseling. (DePaola, DP, Alfano, MC: Dent Clin North Am. 20: 631, 1976)

spent several hours in nutritional analysis and dietary counseling with a patient the cost would be prohibitive. Therefore, the dentist should personally introduce the importance of good nutrition to the patient during the medical/social history and clinical exam and explain the overall nutritional analysis and counseling system used in the office. The patient can then be referred to the appropriately trained auxiliary for further education and qualitative dietary analysis. The diagnosis is then made or additional tests ordered by the dentist who also determines the appropriate dietary management for the patient. The auxiliaries, as well as the dentist, must be very knowledgeable in nutrition and dietetics; and more dentists should consider employing nutritionists, dietitions, and specially trained hygienists to assist in providing nutritional services. The active participation of both the dentist and his staff can ensure that dietary counseling is both effective and affordable for the patient.

It is now appropriate to examine a more specific method for counseling the caries-prone child to improve his diet. In this situation, the nutritional analysis typically need not progress beyond Phase I before the problem, which usually consists of frequent sugar exposures and slight deficiencies in 1 or 2 food groups, can be diagnosed and counseling instituted.

After the child has completed the food diary, he summarizes the information with the assistance of the counselor in a tabular format such as that used at the University of Alabama (Fig. 17-4). At this point, the patient will begin to realize that he may be deficient in one or more food groups. The role of sugar in the dental decay process is then explained by the counselor. The counselor should discuss the relative importance of the *amount*, *frequency*, and *form* of sugar in the diet emphasizing that the frequency of the sugar in the diet is more important than the total amount of sugar consumed. In this regard, it may be easy for the patient to accept the role of sugars in dental caries but not so easy to understand how many sources of sugar are in the daily diet. While sugar by the spoonful is an obvious source, an effort should be made to enlighten the child as to some of the more common sugar-laden products.

During the session, the question of how sugars specifically effect the teeth will arise. To answer this the counselor should point out that sugar is an excellent growth medium for the bacteria living in the dental plaque. When these bacteria are bathed in sugar, they use it for immediate growth and energy needs and store it in the plaque for their long-term metabolic needs. With each sugar exposure the increased metabolic activity of the bacteria results in a spurt in the formation of waste products including acids which can dissolve the tooth enamel. Each time sugar is eaten, acid from the plaque may remain to decalcify the tooth surface for approximately 20-30 minutes. This explanation should make it clear to the child that the more exposures to sugar, the more periods of acid production and more dental decay. When the total sugar in the diet is recorded as in Figure 17-4, the patient will be impressed with the problem if the number of sugar exposures is multiplied by 30 minutes each to give the time each day that his teeth are affected by acids. Once the child and parent realize that ten sugar exposures mean approximately 5 hours of decalcification, they are usually shocked into recognizing the need for dietary modification.

The first suggestion to correct the problem will usually be made by the patient himself. That is, he will note that those sugars recorded in the diet history should be reduced or eliminated. This approach can then be tempered with the aid of the counselor by stipulating certain substitutions which can be made that would both decrease sugar and supply missing foods; for example, celery and cream cheese for a snack instead of a cupcake fulfills both criteria. In addition, condensation of caries promoting foods to during or immediately after a meal when saliva production is high will eliminate many periods of acid production. Once the patient is convinced of both the need to modify the diet and the fact that beneficial changes can be made which are not distasteful, remarkable dietary compliance can be achieved.

Integrating Nutrition into a Preventive Dentistry Program

In view of the discussion in this and the preceding chapter, it is difficult to conceive of a preventive health care program which excludes nutritional analysis and counseling. This is particularly true in the prevention of dental caries, a disease which is the most widespread diet related problem known to

Dates _____   Name _____

| Child reqmt. | Caloric reqmt. for adolescent | | | Adult reqmt. | Food group | Day 1 | Day 2 | Day 3 | Day 4 | Day 5 | Avg. | Diff. |
	1500 to 2000	2000 to 2500	2500 to 3000									
3-4	2-3	3-4	4-5	2	Dairy prods. milk, cheese							
2+ 2-3 oz.	2 3-4 oz.	2 4-5 oz.	2 5-6 oz.	2+ 3-4 oz.	Proteins. meat, fish chicken, egg dried peas dried beans							
1	1-2	2-3	2-3	1-2	Fruits							
3	3	3	3+	3+	Vegetables							
4	4-5	5-6	6-8	4+	Bread, cake cereals							
0	2-3 Tbsp.	3-4 Tbsp.	4+ Tbsp.	+ -	Fats, oils, margarine, butter							
Solid and retentive sugars					During meal							
					End of meal							
					Between meal							
Sugars in solution					During meal							
					End of meal							
					Between meal							

Fig. 17-4. Form used at the University of Alabama, School of Dentistry by the patient and counselor to summarize daily food group and sugar intake.

modern man. Since nutritional modification usually has a preventive rather than a curative effect, it is important to integrate it into a comprehensive preventive dentistry program. A diagrammatic representation of such a program is illustrated in Figure 17-5 in which the preventive needs of the patient are matched to age and oral health status.

Should every patient undergo dietary counseling services? Obviously the answer to this question is no. Only when a specific nutritional problem is identified during nutritional analysis is dietary modification warranted. The nutrition component of a preventive dentistry program, as is the case with all other aspects of the program, must be flexible and personalized to the needs of the patient. Stereotypic programs in which every patient moves from oral hygiene instruction, to prophylaxis, fluoride and sealant therapy, to dietary counseling etc. are expensive for the patient and wasteful of office time of the dentist and staff. Stereotypic programs result in the provision of many services which are not necessary and sometimes harmful. For example, a middle-aged person who uses a hard nylon toothbrush and the roll method of brushing may present in excellent oral health for routine dental care. Even though this patient has no dental caries, periodontal disease, gingival recession or cervical abrasion, many dental offices would "convert" him to a soft nylon brush and the scrub method simply because this technique is part of the "program" in that office. There is no rationale for this conversion, and the change may actually induce oral disease if the patient cannot master the new technique. Similarly, a patient who maintains nutritional balance by consuming 4 or 5 small meals a day should not be arbitrarily converted to the stereotypic three "squares." The key to successful preventive health care is that it be flexible, customized, and constantly reinforced.

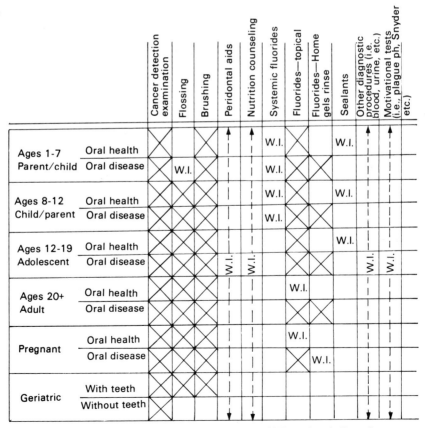

*Oral disease includes caries, gingivitis, periodontitis. W.I. = when indicated.

Fig. 17-5. Incorporation of nutrition counseling into a comprehensive preventive dentistry program. (DePaola, DP, Alfano, MC: Dent Clin North Am 20: 630, 1976)

SPECIAL PROBLEMS

The dentist will confront many special problems in the nutritional management of his patients. As already discussed, those problems which are complicated by systemic or medical implications should be managed by or in consultation with an appropriately trained physician. However, the dentist may play an active role in the dietary management of special problems which relate to the oral tissues. For example, the denture wearer, cleftpalate, orthodontic, or oral surgical patient can all benefit from the dietary recommendations of a knowledgeable dentist. Several of these special conditions which will be encountered by the dentist are outlined in Table 17-4. Although space limitations do not permit a detailed discussion of the special considerations associated with each of the conditions in Table 17-4, the problem of diet and oral health in the elderly will be discussed at greater length to serve as a model for the approach to special dietary problems in general.

In order to appreciate the problems of insuring good nutrition in the elderly, the dentist should first note the pathophysiologic conditions which are common in older patients that may have a bearing on nutritional status.

These factors, which include xerostomia, loss of taste, root caries, ill-fitting dentures, glossodynia, myofascial pain dysfunction, cheilosis, and osteoporosis may be the result of or contribute to a broad range of nutritional problems. At the outset the dentist can do much to treat these problems either directly or symptomatically as outlined in Table 17-5.

The dentist should also take note of the special social, psychological, and behavioral factors associated with ageing that may contribute to nutritional problems. Low income, loss of the mealtime family experience, excessive introspection, inability to get to the market, and long-standing eating patterns are problems which the dentist must carefully consider when counseling older patients. Once again, the authors would like to underscore the fact that simply advising the patient to consume more meals with family, friends and neighbors can have a better effect on the nutritional status of the elderly than can the use of stylized dietary forms. The dentist who appreciates the psychological problems of food intake in the elderly and utilizes his skills to improve the pathophysiologic problems listed in Table 17-5 can have a dramatic impact on the oral health and general well-being of the aged patient.

TABLE 17-4. EXAMPLES OF SPECIAL NUTRITIONAL PROBLEMS ENCOUNTERED IN DENTAL PRACTICE

Problem	Example	Recommendations
Chronic Disease	Diabetes; Ulcers etc.	Diabetes with systemic implications should always be managed by or in consultation with an appropriately trained physician.
Drugs	Contraceptive steroids	Insure adequate folate and ascorbate intake.
	Alcohol	Carefully evaluate overall nutritional status with special attention to thiamin, riboflavin, pyridoxine, folate, zinc, magnesium and protein
	Laxatives	Provide adequate fat soluble vitamins and/or calcium intake.
Congenital defects	Cleft-palate	Instruct parents in special feeding techniques and fabricate obturator as quickly as possible to insure adequate nutrient supply during critical neonatal development. Effect surgical closure at appropriate time.
Oral appliances	Orthodontic bands	Provide careful oral hygiene instruction and emphasize restriction of high sugar products particularly those of the retentive type. Use topical fluorides.
	Fractured jaw	Treat similarly to the orthodontic patient. When the jaws are wired closed provide adequate guidance as to appropriate liquid and semi-liquid diets.
Oral surgery	Periodontal surgery, Tooth extraction	Carefully evaluate the patient's nutritional status for supply of wound healing nutrients, immunological reactivity, and post-surgical negative nutrient balance. Provide liquid diet when necessary. Protect wound from food impaction.
Old age	Ill-fitting dentures	Reline or fabricate new dentures
	Glossodynia	Evaluate for nutritional anemias and B complex deficiencies.

TABLE 17-5. PATHOPHYSIOLOGICAL PROBLEMS WHICH RESULT FROM OR CONTRIBUTE TO MALNUTRITION IN ELDERLY PATIENTS

Problem	Therapy
Xerostomia	Increase consumption of firm, fibrous foods to improve salivary gland function. Increase water intake. Recommend sugarless gum and mints. Evaluate for diabetes, menopause, anxiety and B complex deficiencies
Loss of Taste	Increase salivary output and fluid intake as above. Recommend additional condiments and evaluate for Vitamin A and zinc deficiency. In refractory cases reconstruct prosthetic appliances for minimal palatal coverage.
Root caries	Dietary and hygiene recommendations as for coronal caries. Topical fluoride therapy.
Ill-fitting dentures	Reline or fabricate new prosthesis; increase salivary output. Recommend well-nourishing liquid and soft foods and instruct the patient to cut food into small pieces and chew slowly.
Glossodynia	Evaluate for nutritional anemias, B complex deficiency and endocrine dysfunction. Increase salivary output.
Myofacial Pain Dysfunction Syndrome	Use conventional therapy including occlusal adjustment, bite planes, night guards, muscle relaxants, tranquilizers and psychiatric care. If necessary provide a semi-solid diet to insure adequate nutrition.
Cheilosis	Use topical protective creams. Evaluate for B complex deficiency, particularly riboflavin. Check for bite overclosure and fungal infections.
Constipation	Increase intake of dietary fiber and water.
Osteoporosis	Evaluate calcium, protein and Vitamin D status and calcium/phosphorus ratios. Check for hormonal problems.

DIETARY SUPPLEMENTATION

There are many instances when the dentist should provide dietary supplements to promote rapid changes in nutritional status or to ensure adequate long-term nutrient supply during certain chronic problems. However, supplements should be used sparingly with the emphasis placed on obtaining optimum nutrient intake through diet. Although supplements have a certain amount of "glamour" associated with their use, the patient may soon tire of the novelty and forget to purchase them. In contrast, a careful, slow redirection of the food selection process can provide nutritional balance and will result in behavioral changes consistent with long-term dietary success.

Other than the rapid, short-term correction of vitamin deficiencies, fluoride therapy, and such problems as the nutritional anemias, the most common need for dietary supplements in dental practice relates to supportive therapy for effective wound healing. Navia, based on recommendations of the National Research Counsel, has suggested the following guidelines for the administration of supplemented or therapeutic vitamins:

1. A previously healthy patient with a minor illness expected to last less than 10 days, who is ambulatory and eating well with no history of inadequate nutrition

TABLE 17-6. SUGGESTED DAILY VITAMIN REQUIREMENTS FOR MAINTENANCE OR THERAPY OF SURGERY PATIENTS*

	Mini-mum	Mainte-nance	Thera-peutic
Thiamine hydrochloride (mg)	1.4	3	12
Riboflavin (mg)	1.7	3	12
Niacinamide (mg)	18	20	80
Ascorbic acid (mg)	60	120	350
Calcium pantothenate (mg)	10	20	20
Pyridoxine hydrochloride (mg)	2	4	10
Folacin (mg)	0.1	0.2	0.4
Vitamin B_{12} (μg)	5	10	15
Vitamin A (IU)	5000	5000	5000
Vitamin D (IU)	400	400	400
Vitamin E (IU)	30	60	60
Vitamin K_1 (mg)	2	2	2

* Navia JM: in Menaker L (ed.): Biologic Basis of Wound Healing. P. 170. Hagerstown, Harper & Row, 1975

needs no special consideration in regard to vitamin requirement.

2. When the qualifications in item 1 are not met, the patient is given the maintenance level which is approximately twice the minimum requirement (Table 17-6).

3. The patient receiving all nutrients intravenously should be given the maintenance level with additional supplements of Vitamin C.

4. During serious illness or after severe trauma, requirements for the first few days should be supplied at a therapeutic level. Thereafter, the patient should receive two or three times the minimum daily requirement until recovery is complete.

In addition to the vitamin supplementation regime described above, dietary supplementation or special diets should also be considered. These include a variety of clear liquid, liquid, soft, and regular diets designed for patients with low sodium or low residue needs or nausea, malaise, and gastrointestinal impairment. Recent suggestions that trace minerals, particularly zinc, aid in wound healing are interesting, and these nutrients may be used as nutritional supplements for wound healing in the near future.

SUMMARY

Since diet constitutes one of only a few variables in the etiology of dental caries which an individual may modify, dietary improvement represents one of the most important ways to prevent dental decay. Unfortunately, neither the analysis of an individual's nutritional status nor modification of food intake patterns are easy tasks. Therefore, a comprehensive system of Triphasic Nutritional Analysis has been developed specifically for use in the dental office. This system is based on phases of analysis which become increasingly complex as the needs of the patient dictate. Once enough information is gathered to establish a firm diagnosis the analysis is terminated and appropriate therapy or dietary counseling instituted. The system is designed for participation by both the dentist and auxiliaries trained in nutrition so that optimal service may be provided to the patient at minimal cost. This cost effective team approach is carried through to the dietary counseling phase of the nutrition program. Once again the dentist provides import to the program by introducing the need for dietary intervention and supervising the counseling sessions which are run conjointly by an appropriately trained auxiliary and the patient. Both the dentist and his staff continually reinforce the nutritional program during recall visits.

Behavioral modification is a complex process, and has been discussed at some length particularly in terms of the socioeconomic, cultural, ethnic, religious, and regional variations in food intake patterns. The key to success in dietary behavioral modification as well as success in preventive oral health care in general lies in the flexibility, personalization and, reinforcement built into the program.

GLOSSARY

Appetite. Complex sensations by which an organism is aware of desire for food and anticipates ingestion of a desirable food.

Bioassay. Evaluation of the activity of a substance, such as a vitamin, by measuring the response of test organisms to the substance as compared with their response to a standard (see Oral Bioassay).

Cultural. In study of food habits refers to religious, social, and national habits of a group of people.

Dietary counseling. The process of teaching a patient the importance of nutrition in health and disease, and then formulating conjointly with the patient an improved diet acceptable to both the patient and the counselor.

Essential nutrient. An element or compound which cannot be synthesized by an organism and which is required for life.

Food and Nutrition Board. Established in 1940 by the National Academy of Sciences - National Research Counsel to serve as an advisory body to the government on food and nutrition. Its primary function has been the development and periodic revision of the Recommended Dietary Allowances (RDA).

Glucose tolerance test. A test which demonstrates the efficiency of glucose utilization in the body. Changes are noted in the glucose concentration of the blood at sequential intervals after ingestion of a standard amount of glucose.

Malnutrition. A general term for poor nourishment which may be due to an inadequate diet, an excessive diet, or to some metabolic defect which prevents the body from properly using one or more nutrients.

National Research Council. A group of distinguished scientists appointed by the National Academy of Sciences to coordinate the efforts of major scientific and technical societies of the United States.

Nutrient. Any item of food or nourishment which can be either essential or nonessential for life.

Oral bioassay. A subjective evaluation of the amount of local irritants around the teeth and the degree of periodontal inflammation and/or destruction present. Excessive periodontal breakdown in the absence of significant local irritants is strongly suggestive of nutritional and other systemic problems.

Recommended dietary allowances (RDA). Estimated amounts of specified vitamins, minerals, and protein that have been judged adequate for the maintenance of good nutrition in most U.S. citizens. Determined by the National Academy of Sciences, National Research Council, Food and Nutrition Board.

Triphasic nutritional analysis. A system for determining the nutritional status of an individual by means of progressive phases of evaluation which lead to a definitive diagnosis. The analysis is as simple or sophisticated as the needs of the patient dictate.

SUGGESTED READINGS

Alfano MC: Controversies, perspectives and clinical implications of nutrition in periodontal disease. Dent Clin North Am 20: 519–548, 1976

Alfano MC, DePaola DP: Methods for assessing nutritional status in dental practice. Quint Int 9: 115–125, 1978

Chasens AI: Laboratory medicine in a dental practice. J Oral Med 31: (Special Issue) 13–16, 1976

Clark JW: Nutrition as a therapeutic regime. In Hazen S (ed): Diet, Nutrition and Periodontal Disease. Chicago, American Society for Preventive Dentistry, 1975, pp 28–52

Committee on Dietetics of the Mayo Clinic: Mayo Clinic Diet Manual, 4th ed., Philadelphia, WB Saunders, 1971

DePaola DP, Alfano MC: Triphasic nutritional analysis and dietary counseling. Dent Clin North Am 20: 613–634, 1976

DePaola DP, Alfano MC: Nutrition and oral health. Nut Today 12: 6–32, 1977

DiOrio LP, Madsen KO: A Personalized Program: Educating the Patient in the Prevention of Dental Disease. Chicago, March, 1972

Interdepartmental Committee on Nutrition for National Defense: Manual for Nutrition Surveys. Bethesda, National Institutes of Health, 1963

Madsen KO: Nutritional Basis of Oral Health in Dental Biochemistry. Philadelphia, Lea & Febiger, 1968, pp 158–212

Navia JM: Nutrition and wound healing. In Menaker L (ed): Biologic Basis of Wound Healing. New York, Harper & Row, 1975, pp 157–173

Navia JM: Nutrition and oral disease. In Caldwell RC, Stallard RE (eds): A Textbook of Preventive Dentistry. Philadelphia, WB Sanders, 1977

Nizel AE: Nutrition in Preventive Dentistry: Science and Practice. Philadelphia, WB Saunders, 1972

Nizel AE: Role of nutrition in the oral health of the aging patient. Dent Clin North Am 20: 569–584, 1976

NUTRAN Dietary Analysis: PO Box 15464, Atlanta, GA 30333

Robinson CH: Basic Nutrition and Diet Therapy. New York, Macmillan 1975

Williams SR: Essentials of nutrition and diet therapy. St. Louis, CV Mosby, 1974

Witteman JK: Behavioral implications in successful dietary counseling. Dent Clin North Am 20: 601–612, 1976

18 Antimicrobial Agents for Management of Caries

PAGE W. CAUFIELD

JUAN M. NAVIA

Introduction
Considerations on the Selection and Use of
  Antimicrobial Agents
  Preventive and Therapeutic Trial Strate-
  gies
  Properties of an Ideal Agent
  Delivery Approaches for Antimicrobial
  Agents
  Topical Applications
  Systemically Administered Agents
Specific Plaque Hypothesis
  The Role and Ecology of *Streptococcus
  mutans*
  Intraoral Determinants of Colonization
  Extraoral Determinants of Colonization
  Other Oral Bacteria Associated With
  Dental Caries
  Lactobacilli
  Actinomyces
Selected Antimicrobial Agents Proposed for
  Plaque Control and Management of
  Caries
  Antibiotics
  Penicillins and Analogues
  Vancomycin
  Kanamycin
  Actinobolin
  Summary
  Bis Biguanides
  Characteristics of Chlorhexidine
  Clinical Trials
  Summary
  Fluoride

Antibacterial Properties
  Clinical and Laboratory Investigations
  Combination Therapy—Bis Biguanide
  and Sodium Fluoride
  Summary
Iodine
  Chemical Characteristics and Antimi-
  crobial Properties
  Clinical and Laboratory Investigations
Phosphates
  Types and Specific Properties of Differ-
  ent Phosphates
  Mechanism of Action for Various Phos-
  phates
  Use of Phosphates as Food Additives
  Combination Therapy: Phosphates and
  Fluorides
  Trace Elements
  Quaternary Ammonium Compounds
  Enzyme Preparations
  Vaccines
Prospective Applications of Antimicrobial
  Agents in the Management of Caries
  Longterm Suppression of S. *mutans*
  Replacement with *non-S. mutans* Antago-
  nists
  Replacement with Mutant Effector Strains
  of S. *mutans*
  Antimicrobial Agents and Vaccines
Summary
Glossary
Suggested Readings

INTRODUCTION

Dental caries is an infectious disease of bacterial origin which is influenced in its development by dietary and host factors interacting over a period of time. In view of its bacterial etiology, it seems appropriate that among its proposed remedies, antimicrobial agents should be given careful consideration. In fact, as early as 1890 Miller described in his text the bacterial etiology of dental caries and his subsequent attempts to control the caries process via the application of chemotherapeutic agents. Miller's concept of oral health can be summarized by his introductory statement to caries management:

> ". . . it must be apparent that there are four ways by which we may counteract or limit the ravages of this disease. We may endeavor (1) by hygienic measures to secure the best possible development of the teeth; (2) by repeated, thorough systematic cleansing of the oral cavity and the teeth, to so far reduce the amount of fermentable substances as to materially diminish the production of acid as well as to rob the bacteria of the organic matter necessary to their rapid development; (3) by prohibiting or limiting the consumption of such foods or luxuries which readily undergo acid fermentation to remove the chief source of the ferment products injurious to the teeth; (4) by the proper and intelligent use of *antiseptics* to destroy the bacteria, or at least to limit their number and activity."

Miller tested the antibacterial effectiveness *in vitro* and *in vivo* of more than 20 different antiseptic agents with varied results. For many decades following Miller's observations interest in finding a safe and effective antiseptic for intraoral use was not seriously pursued. It is likely, as Miller himself stated, that the caustic nature of most antiseptics available at that time severely limited their use intraorally.

Aside from the obvious problem of potential toxicity of an agent, several other aspects involving the complex ecologic balance and interaction of oral microflora with the human host may appear at first to make prospects for chemotherapeutic management of dental caries a difficult task to achieve. However, in the last decade or two, with an increased understanding of the ecology of oral microflora, and in particular, recognition and identification of certain organisms associated with dental caries (see Chap. 11), prospects for chemotherapy now appear more promising than ever, notwithstanding the limitations of some of the proposed agents and methods of delivery.

During Miller's time and, in fact, well into the 1900's, dental caries was considered the result of a nonspecific infection arising from the indigenous oral flora as a whole. As a result, attempts for reducing caries using various chemotherapeutic agents were directed against the entire oral flora. The magnitude of the task of reducing the oral flora as a whole was clearly recognized when studies showed the almost infinite number and different types of organisms, both indigenous and transient, that comprise the oral microflora at any given time. Thus, one of the first findings encountered by Miller and some of the scientists who followed was the realization that long lasting suppression or elimination of all of the oral bacteria was an impossible task to achieve.

While it is true that there are difficulties involved in suppressing all bacteria in the oral cavity due to the large numbers and types that exist in the different ecologic niches within the oral cavity, there are some assumptions that could lead to error in evaluating the effectiveness of an oral antibacterial agent. For example, one investigator assumed that plaque organisms divide every 20 to 30 minutes, and therefore, he calculated that if an oral disinfectant was 99.99 per cent effective in killing plaque organisms, then the reduction seen would be apparent for only five hours before the numbers returned to the pretreatment levels. Such calculations are now known to be erroneous (the turnover rate of plaque organisms is 2 to 3 times in 24 hours). Undoubtably, such calculations had a dampening effect on early investigations into this prospective area of caries management, through the use of antibacterial agents.

Another factor which warrants concern is that any antimicrobial agent capable of radically altering the indigenous oral flora for the control of dental caries is likely to interfere with the delicately balanced relationship between the normally nonpathogenic flora and the host. As seen in cases where systemic antibiotics were administered, suppression of the indigenous flora can lead to serious suprainfections by nonsusceptible exogenous pathogens or even by nonsusceptible members of the indigenous flora. For example, yeast or fungi, frequently found in low numbers in the oral cavity, tend to gain prevalence following suppression of the indigenous flora, often to the detriment of the host. This delicate balance between the normally nonpathogenic indigenous flora and the host likely serves an important function in excluding the colonization of potential pathogens. Upsetting this delicate ecologic balance may mean the difference between health and disease; therefore, maintenance of this bacterial equilibrium essential for oral health must be considered when attempts are made to control dental plaque.

Further difficulty has been encountered with chemical prophylaxis of dental caries based on control of total plaque as a whole, without considering the role of specific plaque bacteria which have a direct etiologic role in caries. The concept of nonspecific or total plaque control for prevention of dental caries apparently was adopted by clinicians from early periodontal disease investigations which later was applied to caries prevention. For example, the relationship between plaque and gingivitis has been demonstrated in humans and in experimental animals. When oral hygiene is suspended, the subsequent accumulation of plaque is consistently and predictably followed by gingivitis; removal of this plaque, either chemically or mechanically readily reverses gingivitis. Antiplaque agents, such as chlorhexidine, have been tested and shown to be very effective in preventing formation of plaque and hence in preventing gingivitis. Such a clear and direct relationship between total plaque and dental caries, however, has not been similarly demonstrated. Obviously, if no plaque were present, (i.e., no bacteria on the surfaces of teeth) caries would not develop. However, formation of bacterial plaque is a normal process which occurs in healthy as well as diseased patients. Therefore, complete absence of plaque is not only abnormal but, as previously discussed, unachievable and perhaps even undesirable. In addition, oral hygiene procedures (e.g., brushing and flossing) taught to patients and shown to be effective in controlling certain of the periodontal diseases have been disappointing in terms of their ability to prevent dental caries (see Suggested Readings, WHO, 1972). This finding is likely due to the fact that such mechanical cleansing procedures are not capable of debriding the areas of the dentition most susceptible to dental caries, (i.e., the pits and fissures and the approximal surfaces). Clinical studies where plaque removal was performed at regular intervals by specially trained dental auxillaries have been shown effective in controlling caries, but this approach, although effective, would be difficult to implement on a community or public health basis, at least in this country.

CONSIDERATIONS ON THE SELECTION AND USE OF ANTIMICROBIAL AGENTS

The microbial components of plaque which colonize selected sites of the dentition and which may accumulate in close apposition to the host's gingival tissues are the primary etiologic factor in dental caries and periodontal disease, the two most important diseases of the oral cavity. The microbial composition of dental plaque and its metabolism will determine to a large extent the health status of oral tissues. The enamel surface and the supporting structures of the tooth are therefore constantly being exposed to conflicting influences in the oral cavity, such as the reparative forces of saliva (see Chap. 19) and the destructive activity of bacterial plaque.

The control of plaque-dependent diseases can be achieved either by inhibiting implantation, colonization and metabolic activity of plaque bacteria, and/or by increasing the oral tissue defenses and resistance. To date, no isolated approach has been found to be completely effective in preventing plaque-dependent diseases.

In this chapter, several antimicrobial agents and approaches will be discussed in the light of recent findings which show that only certain bacteria comprising the plaque microflora are cariogenic and against which an agent should be directed. It is clearly understood that there are more than one species of bacteria which have been associated with dental caries, and therefore, the agent selected and methods of application should be versatile enough to be effective against most of these cariogens, yet selective enough so as not to disturb the delicate and beneficial balance between the oral flora and the human host. Similar considerations are observed in the treatment of other infectious diseases afflicting man such as those occurring in the gastrointestinal tract, where therapeutic attempts have been directed toward selectively reducing specific pathogens without attempting to eliminate the entire intestinal microflora.

There is no question that antibacterial compounds can prevent caries. This principle was firmly established more than 25 years ago by incorporating penicillin in the food and drinking water of rats. Many subsequent investigators mostly using antibiotics, have confirmed that continuous oral administration of an appropriate antibacterial agent via food and water can suppress cariogenic bacteria in rodents, reducing their caries scores by 90 per cent or more. Following withdrawal of the agent, a group of animals may remain free of cariogenic organisms and nearly free of caries through a number of successive generations.

The only existing comparable data for humans which show an anticaries effect of some systemic antibiotics have come from patients receiving penicillin by mouth daily, with and without supplemental tetracycline, for rheumatic fever or chronic respiratory diseases. During periods from 2 to 5 years these patients developed from 54 to 69 per cent fewer carious tooth surfaces than comparable, untreated groups. The anticaries effect tended to accrue with increases in length of exposure and dosage of the antibiotic regimen; it persisted to some degree for several years after cessation of therapy.

Preventive and Therapeutic Trial Strategies

The planning and evaluation of trials of preventive or therapeutic agents include choice of drug, type of population to be studied, length of study, mode, frequency of administration, and concentration of the drug to be administered. The efficacy of a drug will differ depending on several possible therapeutic strategies:

1. The agent might be intended for treatment of active dental disease in individual patients under close supervision of a practitioner. Treatment in this case could be varied and adapted to conform with the response of the patient.
2. The agent might be intended for prophylactic application in large population groups. Opportunity to modify the regimen individually would then be minimal. Choice of therapeutic agents would be limited to those that are unquestionably safe and efficacious under all conceivable field conditions, where clinical supervision would be minimal.
3. The agent might be expected to control and eliminate existing disease, to arrest caries, and to avert future disease.
4. The agent might be expected to kill accessible cariogenic organisms and to prevent colonization on existing sound tooth surfaces, but not to eradicate established or deep seated infections. In relation to caries, this would mean that clinical trials should last at least four years. As long as two years may be required for incipient, clinically inapparent lesions to manifest themselves and only the increments of the third and fourth years could be expected to reveal accurately the efficacy of the agent.
5. The agent might be expected only to maintain a therapeutically favorable balance of the oral flora by suppressing it nonselectively to levels that minimize the likelihood of odontopathic activity. This strategy seems particularly applicable to preventing periodontal disease, rather than caries.
6. To prevent caries, the agent might be expected only to suppress selectively the known cariogenic bacterial species. This aim has been achieved in experimental animal caries. Several studies show that it is achievable for several months with respect to *Streptococcus mutans* in humans. Such strategy seems particularly applicable in conjunction with the first stated strategy.
7. The agent might be expected to act by preventing or removing plaque deposits nonselectively with little or no effect on the relative proportions of oral bacteria. Here mainly surface-active, nonantibacterial substances would be concerned.
8. Theoretically, metabolic regulators

could be found that would not affect viability of plaque bacteria but would inhibit or divert their caries-conducive activities, such as utilization of sugars, production of acids, formation of adherent extracellular polysaccharides, and accumulation of intracellular polysaccharides. This is an interesting possibility that might prove to be effective in controlling metabolic activity of plaque cariogens.

Properties of an Ideal Agent

The criteria for selecting a chemotherapeutic agent for use against cariogenic organism depends, to a large extent, upon the identification of the causative organism(s), the ecology of that organism(s), and the effect of the agent on both the organism(s) as well as on the host. While it is unlikely that any one antimicrobial agent can incorporate all the ideal properties listed below, the clinician should keep these properties in mind when selecting and prescribing an antimicrobial regimen for a patient. Since certain of the oral streptococci, notably S. *mutans* have been designated as an important etiologic agent in initiation of dental caries, focus upon this group of bacteria as the "target organisms" seems appropriate, although other bacteria are also known to be cariogenic.

1. The first and most important property of a chemotherapeutic agent is that it should be safe for intraoral use. Agents intended for topical use should not penetrate the oral or gasterointestinal mucosa nor be systemically toxic if accidently swallowed. Moreover, the agent should not induce hypersensitivity to the host or cause local tissue irritation. The agent should not stain or be caustic to the enamel surfaces. Drugs such as phenolic compounds, sodium hypochlorite and mercurial bichlorides, while excellent antiseptics, are too caustic for direct contact with the oral mucosa. The agent should conform to Food and Drug Administration standards for these types of agents.

2. An antimicrobial agent should be rapidly bactericidal so that selection for resistant organisms becomes less probable. Since the contact time between a topically applied agent and oral flora by necessity is limited, a rapid bactericidal action is desirable. Iodine is an example of an antiseptic agent which meets this criteria. Once contact is made between iodine-containing solutions and bacteria, they are immediately killed. High concentrations of fluorides (>1000 ppm) and chlorhexidine also exhibit bactericidal properties. Antibiotics, on the other hand, exhibit bactericidal properties only when the target organisms are actively dividing. Thus, the antibacterial effect is seen primarily in the daughter cells, rather than the parent cell. Therefore, its killing action is a time dependent occurrence.

3. The antimicrobial agent should possess a degree of specificity sufficient to affect the cariogenic organisms without unduly disturbing the delicate balance between indigenous microflora and host.

4. The ideal antimicrobial agent must be able to penetrate dense microbial plaque and be retained in the oral environment for extended periods after application. Molecular charge and size are likely to be important in meeting these two criteria. Since contact time between plaque and antimicrobial agent is likely to be limited, the ability to be retained in the oral cavity (particularly at the plaque-enamel interface) enhances the antimicrobial effectiveness of the agent. Chlorhexidine and fluorides are both known to reversibly bind to enamel surfaces (hydroxyapatite), pellicle, and/or plaque, thus prolonging their retention and antimicrobial effectiveness. Research is currently underway perfecting laminated resins which are capable of slowly releasing fluoride at a predetermined rate and concentration. The prospect of incorporating such a device into acrylic appliances and/or restorations of caries-active patients for the prolonged delivery of an antimicrobial agent is promising.

5. Medically important antibiotics, such as any of the penicillins or tetracyclines, should not be selected for preventing caries since such usage might compromise their effectiveness in treating more serious local or systemic infections.

6. To reduce the likelihood of altering the intestinal flora unfavorably, the agent should be destroyed or inactivated in the

gastrointestinal tract. Similarly, since the agent would possibly find its way into waste disposal systems in considerable quantities, it should be readily biodegradable in the environment.

7. On a practical level if widespread use of a particular chemotherapeutic agent is anticipated, then the agent must be easy to apply and handle, exhibit stability in solution, be active over a wide spectrum of pH and concentrations, and be easily manufactured at a reasonable cost.

8. Lastly, the agent must have an acceptable taste, either by itself or in combination with masking flavoring agents. Experience from clinical trials using high concentrations of stannous fluoride and chlorhexidine amply demonstrate the importance of this last property.

Delivery Approaches for Antimicrobial Agents

The route of administration of an agent to be applied to tooth surfaces is as important as the choice of agent and may be determined at least in part by its characteristics. Simply stated, the aim is to develop adequate means (vehicles, devices, administration schedules) to assure that the agent is delivered to the proper site in sufficient concentration for a sufficient length of time to accomplish its anticipated effects. Theoretically, there might be advantage in prolonged delivery via ingestion, absorption, and excretion from the blood stream in salivary secretions. (Spiramycin would suit this regimen.) The possibilities for systemic side effects, however, offset the possible advantages and make application directly to the teeth (topical application) the method of first choice.

Dental caries is a localized disease confined to the tooth surfaces that is readily accessible to the clinician for direct observation and application of various chemical agents. However, certain areas of the dentition are not as readily accessible as others. For example, the depths of the pits and fissures and the approximal surfaces just below the point of contact with the adjacent tooth are physically well protected. They are also the areas most prone to caries. In contrast, the buccal and lingual surfaces of the teeth are more readily accessible, but they are also the enamel surfaces least affected by caries.

In addition to the physical difficulty in gaining access to certain dental sites, there are problems related to the washing effect of saliva on tooth surfaces. The buffering and/or diluting effect of saliva, while playing an important role in caries inhibition, can also interfere with the application and effectiveness of a particular antibacterial agent.

Another consideration in the use of chemotherapeutic agents is that even though the teeth are quite inert to chemical and physical assault, the gingival tissue surrounding them are very sensitive to chemical or physical effects. Therefore, the agent must be delivered to the teeth in such a way as not to damage the surrounding tissue.

Topical Applications

A wide array of different approaches for topically applying chemotherapeutic agents have been reported, each having its own distinct advantages and disadvantages.

Mouthrinses. Mouthrinsing with solutions containing an antibacterial agent has been one of the first methods employed by early investigators. Today, this method is probably the most common method of introducing antiseptics into the oral cavity and is widely accepted by the public. In terms of ease of application and convenience, mouthrinsing has no rival. However, this particular method has certain inherent disadvantages.

First, its main disadvantage is that it brings the antiseptic agent in contact with oral soft tissues which harbor the largest reservoir of nonodontopathic indigenous flora. Mouthrinses capable of upsetting the entire flora could result in suprainfection by yeast and fungi and/or other abnormalities (i.e., "hairy or black tongue"). The latter abnormality has been associated with prolonged use of chlorhexidine solutions.

Second, agents capable of radically altering the odontopathic flora colonizing the teeth could also be caustic to the oral mucosa. For example, high concentrations of iodine, acidulated fluorides, chlorhexidine, and stannous fluoride have been shown to cause varying degrees of tissue irritation which preclude their application via mouthrinsing, except in dilute concentrations.

Third, dilution and buffering effect of saliva are likely to render the agent in a mouthrinse less effective.

A fourth disadvantage is that even though the rinse is confined to the oral cavity, its ability to penetrate into all retentive sites and through the depth of plaque is primarily governed by the amount of time that the mouthrinse can be held in the mouth, a few minutes at most. (Some agents such as chlorhexidine and fluoride are capable of being retained even after spitting the mouthrinse owing to their previously discussed property of retentiveness.)

Fifth, the potential toxicity of swallowing 5 to 10 ml. of the active agent in a mouthrinse must be considered.

Dentifrices. Like mouthrinses, the use of dentifrices for delivering chemotherapeutic agents has public acceptance, and was the first approach used for applying penicillin and fluoride preparations directly to the dentition. Recently, chlorhexidine has also been incorporated into a dentifrice. Dentifrices intended for patient self application have been evaluated intensively due to the obvious advantage that the patient can apply an agent several times each day as part of routine oral hygiene. Since toothbrushing with a dentifrice conforms to customary practice in most Western societies, the incorporation of an anticaries agent in a dentifrice offers an attractive mode of therapy. Dentifrice gels containing antimicrobial concentrations of fluoride are currently available, however, they can only be obtained with a dentist's prescription or be applied in the dentist's office.

Nonprescription fluoride dentifrices currently available to the public are likely to exhibit little antimicrobial effectiveness since they contain only low concentrations of fluoride. Nevertheless, they are still useful in reducing caries when used regularly.

In addition, the effectiveness of any dentifrice relies on the ability of the patient to use a toothbrush. It is unreasonable to expect most children under the age of 10 to brush their teeth adequately. Moreover, many children or young adults who are caries active often exhibit poor oral hygiene habits. Prescribing the use of chemotherapeutic dentifrice for these patients as the primary preventive measure for controlling dental caries will likely prove disappointing. Even with excellent manual dexterity and patient cooperation, the ability to brush teeth so as to deliver an antibacterial agent to all tooth surfaces including approximal surfaces and pits and fissures is at best uncertain.

In contrast, professionally applied dentifrices containing antimicrobial concentrations of fluoride have been shown to be effective in reducing the incidence of dental caries and in reducing the levels of S. *mutans* on certain tooth surfaces. Two studies have shown that high concentrations of either 5 per cent monophosphate fluoride paste or a 9 per cent stannous fluoride paste were impressive in preventing caries or suppressing cariogenic bacteria.

Applicator Trays and Direct Application. The practice of applying a chemotherapeutic agent in an applicator tray or by directly painting the agent onto tooth surfaces constitutes the most direct method of bringing an agent in contact with the odontopathic bacteria colonizing the tooth surfaces. Applicator trays, either custom made to the patient's dentition or preformed, offer several advantages. First, the technique confines the agent primarily to teeth. This feature allows the clinician to use agents in concentrations which would normally be too irritating to the mucosal tissue. Second, the agent is not diluted or buffered by saliva. Third, patients can retain trays in contact with the teeth for periods in excess of five minutes, which is considerably longer than any of the other modes of application described.

The main disadvantage of custom made tray applicators is that their fabrication is relatively expensive and that they must be constantly remade to conform to the changing dentition in growing children. For this reason, preformed noncustom applicator trays have been made available. They have been reported effective in confining the agent to the tooth surfaces. However, another potential disadvantage of tray applicators is that it is uncertain whether an agent can be adequately delivered to the approximal sites. Two studies, one using vancomycin and the other using acidulated fluoride, reported that the levels of S. *mutans* in the approximal areas were unaffected after one to two weeks of tray-applied therapy. However, daily insertion of tray applicators containing 1.1 per cent NaF gel for two years in a public school system was effective in reducing caries up to 85 per cent. Occlusal, as well as approximal lesions were reduced.

Direct application of an antibacterial agent by swabbing or painting surfaces of teeth involves more labor and time investment and is usually professionally administered, thus expensive, but likely represents the most effective means of applying an antimicrobial agent to the teeth. Not surprisingly, the degree to which the applied agents are effective in reducing plaque bacteria or caries depends not only on properties of the agent but also on the meticulousness of the clinician in the delivery of the agent.

Slow Release Delivery Systems. Perhaps one of the more novel and potentially promising approaches for delivering a chemotherapeutic agent comes from the recent development of polymer-coated microcapsules or laminated polymers capable of slowly releasing antimicrobial agents at a predetermined rate. In the laminar arrangement, (Fig. 18-1) the active agent, a fluoride-containing polymer matrix is sandwiched between two polymer membranes which govern the rate of fluoride ion diffusion out of the matrix and into the surrounding environment, the oral cavity. Laminates have been constructed which are capable of linearly releasing anywhere from 0.02 to 1.0 mg. fluoride per day for periods up to six months. Conceivably, after preliminary testing is completed, the trilaminar wafer will be incorporated into a filling, acrylic prosthesis, or directly attached to the dentition, thus allowing continous release of an optimal amount of fluoride (Fig. 18-2). When depleted of fluoride, the wafer can be replaced. Such a system requires little effort in terms of patient cooperation and expense. Moreover, incorporating this device into orthodontic or prosthetic devices might reduce the caries proneness that these patients exhibit.

Microencapsulation of minute particles of antimicrobial agents such as antibiotics and sodium fluoride to obtain a slow release has also been developed for potential treatment of

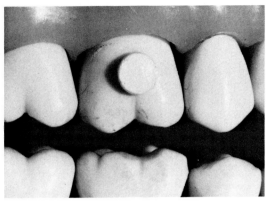

Fig. 18-2. Proposed intraoral application of slow fluoride release wafer. (Courtesy of D. Cowsar, Southern Research Institute, Birmingham, Alabama)

periodontal disease and caries. A predetermined amount of encapsuled substance (for example, antibiotic) could be placed locally into a periodontal pocket for slow release. For caries prevention, a larger capsule containing many small encapsulated particles of NaF could be swallowed enabling the fluoride to be slowly released and absorbed at a predetermined rate.

Varnishes. The apparent inability to retain fluoride on the enamel surface following topical applications has stimulated investigators to devise methods to prolong the contact time between fluoride and enamel. Two products, Duraphat® (Woelm Pharma, Eschwege, West Germany) and Fluor Protector® (Ivoclar, Schaan, Liechtenstein) have recently been introduced in Europe as vehicles for sustained fluoride release. Duraphat® is a fluoride varnish containing 5 per cent sodium fluoride in an alcoholic suspension of natural resins. Fluor Protector® is a polyurethane varnish containing a difluorosilane yielding 0.7 per cent fluoride. Both preparations have been shown to increase uptake of fluoride into enamel *in vitro*. In addition, both preparations have been shown to exert cariostatic effect in limited animal and human clinical trials. The anticaries effect has been shown to last up to one year following a single application of Fluor Protector.

While the antimicrobial effectiveness of fluoride varnishes has not yet been reported, it is conceivable that application of such an agent to the occlusal pits and fissures, for example, might exert a powerful antimicrobial effect on those organisms colonizing these sites. Other investigations have reported that antimicro-

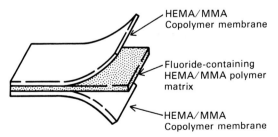

Fig. 18-1. Reservoir–Fluoride–Releasing Device–trilaminar configuration permitting slow, predetermined release of fluoride into the oral cavity. HEMA = hydroxyethyl methacrylate; MMA = methyl methacrylate. (Courtesy of D. Cowsar, Southern Research Institute, Birmingham, Alabama)

bial agents, such as vancomycin, exert a pronounced inhibiting effect against caries and S. *mutans* associated with occlusal fissures, presumably due to the sustained contact these retentive sites seem to afford. Duraphat®, for example, contains around 20,000 ppm. fluoride, part of which is readily available as free fluoride ion and likely capable of exerting a bactericidal effect.

Although the retention of varnish preparations is limited to days or weeks, they theoretically could exert a pronounced and lasting antibacterial effect to treated sites before washing out. Significant reductions in S. *mutans* populations, which lasted up to 12 weeks, have been reported in occlusal fissures following eight to ten daily topical applications of APF (see Fig. 18-8). It is conceivable that once populations of S. *mutans* are reduced, the treated fissures may be expected to remain relatively free of S. *mutans* for an extended period of time.

Prospects for using fluoride-containing varnishes in conjunction with other antimicrobial agents, such as iodine and/or chlorhexidine, also seems promising, since the F varnish could be used to disinfect pit and fissures, and the iodine or chlorhexidine used to disinfect smooth surfaces. The frequency of application would naturally need to be determined to ascertain maximum anticaries effectiveness.

Systemically Administered Agents

While the administration of low concentrations (1 to 5 ppm.) of fluoride in the drinking water constitutes the most effective caries preventive approach to date, it is not clear to what extent, if any, its antibacterial effect determines its cariostatic action. In the past, most investigators favored the concept that low concentrations of fluoride exerted an anticaries effect by altering the crystalline structure of enamel, thus making it less susceptible to decay. If the latter is the principal action of systemically administered fluoride, and many dental researchers feel that it is, then it is not within the scope of this chapter to consider low concentrations of systemically administered fluorides as part of the chemotherapeutic management of plaque. However, the antibacterial effects of higher concentrations of fluorides will be discussed later in this chapter.

The effect of long-term administration of systemic antibiotics solely for control of dental caries in humans has not been reported, nor has it been seriously considered. Several retrospective studies of patients receiving long term regimens of daily doses of either penicillin or tetracycline have shown a decreased incidence of caries in these patients when compared to nontreated controls. In order for a systemically administered agent to be effective in suppressing the odontopathic flora, it must be available within the plaque in a high enough concentration and for a sufficient period of time. Moreover, it has to be selective against cariogenic organisms without upsetting the other nonodontopathic organisms. At present, there is no systemically administered chemotherapeutic agent (besides fluoride) that can be safely and effectively administered for reduction of caries.

THE SPECIFIC PLAQUE HYPOTHESIS

A direct, positive correlation between the *quantity* of plaque colonizing the cervicogingival areas of the dentition and gingivitis has been convincingly demonstrated. In the case of other forms of periodontal disease and caries, however, recent evidence strongly indicates that it is the *qualitative* differences between plaques, *i.e.* the specific bacterial composition of the plaque and the specific intraoral site that the plaque colonizes, that determines which disease, if any, the plaque will cause. These two aspects of plaque ecology (see Chaps. 11 and 12) are fundamental tenets of what Loesche (see Suggested Readings) has described as the *specific plaque hypothesis*. He and others have shown that it is possible to isolate and culture distinct types of microorganisms within plaque obtained from different sites in the mouth associated with the presence or absence of dental disease at the particular site. For example, specific plaques have been associated with dental caries, acute necrotizing gingivitis, and juvenile periodontitis and well as a nondisease associated plaque. In fact, for the case of dental caries, several investigators now feel that caries can be considered as at least three distinct disease processes, characterized in part by the site of attack (pits and fissures, smooth enamel surfaces, or exposed root cementum) and the bacterial flora associated with the lesion.

It is likely, that some or all the above specific plaques and others not yet characterized can exist in different individuals, within a single individual or even adjacent to and on the same tooth site.

In contrast, the *nonspecific plaque hypothesis*, which has held sway in the past, assumes that all plaques are similar in bacterial composition and that the *quantity* of plaque present determines health or disease. In the case of dental caries, the amount of plaque per se does not seem to be the essential parameter influencing whether cavitation will occur or not. This fact is clinically evident in those patients having large plaque accumulation but having little or no evidence of caries. This is not to say that a large accumulation of plaque cannot be cariogenic. Clearly it can be, but plaque quantity itself is not the determining factor as to whether caries will occur or not.

As our knowledge concerning specific bacteria associated with dental caries increases, an approach to caries control based on specifically directed antibacterial regimens seems more tenable. Along these lines, three aspects of dental caries prevention relevant to the use of antibacterial agents in caries management need be considered: identification of the cariogenic organism(s); study of the ecology and metabolic characteristics of these organism(s); and identification and implementation of a chemotherapeutic approach that takes into account the first two variables mentioned.

The Role and Ecology of *Streptococcus mutans*

Intraoral Determinants of Colonization

In recent years a great deal of evidence has accumulated linking *Streptococcus mutans* with the initiation of enamel caries in humans and in laboratory animals. A more detailed description of this organism and its relationship with dental caries is given in Chapters 11 and 13. Knowledge concerning the ecology (see Chap. 12) of odontopathic organisms such as *S. mutans* is critical to the development of a rational approach to chemotherapy. Indeed, much of the renewed interest toward the potential for chemotherapeutic management of dental caries arises from recent knowledge gained from examining the unique ecology of this particular plaque organism. Most pertinent to a chemotherapeutic control of *S.*

mutans is its apparent feeble ability to reinfect the oral cavity following intensive disinfection procedures. This can be explained by several known aspects of *S. mutans* ecology. For example, the colonization of *S. mutans* within the oral cavity is confined to, and dependent on, the presence of nonshedding surfaces such as enamel, metallic restorations, and/or prosthetic appliances. This finding suggests that if teeth could be effectively disinfected, the main intraoral reservoir of this organism would be eliminated. Recolonization of teeth following disinfecting procedures would be limited due to the following aspects of the unique ecology of *S. mutans*. First, soft tissues (i.e., cheek, vestibule, tongue dorsum) and saliva are known to contain only low numbers of this organism (less than 1 per cent of the total cultivable streptococci). This is in part due to the relatively weak ability of *S. mutans* to adhere to the various intraoral surfaces compared to other oral streptococci as shown *in vitro* and *in vivo* by several investigators. In addition, since the epithelial tissues surrounding the teeth undergo constant desquamation, and because *S. mutans* cells show low affinity for epithelial surfaces, the chances for other intraoral surfaces other than the teeth to act as reservoirs from which *S. mutans* could recolonize the disinfected tooth surface is remote.

Another finding which indicates the reduced ability of *S. mutans* to adhere to the tooth surfaces comes from studies which have shown that intraoral spread of this organism from an infected to a noninfected site occurs only to a slight degree, if at all. The feeble ability of this organism to adhere, even to enamel surfaces, and its discrete pattern of microcolonization, partly account for and attest to the slow rate at which this organism is seen to spread from site to site.

Finally, as mentioned previously, the turnover rate of plaque organisms, including *S. mutans*, has been estimated at 2 to 3 generation cycles per 24 hours. For these reasons, it is difficult for *S. mutans* cells surviving disinfection to regain quickly their predisinfection levels.

Extraoral Determinants of Colonization

Another set of factors opposing recolonization following disinfection procedures is the unlikelihood of reinfection of the oral cavity with

S. *mutans* originating from extraoral sources, (i.e., those sources harboring this organism outside the disinfected oral cavity). Unlike several other common infectious diseases afflicting man with natural reservoirs outside the host (tetanus for example) the natural reservoir of S. *mutans* resides almost exclusively within the oral cavity of humans. While it is well documented that certain laboratory and wild animal populations harbor organisms phenotypically similar to those S. *mutans* found in humans, distinct genotypic differences exist between human and nonhuman types of this organism.

Attempts by several investigators to artificially implant in adult subjects S. *mutans* originally derived from either human or animal sources have been accomplished only with great difficulty, if at all. Therefore, it has been assumed that natural transmission of S. *mutans* between adult humans also does not readily occur. In addition, it has also been surmised that the likely vehicle of transmission of S. *mutans* is the saliva from an infected human. Since saliva is known to contain this organism in low numbers this is not an unreasonable assumption. However, the degree or frequency of encountering another person's infected saliva is not known, nor is the role played by indirect vectors such as saliva-contaminated eating utensils or airborne droplets of saliva. In view of the difficulty encountered when attempting to implant artificially highly concentrated inoculums of S. *mutans* into human volunteers, it can be presumed that the low number of S. *mutans* present in saliva would not constitute a potent source for infecting another host.

It must be emphasized that while the difficulty of transmitting S. *mutans* between adults (as seen from limited studies using artificial conditions) presents evidence that transmission and acquisition does not readily occur, it would be erroneous to extrapolate these observations to all human situations. Worldwide epidemiologic surveys reveal that most humans are infected with S. *mutans*, indicating that this organism has been readily transmitted from host to host. The apparent contradiction between the experimental transmission data and the known epidemiologic data can be partially resolved if two parameters influencing acquisition and transmission of S. *mutans* are considered. The first parameter is the age of the recipient host at

time of acquisition. Like most other known infectious diseases, the very young and the very old are usually more susceptible to acquiring a given infection. It has been seen, for instance, that young rodents are more readily infected with S. *mutans* than are their parents or older siblings. The reasons for the apparent resistance to infection by S. *mutans* exhibited by older animals is not known, but is likely due in part to the presence of a stable indigenous flora which provides competition for substrates and/or binding sites, hormonal differences, and also possibly a more advanced degree of host immunity in comparison to younger rats.

The second parameter likely involved in acquisition and transmission of S. *mutans* is the degree of infection present in the source of infection, often the parent(s) of the host. Investigators have shown that in both laboratory animals and in humans, transmission of S. *mutans* tends to be mediated through maternal lines. In one such study, a high percentage of bacteriocin-typed strains of S. *mutans* found in mothers was subsequently recovered from their children, implying either direct transmission through frequent contact with them or with another infected host. The latter possibility seems unlikely in view of the difficulty adults are known to experience in acquiring artificially implanted S. *mutans* as discussed above.

Certain epidemiologic studies have indicated a stronger correlation in caries experience as measured by DMF index between mothers and children than between fathers and their children. In addition, as mentioned previously, transmission of cariogenic organisms such as S. *mutans* have also been shown to follow maternal lines. These observations lead to the speculation that mothers may be a major source of cariogenic flora and that children will tend to reflect the degree of S. *mutans* infection seen in their mothers. This aspect of the ecology of S. *mutans* is relevant to the evaluation of the prospects for chemotherapy since it suggests that if the levels of S. *mutans* present in parents (particularly in mothers) could be reduced, the chances of transmitting S. *mutans* to the child may be reduced. At this time, however, it is obviously premature to assume that reduction of the natural reservoirs in the carrier host will prove to be a feasible method of reducing dental caries in young children.

Other Oral Bacteria Associated with Dental Caries

Lactobacilli

Early investigations initiated forty years ago reported a positive relationship between certain species from the genus Lactobacillus and dental caries. In view of this positive relationship, lactobacilli were considered to be the main etiologic agent of dental caries.

The acidogenic and aciduric properties of this organism, along with its frequent association with carious lesions, strengthened arguments implicating this group of organisms in the caries process. While a direct relationship between the number of carious lesions and the number of lactobacilli present in saliva was found when large numbers of subjects were examined, it is now known that lactobacilli are, for the most part, secondary invaders of already initiated lesions rather than being the primary initiators of caries lesions.

Both *in vivo* and *in vitro* experiments have shown lactobacilli to exhibit only a feeble ability to adhere to intact enamel surfaces. Experiments using germ-free rats infected with lactobacilli indicated that this organism was capable of producing minimal caries, but only in retentive occlusal fissures. When this organism was implanted in pathogen-free hamsters which do not have deep fissures, no carious lesions were produced. It appears, therefore, that this organism requires a stagnant, retentive niche in which to colonize; pits and fissures, enamel and restorative defects, and carious lesions provide ideal habitats for this organism. Once established in a retentive site, lactobacilli may contribute to the progression of a carious lesion. Several investigations involving human subjects show that when all carious lesions are restored, the prevalence of lactobacilli usually fall to undetectable levels.

While the role of this organism in the initiation of caries is not considered to be a primary one, it must not be lightly regarded. Few organisms are as capable to produce acid and survive in a low pH environment as are the lactobacilli. Moreover, a recent preliminary report has indicated that lactobacilli may be important in the initiation of caries in occlusal pits and fissures of humans.

Actinomyces

Certain members of the genus Actinomyces have been associated with cemental or root surface caries. Among these organisms A. viscosus appears to selectively colonize the tooth surface similarly to S. mutans and S. sanguis. While Actinomyces have been shown capable of forming organic acids able to lower the pH in vitro, their acidogenic and aciduric properties are notably less than that of S. mutans and lactobacillus. For this and possibly other reasons, Actinomyces are generally unable to initiate caries lesions on fully mineralized enamel surfaces but are likely capable of contributing to lesions on less mineralized cemental surfaces. Actinomyces have been found associated with cemental caries in both laboratory animals and in man. Current investigations are underway in an attempt to delineate the precise role of these organisms in caries afflicting the cemental surfaces. In addition, more specific information is being gathered linking these organisms with various forms of periodontal disease.

SELECTED ANTIMICROBIAL AGENTS PROPOSED FOR PLAQUE CONTROL AND MANAGEMENT OF CARIES

Antibiotics

Following Miller's initial attempts to find a suitable chemotherapeutic agent for caries control in the late 1800's, disillusionment and/or lack of interest generally prevailed in this area until the 1940's. However with the clinical introduction of the "miracle drug," penicillin, prospects for control of infectious diseases, including dental caries, were revitalized.

Antibiotics are generally described as biologic substances produced by specific microorganisms that are capable of exerting an inhibitory or lethal effect on other microorganisms. Nearly all antibiotics available today, while initially derived from microorganisms, have been chemically modified to enhance antimicrobial efficiency or potency in clinical application.

Prior to the discovery of sulfa drugs and penicillin, bacterial infections were managed primarily by topical application of antiseptics and surgical debridement of infected tissue. Attempts for systemic control of bacterial sepsis at that time were limited. Those agents that were used systemically were highly toxic to all living cells and had to be carefully administered and monitored to allow their antimicrobial effects to occur without harming the patient. In general, antibiotics have had limited use in dental practice even though their oral effectiveness has been demonstrated in animal studies and in some clinical studies.

The initial search for antibiotics to be used in the control of plaque was limited by the uncertainty about the identity of the microorganisms etiologically responsible for plaque dependent diseases. Therefore, broad spectrum antibiotics were among the first to be used, but were later discovered to exhibit certain limitations:

1. Imbalance of the oral and/or intestinal flora with overgrowth of resistant organisms. (Cases of black, hairy tongue, oral moniliasis, enteritis, and diarrhea).
2. Undesirable selection of strains of bacteria resistant to the antibiotic being used, which could cause interference with the use of the antibiotic in systemic, infectious diseases.
3. Development in the host of allergic and even anaphylactic reactions.

With the understanding of the cariogenic properties of specific microorganisms such as S. mutans, this search is now better oriented and may possibly yield a specific type of antibiotic which might control the activity of these specific "target" organisms, without upsetting the ecologic balance in the oral cavity.

Penicillins and Analogues

Penicillin and its numerous analogues are inhibitors of cell wall synthesis and for that reason are bactericidal against growing organisms. They exhibit a narrow spectrum of antibacterial activity, being particularly effective against gram positive streptococci, including those found in the oral cavity. The antibacterial action of penicillin and other cell wall inhibitors is limited to bacterial cells which are actively dividing, hence forming new cell walls.

Topically Applied Penicillins. It was not long after the introduction of penicillin that dental investigators showed the inhibitory effect of this agent on dental caries in laboratory animals. In fact, when penicillin was continuously available in the water supply of rodents, almost total prevention of dental caries was demonstrated.

Clinical trials involving human subjects were conducted soon thereafter testing the caries effectiveness of penicillin-containing dentifrices. Children brushed one to three times daily for varied periods of time and caries increments were recorded. Most studies, except one, reported marginal or no reductions in dental caries scores. A single study reported a 50 per cent reduction in caries increments after one year brushing with penicillin dentifrice. The uneven and conflicting results of these dentifrice studies, coupled with the growing awareness of penicillin-associated host hypersensitivity and bacterial resistance, brought to a halt all but essential uses of penicillin, particularly the topically-applied preparations. In retrospect, the discontinuation of using penicillin-containing dentrifices was warranted, not only because of the possible side effects it might have produced, but also because it was delivered ineffectively via toothbrushing and in suboptimal concentrations.

Systemically Administered Penicillins. Several retrospective studies have been reported evaluating the anticaries effect associated with the long term administration of penicillins. Children taking daily oral doses of penicillin prophylactically, as part of a post rheumatic fever therapy, were reported to have significantly less (18 to 55 per cent) DMFS scores compared to nontreated groups. Likewise, cystic fibrotic patients receiving daily doses of antibiotics mainly from the tetracycline group, were reported to experience significantly less dental caries than their non-afflicted siblings.

Long term systemic administration of antibiotics for the prevention of dental decay in otherwise healthy children is unjustified because comparable reductions can be achieved by simpler, less risky means (i.e., fluoridated water). This does not exclude however, the possible use under highly controlled conditions of a short term regimen of systemic antibiotics as part of the treatment of a patient for an unusually severe dental infection such as seen in the case of rampant "nursing bottle caries" or "radiation caries." Surprisingly, the effects of short-term regimens of systemic antibiotics on odontopathic organisms such as *S. mutans* or on caries have not been reported.

Vancomycin

Vancomycin, a polypeptide inhibitor of cell wall synthesis, has a bactericidal spectrum of action similar to that of penicillin, primarily against gram positive organisms. Vancomycin is poorly absorbed through the gastrointestinal or oral tract, thus having limited use in medicine. In view of the above characteristics vancomycin appeared attractive as a topical anticaries agent.

Extensive testing in both laboratory animals and humans has shown vancomycin capable of exerting an adverse effect of *S. mutans* colonizing the various tooth surfaces and on caries increments. In human studies (Table 18-1) concentrations between 1 per cent and 15 per cent were applied repeatedly by either swab or applicator trays. The net effect of such applications was limited to suppression of *S. mutans* rather than to their elimination. This effect was pronounced on occlusal surfaces, but relatively little effect was noted on *S. mutans* colonizing approximal surfaces. Caries reductions after nine months of near daily applications averaged around 22 per cent or the equivalent of one surface less decay per subject per year.

Although only modest reductions in concentrations of *S. mutans* or in caries increments were obtained in these studies, valuable insight was gained. For instance, cell wall synthesis inhibitors such as penicillin and vancomycin are for the most part only effective against growing, actively dividing bacterial cells. Since mean generation time of plaque microorganisms, including *S. mutans*, is estimated to be low (2–3 times/day), prolonged exposure to cell wall inhibitors is probably required for the drug to decrease appreciably their concentration in the plaque microflora. The clinical data supports this speculation since the most pronounced antibacterial effect was obtained in the retentive sites (i.e., pits and fissures) where prolonged exposure was most likely to occur. Therefore, in order for a cell wall inhibitor to exert more than a temporary suppressive effect on plaque microorganisms, it must remain in contact with an actively multiplying bacteria over an extended period of time.

Another difficulty associated with prolonged use of a narrow spectrum antibiotic such as vancomycin is the possibility of causing a shift in the composition of the plaque from a predominantly gram positive flora to one having increased numbers of gram negative organisms. Such a shift was reported when subjects rinsed three times daily for five days with a 0.5 per cent vancomycin solution. The long and short term consequences of such alteration in the oral flora is not predictable at this time, but it must be viewed cautiously, since several of the gram negative organisms have been associated with periodontal disease.

TABLE 18-1. SUMMARY OF CLINICAL TRIALS USING VANCOMYCIN PREPARATIONS FOR REDUCING POPULATIONS OF *STREPTOCOCCUS MUTANS* AND DENTAL CARIES IN HUMANS

Investigators	Conc.	Mode of Application	Frequency and Duration	Results
Jordan & DePaola, 1974	3%	Custom-tray Applicators	5 days, twice daily for 10 min.	Reduced populations *S. mutans* in sound and carious fissures for one week.
DePaola, *et al.*, 1974	1%	Custom-tray Applicators	5 days, twice daily for 15 min.	Reduction in populations of *S. mutans* in buccal plaque for one week.
Jordan & DePaola, 1977	15%	Custom-tray Applicators	5 days, twice daily for 15 min.	Reductions in population of *S. mutans* in buccal plaque for up to 8 weeks.
DePaola, *et al.*, 1977	3%	Custom-tray Applicators	Average 150 treatments per year; once daily for 5 min.	Reduction in populations *S. mutans* in plaque from fissure and smooth surfaces and reduction in caries increment of one surface per year.

Kanamycin

Kanamycin is an aminoglycan antibiotic (Fig. 18-3.) which is poorly absorbed through the oral mucosa or the gastrointestinal tract. Its principal mode of action involves the inhibition of bacterial protein synthesis, hence its activity includes a relatively broad spectrum of bacteria, (i.e., gram positive and gram negative organisms).

By virtue of its nonabsorbancy and broad spectrum antibacterial activity, kanamycin was originally selected for topical use in reducing plaque associated with periodontal disease. Bacteriologic assay of microorganisms from plaques collected from individuals treated for 5 days with topical application of this agent indicated that kanamycin had its most pronounced effect on gram positive streptococci in supragingival plaque. Based on this observation, kanamycin was then tested for its efficiency in reducing certain of the supragingival streptococci associated with dental caries. A 5 per cent kanamycin-containing gel was applied using applicator trays twice a day for one week to the dentition of children with rampant caries. Following restoration of all carious lesions, these same children were treated again with kanamycin in a manner identical to the initial treatment. After an interval of 14 to 37 months following the last kanamycin treatment, the treated children were found to have 46 per cent fewer caries than a comparable placebo group. At the nine month recall visit after kanamycin treatment, however, the kanamycin-treated group experienced seven times more new lesions compared to the placebo group. The investigators proposed a theoretical model (Fig. 18-4) taking into account both the bacteriologic and clinical findings to explain the initial acceleration of the caries process seen at the nine-month interval. If the model is correct and applies to other antimicrobial agents, then certain deductions can be made concerning chemotherapy and dental caries: (a) to be effective an agent must be capable of penetrating and destroying the odontopathic organisms present in the subclinical or primary lesion. Kanamycin gel evidently was unable to exert its antimicrobial activity on cryptic organisms within the subclinical lesion; (b) overt or clinically detectable caries lesions should be restored prior to applying antimicrobial agents to reduce the reservoirs of odontopathic organisms such as S. mutans and to prevent their enrichment where the competing, nonodontopathic organisms are suppressed; and (c) potentially odontopathic organisms found colonizing sound enamel surfaces can be suppressed for appreciable periods of time by antimicrobial agents if the agent comes in contact with the bacteria at optimal contact time-dose conditions.

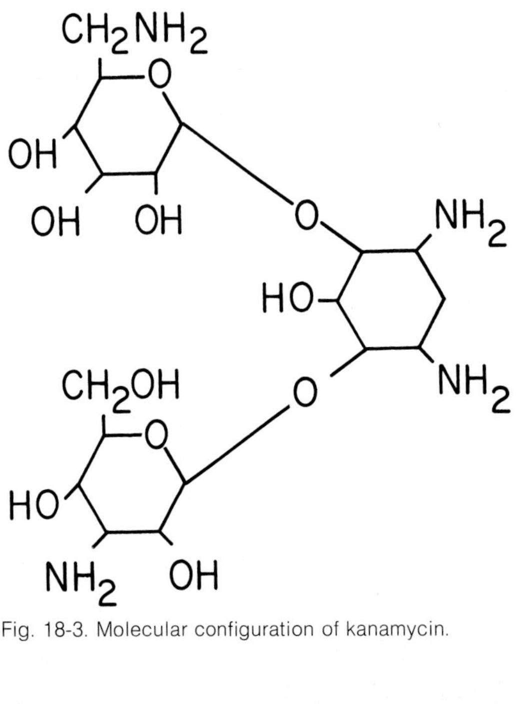

Actinobolin

Actinobolin is an antibiotic produced by *Streptomyces griseoviridis* var. *atrogacieus* which has been shown to inhibit protein synthesis in streptococci, and therefore has been considered as a potentially useful agent in caries control. This antibiotic has also been of clinical interest because of its antileukemic activity, particularly in combination with 1-β-D arabinofuranosylcytosine. Actinobolin has chemical, biologic, and pharmacologic properties which make it potentially useful in the control of caries, and therefore animal studies were conducted to test its effectiveness.

Actinobolin at concentrations of 18.8 or 37.6 ppm in the diet fed to rats was found to reduce their caries scores by 56 and 81 per cent respectively. No undesirable side effects were noted in the rats consuming the caries promoting diet containing the antibiotic. The reductions obtained with actinobolin supple-

Fig. 18-3. Molecular configuration of kanamycin.

mented diets at a level of 37.6 ppm were comparable to caries reductions obtained in this same experiment with 25 ppm fluoride in the drinking water.

While actinobolin is effective in controlling the growth of streptococci and the development of caries it does not interfere selectively with acid production or with glucosyl transferase activity in streptococci exposed to con-

centrations of actinobolin as high as 500 μg/ml. Actinobolin is an antibiotic which shows promise because it is not absorbed in the intestine and also because it has the ability to bind calcium which would facilitate adsorption to the enamel surface.

Effective use of this antibiotic as a cariostatic agent is predicated on full understanding of its physiologic and pharmacologic proper-

Fig. 18-4. Theoretical model explaining the observed effect of an antimicrobial agent (kanamycin) on bacterial populations associated with precarious and sound enamel surface. **A.** Subclinical lesion (1) initial demineralization and penetration of enamel by odontopathic organisms with some non-odontopathic organisms in surface plaque competing for substrates and attachment sites. (2) Topical kanamycin application destroys accessible bacteria in outer layers of plaque, mostly non-odontopathic organisms. (3) Non-affected odontopathic organisms from depth of precarious lesion grow out and become dominant in overlying plaque. (4) Hence plaque becomes more cariogenic and cavitation process is accelerated. **B.** Sound enamel surface, (1) Both odontopathic and non-odontopathic organisms compete for substrate and binding sites on sound enamel surface, each keeping the other in balance. (2) Kanamycin application destroys both odontopathic and non-odontopathic organisms in surface plaque. (3) Since non-odontopathic organisms are more numerous in saliva and adhere better to enamel surfaces than do odontopathic organisms, non-odontopathic organisms dominate reformed plaque. (4) Consequently, the tooth surface remains non-carious. (Adapted from Loesche, *et al.*, J. Dent. Res. 56: 254, 1977)

O-non-odontopathic organisms

■-odontopathic organisms

A. Subclinical (Precarious) Lesion

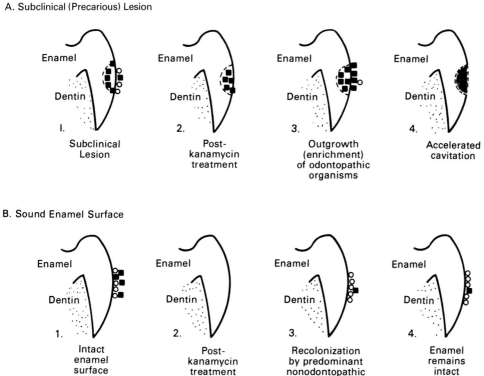

ties and its effect on streptococci metabolism. At this time, there is no FDA clearance in the U.S.A. for actinobolin and no clinical studies have yet been performed using this potentially useful agent.

Summary

Limitations inherent to many of the antibiotics discussed such as: instability in solution; inability to penetrate into plaque and inaccessible surfaces; expense; ineffectiveness against slowly growing bacteria; possible host sensitivity; and bacterial resistance, collectively restrict their potential usefulness for management of dental caries. Less restricted antimicrobial agents such as chlorhexidine, iodine, and fluoride, along with other antimicrobial agents yet to be tested may accomplish the same end result without undesirable side effects and complications.

Bis Biguanides

The two most common, commercially available bis biguanides are chlorhexidine and alexidine. These topical antiseptics are characterized by a molecular structure having both hydrophobic and hydrophilic constituents (amphipathic) and possessing a net positive charge at physiologic pH (Fig. 18-5). Bis biguanides exhibit properties similar to cationic detergents, therefore their antimicrobial properties are intimately associated with their ability to form polar-nonpolar complexes. Their principal mode of action against bacterial cells likely involves ionic adsorption to the negatively charged bacterial surface; interaction with and damage to the permeability barrier of cytoplasmic membranes; penetration into cells and subsequent precipitation of cytoplasmic constituents; and culmination in membrane leakage and cell death. Bis biguanides are considered bactericidal against a wide spectrum of microorganisms including

gram positive and gram negative bacteria, fungi and yeast. Several studies have demonstrated chlorhexidine to be poorly absorbed through intact mucosal epithelium lining the oral and gasterointestinal tracts. The small amounts that may enter the body are subject to minimal degradation. The most available and extensively tested bis biguanide is chlorhexidine, 1,1′-hexamethylene bis [5-(p-chlorophenylbiguanide)] available outside the U.S. in solution as a digluconate salt (Hibitane®).

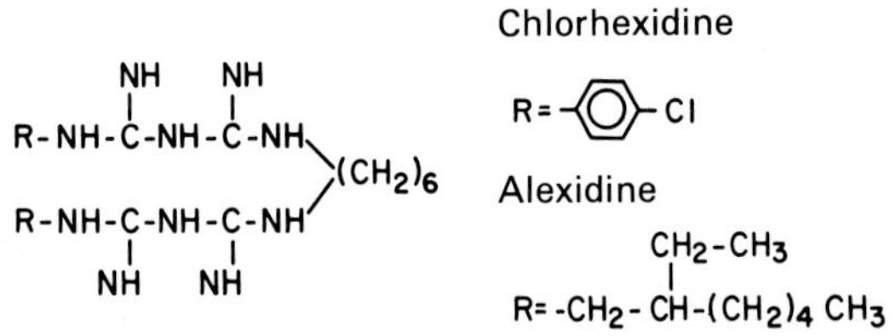

Chlorhexidine has been used widely outside the U.S. for over 20 years as an environmental disinfectant and a topical antiseptic. Some of its therapeutic uses include control of infections secondary to burns, wounds, skin, and eye injuries, and for pre- and postsurgical antisepsis. In view of the remarkably low toxicity this agent is known to exhibit, as evident from its wide clinical use during the last two decades, it is not surprising that its use as an oral antiseptic was proposed. Today chlorhexidine is perhaps the most extensively tested oral antiseptic available; in spite of this, it has yet to be approved by the Food and Drug Administration for use in the U.S.

Chlorhexidine and alexidine are best known in dentistry as antiplaque agents. While initially proposed for use in humans as only an investigative tool for studying plaque formation, chlorhexidine was soon adopted as a promising, clinically acceptable antiplaque agent. Löe and coworkers (see Suggested Readings) used chlorhexidine to demonstrate the relationship between plaque accumulation and gingivitis. Plaque formation and gingivitis could be totally prevented in the absence of mechanical hygiene with two daily mouth rinses containing either 0.2 per cent or 2.0 per cent chlorhexidine. The test periods ranged from 15 days for topical applications to 40 days for mouthwashes. Based on these observations and the increased understanding concerning the association between plaque and dental diseases, chlorhexidine was proposed as an anticaries agent. Before discussing the potential anticaries effectiveness of this agent, however, certain characteristics and clinical properties should be discussed.

Characteristics of Chlorhexidine

Studies have indicated that chlorhexidine's remarkable antiplaque capacity is related to its ability to be retained in the oral cavity by forming reversible complexes with macromol-

Chlorhexidine

$$R = \langle\bigcirc\rangle - Cl$$

Alexidine

$$R = -CH_2 - CH - (CH_2)_4\, CH_3$$
$$\qquad\qquad |$$
$$\qquad\qquad CH_2 - CH_3$$

Fig. 18-5. Molecular configuration of bis biguanides.

ecules lining the epithelial and tooth surfaces rather than to any innate superiority as an antibacterial agent. In fact, up to 30 per cent of a chlorhexidine rinse is retained in the oral cavity following a single mouthrinse; its retention halflife is calculated to be 63 minutes and residuals are still detected up to one week later. The acquired pellicle (see Chap. 5), comprised largely of glycoproteins of salivary gland origin, can reversibly bind chlorhexidine and hence compete for or alter potential binding sites for bacterial attachment. Thus, the acquired pellicle possibly serves as a reservoir that facilitates a prolonged contact between chlorhexidine and the already attached bacteria (Fig. 18-6).

Binding between chlorhexidine and macromolecules such as glycoproteins appears to be ionic in nature, chlorhexidine being highly positively charged and terminal groups of glycoproteins being negatively charged (Fig. 18-6). The ionic nature of this binding is supported by data showing that a decrease in pH leads to a reduction in the amount of chlorhexidine retained in the oral cavity.

Theoretically, if the interaction between chlorhexidine and cytoplasmic membranes is nonspecific, then questions concerning the possible toxicity to mammalian cell must be raised. When low concentrations of chlorhexidine (0.02%) were introduced into human-derived HeLa cell cultures, cytotoxicity was observed. However, repeated animal and human clinical studies and isotope-labeled chlorhexidine solutions have shown this agent to be unable to penetrate or damage intact epithelium. This apparent inability of chlorhexidine to penetrate epithelium may be related to the presence of a protective layer of glycoproteins or mucopolysaccharides covering the epithelium that can bind chlorhexidine.

The most clinically undesirable side effect of repeated chlorhexidine applications is its ability to stain the teeth and the dorsum of the tongue. The exact mechanism explaining this staining effect is not entirely known, but is thought to involve the formation of pellicle-chlorhexidine complexes, the denaturation of proteins, or an interference with the normal bacterial degradation of macromolecules. The discoloration, however, is not permanent, so that the dark brown stain can be easily removed with an abrasive dentifrice.

Evidence of bacterial resistance associated with prolonged use of chlorhexidine has been reported. Six to eighteen months of contin-

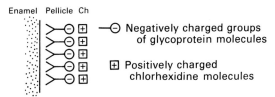

Fig. 18-6. Postulated interaction between chlorhexidine, pellicle, and enamel surface. Positively charged chorhexidine molecules reversibily bind to negatively charged terminal groups of the glycoproteins comprising the acquired pellicle covering the enamel surface. CH-chlorhexidine molecule, ⊖ negatively charged groups of glycoprotein molecules, ⊞ positively charged chlorhexidine molecules.

uous use in Beagle dogs resulted in the appearance of a chlorhexidine resistant plaque comprised primarily of gram negative organisms accompanied by the return of plaque associated gingivitis. Moreover, prolonged human clinical trials using chlorhexidine mouthrinses and dentifrices report the appearance of a chlorhexidine resistant strain of S. sanguis. In vivo and in vitro studies have not demonstrated chlorhexidine resistant strains of S. mutans even after exposure of this organism to different concentrations of chlorhexidine.

Another characteristic which might hinder general use of chlorhexidine for personal oral hygiene is its bitter taste which can be partially masked by using flavorants and lower concentrations of the agent. Other infrequently reported side effects include a transient diminuation of taste sensation, parotitis, and mucosal irritation and desquamation. Allergic reactions to chlorhexidine have been reported, but are considered rare.

Clinical Trials

The anticaries effectiveness of topically applied chlorhexidine solutions or gels has recently been demonstrated in several animal models (Table 18-2). In general, anticaries effectiveness of chlorhexidine is more pronounced for smooth surface caries than for sulcal or fissure caries.

Considering its excellent potential as an antibacterial agent, only limited clinical data is available concerning chlorhexidine's ability to reduce caries in humans. Under conditions designed to stimulate caries (frequent rinses with sucrose solutions and suspension of oral hygiene), smooth surface lesions were shown to be completely inhibited by repeated rinses

TABLE 18-2. ANTICARIES EFFECTIVENESS OF TOPICALLY-APPLIED CHLORHEXIDINE SOLUTIONS IN ANIMAL MODELS

Investigators	Animal	Concentration	Frequency, Duration & Mode of Application	Results
Regolati, et al. 1969	Osborne-Mendel rat	0.12–0.5%	Once daily for 20 days via brush	22–56% reduction in sulcal caries 57–86% reduction in smooth surface caries
Regolati, et al. 1974	Osborne-Mendel rat	1.0%	Once daily for 20 days via syringe	48% reduction in sulcal caries 69% reduction in smooth surface caries
Emilson, et al. 1976	Albino hamster	0.2%	Twice daily for 4 wks	42% reduction in smooth surface caries
		2.0%	Once daily for 4 wks via syringe	88% reduction in smooth surface caries
Brayer, et al. 1977	Syrian hamster	0.2%	Drinking water ad libitum for 50 days	52% reduction in smooth surface caries
McDonald et al. 1978	Wister rat	0.2%	Once and twice daily for 7–8 wks via swab	10–20% reduction in sulcal caries 53–84% reduction in smooth surface caries
Caufield, et al. 1979	Sprague-Dawley rat	0.5%	Twice daily for 21 days via swab	45–95% reduction in sulcal caries 34–71% reduction in smooth surface caries

with 0.2 per cent chlorhexidine solutions. In this study, caries inhibition was similarly achieved by eliminating the sucrose rinses and reinstituting normal oral hygiene. Other investigators have shown that S. mutans could be reduced to undetectable levels after two weeks of intensive treatment consisting of applications of chlorhexidine gel using applicator trays. S. mutans cells did not reappear in plaque samples until after 11 weeks post treatment. Whether such notable reductions in populations of S. mutans will result in caries reductions is yet to be demonstrated, but they are expected to be cariostatic.

In a long term clinical trial, a 0.5 per cent chlorhexidine gel was applied via applicator trays biweekly, without eliminating mechanical cleansing, to evaluate its ability to chemically remove plaque from the teeth of children. After one year of bi-weekly applications, investigators failed to observe any anticaries effect. In fact, it was reported that the chlorhexidine treated children experienced more new caries formation than did children not participating in the treatment program. Likely, the mode, duration, intensity, and/or frequency of application were inadequate for achieving the desired reduction in caries. Moreover, the investigators appear to be operating upon the assumption that the quantitative alterations in plaque would result in a reduction in caries. Such an approach, under the nonspecific plaque hypothesis discussed earlier in this chapter, is likely to lead to disappointing results in terms of caries reduction.

Summary

Repeated clinical trials have shown bis biguanides, notably chlorhexidine and alexidine, to be effective antiplaque agents. Moreover, the ability of chlorhexidine to reduce significantly populations of S. mutans in humans also makes this agent particularly attractive as an anticaries agent. However, surprisingly little data are presently available concerning their long-term effectiveness in preventing dental decay in humans. Such studies are needed to define the proper dosage, vehicles of delivery, mode of application, and duration and frequency of treatment necessary to exert the maximum anticaries effect. In addition, several of the negative effects accompanying chlorhexidine treatment, such as its bitter taste, staining of teeth, and possible selection for bacterial resistance, while not significant obstacles, do nonetheless, require a great deal more research, assuming that F.D.A. approval for testing will be forthcoming in the future.

The selective adsorption of an antibacterial agent, such as chlorhexidine, to the tooth surface and its subsequent release suggests a novel concept in the prevention of plaque-dependent diseases. Only on the basis of more research in this area will it be possible to know to what degree this concept can be applied clinically and can aid in the development of antibacterial agents to control plaque and help in the prevention of caries.

Fluoride

The proven anticaries effects of systemically administered fluoride and of topically applied fluoride preparations have been well documented and are reviewed in Chapter 20. Fluoridation of public water supplies or the administration of fluoride supplements to young children constitutes the most effective caries preventive procedure yet implemented.

Antibacterial Properties

The exact mechanism of systemically administered fluorides' anticaries effect is not precisely known. There is a growing amount of evidence to suggest that in the case of topically applied preparations containing high concentrations of fluoride (>1000 ppm F^-), a direct antibacterial effect is involved. The ability of fluoride to inhibit enolase activity, a key enzyme in the glycolytic pathway, has been known for some time. The inhibition of enolase activity has three important sequelae in terms of altering the potential cariogenicity of oral microorganisms, particularly the homofermentative streptococci and lactobacilli (see Fig. 18-7). Intermediates and end-products formed distal to the inhibited enolase enzyme such as phosphoenol pyruvate (PEP) and lactic acid will no longer be produced. Decreased lactic acid production should render the affected organisms less cariogenic. The subsequent decrease in PEP formation also results in a decrease in the amount of glucose transported across the cell membrane since PEP is an essential donor of the activated phosphate moiety in a glucose transferase system. In addition, a decreased glucose uptake will lead to decreased formation of intracellular polysaccharides (IPS). These glucose polymers are important sources of energy reserve for use when glucose is unavailable from external sources (see Chap. 14).

In vitro experiments have shown that one to ten parts per million (ppm) fluoride are capable of reducing acid production by oral microorganisms, 250 ppm fluoride can inhibit

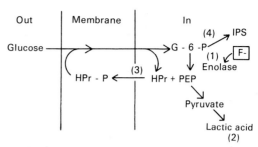

Fig. 18-7. Antimetabolic action of fluoride on hexose fermenting bacteria (e.g., *Streptococcus mutans*). (1) F⁻ exerts a direct inhibition on enolase enzyme, (2) resulting in decreased lactic acid production and (3) decreased formation of phosphoenol pyruvate (PEP). PEP is an essential donor of activated phosphate moiety necessary for transportation of glucose across the cell membrane. Hence, decreased glucose uptake leads to a decrease in metabolism and (4) decreased formation of intracellular polysaccharides (IPS) stores.

growth and 1,000 ppm fluoride can be bactericidal. A 10 per cent stannous fluoride solution (24,000 ppm) applied directly to colonies of S. *mutans* on agar plates for one minute resulted in a 95 to 100 % cell mortality.

Fluoride in antibacterial concentrations may be available against oral microorganisms present in plaque from two sources. Plaques isolated from subjects living in different communities have been reported to contain 6 to 150 ppm total fluoride; of this amount, seven to ten per cent is probably unbound and available in ionic form. The enamel surface of teeth also may contain fluoride in concentrations ranging from 1,500 to 4,500 ppm. Thus, the enamel mineral may serve as a reservoir which concentrates and releases fluoride into the acid producing plaque, possibly exerting an antibacterial effect.

Surface-bound fluorides have also been reported to interfere with attachment of pellicle and bacteria to enamel. Negatively charged fluoride ions presumably react via reversible ionic bonding with positively charged Ca^{++} in enamel or acidic groups of glycoproteins of pellicle. It is possible that they competitively inhibit initial ionic adsorption of negatively charged bacteria to enamel and/or pellicle.

Clinical and Laboratory Investigations

Several large scale clinical trials confirming the anticaries effectiveness of topical fluorides have been reported. One such study involved daily applications of sodium fluoride (NaF) to the teeth of children for two years. A 75 to 80 per cent reduction in DMFS increments was reported with a residual anticaries effect lasting two years after discontinuation of treatment. Some investigators have suggested that the effect is the result of antibacterial properties of fluoride. Others have ascribed this residual effect of topical fluoride administration to a reduction in enamel susceptibility to demineralization, since no significant difference in the levels of S. mutans and other suspected odontopathic organisms could be found between treated and control groups. However, other studies have reported specific effects of topically applied fluorides on concentrations of S. mutans on various tooth surfaces. Reductions in percentages of S. mutans colonizing smooth buccal surfaces, approximal sites and occlusal fissures have been reported one week following topical applications of fluoride. Sustained reductions in the levels of S. mutans in occlusal fissures was reported for up to twelve weeks in one study (Fig. 18-8).

A study has been conducted evaluating the effect of daily topical fluoride applications (4,500 ppm F⁻) on concentrations of S. mutans in plaque and on the incremental rate of new caries lesions in patients with radiation-induced xerostomia. While increases in the levels of S. mutans in saliva and plaque were shown to be only temporarily delayed in the fluoride treated group, new caries increments were remarkably low in this group when compared to the control group. These data suggest, among other possibilities, that the effectiveness of topical fluoride in preventing caries seen in radiation-treated patients was the re-

sult of its interference with the metabolism of S. mutans rather than the result of a permanent reduction or an elimination of this organism. The assumption that S. mutans was responsible for the initiation of caries is based on the observation that caries increment of the control rose as the levels of S. mutans in plaque and saliva increased. Support for the notion that certain concentrations of topical fluorides may be antimetabolic rather than bactericidal has been previously stated.

The restoration of existing caries lesions prior to the application of topical fluorides has been shown to be effective in reducing populations of S. mutans. In view of what is known about the potential for caries lesions to serve as a reservoir of S. mutans, mechanical debridement and restoration of lesions appears a logical and essential approach to reduce the severity of this infection.

The combination of biweekly prophylaxis with fluoride-containing paste, comprehensive oral hygiene instruction, and restoration of all existing caries lesions was shown to be effective in preventing virtually all new dental caries in children. The effect of this regime on S. mutans levels was not assayed, but the authors ascribe the reduction in caries mainly to the mechanical removal of odontopathic plaque.

Combination Therapy—Bis Biguanide and Sodium Fluoride

The feasibility of combining two or more anticaries agents to yield an additive or synergistic anticaries effect has also been reported. The combination of chlorhexidine and sodium fluoride shows considerable promise. Preliminary studies indicate that the two agents are compatible in aqueous solutions at clinically effective concentrations in vivo and in vitro. One study showed that combined one per cent chlorhexidine diacetate and 0.13 per cent sodium fluoride solutions could substantially reduce dental caries in rats when topically applied daily for 20 days. The caries reduction for smooth surfaces caused by the combined agents was greater than that seen by either of the agents alone, but the effect was not strictly additive. The caries reductions observed in sulcal lesions, however, were additive. This observation is of particular interest since most known antibacterial agents, including systemically-administered fluorides, have failed to re-

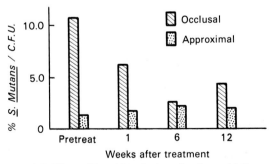

Fig. 18-8. Effect of 8 to 10 topical applications of 1.2 per cent acidulated phosphate fluoride gel (APF) on populations of S. mutans in occlusal fissure and approximal surface plaques. Anti-S. mutans effect was more pronounced in occlusal fissure plaques than for approximal surface plaques, lasting up to 12 weeks after application. (Data from Loesche et al., Caries Res. 9: 139, 1975)

duce substantially the progress of pit and fissure lesions. Lower caries scores were also reported in hamsters receiving chlorhexidine and sodium fluoride in their drinking water compared to nontreated animals or those receiving only one agent.

The effect of topically-applied chlorhexidine-sodium fluoride (CH-NaF) gel on populations of S. *mutans* has been investigated in humans who received intensive daily applications. In these subjects populations of S. *mutans* were suppressed to undetectable levels up to three months. While only a preliminary report, the CH-NaF treatment used in this study probably constitutes one of the most potent antimicrobial assaults to date when concentrations and duration of effect in humans is considered.

The prospect of combining two or more chemotherapeutic agents, hence capitalizing upon differences in affinity, sites, and/or modes of action against caries certainly merits further investigation. Such an approach has been employed successfully in medicine, for example, by combining three different sulfa drugs to yield a more potent regimen. While one agent may be effective in being retained in the oral cavity for a more prolonged antibacterial effect, another agent could enhance remineralization and repair of damaged tooth substance. Perhaps one or both agents have side effects at high concentrations, but in combination at lower concentrations, they may exhibit an anticaries effect that is additive but causing only minimal side effects. It is also possible that one agent may be more effective in preventing pit and fissure lesions, while the other agent is more effective in preventing smooth surface lesions. The possible combinations are numerous, and with time and increasing knowledge concerning the identification and ecology of the cariogenic flora, combinations may evolve which best fulfill the ultimate objective, the elimination of dental caries.

Summary

Of all trace elements that have been suggested as having cariostatic properties, only fluoride has been found to be unquestionably effective. The exact cariostatic mechanism of fluoride is not known but the following effects of fluoride have been proposed as factors influencing its anticaries effect:

1. interference in enzymatic processes of bacteria,
2. direct bactericidal action,
3. interference with attachment of odontopathic organisms to the teeth, hence reduction of plaque formation,
4. enhancement of enamel remineralization,
5. stimulation of the formation of large apatite crystals, and
6. lowering the solubility of enamel.

In view of all these properties fluoride is undoubtedly the best ally dental disease prevention has. Only recently has topically applied fluoride been investigated for its usefulness as an antibacterial agent. Further attention will most likely focus on devising ways to maximize this antibacterial effect (i.e., increasing the exposure time between the agent and the oral microflora, or combining it with other cariostatic agents such as phosphates or bis biguanides). The proven safety of fluoride delivered as topical applications makes it a very attractive cariostatic agent.

Iodine

The antibacterial effectiveness of iodine is well documented. Its use in medicine dates back at least 150 years. Prior to the introduction of antibiotics, iodine preparations enjoyed widespread acceptance as a topical antiseptic, particularly for the treatment of wound sepsis, and as a surface disinfectant. Incidents of allergy and poisoning secondary to accidental ingestion of iodine preparations have been reported but are considered rare. This is a remarkable finding considering the widespread availability of iodine as a common household remedy.

Intraoral usage of iodine solutions dates back to Miller (1890) who reported the use of this agent as an antibacterial mouthrinse. Prior to the introduction of antibiotics, iodine solution was topically applied to the tonsils and pharynx for treatment of acute and chronic tonsilitis. Iodine preparations have been used in dentistry as a presurgical and preinjection antiseptic, root canal disinfectant, antiplaque agent, and in the treatment of various forms of periodontal disease.

Aside from its low tissue and host toxicity, one property of iodine solution that makes it particularly attractive as an oral disease preventive agent is that its bactericidal effectiveness is not time dependent; that is, its ability to kill microorganisms is immediate once contact with the organism is established. This property makes iodine unique among other known antiseptics.

Studies done *in vitro* have shown that I_2-KI solutions (0.04–0.2%) are effective in penetrating and killing oral microorganisms (including S. *mutans*) within dense, preformed plaques.

Among the disadvantages of iodine solutions are their metallic taste and their tendency to stain silicate and/or composite restorations with prolonged use (over 10 applications). While complexed iodine preparations, such as polyvinylpyrrolidone-iodine (PVP-I_2), are more acceptable in terms of taste, they exhibit less bactericidal activity compared to inorganic I_2-KI preparations.

Chemical Characteristics and Antimicrobial Properties

Elemental iodine, a diatomic molecule (I_2), is a member of the halogen family which also includes two other known antibacterial agents, fluorine and chlorine. Studies indicate that the antimicrobial effectiveness of iodine preparations is directly related to the amount of free I_2 available in solution. Iodide (I^-) found in equilibrium with I_2, however, exhibits little or no antimicrobial properties and is usually added as a common ion stabilizer. I_3 and HIO, found only in low concentrations because of their instability in solution, have also been reported to exhibit antimicrobial action. Iodine's antimicrobial properties relate to its high reactivity with proteins, unsaturated lipids, and organic macromolecules via oxidative halogenation reactions which, in the case of bacterial cells, cause denaturation and precipitation of cytoplasmic constituents leading to rapid cell death. In view of iodine's mechanism of action it is considered germicidal against a wide spectrum of microorganisms including gram-positive and gram-negative bacteria, fungi and yeast, spores and viruses. Iodine is active against bacteria over a wide range of pH values and concentrations. In aqueous solutions containing inorganic iodine-KI at a pH less than 6, the predominant species will be the bactericidal I_2. This is of particular significance if combinations of I_2-KI and NaF are to be considered since NaF also exhibits greater bactericidal properties at a pH below 5.8.

Iodine complexed with solubilizing agents such as polyvinylpyrrolidone (PVP-I_2) is commercially available and commonly used in medicine and dentistry as a skin and oral mucosal disinfectant. Part of I_2 in PVP-I_2 preparations is complexed and unavailable for reaction with microorganisms; only about 1 per cent I_2 from 10 per cent PVP-I_2 solution is available as free iodine. *In vitro* and *in vivo* testing indicates that PVP-I_2 is less effective in killing plaque microorganisms than are lower concentrations of inorganic iodine solutions.

Clinical and Laboratory Investigations

The use of topically applied iodine to investigate certain ecologic aspects of S. *mutans* infections has been reported. Following a single application of a 0.2 per cent I_2-KI solution to selected approximal sites, over 50 per cent of the previously S. *mutans* infected sites remained free of detectable numbers of this organism for up to 13 weeks. A 2 per cent aqueous I_2-KI in 53 per cent glycerin solution applied to the teeth of young adult subjects significantly reduced the populations of S. *mutans* in occlusal fissures, approximal surfaces, and saliva for several weeks after application. Approximal surfaces remained significantly reduced of S. *mutans* (85%) up to 24 weeks following application. Occlusal fissures regained their pretreatment levels of S. *mutans* 24 weeks after treatment possibly as a result of the ease with which fissures are initially colonized by S. *mutans* compared to smooth surfaces, or as a result of the ability of S. *mutans* cells located in the inner depth of the fissure to survive disinfection and grow out of the fissure. This study also showed the statistical relationship between numbers of S. *mutans* in saliva and numbers colonizing the teeth, indicating the potential usefulness of assaying the effect of a disinfecting agent on populations of S. *mutans* colonizing the teeth by monitoring their concentration present in saliva.

A 2 per cent I_2-KI glycerin-H_2O solution, identical to that used in humans has been also tested in a rat model. The solution was topically applied twice daily for three weeks to the molar teeth of rats previously infected with S. *mutans*. The iodine solution significantly reduced buccal surface caries 68 to 100 per cent and sulcal caries 20 to 74 per cent compared to water-treated control animals. In addition, bacteriologic assay showed that reductions in smooth surface (buccal) caries were related to reductions in S. *mutans*, while reductions in sulcal lesions corresponded with reductions in total streptococcal and total anaerobe counts. Just as in the human studies, iodine tested in a rat model was more effective on populations of S. *mutans* colonizing smooth surfaces than in fissure sites.

Collectively, these findings indicate that smooth surface caries can be controlled through reduction of populations of S. *mutans* colonizing their surface, but that occlusal fissures or sulci, due to their unique anatomy, may be more resistant to disinfecting procedures.

Phosphates

Phosphates have been proposed as agents that exhibit cariostatic properties when added to sugar-containing diets or food. Studies done using animal models, especially rodents, have been successful in demonstrating their cariostatic effect, while results obtained in human clinical studies have been inconsistent.

Types and Specific Properties of Different Phosphates

Even though the generic term "phosphates" is used to designate compounds containing the phosphate group, they are a variety of compounds with distinct and different properties. Among those tested for their cariostatic properties are mainly the inorganic simple monophosphates such as sodium and potassium phosphate, and the calcium phosphate dihydrate (DCP). Among the linear polyphosphates also tested for their cariostatic properties are pyrophosphate, tripolyphosphate, and hexametaphosphate. The cyclic forms such as sodium trimetaphosphate (TMP) have been found to have excellent cariostatic properties when tested in rodents and have even been shown to yield significant reductions in caries in one clinical study where the TMP was added to a chewing gum base. Results of this study show not only a caries reduction, but also a reduction in the number of S. *mutans* on tooth surfaces of children in the experimental group in comparison to the control group. There are also some organic phosphates such a phytates (inositol phosphates), sucrose phosphates, and glycerophosphates which also have cariostatic properties. Thus,

there are a variety of different phosphate compounds with widely different chemical properties (solubility, degree of ionization, solution *p*H, chelation ability, stability) and cariostatic properties (significant differences between these phosphates in their ability to reduce caries are seen depending on animal models and experimental procedures used by investigators).

Mechanism of Action for Various Phosphates

Because there are many different types of compounds containing phosphates, no single mechanism can explain the cariostatic action of all phosphates. The action of some could be directed to maintaining the integrity of the enamel surface, while the action of others could involve direct effects on the metabolism and attachment of bacteria in plaque. The following mechanisms of action have been suggested to explain the local cariostatic action of phosphate compounds:

1. Providing a common ion effect which slows down enamel dissolution,
2. Contributing a buffer effect to prevent low *p*H drops in plaque,
3. Exchanging enamel carbonate for phosphates,
4. Fostering the remineralization of enamel affected by caries,
5. Stimulating posteruptive maturation of enamel,
6. Making phosphates available for bacterial metabolism in plaque, thus sparing enamel phosphates,
7. Acting synergistically with contaminating F found in some phosphates (or in plaque),
8. Desorbing and/or specific adsorption of proteins to enamel (pellicle), and
9. Reacting with lipids or proteins of cell walls and also extracellular materials to change the agglutination and attachment capability of cariogenic bacteria.

It should be pointed out that some of these mechanisms involve action on bacterial plaque and not on enamel repair and maintenance.

Use of Phosphates as Food Additives

Assuming that cariostatic properties of individual phosphates were to be fully demon-

strated in animal and clinical studies the probable delivery systems would either be a
mouthrinse or fortification of a sugar-containing food. Because phosphates are nutrients,
fortification of foods would be the first choice.
In the implementation of phosphate fortification of sugar-containing foods careful consideration should be given to the following:

1. The phosphate used should be stable to
   ensure that the structure of the phosphate compound essential to its cariostatic property is maintained.
2. Assurance should be made that the supplemented phosphate does not interfere
   with intestinal absorption of trace elements or induce calcium: phosphorous
   imbalances.
3. Care should be taken to determine that
   increased consumption of the phos-
   phate-fortified foods does not produce
   undesirable nutritional effects, particularly in bone metabolism.

Combination Therapy: Phosphates and Fluorides

Whether specific phosphates act on plaque
bacteria and/or enamel surface is not clearly
understood at this time. However, dicalcium
phosphate and sodium trimetaphosphate are
two phosphates for which there is enough information from animal and clinical studies to
consider then promising agents to be used in
caries control. Further work is necessary to establish the best delivery system and conditions
of these potentially useful cariostatic agents
for humans.

One aspect that deserves special attention is
the possible synergistic effect of certain phosphates, such as the dicalcium phosphates
(DCP), and the trimetaphosphate with fluoride. Some studies have reported that DCP
normally contains 50 or more ppm of F and
that the presence of such fluoride concentrations may enhance the cariostatic action of
the phosphate. Other well known combinations of fluorides and phosphates include acidulated phosphate fluoride (APF) and mono-
fluoro phosphate (MFP), both known to exert
an anticaries effect.

Trace Elements

Besides the elements and inorganic compounds
previously discussed, there are a large number
of elements which are found in trace concentrations in human dental tissues that could
play an antibacterial role at low concentrations. Many of these elements are nutritionally essential, while others are nonessential
and enter the body in an adventitious manner
with the food and water consumed. While the
essential trace elements (Fe, Cu, Zn Mo, Mn,
Cr, Co, I, Se) have definite biologic and biochemical roles in the body, other proposed essential elements (Si, Ni, F)have yet to be
clearly defined in terms of metabolic function
in human tissues.

Trace elements, however, may have other
beneficial effects on oral health, particularly
caries prevention. The importance of fluoride, for example, has been discussed (see
Chapter 20), but it should be recognized that
other trace elements might interact with fluoride to produce additive or synergistic cariostatic effects. Some of the elements that are
considered to be of possible importance in the
control of caries are boron, lithium, molybdenum, strontium, and vanadium. Some elements such as zinc have been shown to have a
definite antibacterial effect at low concentrations ranging from 8 to 32 ppm Zn^{++}. *In vitro*
tests where *S. mutans* was grown in chemically defined media of known trace element
composition showed these effects, but *in vivo*
tests in animal studies did not show a clear
cariostatic effect for this element. Selenium
has been suggested as a trace element which
probably has a caries stimulating effect when
present in the drinking water.

The evidence for the cariostatic effect of
lithium is convincing and comes from the inverse relationship between lithium concentrations in oral tissues and fluids and caries seen
in epidemiologic studies done in Papua, New
Guinea. The evidence for the possible cariostatic effect of strontium comes from studies
in northwestern Ohio where people show low
caries and high concentrations of strontium in
enamel. This epidemiologic finding, together
with other laboratory studies, indicates that
strontium is possibly a promising element to
be considered in caries control alone or in
combination with fluoride.

In general, the effects of trace elements on
plaque bacteria and caries have been con-
founded because of differences in the experimental conditions used to investigate these effects. Some of the major differences between
studies include the following:

1. Characteristics of different animal species and strains used to test the elements
2. Routes of administration
3. Time (age) of administration, particularly in reference to development of the dentition
4. Chemistry and availability of the element depending on type of compound used in the experiment
5. Amount required vs. toxicity levels (this problem is further complicated by the existence of biological reserves)
6. Composition of experimental diets used to test the element (natural vs. purified diets)
7. Trace element contaminants, interactions or interferences, and
8. Experimental design: methods and procedures.

The search for trace elements or minerals for possible use against the cariogenic microflora continues since it is well established that bacteria either require these elements for essential metabolic procedures or can be inhibited by these agents. Their effect can be a direct one or an indirect one as a result of an action in combination with fluoride or other minerals. Regardless, trace elements still constitute a viable research option that could contribute to caries control.

Quaternary Ammonium Compounds (QAC)

Several quaternary ammonium compounds that are known to have bacteriostatic and bactericidal properties have been tested. A mixture of "domiphen bromide", a quaternary ammonium salt, and a surface active agent (cetylpyridinium chloride), has been tested on 27 adults showing a 38 per cent decrease in plaque. In a comparison of QAC (benzalkonium) with chlorhexidine and a surface active compound in their ability to inhibit *in vitro* plaque formation by S. *mutans* and gram negative filamentous rods, QAC was found to be more effective than the other test compounds. These compounds offer possibilities as control agents for plaque, but again insufficient research data is yet available to recommend their use for human trials.

A group of compounds which are not included in the QAC group, but which also contain ammonia, are the albyl and aromatic amines and their salts. *In vitro* studies indicate that albylamines are active against S. *mutans* 6715. Some of the more active compounds are decylamine, dodecylamine, tetradecylamine, and hexadecylamine. These agents seem to have promise as antiplaque agents, and further studies are required to ascertain their clinical effectiveness and possible toxic side effects.

Enzyme Preparations

The possibility of controlling plaque by enzymatic digestion of the interbacterial matrix, which holds plaque organisms together and contributes to their attachment to tooth surfaces, has been explored. Acting on the assumption that this matrix is mucoprotein in nature, early trials were made with various hydrolytic enzymes including proteases, mucinases, carbohydrases, amylases, muramidase (lysozyme), esterases, and lipases. Despite some evidence that such preparations inhibited plaque and calculus formation in humans and caries formation in animals, none of them was sufficiently outstanding to warrant general acceptance. In response to the discovery that glucans synthesized by plaque bacteria from sucrose are significant components of plaque matrix (see Chapter 14), attention has been focused on glucanases, (i.e., dextranase (hydrolyzes $\alpha(1 \rightarrow 6)$ glucosidic linkages), and "mutanase" (hydrolyzes $\alpha(1 \rightarrow 3)$ linkages)). Some of the anticaries trials run with hamsters and rats being fed a diet supplemented with glucanase additives yielded promising results.

A dextranase obtained from *Penicillium funiculosum* was reported capable of disintegrating plaque. Several other studies done with experimental animals under control conditions indicated a useful potential for dextranase. Based on these data, a study was conducted with 47 dental students, but no statistical differences were found in amount of plaque formed between the treated group with the dextranase mouthwash and the control group at the end of one week. Another study with ten human subjects who formed plaque containing S. *mutans* gave positive results. Plaque removal or prevention in humans using mouthrinses containing dextranase has not been impressive, partly because, as was learned subsequently, $\alpha(1 \rightarrow 6)$ linkages are not the only linkages of plaque glucan, and partly because bacterial glucan does not predominate in human dental plaque, as it does in the animal analogues.

Recent efforts have been directed to the isolation of different dextranases having different *p*H stability, molecular weight, and specificity of action on dextrans containing varying proportions of different linkages. One of them, an enzyme produced by *P. funiculosium* NRRL 1768 seems to be fairly active in plaque control.

Certain logistic difficulties restricting the clinical usefulness of dextranase preparations remain, i.e., retaining these relatively slowly acting hydrolases in contact with plaque long enough to be effective, and overcoming their inability to penetrate dense microbial plaques. Other enzymes to consider in this approach are levanases to hydrolyze bacterial levan and invertases to hydrolyze sucrose before it reaches the plaque bacteria. Combinations of polysaccharases with proteases and antibacterial chemicals might exert a synergistic effect in disrupting aggregates of plaque microorganisms.

Vaccines

Success in preventing many infectious diseases by active immunization has stimulated the hope that a similar approach could be devised for preventing dental caries and periodontal disease. The likelihood of inducing effective resistance to caries by injecting cariogenic bacteria or their cell components parenterally has been analyzed thoroughly but found to be clinically unacceptable for use in humans. Nevertheless, caries reduction in rats and monkeys following oral administration of whole cells of S. *mutans*, its cell walls, glucosyl transferases, or miscellaneous glucosidases continues to be reported often enough to encourage further research.

Development of a caries vaccine faces a combination of formidable problems. In caries, an essentially unreactive tissue, dental enamel, is colonized constantly by acidogenic bacteria, which under suitable conditions initiate progressive demineralization and cavitation. The areas most often involved, the crowns of the teeth, are physically isolated from the most common source of antibodies, the blood-vascular system. Accordingly, it is hardly surprising that an attack of caries, unlike an attack of most infectious diseases, confers no resistance to a subsequent attack.

Likewise, caries has not been shown to engender a characteristic serum antibody response. Even if it did, we would not have an indicator of the anticaries status of the oral cavity. Except for a minor contribution from plasma proteins via gingival crevice exudate, the predominant type of antibody operative in the oral cavity designated as secretory immunoglobulin A (sIgA), is derived mostly from salivary glands. Antibacterial effects of antibodies, in any case, depend frequently on adjuvant reactions with components of complement or on phagocytosis, or on both; neither seems to function more than minimally in the lumen of the oral cavity. Though phagocytic cells capable of engulfing oral bacteria enter the mouth continuously in considerable numbers, few localize on the teeth. Furthermore, saliva promotes their rapid degeneration into a physiologically inert state. Another protective mechanism ascribed to sIgA, is its apparent ability to interfere with the initial attachment of bacteria to host tissues. Hence, stimulation of this mechanism by inducing specific sIgA formation with local injections of bacterial antigens or through other systemic routes could effectively prevent the colonization of certain odontopathic bacteria. Progress will require further studies on identification of cariogenic bacteria and their serological grouping; immunochemical analysis of their cell wall antigens and extracellular products; local antibody formation in regional lymph nodes, other lymphoid tissues, and salivary glands; consequences of local administration of antigens; possible protective functions of salivary IgA; and, eventually, more exactly aimed attempts to immunize against caries.

Seemingly, the chances are much better for immunologic prevention of periodontal disease, for the tissues involved are accessible to the classical immune mechanisms. In addition, the soft tissues generally manifest a characteristic local resistance, which is as yet very incompletely explained. The oral mucosa, in general, and the ginvival sulcus in particular, are constantly exposed to a large variety of bacteria (possibly as many as 100 species) of potentially great virulence in concentrations ranging from 10^8 per milliliter of saliva to 10^{11} per gram wet weight of dental plaque. These bacteria regularly find their way into the subjacent tissues, yet rarely establish infection there. In contrast, when introduced elsewhere in the body, as in bite wounds or the lower respiratory tract, serious, even fulminating disease develops. The exposed surfaces of the gingivae are bathed constantly by saliva whose sIgA may hinder adherence of bacteria to the epithelium. The blood stream commonly bears antibodies to at least some members of the gingival sulcus flora. These antibodies, along with components of complement and actively phagocytic neutrophils, are exuded into the gingival crevice in response to the degree of inflammation normally present in the gingivae of most persons. The deeper periodontal tissues are of course readily accessible to the blood-vascular system. Thus, progress in this area depends on obtaining greater knowledge of the source, structure, immunogenicity, tolerance, and functions of bacterial antigens in periodontal disease.

Caries vaccines produced against bacterial enzymes such as glucosyl transferase, which is essential for the production of extracellular dextrans and mutans, have been developed and shown to interfere with the accumulation of cariogenic organisms such as S. mutans. It remains to be shown that immunization of humans prevents plaque formation and dental caries, and considerable research efforts are under way today to explore and develop this possibility.

PROSPECTIVE APPLICATIONS OF ANTIMICROBIAL AGENTS IN THE MANAGEMENT OF CARIES

Renewed optimism concerning the prospects for antimicrobial management of dental caries as described in this chapter evolved, for the most part, from the designation of specific "target" organism, *Streptococcus mutans*. Many of the methods described for its suppression are based largely on known aspects of its unique ecology. It should be emphasized that other bacteria are known to be involved in the caries process. Unfortunately, their exact role has not as yet been as precisely defined as that of *S. mutans*. As more information becomes available concerning the role of other bacteria in the caries process, methods for interfering with their colonization and/or metabolism will likely be forthcoming. Nevertheless, current methods described in this chapter as well as future methods devised for controlling *S. mutans* in-

fections will continue to be germane since they serve as valuable model systems if and when other cariogenic organisms and their ecology become known. Clearly, many of the basic principles and findings outlined in this chapter, such as properties of the ideal agent and methods of delivery of antimicrobial agents, will also continue to be relevant as more information becomes available.

In spite of the fact that we are still in the early stages of the chemotherapeutic management of caries it is appealing, nonetheless, to speculate on some of the potential applications of an antimicrobial approach, solely, and in conjunction with other proposed methods of prospective caries control.

Longterm Suppression of S. mutans

Based on the available clinical and ecologic data, it now appears possible to suppress effectively populations of S. mutans colonizing certain tooth surfaces in humans for relatively long periods of time (months), depending on appropriate selection of the agent, method of delivery, and subject population studied. That such suppression of S. mutans populations will lead to reduction in dental caries has been demonstrated in the animal model, but is yet to be convincingly demonstrated in humans. Naturally, the working hypothesis of many investigators involved in developing an antimicrobial approach to caries control is that reductions of populations of S. mutans will ultimately lead to a concomitant reduction in caries in humans.

Replacement with non-S. mutans Antagonists

The ability to reduce intraoral populations of S. mutans also opens several other interesting and theoretically worthwhile channels for potential caries control. One such channel might involve the manipulation of the naturally occuring ecologic balance between S. mutans and a relatively nonodontopathic organism *Streptococcus sanguis*. Both groups of organisms colonize the tooth surfaces, hence compete with each other for the same ecologic niche, for substrates, and perhaps even for the same binding sites. Ecologic studies have shown that a definite relationship between the prevalence of S. sanguis and S.

mutans exist. This relationship can be expressed by the S. *mutans*: S. *sanguis* ratio. The higher the numerical value of the ratio, the more S. *mutans* are present, hence the more odontopathic the plaque is presumed to be. Conversely, the lower the numerical value, hence higher prevalence of S. *sanguis*, the less odontopathic the plaque is considered. Several investigators have shown that reducing populations of S. *mutans* by applying to the teeth antimicrobial agents such as kanamycin, chlorhexidine, fluoride, or iodine is accompanied by a notable shift in the S. *mutans*: S. *sanguis* ratio in favor of S. *sanguis*. This shift would be expected based on several *in vitro* and *in vivo* experiments demonstrating that S. *sanguis* is more capable of adhering to both teeth and soft tissue than is S. *mutans*. For that reason, S. *sanguis* has appreciable reservoirs colonizing the soft tissues. While disinfecting of the teeth would adversely affect all bacterial populations colonizing the teeth including both S. *mutans* and S. *sanguis*, the latter microbe would be favored to recolonize due to its better ability to adhere and the ready availability of an intact intraoral reservoir residing on the soft tissue and in saliva. Once recolonization of the teeth by S. *sanguis* occurs, it could theoretically exclude the recolonization of S. *mutans* for an as yet undefined period of time.

Another possible mechanism that might be devised to exploit the natural ecologic antagonism between S. *mutans* and S. *sanguis* involves the reduction of populations of S. *mutans* using disinfecting procedures followed by artificially introducing a concentrated culture of S. *sanguis* into the oral cavity. The S. *sanguis* inoculum would be derived from the individual being disinfected so as not to introduce an exogenous strain into the oral cavity, a factor also favoring its implantation. The slurry of concentrated cells might be painted on the surfaces of the teeth in a manner similar to the application of disinfectant. To date, no attempts such as the ones just described have been reported, only postulated.

Replacement with Mutant Effector Strains of S. *mutans*

Investigations are currently under way in several laboratories using mutants of S. *mutans* for delineating those characteristics of this organism which contribute to its virulence in the caries process. Mutants with decreased cariogenic potential are also being selected for possible introduction into humans with the hope that these mutant strains might compete with or preclude the colonization of the "wild type" (naturally acquired) strains of S. *mutans*. One such mutant strain designated as JH145 (Hillman, see Suggested Readings) exhibits an alteration of a terminal enzyme in the glycolytic pathway (lactate dehydrogenase or LDH) which normally converts pyruvate to lactic acid. This LDH-deficient mutant produces primarily ethanol instead of lactic acid. For this reason animals infected with the LDH deficient mutant exhibit few caries lesions compared to animals infected with the original parent strain of the mutant. Moreover, preliminary investigations have shown that these LDH deficient mutants compete successfully with the wild type in terms of adherence, infectivity, and biochemical characteristics. This indicates that the LDH strains tested appeared identical in characteristics tested to the parent strain except for altered gene coding for the structural enzyme LDH. Plans are currently being formulated in an attempt to suppress indigenous populations of S. *mutans* with topically applied disinfectant followed by oral inoculations of the LDH defective mutant strain. If the LDH defective strain can become established in the human oral cavity, and animal studies indicate that this is likely, then it is expected to compete successfully for colonization sites on the tooth surfaces, possibly excluding recolonization of the more virulent wild type organism.

One potential problem faced by studies using mutants is the probability of the mutant undergoing a "back mutation" or reversion to the original, more virulent parent strain. The probability of a revertant appearing depends in part on the total number of mutants in the oral cavity; theoretically 1 in 10^7 mutants could revert back to the parent strain. In fact, reversion was observed occurring in mutant-infected gnothobiotic rats but not in conventional rats, presumably due to the greater total number of innoculated organisms that a mono-infected animal can harbor compared to a conventional animal with an already present, naturally acquired flora (higher numbers of organisms favor back mutations).

Antimicrobial Agents and Vaccines

Interest in developing a vaccine (see Chap. 15) effective in preventing dental caries has also evolved as a result of the identification of specific organisms, such as *S. mutans*, as important pathogens in caries. The potential usefulness of combining antimicrobial agents with a vaccine arises from several studies in primates which indicate that an IgA mediated, and vaccine stimulated, immune response functions primarily by preventing initial colonization of organisms such as *S. mutans* rather than by a direct antimicrobial action on "target" organisms already established in the oral cavity. Therefore, one approach to caries prevention might include reducing the already established populations of *S. mutans* with an antimicrobial agent followed by oral immunization to prevent recolonization of the disinfected oral cavity by either endogenous or exogenous sources of *S. mutans*. Again, speculation as to the efficacy of such a combined treatment regimen is premature. Nonetheless, the multifactorial nature of dental caries may dictate that its ultimate prevention requires multiple approaches, including boosting host resistance and reducing microbial challenge.

SUMMARY

The use of antimicrobial agents in the management of dental caries is an idea that dates back to the origins of dental research. The rebirth of this concept is a reflection of recent advances that have led to a further understanding of the etiology of this complex disease process. The reader cannot but be impressed by the multiplicity of approaches that have been attempted in an effort to attack the bacterial component in the etiologic triad underlying dental caries. It is not the intention of this chapter, nor would it be possible, to give the dental clinician specific recommendations at this time as to which antimicrobial agent to use in a given situation. The science is too new; the full clinical implications as yet untested. It is, rather, the intention of this chapter to provide the reader with a sound background into the history and rationale of chemotherapy so as to equip the clinician with the knowledge necessary to evaluate and use new techniques as advances are reported. It is almost a certainty that in the next decade of dental research the area of antimicrobial control of dental caries will receive much deserved attention.

GLOSSARY

Antibiotics. Antimicrobial agents of microbial origin.

Bactericidal agent. An agent whose effect on microbes is irreversible and lethal.

Bacteristatic agent. An agent which exerts an inhibiting effect on the growth and metabolism of microorganisms. This effect can be reversed when the agent is no longer present.

Chemotherapeutic agents. Chemicals that can interfere directly with the proliferation of microorganisms and neoplastic cells at concentrations that are tolerated by the host. (In recent years, anti-cancer drugs have been included as chemotherapeutic agents.)

Dextranases. Enzymes capable of hydrolyzing specify dextran linkages.

Ecology. That aspect of biology dealing with the interaction of an organism with its environment and with other organisms.

Homofermentative bacteria. Those bacteria that catabolize sugars via anaerobic glycolysis yielding principally lactic acid.

Indigenous oral flora. Those microorganisms found in the oral cavity of most individuals in relatively high numbers.

Infection. The habitation of a host by another smaller organism or parasite. While disease may be the result of certain infections, the term infection does not imply disease.

Infectious disease. Those diseases caused by parasites capable of being transmitted from host-to-host. All bacterial infections are infectious.

Non-specific plaque hypothesis. The notion that all dental plaques are equipotent in causing dentomicrobial diseases such as caries and periodontal disease. Implied is that the quantity of plaque colonizing the tooth is the determining factor as to health or disease.

Odontopathic flora. Those members of the oral flora associated with and capable of producing demineralization of tooth substance.

Specific plaque hypothesis. The notion that various dental diseases are the result of specific bacterial infections and that dentomicrobial plaque associated with each disease can be characterized by its bacterial components as well as by the anatomical site from which it was isolated. In short, this hypothesis implies that qualitative differences exist between plaques associated with different oral diseases.

Suprainfection. Suprainfections are usually associated with antimicrobial therapies in which the "target" pathogen as well as the susceptible indigenous flora are suppressed, allowing for overgrowth of nonsusceptible organisms.

Vector. An object or another organism capable of trans-

mitting a parasite from host to host. Eating utensils or dental instruments may act as vectors transmitting oral microorganisms.

Vehicle of transmission. The medium in which an infectious agent is transmitted. Oral disease may be transmitted to other humans via saliva or droplets of oral fluids containing oral microbes.

SUGGESTED READINGS

Axelsson P, Lindhe J: The effect of a preventative programme on dental plaque, gingivitis and caries in schoolchildren. Results after one and two years. J Clin Periodontol 1: 126–138, 1974

Beighton D, McDougall WA: The effects of fluoride on the percentage bacterial composition of dental plaque, on caries incidence, and on the *in vitro* growth of *Streptococcus mutans*, *Actinomyces viscosus*, and Actinobacillus sp. J Dent Res 56: 1185–1191, 1977

Berkowitz R, Jordan H: Similarity of bacteriocins of *Streptococcus mutans* from mother and infants. Arch Oral Biol 20: 1–6, 1975

Berkowitz R, Jordan H, White G: The early establishment of *Streptococcus mutans* in the mouths of infants. Arch Oral Biol 20: 171–174, 1975

Berliner A: A clinical investigation of the effect of aqueous iodine solutions. J Dent Res 34: 402–412, 1955

Bibby BG: Antibiotics and dental caries. In "Dietary Chemicals vs. Dental Caries. Advances in Chemistry Series #94, American Chemistry Society, Washington DC, 1970

Bibby, BG, Van Kesteren M: The effect of fluoride on mouth bacteria. J Dent Res 19: 391–402, 1940

Birkeland JM, Charlton G: Effect of pH on the fluoride ion activity of plaque. Caries Res 10: 72–80, 1976

Bowen WH: Nature of plaque. In Melcher AH, Zarb GA (eds): Preventive Dentistry: Nature, Pathogenicity and Clinical Control of Plaque. Oral Science Reviews, Munksgaard, Copenhagen, 1975, pp 3–21

Bratthall D, Kohler B: *Streptococcus mutans* serotypes: Some aspects of their identification, distribution, antigenic shifts and relationship to caries. J Dent Res 55: C15–C21, 1976

Bayer L, Gedalia I, Gover A: Chlorhexidine and fluoride in prevention of plaque and caries in hamsters. J Dent Res 56: 1365–1368, 1977

Brown AT, Patterson CE: Ethanol production and alcohol dehydrogenase activity in S. *mutans*. Arch Oral Biol 18: 127–131, 1973

Brown LR, Dreizen S, Handler S: Effects of selected caries preventive regimens on microbial changes following irradiation-induced xerostomia in cancer patients. In Stiles HM, Loesche WJ, O'Brien TC (eds): Microbial Aspects of Dental Caries, Vol I. Washington DC, Information Retrieval, 1976, pp 275–290

Caldwell RC, Sandham HJ, Mann WV, Finn SB, Formicola AF: The effect of a dextranase mouthwash on dental plaque in young adults and children. J Am Dent Assoc 82: 124, 1971

Carlsson J, Grahnen H, Jonsson G: Lactobaccilli and streptococci in the mouth of children. Caries Res 9: 333–339, 1975

Caufield PW, Gibbons RJ: Suppression of *Streptococcus mutans* in the mouth of humans by a dental prophylaxis and topically applied iodine. J Dent Res 58: 1317–1326, 1979

Caufield PW, Navia JM, Rogers A, Alvarez C: Effect of topically applied antimicrobial agents on caries and on populations of *Streptococcus mutans* in rats (abstr). J Dent Res 58: 184, 1979

Cole JA: A biochemical approach to the control of dental caries. Biochem Soc Trans 5: 1232–1239, 1977

Cowsar DR, Tarwater OR, Tanquary AC: Controlled release of fluoride from hydrogels for dental applications. ACS Symp Ser 31: 180–197, 1976

Coykendall AL, Lizotte PA: *Streptococcus mutans* isolates identified by biochemical tests and DNA base contents. Arch Oral Biol 23: 427–428, 1978

DePaola PF, Jordan HV, Berg J: Temporary suppression of *Streptococcus mutans* in humans through topical application of vancomycin. J Dent Res 53: 108–114, 1974

DePaola PF, Jordan HV, Soparkar PM: Inhibition of dental caries in school children by topically applied vancomycin. Arch Oral Biol 22: 187–191, 1977

Edgar WM: The role of saliva in the control of pH changes in human dental plaque. Caries Res 10: 241–254, 1976

Emilson CG, Krasse B, Rölla G: The effect of some bisbiguanides on experimental dental caries in hamsters. Caries Res 10: 352–362, 1976

Emilson CG, Krasse B, Westergren G: Effect of a fluoride-containing chlorhexidine gel on bacteria in human plaque. Scand J Dent Res 84: 56–62, 1976

Englander H, Carlos J, Senning R, Mellberg J: Residual anticaries effect of repeated topical sodium fluoride applications by mouth pieces. J Am Dent Assoc 78: 783–787, 1969

Englander H, Keyes P, Gestwicki M, Sultz H: Clinical anticaries effect of repeated topical sodium fluoride applications by mouth pieces. J Am Dent Assoc 75: 638–644, 1967

Ericsson S: Cariostatic mechanisms of fluorides: clinical observations. Caries Res 11: 2–41, 1977

Etiology and prevention of dental caries. Technical Report Series No. 494, Geneva, World Health Organization, 1972

Fitzgerald RJ: Inhibition of experimental dental caries by antibiotics. Antimicrob Agents and Chemotherapy 1: 296, 1972

Fitzgerald RJ: The potential of antibiotics as caries-control agents. J Am Dent Assoc 87: 1007, 1973

Fitzgerald RJ, Spinell DM, Stauelt TH: Enzymatic removal of artificial plaque. Arch Oral Biol 13: 125, 1968

Gershenfeld L: Iodine. In Reddish G: Antiseptics, Disinfectants, Fungicides and Chemical and Physical Sterilization, 9th ed. Philadelphia, Lea & Febiger, 1957, pp 223–277

Gibbons RJ, DePaola PF, Spinell D, Skobe Z: Interdental localization of *Streptococcus mutans* as related to dental caries experience. Infect Immunity 9: 481, 1974

Gibbons RJ, van Houte J: Selective bacterial adherence to oral epithelial surfaces and its role as an ecological determinant. Infect Immunity 3: 567–573, 1971

Gibbons RJ, van Houte J: Dental caries. Annu Rev Med 26: 121–136, 1975

Gjermo P: Chlorhexidine in dental practice. J Clin Periodontol 1: 143, 1974

Goldstein-Lifschitz B, Bauer B: Comparison of dextranases for their possible use in eliminating dental plaque. J Dent Res 55: 886–892, 1976

Handelman SL, Mills JR, Hawes RR: Caries incidence in subjects receiving long term antibiotic therapy. J Oral Ther 2: 338–345, 1966

Henry C, Navia JM: Sodium trimetaphosphate influence on the early development of rat caries and concurrent microbial changes. Caries Res 3: 326, 1969

Hillman JD: Lactate dehydrogenase mutants of *Streptococcus mutans*: isolation and preliminary characterization. Infect Immunity 21: 206–212, 1978.

Holmberg K, Hollander H: Interference between grampositive microorganisms in dental plaque. J Dent Res 51: 588–595, 1972

Jenkins GN: Recent advances in work with fluorides and the teeth. Br Med Bull 31: 142–145, 1975

Johnson CP, Hillman JD: Competitive properties of LDH - deficient mutants of *Streptococcus mutans* (abstr). J Dent Res 58: 103, 1979

Jordan HV: A systematic approach to antibiotic control of dental caries. J Can Dent Assoc 39: 703, 1973

Jordan HV: Cariogenic flora: establishment, localization and transmission. J Dent Res 55: C–10, 1976

Jordan HV, DePaola PF: Effect of a topically applied 3% vancomycin gel on *Streptococcus mutans* on different tooth surfaces. J Dent Res 53: 115, 1974

Jordan HV, DePaola PF: Effect of prolonged topical application of vancomycin on human oral *Streptococcus mutans* populations. Arch Oral Biol 22: 193, 1977

Keene HJ, Shklair IL, Hoerman K: Partial elimination of *Streptococcus mutans* from selected tooth surfaces after restoration of carious lesions and SnF$_2$ prophylaxis. J Am Dent Assoc 93: 328–333, 1976

Keene HJ, Shklair IL, Mickel GJ: Effect of multiple dental floss-SnF$_2$ treatment on *Streptococcus mutans* in interproximal plaque. J Dent Res 56: 21, 1977

Kelstrup J, Funder-Nielsen TD: Adhesion of dextran to *Streptococcus mutans*. J Gen Microbiol 81: 485–489, 1974

Keyes PH, Englander HR: Fluoride therapy in the treatment of dentomicrobial plaque diseases. J Am Soc Prev Dent 5: 17–26, 1975

Keyes PH, Hicks MA, Goldman BM, McCabe RM, Fitzgerald RJ: Dispersion of dextranous bacterial plaques on human teeth with dextranase. J Am Dent Assoc 82: 136, 1971

Keyes PH, McCabe RM: The potential of various compounds to suppress microorganisms in plaques produced *in vitro* by a streptococcus or an actinomycete. J Am Dent Assoc 86: 396–400, 1973

Kleinberg I: Formation and accumulation of acid on the tooth surface. J Dent Res 49:1300–1316, 1970

Krasse B: Approaches to prevention. In Stiles HM, Loesche WJ, O'Brien TC (eds): Microbial Aspects of Dental Caries, Vol. III Washington DC, Information Retrieval, 1976, p 867

Krasse B, Edwardsson S, Svensson I, Trell L: Implantation of caries-inducing streptococci in the human oral cavity. Arch Oral Biol 12: 231–236, 1967

Kraus FW, Mestecky J: Salivary proteins and the development of dental plaque. J Dent Res 55: C149–C152, 1976

Lehner T: Immunological aspects of dental caries and periodontal disease. Br Med Bull 31: 125–130, 1975

Levine RS: The action of fluoride in caries prevention: a review of current concepts. Br Dent J 140: 9–14, 1976

Löe H: Symposium on chlorhexidine in the prophylaxis of dental disease. J Periodontol Res [Suppl] 8, (12): 5–6, 1973

Löe H, Schiött CR: The effects of mouthrinses and topical application of chlorhexidine on the development of dental plaque and gingivitis in man. J Periodontol Res 5: 79–83, 1970

Löe H, Schiött CR: The effects of suppression of the oral microflora upon the development of dental plaque and gingivitis. In McHugh WD (ed): Dental Plaque. Edinburgh, E & S Livingstone, p 247, 1970

Loesche WJ: Topical fluorides as an antibacterial agent. J Prevent Dent 4: 21, 1977

Loesche WJ: Chemotherapy of dental plaque infections. Oral Sci Rev 9: 65, 1976

Loesche WJ, Bradbury DR, Woodfolk MP: Reduction of dental decay in rampant caries individuals following short-term kanamycin treatment. J Dent Res 56: 254, 1977

Loesche WJ, Rowan J, Straffon LH, Loos PJ: Association of *Streptococcus mutans* with human dental decay. Infect Immunity 11: 1252–1260, 1975

Loesche WJ, Syed SA, Murray RJ, Mellberg JR: Effect of topical acidulated phosphate fluoride on percentage of *Streptococcus mutans* and *Streptococcus sanguis* in plaque. Caries Res 9: 139, 1975

Luoma H, Murtomaa H, Nuuja T et al: A simultaneous reduction of caries and gingivitis in a group of school children receiving chlorhexidine-fluoride applications. Caries Res 12: 290, 1978

Marthaler TM: Caries inhibition after several years of unsupervised use of amine fluoride dentifrice. Br Dent J 124: 510, 1968

McDonald JL, Stookey GK: Antimicrobial agents and dental caries in the rat. J Dent Res 57: 349, 1978

McGhee JR, Michalek SM, Webb J, Navia JM, Rahman AFR, Legler DW: Effective immunity to dental caries: protection of gnotobotic rats by local immunization with S. mutans. J Immunol 114: 300–305, 1975

Miller CH, Kleinman JL: Effect of microbial interactions on in vivo plaque formation by *Streptococcus mutans*. J Dent Res 53: 427–434, 1974

Miller WD: The Microorganisms of the Human Mouth. Philadelphia, SS White Dental Manufacturing Co, 1890

Mirth DB, Bowen WH: Chemotherapy: antimicrobials and methods of delivery. In Stiles HM, Loesche WJ, O'Brien TC (eds): Microbial Aspects of Dental Caries, Vol 1. Washington DC, Information Retrieval, 1976, p 249

Mukasa H, Slade HD: Mechanism of adherence of *Streptococcus mutans* to smooth surfaces. Infect Immunity 9: 419–429, 1974

Navia JM: Effect of minerals on dental caries. In Harris RS (ed): Dietary Chemicals vs. Dental Caries. Washington DC, Advances in Chemistry Series #94, American Chemistry Society, 1970

Navia JM: Fortification of sugars. In Handbook Series in

Nutrition and Food. W Palm Beach, CRC Press, 1980

Navia JM, Harris RS: Longitudinal study of cariostatic effects of sodium trimetaphosphate and sodium fluoride when fed separately and together in diets of rats. J Dent Res 48: 183, 1969

Navia JM, Lopez H, Harris RS: Cariostatic effects of sodium trimetaphosphate when fed to rats during different stages of tooth development. Arch Oral Biol 13: 779, 1968

Newburn E: Cariology. Baltimore, Williams & Wilkins, 1978

Parsons JC: Chemotherapy of dental plaque. A review. J Periodontol 45: 177–186, 1974

Poole EFG, Newman HN: Dental plaque and oral health. Nature 234: 329–331, 1971

Regolati B, König KG, Mühleman HR: Effects of topically applied disinfectants on caries in fissures and smooth surfaces of rat molars. Helv Odontol Acta 13: 28–31, 1969

Regolati B, Schmid R, Mühleman HR: Combination of chlorhexidine and fluoride in caries prevention. An animal experiment. Helv Odontol Acta 18: 12–16, 1974

Rölla G: Effects of fluoride on initiation of plaque formation. Caries Res 11: 243, 1977

Rölla G, Loe H, Schiott CR: The affinity of chlorhexidine for hydroxyapatite and salivary mucins. J Periodont Res 5: 90, 1970

Rölla G, Melsen B: On the mechanism of the plaque inhibition by chlorhexidine. J Dent Res 54: B57–62, 1975

Schachtele CF, Loken Ae, Knudson DJ: Preferential utilization of the glucosyl moiety of sucrose by a cariogenic strain of *Streptococcus mutans*. Infect Immunity 5: 531–536, 1972

Schamschula RG, Agus H, Bunzel M, Adkins BL, Barnes DE: The concentrations of selected major and trace mineral in human dental plaque. Arch Oral Biol 22: 321–325, 1977

Shiota T: Effect of sodium fluoride on oral lactabacillus isolated from the rat. J Dent Res 35: 939, 1956

Sims W: The concept of immunity in dental caries. I. General considerations. II. Specific immune responses. Oral Surg 30: 670–677, 1970; 34: 69–86, 1972

Singer L, Jarvey B, Venkateswarlu P, Armstrong W: Fluoride in plaque. J Dent Res 49: 455–460, 1970

Stralfors A: Disinfection of dental plaques in man. Sartryck Odontologisk Tidskrift 70: 183–203, 1962

Swing WK, Crawford JJ: Inhibition of plaque forming streptococci and diphteroids by organic compounds (abstr). J Dent Res 1971

Tannebaum PJ, Posner AS, Mandel I: Formation of calcium phosphates in saliva and dental plaque. J Dent Res 55: 997–1000, 1976

Tanzer JM, Reid Y, Reid W: Methods for preclinical evaluation of antiplaque agents. Antimicrob Agents Chemother 1: 376, 1972

Tanzer JM, Slee AM, Kamay BA: Structural requirements of guanide, biguanide and bisbiguanide agents for antiplaque activity. Antimicrob Agents Chemother 12: 721–729, 1977

Tanzer JM, Slee AM, Kamay BA, Scheer ER: In vitro evaluation of three iodine-containing compounds as antiplaque agents. Antimicrob Agents, Chemother 12: 107, 1977

Tanzer JM, Slee AM, Kamay BA, Scheer ER: *In vitro* evaluation of seven cationic detergents as antiplaque agents. Antimicrob Agents, Chemother, 15 408–414, 1978

Taubman MA, Smith DJ: Effects of local immunization with *Streptococcus mutans* on induction of salivary immunoglobulin A antibody and experimental dental caries in rats. Infect Immunol 9: 1079–1091, 1974

Taubman MA, Smith DJ: Immune components in dental plaque. J Dent Res 55: C153–C162, 1976

van Houte J: Oral bacterial colonization: mechanisms and implications. In Stiles HM, Loesche WJ, O'Brien TC (eds): Microbial Aspects of Dental Caries, Vol 1. Washington DC, Information Retrieval, 1976, p 3

van Houte J, Gibbons RJ, Banghart SB: Adherence as a determinant of the presence of *Streptococcus salivarius* and *Streptococcus sanguis* on the tooth surface. Arch Oral Biol 15: 1025–1034, 1970

van Houte J, Green D: Relationship between the concentration of bacteria in saliva and the colonization of teeth in humans. Infect Immunity 16: 624–630, 1974

van Houte, Upeslacis V, Edelstein S: Decreased oral colonization of *Streptococcus mutans* during aging of Sprague-Dawley rats. Infect Immunity 16: 203–212, 1977

Weerkamp A, Bongaerts-Larik L, Vogels GD: Bacteriocins as factors in the *in vitro* interaction between oral streptococci in plaque. Infect Immunity 16: 773–780. 1977

Woods R: The short-term effect of topical fluoride applications on the concentration of *Streptococcus mutans* in dental plaque. Aust Dent J 16: 152–155, 1971

19 Dynamics of Biologic Mineralization Applied to Dental Caries

THEODORE KOULOURIDES

Introduction—The Enamel Remineralization Concept
Biologic Mineralization
    Historic Background
    The General Problem of Calcification
        Effect of pH on the Ionic Product
        Chelation of Calcium Ions
        Ionic Strength
        Activity Coefficients
    Biological Complexities of Mineralized Tissues
        Variability of Mineral Phase
        Organic-Mineral Bonding
        Unattainable Equilibrium
    Mechanisms of Calcification
        Booster Mechanism or Alkaline Phosphatase Theory

        Template Mechanism
    Lability of Bone-Tooth Mineral
Enamel Adaptation to the Cariogenic Challenge
Implications of the Adaptation Concept in Dental Science
Experimental Evidence Supporting Remineralization
The Remineralization Process in the Treatment of Caries
The Possible Impact of Remineralization on Oral Health Programs
Summary
Glossary
Suggested Readings

INTRODUCTION—THE ENAMEL REMINERALIZATION CONCEPT

In cariology, remineralization of enamel is analogous to wound healing in the soft tissues of the body. *Remineralization* is the result of arrestment or reversal of a carious lesion through decreased cariogenic attack, increased resistance of the tooth surface, or a combination of both of these processes. These changes are associated with redeposition of mineral in the microspaces created in the dental tissues by the mineral dissolution (see Chap. 9) that resulted from earlier cariogenic activity. Because the process involves reactions other than mineral incorporation in the lesion (such as deposition of staining and extrinsic organic material), the lesion arrestment, or reversal, is best referred to as lesion consolidation or remineralization; and for practical purposes the two terms are synonymous.

The concept of remineralization was described at the beginning of this century, with some authors claiming success in clinical applications. In general, however, for many years the dental profession felt that the evidence was not sufficient to warrant the adoption of therapeutic disciplines of remineralization for routine patient care. In fact, until recently the term was not even mentioned in operative dentistry text books, and arrestment of caries was presented as an accidental phenomenon beyond the control of the dentist. Today, extensive laboratory and clinical research has established the remineralization concept as an indisputable fact and has demonstrated that the process of lesion consolidation can be enhanced therapeutically.

Thus far in this text we have explored several areas relevant to dental caries from the perspective of host, environment and agent factors involved in the disease process. As our attention focuses on preventive aspects of this disease, it will be our objective in this chapter to describe 1) some general principles of biologic mineralization as background for understanding tooth remineralization, 2) the experimental and clinical evidence supporting the remineralization concept, and 3) our recommendations for applying existing knowledge about remineralization in the practice of dentistry.

It should be pointed out that aspects of remineralization are currently under intensive study by many investigators and, in the near future, more advanced approaches in clinical management will surely become available. Nevertheless, we feel that procedures which have evolved from significant breakthroughs in the field of cariology during the past 70 years of research can now be applied with distinct advantage as therapeutic modalities in present day dentistry.

BIOLOGIC MINERALIZATION

Biologic mineralization or calcification can be defined as the process during which certain tissues accumulate large amounts of minerals and form complex crystals, hence making these tissues (bones and teeth) rigid.

All tissues contain minerals, but there are two important differences between the minerals in soft and hard tissues: (1) the quantity and type of the minerals, and (2) their spatial arrangement. Whereas the various soft tissues contain minerals in the order of less than 1 per cent, the hard tissues of the body can reach levels up to 98 per cent as is the case in enamel. Not only the quantity, but also the form of minerals is different in the soft and hard tissues. In the soft tissues, the minerals are dissociated into ions dispersed randomly in the body fluids and the organic phases. In the hard tissues, however, the minerals form crystalline lattices which, in the case of bone and tooth minerals, have been characterized as apatites. The mineral apatites have the approximate formula $[Ca^{++}]_{10}[PO_4^{\equiv}]_6[OH^-]_2$ (see Chap. 7). The word apatite, derived from the Greek verb "apato" meaning deceive, was given to certain minerals mistakenly thought to be precious stones. Apatite proves to be an appropriate term even today, because after two centuries of research, the true nature of these crystals still remains partially unclear.

Historic Background

Experimental studies concerning the calcification of bones and teeth date back to 1760 with the work of the famous Scottish scientist, John Hunter. Hunter fed madder (a plant containing alizarin red, a dye exhibiting selective affinity for the bone crystals) to pigs and studied the uptake of the pigment by the bone, dentin, and enamel in relation to the age of the animal. He reported that if madder was fed to the animals during the period of tooth calcification it will be deposited in the teeth, but not if it was fed after the completion of tooth development. By following changes of the intensity or the coloration of bones with the timing of the feeding period, he concluded that the bone mineral, as well as the organic matrix, was continuously changing. He observed that the stain in bone gradually disappeared after the dye had been withdrawn from the diet, indicating active metabolic turnover in contrast to the tooth mineral, particularly enamel, which did not exhibit turnover except at the surface. The concept of mineral turnover has been confirmed by radioisotope studies. This is one example of ingenious research conducted with inexpensive and unsophisticated means which has been confirmed using modern laboratory procedures.

Numerous cases exist in medicine and dentistry related to calcification problems, and for this reason it is obligatory that we gain knowledge in this area. For example, pathologic states such as deficient calcification due to lack of vitamin D, or a diet deficient in Ca, P, or abnormal Ca/P ratios present serious clinical entities. Generally, when the bone is less than normally calcified we observe either rickets (occurring during growth), osteomalacia (occurring after cessation of growth), or osteoporosis (occurring during later adult years). However, there also exist those instances of abnormal calcification where the formation of calcific materials appear in organs that usually do not calcify. Examples of these pathologic states include arteriosclerosis and myositis ossificans. Formation of stones in different cavities, such as urinary stones, sialoliths and dental calculus are other examples of abnormal calcification. Even aging has been described as a process involving excessive mineralization of the normally uncalcified connective tissues.

In dentistry we are confronted with two major disease states: dental caries and periodontal disease. Both diseases are intimately linked with dysfunction in biologic mineralization. Caries can be considered as the reverse of calcification, namely demineralization of enamel and dentin. Calculus formation, one of the most important causative factors in periodontal disease, is the result of the precipitation of minerals into the bacterial plaque, hence causing mechanical damage as well as favoring further bacterial accumulation. Moreover, the resorption of the alveolar bone is a more serious sequelae of periodontal disease and also represents a manifestation of mineralization dysfunction. The orthodontic movement of teeth through alveolar bone involves the resorption of bone on one side of the tooth and bone deposition on the other side. The oral surgeon is concerned with bone healing as it pertains to calcification of the reparative callus. The prosthodontist is concerned with the adequacy of the bone supporting the teeth of bridge abutments, or with the alveolar bone underlying the mucosa. Bony support is a major determinant in the success or failure of the bridge or removable appliance. For all of these reasons dentists will be much better qualified to understand specific problems of their patients if they know the principles of biologic mineralization.

The General Problem of Calcification

As with all other biologic functions, calcification can be seen as a wonderfully complex reaction of living organisms. Considering that the blood and the interstitial (tissue) fluid circulate rather rapidly through all tissues of the body, the question of why some of the tissues at a specific time of their development calcify while other tissues do not is of particular interest. The calcification problem can be expressed in two ways:

(a) Why do not all tissues in which the interstitial fluid circulates become calcified?

(b) What local mechanisms are responsible for initiating and stopping calcification in bones and teeth?

The formation and dissolution of every crystalline solid depends upon the equilibrium of two forces. In the case of hydroxyapatite, the balance of these two forces depends upon the concentration of calcium, phosphate, and hydroxyl ions in the surrounding fluid. The ionic activity at equilibrium (when hydroxyapatite neither forms or dissolves) is a constant, as with every other crystalline solid in a solvent containing the ionic components of the solid. This constant is expressed as the product of concentrations of calcium × phosphate × hydroxyl ions and is referred to as the *solubility product constant* (K_{sp}). When the ionic concentration in the surrounding fluids equals the K_{sp} product, the exchange of ions between solid and solution is equal in both directions with a zero net change. At the interface between solid and solution the ions of the solid exhibit thermal motion, constantly crossing the interfacial plane, with some ions migrating to the solution while an equal number replaces them by incorporation into the solid. This dynamic equilibrium between the crystals and their fluid environment is influenced by several factors including pH, chelation, and concentration of all types of ions in the solution.

Effect of pH on the Ionic Product

The value of the ionic product of calcium and phosphate ions in solution is affected by the presence of hydrogen ions because hydrogen ions determine the pH and the pH defines the dissociation of phosphoric acid, which is the totally protonated form of the orthophosphate ion. From pH 0 to pH 14, H_3PO_4 successively dissociates at 3 levels:

		pKa
1. $H_3PO_4 \rightleftarrows H^+ + H_2PO_4^-$ or P_1	(Primary)	2.16
2. $H_2PO_4^- \rightleftarrows H^+ + HPO_4^=$ or P_2	(Secondary)	7.16
3. $HPO_4^= \rightleftarrows H^+ + PO_4^\equiv$ or P_3	(Tertiary)	12.4

In solutions of pH lower than 1.0 almost all the phosphate will be in the undissociated form of phosphoric acid due to the extremely high concentration of hydrogen ions. If the pH is raised by addition of a base such as NaOH, an increasing proportion of H_3PO_4 will be converted by dissociation of one hydrogen to the primary phosphate ion $H_2PO_4^-$. The ratios of the two types, H_3PO_4 and $H_2PO_4^-$, will be unity at the pH of the first dissociation constant (pKa) 2.16. Further increase in the pH will shift the concentrations of the two phosphate species so that the $H_2PO_4^-$ becomes predominant. This form dissociates in increasing proportions giving rise to the secondary phosphate, $HPO_4^=$. Finally, with the third stage of dissociation, all the phosphate is converted to tertiary phosphate, $PO_4^\equiv$, which is the ionic component of hydroxyapatite crystals. At pH 2.16, 50 per cent of the total phosphate is H_3PO_4 and 50 per cent is $H_2PO_4^-$; at pH 7.16 50 per cent is $H_2PO_4^-$ and 50 per cent is $HPO_4^=$; at pH 12.4 50 per cent is $HPO_4^=$ while 50 per cent is $PO_4^\equiv$.

The three types of phosphate anions, the primary, secondary, and tertiary species, behave as different molecules. The only characteristic they have in common is that they can be converted from one to the other under the pH conditions as defined by the acidic dissociation constants. Even at neutrality, the main ionic species in the solution are the primary and secondary phosphates. The tertiary form exists only in trace amounts. The fact that bone and tooth crystals consist of tertiary phosphate indicates an extreme affinity of calcium for that ion. As the tertiary phosphate is used up in the formation of hydroxyapatite, it is replenished by the dissociation of the secondary phosphate. Alternatively, a precursor salt of the secondary phosphate ($CaHPO_4$) can be rapidly hydrolyzed to hydroxyapatite.

With these reactions in mind, we can understand why at low pH the levels of $PO_4^\equiv$

ions in the solution will approach 0. One factor of the ionic product (i.e., $PO_4^\equiv$) is nonexistent at low pH, while at the same time the hydroxyl ion concentration is very low. Thus low pH causes dissolution of hydroxyapatite.

Another way that we can conceptualize the influence of low pH on hydroxyapatite crystal dissolution is to consider the reaction as a competition between hydrogen ions and calcium ions for the phosphate bonds. High hydrogen ion concentration will dissociate calcium phosphate bonds and liberate these ions for migration to the surrounding fluid. In this competition the hydrogen ion has a unique migrating advantage. Since hydrogen is part of the water molecule its migration is not retarded by the hydration shell (the layer of water molecules bound to all ions) as is the case with the calcium or the phosphate ions. This concept of ionic competition and the involvement of migrating velocities enables us to understand the profound effect of hydrogen ion in cases of oscillating acidities such as those encountered in dental plaques. With the introduction of fermentable substrates the plaques develop high acidities to be neutralized within 10 to 30 minutes by the salivary flow or neutralizing microbial fermentation. If the process is repeated frequently the hydrogen ion with its migrating advantage will penetrate through microporosities into deep layers of enamel, possibly inaccessible to calcium ions due to the hydration shell retardation. Actually these differences in migrating velocities could provide at least a partial explanation for the development of subsurface lesions (see Section V). The apparently intact surface acts as an ionic sieve in essence slowing down the calcium and phosphate migration to a greater extent than that of hydrogen ion. A diagrammatic illustration of this concept is presented in Figure 19-1. From this figure it can be seen that case I presents the state of equilibrium with no change in the enamel structure. Case II presents the case leading to caries. The demineralizing (D) activity is higher in intensity, frequency or duration than the mineralizing (M). Enamel dissolves at the subsurface more than at the surface because the relative activity of the hydrogen ion is higher at the subsurface

Ionic diffusion as a factor in the development of subsurface lesion

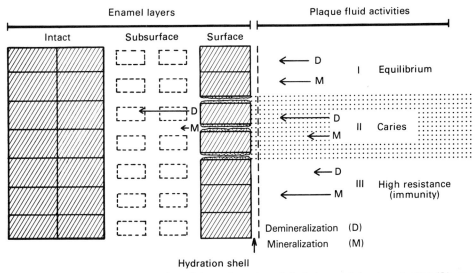

Fig. 19-1. A diagrammatic illustration of the cariogenic activity in terms of demineralization (*D*)–remineralization (*M*) reactions.

due to the ionic permselectivity of the surface. Two factors favor this type of dissolution: (a) the high velocity of hydrogen ion diffusion through water molecules in the diffusion channels of the surface layer, and (b) the self-limiting nature of the remineralization process through formation of solid which blocks the channels for ionic diffusion, particularly of the calcium and phosphate ions, into the body of the lesion. These two factors become more important with the frequency of oscillations from the supersaturated to the undersaturated state. Selective mineral retention may convert the enamel surface into a more effective barrier of diffusion even for the hydrogen ion, in which case the acid resistance of the surface increases. Case III presents the state of high caries resistance when the *M* activity (mainly influenced by the rate of flow and composition of saliva) is never overcome by the *D* activity. This case refers to persons who are immune to caries from the point of view of *D/M* equilibrium.

Chelation of Calcium Ions

Another parameter which influences the dynamic equilibrium at the tooth surface is the presence of chelating compounds. Certain organic molecules called chelators are able to eliminate calcium ions from the solution by forming compounds known as metal chelates.

Chelators are characterized by a large number of polar moieties such as carboxyl, hydroxyl, and amino groups. These molecules, in addition to forming *ionic* bonds between negative organic ions (anions) and calcium ions, form multiple *coordination* bonds which increase the stability of the binding. Essentially, the formation of a chelate involves displacement of the hydration shell of the metal ion by the chelator molecule or molecules through the formation of multiple coordination bonds between the polar groups (ligands) of the organic molecule. The main ligands are carboxyl, hydroxyl, and amino groups of organic molecules. Thus, the metal ion surrounded by the chelator is not part of the activity product of the ions in solution. Since it lowers the value of the solubility product, chelation contributes to mineral dissolution.

Actually the term *chelation* is derived from the Greek word "χηλη" (*chele*) for "claw" to indicate the grasp of the metallic ion by an organic molecule surrounding the calcium ion with rings of carbon chains as the several negative organic groups bind to the ion. The distance of these polar groups in terms of units of carbon atoms in a ring formation is an important factor. The favored ring structure has five, six, or seven atoms. These rings are favored by the carbon to carbon angle which at its optimum is 109.5°. A square ring would have a 90° angle which would strain the bond angle. On the other hand, if the ring had more than seven atoms, the polar groups would be too far apart and the probabilities of their approaching the same spot (the Ca^{++}) would be minimal.

Ionization of carboxyl groups increases the number of possible polar groups in an organic molecule and at the same time creates conditions of electrostatic attraction between the positive calcium ion and the negative organic ions. Since the dissociation of carboxyl groups requires a rise in pH, the chelation effect is greater under alkaline conditions when an organic molecule with two or more carboxyl groups will have several groups in anionic form available for the binding of Ca^{++}.

An example of a common chelator is the citrate anion. At the low pH of 2, most molecules of a citric acid solution will be in the undissociated form. This situation changes at higher pH levels. One can picture the H^+ of the three carboxyl groups dissociating one after another as the environment becomes poor in H^+ (as the pH is raised). The dissociation constants for the three carboxyl groups of citric acid expressed as pKa's are 3.08, 4.39, and 5.49.

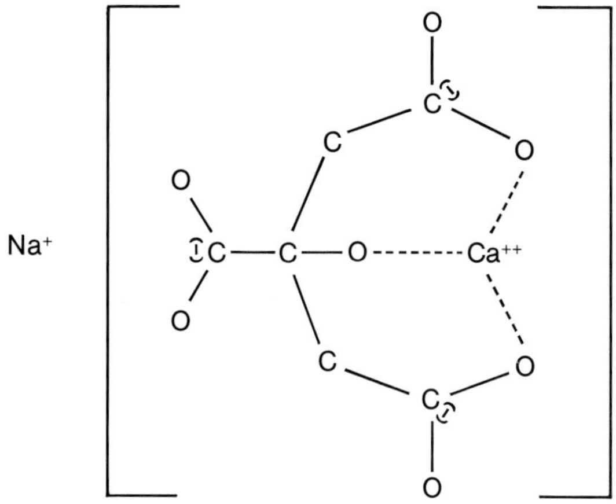

Fig. 19-2. Example of calcium citrate chelate.

ing characteristic of metal chelates. The chelate with a trivalent citrate blocks the activity of the calcium ion and behaves as a monovalent anion.

Most amino acids, peptides and anions of organic acids can form chelates with calcium ions, thus reducing the effective ionic concentration and the ionic product of $[Ca^{++}]^{10}[PO_4^{\equiv}]^6[OH^-]^2$ in the solution. As

Forms of Citrate

pKa$_1$ = 3.08   pKa$_2$ = 4.39   pKa$_3$ = 5.49

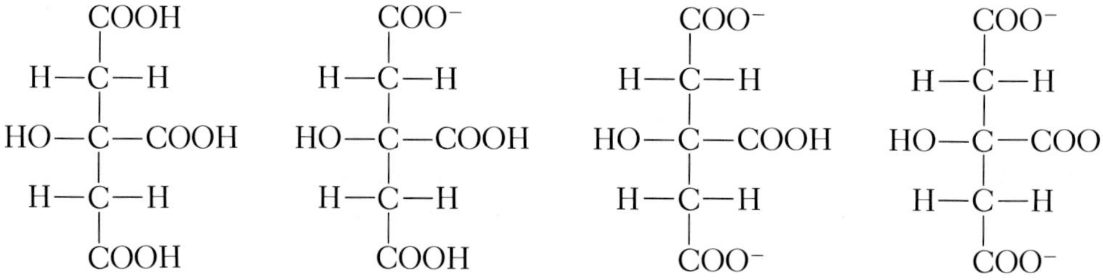

COOH	COO$^-$	COO$^-$	COO$^-$
H—C—H	H—C—H	H—C—H	H—C—H
HO—C—COOH	HO—C—COOH	HO—C—COOH	HO—C—COO$^-$
H—C—H	H—C—H	H—C—H	H—C—H
COOH	COOH	COO$^-$	COO$^-$
Undissociated	Monovalent	Divalent	Trivalent

Thus, at neutrality the major proportion of citrate is in the trivalent form. The three types of citrate anions have different reactivities with other molecules or ions. In fact, the different ionic forms of citrate can be considered as different molecules. In terms of chelation, the trivalent citrate with the four polar groups (3 ionized carboxyls and 1 hydroxyl), forms a most stable chelator with the calcium ion, an organic metalic complex with one negative charge as shown below (Fig. 19-2).

This two-dimensional illustration of calcium citrate demonstrates the claw-like bond-

with citric acid, high pH favors chelation of calcium with the other organic molecules also.

Actually, one theory of the etiology of caries suggests chelation to be the primary mechanism of mineral dissolution (see Chap. 8). However, the concentration of chelators in the dental plaque is too low to account for a strong demineralizing effect and the acid pH caused by the fermentation of sugars does not favor chelation. The majority of dental investigators feel that the hydrogen ion is the main culprit causing enamel dissolution while chelators are possible contributors by reducing the concentration of free calcium ions in the above described dynamic equilibrium at the interface between solid and solution.

Ionic Strength

The value of the ionic product of calcium and phosphate necessary to resist dissolution of hydroxyapatite is also affected by the ionic strength which takes into consideration all types of ions in the solution. The calculation of ionic strength (μ) is given below, where C = molar concentration and V = valence of the ion.

$$\mu = \tfrac{1}{2}(C_1V_1{}^2 + C_2V_2{}^2 + C_3V_3{}^2 + \cdots + C_nV_n{}^2)$$

Because of the extremely low solubility of hydroxyapatite, the contribution of calcium, phosphate, and hydroxyl ions to the ionic strength of the surrounding biological fluids is minimal. The main value in this expression comes from ions foreign to the apatite lattice such as Na^+ and Cl^-. Thus, where ionic strength is high due to many "foreign ions", the net effect is to interfere with effective collisions of calcium and phosphate ions. This interference tends to reduce the degree of saturation and consequently the likelihood of growth of existing crystals or the formation of new crystals.

Just as the presence of foreign ions reduces the rate of effective collisions leading to solid formation, so too does the presence of charged molecules in a system of a crystalline solid immersed in a given solvent (like H_2O) as they shift the equilibrium towards solid dissolution. By attracting the calcium and phosphate ions these charged molecules compete with ionic attractions that lead to the formation or maintenance of the solid. The shift in the effective collisions can be counterbalanced by an increase of the calcium × phosphate × hydroxyl ion product in the solution. However, if this increase is not provided from an outside source, then ions from the solid hydroxyapatite will migrate towards the fluid until the requirements of the solubility product are met. In other words, under conditions of an ionic product below the Ksp, enamel or bone crystals will dissolve. In essence this mineral dissolution describes the initiation of dental caries.

Activity Coefficients

The effects of pH, chelation, ionic strength, and charged ions can be accounted for in systems where all the above variables are known. In these systems, instead of formulating a different Ksp for each value of the variables, the science of physical chemistry has introduced the concept of *activity coefficients*. These are correction factors calculated from data on the composition of solutions, electrical conductivity, change in the boiling or freezing point, etc. The analytical value of the calcium × phosphate × hydroxide product corrected by the activity coefficient of each ion always gives a constant Ksp value for a certain salt in a given solvent at the same temperature and it is called the activity product. For a sparingly soluble salt such as hydroxyapatite the activity product is an extremely small number. For this reason it is expressed as pKsp, (i.e., the logarithm to the base 10), similar to the calculation which describes the pH. The activities of the ionic components $[Ca^{++}]^{10}$ $[PO_4]^6[OH^{-2}]$ yield an equilibrium Ksp = 10^{-118} or pKsp 118.

Perhaps one simple way to bring together the above concept is to consider the interface between solid crystals and solution as a very active plane of ionic migration. At the surface of the solid the ions exhibit the thermal motion or vibration toward the solid and the solution across the interfacial plane. Some of these ions escape to the solution while others from the solution are incorporated in the solid. The tendency of ions to escape is called *fugacity* from a Greek word "$\phi\epsilon\nu\gamma\omega$" (fevgo) meaning "to leave." When the fugacity of the ions at the surface is counteracted by the tendency for incorporation of the ions of the solution, an equal number of ions will migrate in both directions across the interface causing no net change in the ionic concentration of the solid or the solution. This constitutes the equilibrium. On the other hand, when the force for ionic incorporation into the solid is diminished because of low ionic concentration in the solution (or low activity product), fugacity predominates and more ions migrate to the solution than are incorporated into the solid. This situation describes the process of dissolution. The opposite situation involves more mineral incorporation in the solid. A high product of calcium, phosphate, and hydroxyl ions in the solution will overcome the fugacity and lead to new solid formation or the growth of existing solid. The dividing line between the two situations is the Ksp, the ionic product at equilibrium. Above the Ksp solid forms (supersaturation), while below the Ksp solid dissolves (undersaturation).

Biological Complexities of Mineralized Tissues

What we have described thus far refers to relatively simple systems of a salt in equilibrium with solutions of known composition. However, there are important differences between the simple model of a sparingly soluble inorganic salt (such as hydroxyapatite) in water and the interactions between the hard tissues and the serum or saliva in the human body.

Variability of Mineral Phase

Calcium and phosphate ions form an array of salts. Depending on the pH of the solution, the solid can be hydroxyapatite, $Ca_{10}(PO_4)_6(OH)_2$, octacalcium phosphate, $Ca_8H_2(PO_4)_6$, dicalcium phosphate, $CaHPO_4$, or monocalcium phosphate $Ca(H_2PO_4)_2$. The various calcium phosphate salts are characterized by different x-ray diffraction patterns (see Chap. 7) and calcium to phosphorus ratios. Those ratios vary from 1.67 for hydroxyapatite to 0.5 for monocalcium phosphate. At neutral pH the predominant salt is hydroxyapatite, but since the plaque can develop low pH's some of the other salts could also be formed.

Ionic substitutions in the apatite crystalline phase can change the composition of bone and tooth mineral (see Chap. 7) to such an extent that it cannot be considered as a stoichiometric compound such as the secondary calcium phosphate ($CaHPO_4$) or most inorganic crystalline solids. Therefore, the solubility product for the mineral of bones and teeth is not precisely defined. As a result, the solubility product of enamel is usually considered an approximation of the solubility product of hydroxyapatite, with variations imposed by irregular amounts of other minerals. It is logical that such variable factors in the composition of the mineral, at least in part, influence the differing caries susceptibility seen between different patients. Furthermore, knowledge of reactions affecting the solubility of enamel mineral may enable us to convert the susceptible enamel surfaces into resistant ones.

Organic-Mineral Bonding

The relationship between the organic and mineral components of the teeth is another area which has received considerable attention by dental researchers in recent years. Out of this interest has evolved the concept of heterogeneous nucleation to explain the process responsible for the initiation of calcification of bones and teeth. According to this theory the organic matrix seems to act as a nucleator which brings about the formation of crystals at lower concentration values than those required for spontaneous precipitation. It would seem likely that the bonds between the minerals and the organic material influence the various chemical properties of the crystals, one of which is solubility. This relationship is particularly important at the enamel surface with its developmental or acquired organic membrane-like structures (see Chap. 5). Undoubtedly such films influence the properties of the underlying crystals, one of which is solubility in acids, and add to the complexity involved in describing the biological process for the mineralization of tissues.

Unattainable Equilibrium

A third dissimilarity between the ideal system of crystals in water and the case of biologic hard structures and their environment is the *unattainable equilibrium*. The compositions of both the crystals and their fluid environment are subject to continual change which affects the stability of the system. When the conditions for crystal formation predominate, the result is accretion of minerals, while in the opposite case the result is mineral dissolution. The composition of tissue fluid is maintained at relatively constant levels of pH and mineral concentrations through the mechanisms of homeostasis. However, the composition of the fluid next to the tooth surface is subject to a variety of influences. Because salivary gland secretions vary, the tooth surface fluid may differ according to the location of the tooth in the mouth with respect to the gland ducts. Furthermore, extreme variations of the oral fluid are introduced when food comes in contact with the tooth surfaces, or when the food supplies the substrate for the enzymatic degradations which occur in bacterial plaques. Thus with these varying chemical reactions and the effects of external environment on the oral fluids the ionic product of calcium, phosphate, and hydroxyl ions at different locations of the interface between the tooth surface and the dental plaque frequently oscillates between widely different values. As an example, with a sucrose rinse the pH of the dental plaque will be lowered from neutrality to a value of 4.0 indicating a thousand times higher concentration of hydrogen ion and less concentration of hydroxyl ions. Even for a very short period of time this situation will be a severe stress causing mineral dissolution. With subsequent acid neutralization the ions in the proximity of the interface will tend to replace the mineral lost. In the process inorganic ions foreign to the composition of pure hydroxyapatite, organic molecules, and stains present in the vicinity of the interface are incorporated in the enamel altering its chemical composition. This reconstituted surface may have different physical and chemical properties than the original enamel formed from the tissue fluid which is very different than the plaque fluid that contributes to the repair process. Since the new solid is different, and essentially undefined due to the wide variation in plaque fluid compositions, its resistance to acid is also undefined. Considering all these possibilities we can understand the reasons for the difference between the world of pure chemistry and the complex biologic reactions at the tooth surface.

Although the biologic system cannot be precisely defined in terms of the physicochemical principles of the solubility product, the concept is useful for our understanding of the physiologic phenomena and the abnormalities of mineralization. For example, there is little doubt that acid production under microbial plaques formed on the enamel surface will contribute to demineralization, or that enamel with high fluoride content will resist a stronger acid attack because of reduced solubility. Furthermore, as we shall see in this chapter, the concept can be utilized therapeutically with the administration of mineralizing mouthwashes for the reversal of incipient lesions.

Mechanisms of Calcification

Two mechanisms have been suggested to account for the calcification of bones and teeth—the booster mechanism and the template mechanism.

Booster Mechanism or Alkaline Phosphatase Theory

The booster theory for hard tissue mineralization suggests that in the tissue fluid of bones and teeth the calcium $\times$ phosphate $\times$ hydroxyl product is increased over the values of serum thus causing crystallization of the bone salt. The main evidence in support of this mechanism is the localization of the enzyme alkaline phosphatase in calcifying cartilage. According to the theory alkaline phosphatase acts on the hexose monophosphate provided by the breakdown of glycogen to liberate inorganic phosphate. The inorganic phosphate thus added to the normal concentration in the tissue fluid locally increases the ionic product to the point of crystallization of bone salt.

However, alkaline phosphatase is not uniquely found in calcifying cartilage, but is also seen in noncalcifying tissues. Generally, the enzyme is associated with high metabolic activity. On the other hand, the search for the expected elevated sugar phosphate substrate in areas of calcification has not been successful. A significant boost of the solubility product would require higher concentrations of sugar phosphates than are found in the calcifying cartilage. An additional inconsistency of this theory is the evidence that alkaline phosphatase is found not only in structures that accumulate phosphate salts, but also in hard structures accumulating carbonate salts like the shells of some marine animals. In the face of all these difficulties, even the supporters of this theory suggest that in addition to the alkaline phosphatase there must be another "local" mechanism involved in biologic mineralization.

Template Mechanism

The template theory of tissue calcification emphasizes the role of the changes occurring in the organic matrix of bones and teeth just before calcification. Calcifying cartilage is known to be rich in enzymes. This theory suggests that metabolic activity that occurs results in the rearrangement of molecules and reactive groups towards a spatial configuration appropriate to trigger crystal formation. This configuration is termed the *template*. We can better understand the role of the template if we remember that the initiation of crystal nuclei proceeds over a higher energy barrier than the subsequent growth of the crystals. Thus, the suitable spatial arrangement of active groups in the template is needed mainly to start calcification; from then on the actual growth of the crystal demands less energy.

Strong evidence for the template theory was provided in studies of the reversible inhibition of calcification by specific ions like beryllium, magnesium, and copper. Treatment of rachitic cartilage with these ions prevents calcification, presumably by blocking the active groups of the template. This poisoning can be reversed by treatment with calcium chloride which apparently displaces the blocking ions and thus liberates the template for the hydroxyapatite crystal formation. Attempts have been made to define the template and to correlate it with the presence of a specific molecule. A specific arrangement of collagen, or combination of collagen with muccopolysaccharides, or the presence of a specific protein such as a phosphoprotein, have been suggested as important characteristics of the template. At present, we can only state that calcifying templates can be provided by various biologic molecules contained in the organic matrices of the bones, enamel, dentin, and other calcifying structures. Furthermore, in abnormal calcification the template could be provided by molecular reorganizations in tissues that do not usually calcify. Abnormal calcification can be induced in many tissues as a hypersensitivity reaction called *calciphylaxis*. Compounds like Vitamin D and parathyroid hormone and others (called sensitizers) when administered systemically in excessive amounts cause calcification of tissues that usually do not calcify (such as skin and the tissues of the cardiovascular system). Calcification of sensitized animals can be directed to specific tissues by injecting into these tissues other chemical substances such as salts of iron, chromium, aluminum, and other substances called *direct challengers*. On the other hand, injection of compounds like dextran, polymyxin, or glucocorticoids cause calcification of tissues at sites distant from the sites of injection. These compounds are called *indirect challengers* (see Figs. 19-3, 19-4).

In conclusion, at present the evidence on the mechanism of calcification suggests that two major factors are involved, (1) the calcifiability of the tissue, and (2) the calcifying potential of the fluid bathing the tissues. The magnitude of these two factors regulates and

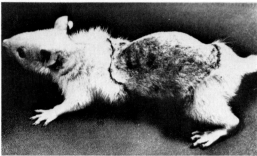
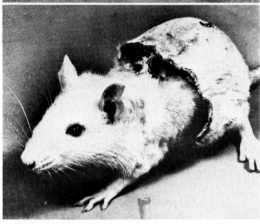

Fig. 19-3. Experimental calciphylaxis showing abnormal hardening and cracking of the skin of a rat. The animal was sensitized systemically with the indirect calcifier dihydrotachysterol and challenged locally in the skin with infiltration of ferric dextran. (Selye, H: Calciphylaxis Chicago, University of Chicago Press, 1962.)

directs calcification in specific tissues like bones and teeth. Given a certain calcifying potential of the serum, the tissues with the highest calcifiability will calcify preferentially. Calcifiability is imparted to a tissue by certain types of spatial arrangements of active groups which constitute the calcifying template. The template, functioning as a nucleator, binds mineral components and triggers precipitation. After nucleation the crystals will grow until they fill the available space in the matrix of the hard tissues. Even after their formation, the crystals are subject to possible changes influenced by their fluid environment as will be described in the next section of this chapter.

Lability of Bone-Tooth Mineral

Ionic exchanges between crystals and their fluid environments can be *isoionic* when one ion is replaced by the same type of ion (as Ca

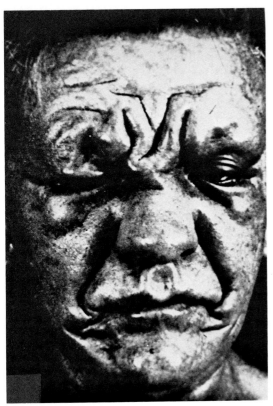

Fig. 19-4. Human condition resembling experimental calciphylaxis. It is a case of scleromyxederma in which the skin became hard and fragile due to high accumulation of minerals. (Selye, H: Calciphylaxis. Chicago, University of Chicago Press, 1962)

partments, or pools, from which the organism can draw ions as they are needed for the metabolic activities and the maintenance of the hard tissues (see Fig. 19-5).

A large number of ions and molecules can be found in the hydration shell and on the crystal surface, but only those compatible with the hydroxyapatite lattice can be found in the crystal interior. The skeleton is a storehouse of minerals. In addition to calcium and phosphate, a significant amount of strontium, magnesium, lead, and other ions can be stored in the skeletal system. Because of its large size citrate can only be found on the surface of the crystals, while carbonate is found both at the surface and within the crystal interior.

The rate of exchange reactions varies according to the involved pools. For instance, it takes longer for ions to exchange from the serum pool to the crystal interior than to the pool of the hudration shell. Similarly, the loss of ions from the crystal interior is slow. As an example, it has been postulated that if an individual is exposed to radioactive Sr^{90}, a byproduct of nuclear reactions that can be found in milk, the radioactivity damage to the bone marrow can be very serious because Sr^{90} can enter the crystal interior of bone and remain there for a long time.

Here we interject a principle of ancient wisdom related to the importance of body fluids in health. Embedocles (c. 500 B.C.) considered that all diseases were caused by disturbances in

Fig. 19-5. Diagrammatic representation of the various ionic pools around a crystal. Ions are found in: the interior of the crystal, the crystal surface, the hydration shell, or the tissue fluid surrounding the crystal. The size and charge of the ions determine their accessibility to the various pools.

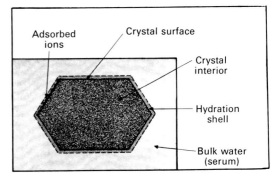

with Ca^{45}), or *heteroionic* when the replacing ion is of different type (as F for OH). These ionic exchanges are governed by two factors, the size and charge of the ions. Ions of similar size and charge are more apt to exchange for each other than are dissimilar ones. It is also known that some of the bone minerals are more labile than others, apparently existing in a more soluble form. It has been postulated that the labile minerals are amorphous solids in contrast to the more stable, crystalline solid. Another view suggests that the carbonate mineral is more labile than phosphate, especially at low pH.

The bone and tooth crystals can be considered to be one end of a continuum of ionic pools with the serum being the other end. An ion can be in one of five positions, the crystal interior, the crystal surface, adsorbed on the crystal surface, in the hydration shell that surrounds the crystals, and finally, in the serum. These positions can be considered as comthe proportions of the body fluids. With the knowledge of his time he theorized that when the body fluid has the appropriate composition in terms of the four humors, phlegm, blood, black, and yellow bile, the organism remains healthy. Manifestation of disease was indicative of a disturbance in the proportions of the four humors of the body. The mineral equilibrium between the biologic crystals and their fluid environment presents a comparable interdependence. While health reflects the proper ionic compositions of the parent fluid at the tooth surface, dental disease can be attributed to either an excess or a deficiency of certain constituents of the fluid such as hydrogen, hydroxyl, calcium, phosphate, and fluoride ions. This is contrary to the simplistic view that the tooth surface has a more or less standard resistance to caries attack, depending on hereditary conditions, and that it will decay as soon as the fluid environment of the dental plaque exceeds the critical level of acidity. The expression "my teeth have cavities because they are soft like my mother's" does not represent a valid fact. The similarity of their lifestyle, rather than genetics, offers a better explanation of the similarity in caries susceptibility.

An example of an heteroionic exchange that is of interest to us in preventive dentistry is the replacement of F⁻ for the OH⁻ of hydroxyapatite. Fluoride ion is compatible with the requirements of the apatite lattice (see Chap. 20) so that it can be found in any of the five ionic pools. Incorporation of fluoride in the crystals reduces their solubility, while the presence of fluoride in the hydration shell or the surrounding fluid enhances remineralization.

The availability of fluoride in all of the ionic pools, the factors influencing its position, and its functions in the demineralization - remineralization reactions are of more than mere academic interest. A dentist's understanding of these factors will influence the choice of methods to be employed for therapy. For example, the fluoride-enriched crystal is relatively stable; this state can be reached clinically by one or two topical applications of fluoride solution a year. However, fluoride enrichment of the hydration shell is a relatively transitory phenomenon, so that clinical success in affecting caries resistance using this pool requires frequent application, such as using a daily fluoride mouthwash or one of the fluoridated dentifrices. The presence of fluoride in the oral fluid modifies the fluid of the

bacterial plaques so that the oscillating states of undersaturation and supersaturation will tend to convert more hydroxyapatite crystals to fluoroapatite and thus increase the tooth's resistance to acid dissolution. It has been demonstrated that microbial plaques accumulate fluoride and that fluoride accelerates the process of remineralization. It has also been shown that remineralized lesions contain higher concentrations of fluoride which can be considered as the marker of the remineralization reaction.

The demonstration of fluoride's involvement in enamel remineralization resulted in the use of fluoride through the vehicle of mouthwashes. The new rationale explains a long standing question of why topical applications of *concentrated* fluoride solutions to erupted teeth have not been as cariostatic as the consumption of very dilute one ppm fluoride in communal water supplies throughout life. It is now known that drinking fluoridated water supplies fluoride to the microbial plaque, with the result that fluoride is available at the site where it is needed most, (i.e., at the tooth surface sites under cariogenic attack). It is at these sites that the fluoride should be available for participation in the remineralization phase of the dynamic equilibrium between the enamel and its fluid environment.

In contrast, infrequent topical application of concentrated fluoride solutions will convert a relatively small number of the surface crystals to fluorapatite thereby reducing the surface solubility. This fluoride incorporation is not as dynamic as that seen with frequent plaque enrichment since surface fluoride is lost with time and the loss is predominant in the areas of cariogenic activity. We thus come to the explanation of the paradox: frequent fluoride supply to the fluid environment of the microbial plaques will depress the rate of demineralization, thus shifting the equilibrium towards higher stability of tooth minerals and offering greater protection against caries than the infrequent use of higher concentrations of fluoride.

ENAMEL ADAPTATION TO THE CARIOGENIC CHALLENGE

Biologic adaptation is the response of living beings, organs, or tissues to a damaging environmental challenge resulting in a higher resistance to that challenge. Two types of adaptation to the cariogenic conditions can be considered, one that concerns the tooth surface and a second that is related to the individual's behavior. The first involves a change in the composition of the tooth surface, the second refers mainly to the practice of disciplines of oral hygiene and diet. As we discuss tooth remineralization we are focusing mainly on the adaptation of the tooth surface to the cariogenic challenge. As the teeth erupt into the oral cavity they leave the homeostatically controlled environment of the tissue fluid to encounter the strong challenges of the oral fluid. Similar to other cases of biologic adaptation to any type of stress, the intensity and frequency of the challenge are critical factors. While strong repeated challenges will start lesions, weak infrequent challenges will allow time for equilibration, in the specific case of caries, with the preferential replacement of soluble minerals by insoluble ones. The conditions for enamel's adaptation to the cariogenic challenge are diagrammatically illustrated in Figure 19-6. Each mineralization cycle involves a period of fluid supersaturation when the driving force is for mineral deposition. A period of undersaturation will cause mineral dissolution if the tooth surface at that site is soluble in a solution of that degree of undersaturation. The most soluble minerals

in the enamel are the first to dissolve during the undersaturation period, while the most insoluble minerals from the plaque fluid will be preferentially deposited during the supersaturation period. For example, undersaturation would preferentially dissolve calcium and magnesium carbonate in the enamel, while supersaturation will deposit fluoroapatite if the plaque fluid contains appropriate concentrations of fluoride ion at the time of mineral formation.

Under ideal composition of the fluid environment each cycle may increase the resistance of the tooth surface to subsequent episodes of mineral dissolution. When the tooth resistance reaches a level sufficient to withstand the dissolving potential of the undersaturation periods, the surface will become immune to caries at least as long as the undersaturation remains at similar levels regarding intensity, duration and frequency of challenge. Conceptually we can see tooth surface adaptation as the result of a fortuitous response to the stress of undersaturation, while the development of a lesion is the result of excessive stress beyond the limits of tolerance and adaptation of the system. Even though the rest of the tooth surface may remain relatively soluble, so long as it is beyond the areas of cariogenic challenge it will not develop carious lesions. Thus the interplay between the

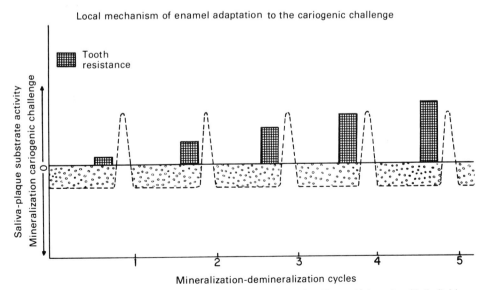

Local mechanism of enamel adaptation to the cariogenic challenge

Fig. 19-6. Diagrammatic representation of the adaptation reaction. Enamel interacts with its fluid environment in periods of undersaturation and supersaturation presented here as periodic cycles. The undersaturation periods dissolve the most soluble mineral at the site of cariogenic attack, while the periods of supersaturation deposit the most insoluble minerals if their ionic components are present in the immediate fluid environment. As a result, under favorable conditions of remineralization, each cycle could lead towards higher enamel resistance to a subsequent challenge.

demineralization and mineralization phases of the cycle can lead to two outcomes. *Intense, prolonged and frequent undersaturation will result in a carious lesion. Less intense, short, and infrequent periods of undersaturation, interrupted by periods of supersaturation, will not only maintain the tooth surface intact but also may improve its resistance to subsequent caries attack, provided that the composition of the "parent fluid" during the remineralization phase is favorable.* This favorable composition of the parent fluid has not yet been completely defined, but it is established that normal saliva is a natural, healthy fluid in which caries cannot develop; frequent plaque removal will increase the time available for the intimate contact between the enamel surface and saliva; frequent plaque, removal will decrease the opportunities for cariogenic plaque to develop; and fluoride in the plaque fluid will reduce the rate of demineralization and increase the rate of remineralization, thereby improving the stability of the enamel surface and protecting against subsequent caries attack. Figure 19-7 presents a diagrammatic illustration of the effect of local adaption reactions. With a series of demineralization and remineralization cycles, change in the composition of the tooth can occur into the deep layers of enamel, sometimes as far as the DEJ. The specific nature of the adaptation reactions are by definition localized to those areas most susceptible to cariogenic challenge. The degree of the cariogenic challenge can be directly related to the lifestyle of an individual, taking into consideration such factors as the quantity and frequency of intake of fermentable carbohydrates (see Chap. 16), the practice of oral hygiene procedures, the frequent availability of fluoride, and perhaps other habits associated with the customs of an individual's social environment.

IMPLICATIONS OF THE ADAPTATION CONCEPT IN DENTAL SCIENCE

The concept of adaptation of enamel to caries attack can explain several phenomena of dental science in a manner that is compatible with the available experimental evidence. For example, it has been a riddle as to why some mouths harboring cariogenic organsims do not develop caries. This can now be explained in terms of the stress of the cariogenic challenge being met by the appropriate remineralizing conditions. The result is a relative immunity acquired because the areas at risk have become areas of resistance through the previously described demineralization and remineralization reactions. Sometimes persons with poor oral hygiene, and/or uncontrolled dietary intake, also do not develop caries. The local increase in resistance of the challenged areas of enamel provides at least part of the explanation for the lack of dental decay in these cases.

The adaptation concept is represented in several other dental situations. Fluoride (see Chap. 20) has a most profound cariostatic effect at extremely low concentrations, such as the 1 ppm addition to the drinking water supplies. Apparently the frequent presence of fluoride in the fluid environment of the tooth converts the tooth surfaces at risk into areas of high resistance. The result is an adaptation of the challenged and remineralized enamel surface to the cariogenic challenge before a lesion can advance to the stage of frank cavitation. Post eruptive tooth maturation, combined with the uptake of fluoride, particularly in areas of cariogenic challenge, also results in caries resistance. The immunity to caries around silicate restorations with faulty margins is yet another example. Because silicate restorations leach small quantities of fluoride, which could continuously counteract the existing cariogenic challenge, a more caries resistant tooth surface evolves due to local remineralization. These observations give strong support to a concept of dynamic adaptation constantly occurring in the oral cavity

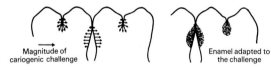

Magnitude of cariogenic challenge

Enamel adapted to the challenge

Factors in Adaptation Reaction:

1. Frequency, duration, intensity of cariogenic challenge
2. Frequency, duration, intensity of mineralizing activity
3. Composition of mineralizing fluid

Fig. 19-7. Illustration of the local effect of adaptive reactions. Areas of tooth enamel under alternating cariogenic challenge and remineralization reactions may develop into areas of high resistance. The phenomenon can be enhanced therapeutically with frequent fluoride applications.

through the interaction of the tooth surface with its fluid environment.

The above statements may mistakenly be taken as an attempt to explain *everything* in dental caries on the basis of the adaptation concept. This is far from the intent. Dental caries is a multifactorial disease (see Chap. 8) and any attempt to explain it on the basis of a single factor or concept is both futile and inaccurate. One factor or condition may have a tendency to enhance or reduce the challenge, or to increase or reduce the tooth resistance to the challenge. However, there are many factors or conditions with separate contributions to the etiology of disease. The main goal of dental science is to take all factors and concepts into consideration and synthesize a better understanding of both the etiology and prevention of dental disease so as to arrive at recommendations for the therapeutic management of caries by the practitioner. Only in this context do we feel that the adaptation concept offers an important contribution to the understanding of caries. Specifically the adaptation concept will suggest to the dental practitioner a new approach in managing incipient caries. Instead of placing conventional restorations based on the assumption that the cariogenic process will result in open cavities, the dentist will observe these lesions at the 6-month recall appointment. At the same time an attempt will be made to enhance the probabilities of adaptation through improved oral hygiene and frequent fluoride applications.

EXPERIMENTAL EVIDENCE SUPPORTING REMINERALIZATION

In an effort to stimulate further understanding and research both by laboratory scientists and clinicians, the experimental findings that led to the development of the adaptation concept through consolidation of enamel lesions will be reviewed briefly.

The initial findings supporting this concept came from clinical observations. It has been noted that extracted teeth frequently exhibit stained areas or spots indicative of previous cariogenic activity which have become arrested for various, oftentimes unknown, reasons. Chemical analysis of material excised from yellow or brown spots reveals that interactions with elements of the plaque fluid have changed the local composition of enamel. These areas, which have a high content of organic material and fluoride, and small quantities of carbonate and other exogenous trace elements, are softer than unaltered sound enamel, but are nonetheless more resistant than sound enamel to acid dissolution. As indicated by the high concentration of fluoride in the areas of consolidated lesions, selective demineralization and remineralization activities have apparently replaced the most soluble with more insoluble minerals. Actually, the difference in fluoride concentration in the areas of consolidated lesions from that in the adjacent normal enamel can be taken as a marker of remineralization because fluoride is the component of the most insoluble apatite mineral, fluorapatite. Normally the outline of the tooth surface remains intact after the mineral exchange of demineralization and remineralization since the incipient enamel lesions (see Chap. 10) are characterized by *subsurface* rather than surface mineral dissolution (Fig. 19-8). Such observations on extracted teeth show that lesion consolidation is a natural defense of the oral cavity against caries.

The concept of enamel remineralization has also been investigated using various experimental models. *In vitro* experiments have demonstrated that exposure of enamel surfaces to mild acid will induce softening similar to that seen in a subsurface lesion. When enamel surfaces softened by exposure to mild acids (such as acetic or lactic acids buffered to pH 4.0–5.0) are placed in solutions supersaturated with hydroxyapatite, rehardening occurs; experiments in which the synthetic mineralizing solution is replaced with saliva produce similar results. Chemical analysis shows that the softening and rehardening phenomena are paralleled by mineral loss or gain. In addition, animal experiments have revealed that, under conditions that favor remineralization (such as elimination of sucrose from the diet), incipient enamel lesions will actually regress.

In humans, intraoral experimental cariogenic conditions have been produced by increasing the stagnation of microbes and foods at the enamel surface. This has been accomplished through the development of the Intraoral Cariogenicity Test (ICT) and used to study the demineralization-remineralization reaction. For this test, a slab of human or bovine enamel cut from extracted teeth is mounted in prosthetic or orthodontic devices

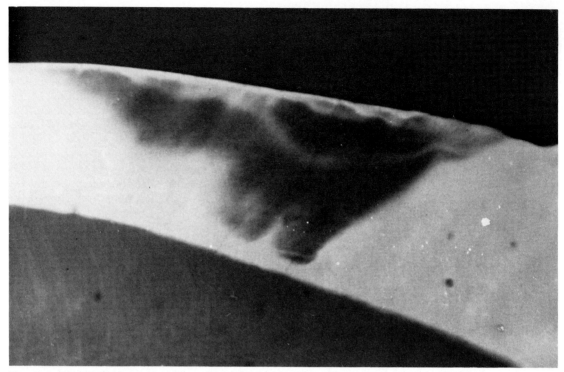

Fig. 19-8. Microradiograph of a carious lesion in human dental enamel. The radiolucent region is positioned in the subsurface enamel deep to a well mineralized surface layer. Well mineralized laminations can be seen passing through the subsurface region reflecting zones of remineralization. (Courtesy of Dr. LM Silverstone)

and exposed to the environment of the human mouth under controlled conditions (Fig. 19-9). The microbial retention associated with natural caries development is replicated in the ICT by placing a cover of Dacron gauze of defined mesh on the test enamel. In order to avoid harmful effects of cariogenic test substrates on the volunteer's natural teeth, the subjects immerse the experimental sites in solutions of the test substrates extraorally (Fig. 19-10.

The effects of the experimental conditions on the test enamel are evaluated by microscopic observations of the test surface and by measurement of changes of surface microhardness. The microhardness test is particularly applicable for such studies because caries lesions leave an apparently intact surface under which the typical subsurface lesion develops. With the increased porosity due to subsurface demineralization the mechanical indenter (Fig. 19-11) meets less resistance from the affected enamel and penetrates down to the unaffected sound enamel. The difference in penetration between a set of initial and a set of final indentations provides a good measurement of the demineralizing ac-

tivity. Essentially this difference approximates the thickness of the enamel layer that suffered experimental decay. The principles of the microhardness test are illustrated in Figure 19-12. The partially demineralized layer is illustrated as a dotted area. The maximum depth of penetration is calculated from the measured length of indentation on the basis of indenter geometry. The ratio of length to the penetration of the indenter tip is 30.5. The indenter penetrates about 5 microns into the enamel and increasingly deeper (for precise measurements up to 20 microns) into the softened enamel. Since the resistance to penetration of the softened layer is considerably less than that of sound enamel, the difference between the final and the initial penetration gives an approximation of the thickness of the affected (softened) layer of enamel.

Figure 19-13 shows an example of an enamel surface indented before and after exposure to the ICT. The cracks around the margins of the large, final indentations indicate that the indenter has crushed through an apparently intact surface layer into the subsurface lesion and the underlying enamel.

The ICT has several advantages over other

experimental models used in caries research for the study of the demineralization—remineralization reactions. First, the measured alteration of the test enamel is due to microbial interactions with the diet and saliva in the human mouth under conditions very similar to those causing natural caries. Secondly, a major problem seen with testing a patient's real teeth is avoided. The prosthetic appliances carrying the test enamel can be im-

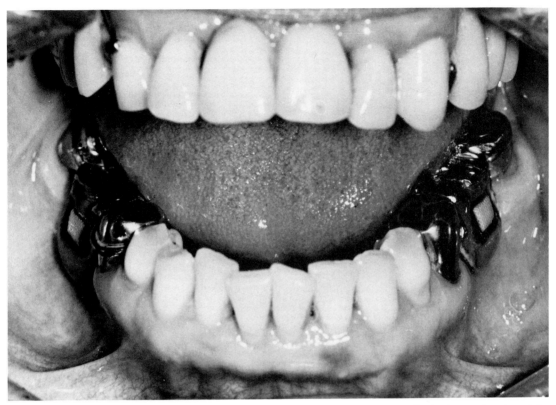

Fig. 19-9. Picture of a partial denture carrying tooth enamel with its dacron gauze cover for the intraoral cariogenicity test (ICT).

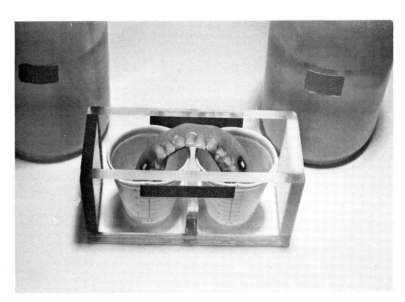

Fig. 19-10. The immersion apparatus with a full denture for the controlled extraoral supplementation of two substrates.

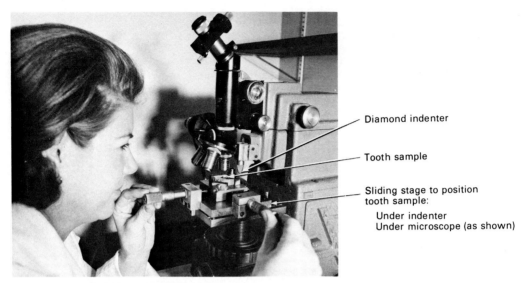

Diamond indenter

Tooth sample

Sliding stage to position
tooth sample:

Under indenter
Under microscope (as shown)

Fig. 19-11. The KENTRON Microhardness Tester. The stage of the tester moves the sample in two positions: under the indenter which is released to indent the enamel under conditions of standardized pressure, and under the microscope for the measurement of the indentation with a vernier microscale. Essentially the principle of the microhardness testing is similar to that of a dental explorer which will penetrate deeper in softened than in hard enamel. The microhardness measurements are extremely sensitive to subsurface enamel demineralization under mildly acidic conditions similar to those involved in natural and experimental caries.

The microhardness technique for measuring
subsurface enamel demineralization

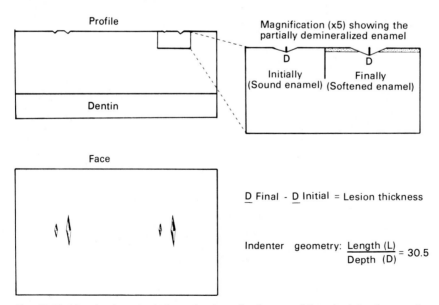

Profile

Dentin

Face

Magnification (x5) showing the
partially demineralized enamel

D   D

Initially   Finally
(Sound enamel) (Softened enamel)

D Final - D Initial = Lesion thickness

Indenter geometry: $\dfrac{\text{Length (L)}}{\text{Depth (D)}} = 30.5$

Fig. 19-12. Microhardness technique. A schematic diagram of the principle of measuring experimental caries on enamel surfaces on the basis of indenter penetration. The initial state represents the picture of indenting sound enamel, while the final is a picture on enamel softened either in the ICT or acid buffers. The magnitude of indenter penetration is enlarged in order to illustrate the principle.

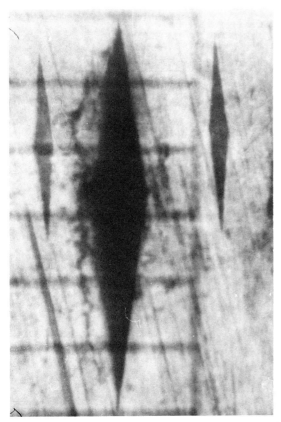

Fig. 19-13. Enamel indented before and after exposure to the ICT for one week. The two small indentations reflect the surface hardness of sound enamel, while the large middle one reflects the effect of ICT cariogenic activity. The cracking in the margin of the large indentation is indicative of a subsurface lesion under the apparently intact test surface.

mersed in solutions of fermentable substrates or mineralizing compositions under specified conditions of temperature and time. Since the appliance can be rinsed before reinsertion to the mouth, the damage from the effect of substrates to the natural teeth of the test volunteer is avoided. Thirdly, the test depicts cariogenic activities over a short time period. Caries develop with a number of intermittent demineralization and remineralization activities over long periods of time, months and sometimes years. Thus the commonly used DMF index and DMF increment (see Chap. 23) for a given period reflects the predominance of cariogenic activities during the time of observation, but it is past history in relation to the subjects' current activity. The ICT reflects the cariogenic activity of a specified time, usually one week, and thus it is more closely related to the current activity of the subject. In addition, one week is a convenient time period to evaluate factors such as diet, the use of mouthwashes, and other items of oral hygiene. Fourthly, the ICT simplifies the problems of caries studies based on natural human teeth which vary widely in their resistance to decay, particularly because of the variable composition of the outer enamel layer that has been subjected to mineral exchanges from the oral fluids, saliva, and diet. Bovine test teeth of which the outer surface is removed, present a much more standard surface for the evaluation of the intraoral cariogenic attack or the degree and quality of remineralization of presoftened surfaces. Furthermore, since the ICT experiments can be replicated, the effect of a single factor, such as the cariogenic contribution of a dietary item or the protective effect of a preventive treatment, can be tested a sufficient number of times for statistical evaluation. Such evaluations are extremely difficult in longitudinal epidemiologic studies because of the superimposition of many other uncontrollable factors related to the variable lifestyle and to the progressive elimination of the most susceptible tooth surfaces of the participants. After the decay of the most susceptible pits and fissures and proximal surfaces, it will take a much stronger cariogenic activity to produce lesions on the remaining natural teeth, whereas in the ICT the resistance of another test slab is quite similar to a previous one.

The ICT has been used extensively to study the demineralization-remineralization equilibrium. It has been found that individuals differ in their propensity to develop ICT caries. This propensity is not always directly correlated with their DMF which is a measure of the past caries activity. It appears that the demineralization-remineralization equilibrium changes throughout the life of the subject, possibly related to changes in the diet, oral hygiene, maturation of the teeth or perhaps other factors. Among the substrates which have been evaluated with the immersion system of the ICT, xylitol, xylose, maltitol, and lycasin have been found to be noncariogenic, while others such as sorbitol and mannitol seemed to be less cariogenic than sucrose. There was no detectable difference between the high cariogeneity of sucrose, glucose, and fructose. However, the effect of supplementary 3 per cent sucrose has been shown to be neutralized by the addition of 1 ppm fluoride to the sucrose solution. Apparently the presence of 1 ppm fluoride shifted the demineralization-remineralization equilibrium in the direction of remineralization to such an extent that it negated the demineralization caused by 3 per cent sucrose immersion. One hundred ppm fluoride concentration added in the sucrose solutions (used for the four 10 minute immersions daily) had an even stronger effect. Fluoride analysis of the enamel samples recovered from such experiments indicated that cariogenic (demineralization) activity contributed to a higher fluoride uptake by the enamel. We can thus conclude that fluoride's presence in the fluid environment of enamel surfaces under cariogenic attack not only diminishes the effect of demineralizing activities, but also increases the resistance of enamel, probably by selectively replacing the most soluble minerals by more insoluble ones. In other words, the ICT has demonstrated experimentally in the human mouth that fluoride has a triple effect: it decreases demineralization; it increases remineralization; and it increases the resistance of the remineralized surface to a subsequent attack. These findings agree with the background information of earlier observations on the high fluoride content and the high acid resistance of arrested carious lesions.

Topical treatments have been evaluated in the ICT by applying the fluoride solution on the test enamel prior to its insertion into the ICT in a way similar to that used in clinical dental practice. The effect of such treatments is measured both from the changes in enamel microhardness and from microradiographic pictures of sections from the test surfaces. Such experiments have been in agreement with the earlier *in vitro* and epidemiologic studies showing that topical fluoride treatments are effective cariostatic agents. Furthermore, it has been clearly demonstrated that the benefit of the fluoride treatments depends greatly on the condition of enamel prior to the treatment. Enamel primed by presoftening in acid, or by earlier cariogenic activity in the ICT, receives considerably greater benefit from the fluoride application than sound enamel. Apparently cariogenically primed enamel offers microspaces for the deposition of fluoride salts in contrast to the dense, sound enamel. The demonstration of this effect is shown in Figure 19-14. The left half of the enamel slab was presoftened by a 4-hour exposure to an acid buffer, while the

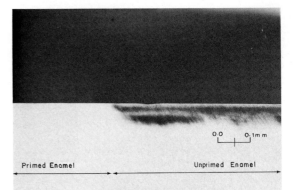

Fig. 19-14. Microradiography of a subsurface enamel lesion produced on a bovine enamel slab treated with SnF_2 and then exposed to the 7-day ICT and to a subsequent 7-day immersion in acid buffer. Prior to fluoride treatment the left side of the test surface was primed by a 4-hour exposure to 0.01 M lactic acid buffer, pH 4.5, while the right side was protected with varnish.

right half was protected with nail varnish. After the acid priming the varnish was removed and the entire surface was treated with 2 per cent SnF_2 for 4 minutes. Then the slab was mounted in the ICT for 1 week intraoral exposure involving demineralization and remineralization reactions. The recovered slabs were subsequently exposed for 7 days to the pH 4.0, 0.01 M lactic acid buffer enriched with 3 mM calcium and 1.8 mM phosphate ion to simulate demineralizing conditions in the oral environment. The picture shows extensive demineralization of the right side in contrast to the left. This difference is attributed to the increased intraoral remineralization and fluoride retention on the presoftened side in contrast to the sound side of the enamel slab. Similar results were obtained with NaF and APF treatments. Thus, incipient demineralization primes the enamel surface for higher fluoride uptake and subsequent intraoral remineralization with the end result of high resistance to the subsequent cariogenic challenge.

This experimental demonstration has profound implications for our approach in the clinical treatment of caries. It is now generally accepted that incipient enamel lesions can be arrested and become areas of resistance if given fluoride treatments. Such a therapeutic regimen, particularly for patients motivated towards practices of better oral hygiene, will avoid the possible iatrogenic sequellae of restorative dentistry such as removal of tooth tissue, possible leakage of the margins of a restoration, fracture of a tooth, or gingival irritation. It should be emphasized, however, that such treatments are not indicated in patients with continuous neglect of their oral hygiene because in such cases the overwhelming cariogenic attack is not likely to be counterbalanced by lesion arrestment through remineralization.

THE REMINERALIZATION PROCESS IN THE TREATMENT OF CARIES

Lesion consolidation entails incorporation of fluoride, and possibly other extrinsic dietary elements that contribute to increased acid resistance of the tooth surface. Due to the inclusion of organic material in the lesion, the consolidated surface remains softer than the original enamel, although it is more resistant to further acid dissolution. These areas appear as white, yellow, or brown spots at the sites at risk for caries initiation such as the pit, fissure, interproximal, and cervical areas of teeth. Since physical demands for hardness in these areas are minimal, the relative softness of a consolidated lesion is not a significant disadvantage. The same consideration applies to tooth discoloration; since the consolidated lesions are not normally visible, esthetics is not a problem.

Many data have been gathered on the remineralization process through clinical observations. When student volunteers interrupted their oral hygiene procedures and used a mouthrinse of 50 per cent sucrose nine times daily, incipient caries lesions were observed within three weeks. However, when the usual oral hygiene procedures were resumed in conjunction with fluoride treatments, most of these lesions regressed and finally disappeared. The regression of incipient caries lesions has been observed in several epidemiologic studies. The phenomenon is more prevalent when persons who have habitually neglected their oral hygiene are trained to improve their home care procedures and their dietary habits.

The concept of lesion consolidation just described can be used in the treatment planning for the management of caries. Since caries is an imbalance between demineralization and remineralization activities, the disease process can be corrected in several ways depending also upon the behaviour of the individual patient. Reduction or elimination of refined carbohydrates, training in thorough plaque removal, and fluoride rinses, will each shift the balance towards consolidation of incipient lesions.

One pertinent question in treatment planning is how far can a lesion be allowed to advance in anticipation of successful physiologic defense before dental surgery is recommended? The answer to this question is not yet clear. The pathogenesis of clinical caries advances through three stages: (1) subsurface demineralization without a macroscopic break of the enamel; (2) cavitation with the lesion advanced to or beyond the DE junction; and (3) advancement of the lesion towards the dental pulp. Since cavitation increases the microbial accumulation, it is logical to assume that it introduces a disadvantage in the consolidation mechanism. In addition to the severity of the lesion itself, the response of the patient to the consultation by the dental team should also be considered in the decision as to whether the lesion should be treated therapeutically or surgically. The first realization by the clinician is that no risk is involved in planning a six month period of observation for an enamel-only lesion in a patient who is motivated toward an improved diet, good oral hygiene, and fluoride treatments. If, after the observation period, the lesion shows no signs of progress the chances are good for its consolidation into a resistant area. On the other hand, if a lesion progresses during this time and there is evidence of lack of patient cooperation, the lesion should be treated with conventional restorative procedures. The advantages of the conservative treatment over the conventional restorative approach are obvious.

In the examination of incipient lesions considered for arrestment, the clinician should be cautious about using sharp explorers applied with pressure because it is quite possible that the explorer will penetrate a subsurface lesion and actually cause a frank cavitation. Light pressure of the explorer to sense the surface continuity will be sufficient for the purpose of identifying macroscopically open caries. It should always be remembered that if the patient accepts the preventive approach, the initial thrust of the dental team aims at teaching the etiology of dental disease, correcting detrimental dietary habits and training in the skills of plaque removal rather than starting with the restorative treatment.

Occlusal pits and fissures will be the most difficult types of lesions to assess as to the need for restoration since their deeper surfaces are relatively inaccessible to both direct visual examination and radiographic diagnosis. In these cases, clinical judgment and the patient's response will be the main criteria for determining treatment. Normally, active lesions appear to be surrounded by a white frame in the adjacent enamel, which reflects the incident light giving the picture of white spots; consolidated lesions blend directly with the translucent sound enamel and may show yellow or brown coloration attributable to the incorporation of stains in the porous enamel during the process of lesion consolidation.

Smooth surface (buccal and lingual) lesions are easily accessible for direct visual and light tactile examination with an explorer. However, the principal criterion for judging the severity of interproximal lesions is their appearance in a bitewing radiograph. In some instances, when the explorer is of limited use, the surface continuity can be assessed with dental floss. Consolidation of interproximal lesions is particularly desirable because of the difficulty in the placement of perfect Class II restorations, the necessity for sacrificing a considerable amount of sound tooth structure thereby weakening the tooth and the possibility of increasing the risk of future periodontal problems.

Cemental-dentinal lesions are encountered in advanced age when the gingiva retreats and leaves the root surface exposed to the cariogenic challenge. The arrestment of these lesions has not been sufficiently studied, but it is reasonable to believe that similar demineralization and remineralization reactions would produce the same beneficial results seen in the enamel. Of course, one important characteristic in this case is the presence of a considerable amount of organic material in these tissues that might be attacked by proteolysis as well as acid demineralization. At present there is no doubt that thorough plaque removal and establishment of contact with saliva, the natural "parent fluid" of the oral cavity, will enhance the chances of lesion consolidation. Furthermore the resistance of remineralized root surfaces will be higher if fluoride is present in the parent fluid from which new crystals are formed. Since the timing of cariogenic attacks is unpredictable, the more fre-

quently the fluoride is supplied to the oral fluid the better are the chances of fluoride incorporation into the remineralized cementum and dentin. Epidemiologic evidence indicates that frequent use of fluoride-containing mouthrinses is an excellent means of caries prevention. Such mouthrinses are used extensively in Scandinavian countries either under supervision in schools once a week (0.2% NaF) or for daily use at home (0.01%–0.05% NaF). In the preventive dentistry clinic of the University of Alabama in Birmingham we recommend the daily use of 0.02% NaF, preferably before retiring so that the fluoride-enriched pellicle will interact undisturbed for several hours with the underlying precarious tooth surfaces. Such surfaces will most likely tolerate subsequent attacks, particularly in patients demonstrating excellent oral hygiene. With an understanding of the role of remineralization in dental caries and the clinical judgment gained through experience, the treatment of our patients can more clearly approach the ideals of preventive and conservative therapy.

THE POSSIBLE IMPACT OF REMINERALIZATION ON ORAL HEALTH PROGRAMS

Incorporation of remineralizing treatments into routine dental care programs could have a strong impact on the public health aspects of caries control, particularly with reference to early interproximal lesions. For example, the placement of a Class II restoration may lead to ginvival irritation, recurrent caries at the margins of the restorative material, fracture of the buccal or lingual plate of the tooth, or a general weakening of the tooth's resistance against other physical and chemical assaults. Similar possible hazards can be described for cervical lesions that extend to involve areas on the mesial or distal surfaces, or occasionally around the entire cervix of the tooth. Undoubtedly the patient would benefit immeasurably if given interceptive therapeutic remineralizing treatment as the preferable option to having dental surgery performed.

Therapeutic remineralization will exert an obvious influence on the economics of public and private dental health care when the presently inadequate number of dentists are further pressed by the growing demands for dental treatment. Such an approach will be particularly expedient for public health dentistry in developing countries with a low dentist to population ratio. If these countries adopt the lifestyle of western culture, the potential increase in the demands for dental care cannot conceivably be met by the prospectively limited resources in dental manpower.

SUMMARY

Enamel remineralization is a natural defense reaction of the tooth surface against caries. Incipient caries lesions could reach a healthful equilibrium with the local cariogenic challenge under appropriate conditions determined by the parent fluid, plaque, and saliva that contribute to remineralization and a consolidation of the lesion. When the challenge is not overwhelming, remineralization frequently fills the porous enamel of the incipient lesions with minerals and organic material. Consolidated lesions are more resistant to a subsequent cariogenic challenge if the parent fluid of the remineralization reaction contains ions conducive to insoluble mineral formation. One such ion that is intimately associated with the consolidation of incipient carious lesions is fluoride. With lesion consolidation of the tooth surfaces at risk the individual may adapt to the cariogenic challenge. Such persons may withstand a higher level of challenge than others who have not had the experience of the challenging conditions. Enamel adaptation to the cariogenic challenge will be facilitated by the dental practitioner when the factors or conditions which enhance adaptation reactions are applied during patient care. It is hoped that this chapter will serve as a guide for attaining that goal.

GLOSSARY

Activity Coefficient. A correction factor needed for the calculation of the solubility product which is determined under the ideal conditions of infinite dilution and absence of ions foreign to the salt composition. Under ideal conditions the value of the activity coefficient is unity. In the case of hydroxyapatite other types of ions than calcium, phosphate, and hydroxyl interfere with the formation or growth of the solid thus decreasing the value of the activity coefficient.

Adaptation to a challenge. Adaptation to a challenge is a general phenomenon in biology. Specifically, for dental tissues it indicates an increase in the chemical stability of the tooth surface sufficient to withstand the cariogenic challenge which initiated the adaptive reaction. Chemically, adaptation involves demineralization and remineralization reactions resulting in selective retention of insoluble minerals. Possibly, incorporation of organic molecules within the lesion contributes to the process of adaptation.

Apatite. The mineral of bones and teeth belongs to the crystallographic family of apatites. Apatites are salts of calcium phosphate with a Ca/P ratio of 1.67, but numerous possible ionic substitutions could change the ratio of the ionic components of apatite. Substitution of hydroxyl with fluoride ions will change the hydroxyapatite to fluoroapatite, a most acid resistant mineral, while replacement of phosphate with carbonate will decrease the acid resistance of apatite.

Areas at risk. Because of their anatomy, some areas of the tooth surface are particularly conducive to plaque accumulation. These areas are the most likely to decay because they suffer stronger cariogenic challenge and are relatively inaccessible to the remineralization factors which increase resistance to caries.

Booster theory of calcification. The theory suggesting local supersaturation as the explanation of mineralization in bones and teeth. Such supersaturation could be caused mainly by an increase in the concentration of the calcium, phosphate, or hydroxyl ions in the tissue fluid. It has been postulated that the presence of alkaline phosphatase in the calcifying cartilage acting on hexose monophosphate increases the product of calcium and phosphate ions to levels of spontaneous precipitation.

Calciphylaxis. A hypersensitivity reaction causing calcification of tissues that normally do not calcify, such as skin, muscles, or connective tissue. Experimental calciphylaxis can be either systemic or local and suggests that each tissue has a certain calcifying potential, and that the calcifying potential of both the tissues and the tissue fluid can be altered with various chemicals. It is believed that the mechanism of calciphylaxis in animals is similar to human problems of abnormal calcification such as scleroderma, myositis ossificans, and arteriosclerosis.

Calcium phosphates. Salts of calcium with the various types of phosphate ions. The monovalent $H_2PO_4^-$, the divalent $HPO_4^=$, and the trivalent $PO_4^=$ phosphate form respectively monocalcium $Ca(H_2PO_4)_2$, dicalcium $CaHPO_4$, and tricalcium $Ca_3(PO_4)_2$ phosphate. At the pH and calcium and phosphate concentrations of the tissue and oral fluid, the most common calcium phosphate salt is hydroxyapatite $Ca_{10}(PO_4)_6(OH)_2$, although octacalcium phosphate $Ca_8H_4(PO_4)_6$, and dicalcium phosphate $CaHPO_4$ are suggested as possible precursors. The various calcium phosphates are characterized by their x-ray diffraction patterns and the Ca/P ratios.

Carious demineralization. The interaction between microbial plaques, substrates, and the underlying enamel under conditions of limited saliva contact. Acids that stem from microbial metabolism dissolve enamel minerals and thereby produce a characteristic subsurface lesion. If the process is not intercepted at an early stage it leads to cavitation.

Chelate. The bonding of a metal ion to an organic molecule with many electronegative groups. The organic molecule surrounds the metal, forming both ionic and coordination bonds. Because it is not easily ionized, chelated calcium does not contribute to the solubility product; it is not free to combine with the phosphate or to exchange with calcium at the interface between hydroxyapatite crystals and the equilibrating fluid.

Chemical bonds. There are three main types of bonds, ionic, covalent and coordination. In the *ionic* bond one or more electrons from the electronegative atom are transferred to the positive atom of the compound. In the *covalent* bond the two atoms share one or more pairs of electrons contributed by both bonded atoms, while in the *coordination* bond certain excessively electronegative atoms contribute their own electrons to interact with a positive ion.

Degree of saturation. According to the principle of mass action there is an equilibrium between the solid phase of a salt dispersed in a fluid that contains the ionic components of that salt. Supersaturation indicates ionic concentrations in the fluid higher than those required for equilibrium, while undersaturation indicates concentrations lower than the equilibrium value. Supersaturation causes salt formation and/or growth; undersaturation causes salt dissolution.

Fluoride mouthrinses. Dilute fluoride solutions of either NaF or SnF$_2$, normally below the level of 0.2 per cent, used as a homecare procedure or at schools under supervision. Mouthrinses used daily or weekly are effective cariostatic regimens. The usual concentration range for a daily mouth rinse is between 0.01 to 0.03% fluoride ion.

Heterogeneous nucleation. The formation of crystal nuclei on or within a molecule that is not part of the salt composition. It has been postulated that in certain locations of the organic template the stereochemical arrangement of electric charges is conducive to the formation of mineral salts at lower concentrations than those required by the solubility product of hydroxyapatite.

Hydration shell. The hydration shell is a water jacket around ions or charged surfaces such as hydroxyapatite crystals. Water, being a dipolar molecule with a positive and negative pole, bonds to either the positive or the negative points of the surface of the salt or around the ions in solution. While the bulk water molecules are free to move, the monolayer of bonded water molecules of the hydration shell are restricted.

ICT. (Intraoral cariogenicity test) An intraoral model designed for studies of experimental caries in humans. ICT caries is produced on sample tooth surfaces mounted in prosthetic or orthodontic appliances under conditions favoring microbial retention.

Ksp. The concentration value of the ionic components of a salt in the fluid environment that is necessary for equilibrium. At the Ksp value (constant solubility product) the number of ionic migrations from the solution to the solid and vice versa is equal in both directions. When the ionic concentration in the fluid environment is below the Ksp value (undersaturation) the solid dissolves; when it is above the Ksp value (supersaturation) new solid forms. Each salt has a specific Ksp for a given solvent at the same temperature under the ideal conditions of infinite dilution and lack of interference from ions foreign to the salt composition. For biological fluids the calculation of Ksp needs correction factors called activity coefficients.

Lesion consolidation. A term almost synonymous with remineralization of a caries lesion. Lesion consolidation involves deposition of minerals, organic material, and stains from saliva and diet into the microspaces of the lesion; it is the dental equivalent to wound healing of the soft tissues. Areas of consolidated lesions are more resistant to subsequent cariogenic challenge than sound enamel.

Maturation. The last stage of normal enamel mineralization which occurs during the interaction of the erupted tooth with the oral environment. After maturation enamel is more resistant to cariogenic attacks.

Parent fluid. The fluid from which the crystals of bones and teeth are produced. The tissue fluid is the parent fluid that determines the composition of the crystals of enamel and dentin formed before tooth eruption. After eruption, parent fluid for the tooth surface is the saliva as influenced by the diet and microbial fermentation products. Under bacterial plaques the parent fluid is extremely variable, influenced by limited saliva flow and the enzymatic breakdown of dietary substrates.

Remineralization. The redeposition of minerals in an incipient carious lesion. Actually, the pathogenesis of enamel caries involves a succession of demineralizing and remineralizing activities. The net effect can result in lesion consolidation when the redeposited minerals improve the resistance of the surface to the extent that the usual level of cariogenic activity cannot cause mineral dissolution. Remineralization of incipient lesions does not reconstitute enamel to the original structural and chemical composition. Depending on the parent fluid, consolidated lesions may be more resistant to the cariogenic challenge than sound enamel, thus contributing to the local adaptation of the surface to subsequent cariogenic challenge.

Stoichiometry. Derived from the Greek words which mean "element" and "to measure or count". Expresses the quality of a compound which has defined proportions of its component elements. Hydroxyapatite is not a stoichiometric compound because various ionic substitutions can change the composition of the crystal without appreciably changing the characteristic x-ray diffraction pattern.

Subsurface lesion. Characteristic mineral loss caused on enamel surfaces subjected to mild acid treatment by submersion in partially saturated acid buffers, acid gels, or under the influence of microbial plaques in the human mouth. When examined histologically these lesions show demineralization in considerable depth under an apparently intact surface. The phenomenon has been attributed to the formation of a more acid resistant mineral at the surface than in the subsurface layers of enamel. Most likely the mechanism involves selective loss of the most soluble minerals and their replacement by insoluble ones if the components of the latter are found in the plaque fluid during remineralization.

Template theory of calcification. The postulate that a certain stereochemical arrangement of charged groups of organic molecules induces crystal nucleation by forming a template on which the components of the mineral crystals form the initial nuclei. These nuclei trigger crystal growth as a second stage of biologic mineralization.

Thermal motion. The surface ions of ionic salts in a fluid environment oscillate across the interface between solid and fluid unlike the bulk ions that are surrounded from all directions. Oscillating ions may migrate from the solid to the solution, while other ions from the solution may replace them. Thermal motion offers a useful physical concept for the state of dynamic equilibrium between ionic solids and equilibrating solutions.

Topical fluoride treatment. The professional application of concentrated fluoride solutions. Normally 2 per cent NaF, 8 per cent SnF_2, or APF (acidulated phosphate fluoride containing 1.3 per cent fluoride ions) are painted on the teeth for 4 minutes. Some topical fluorides may be applied in gel form with special trays (see Chapter 20).

SUGGESTED READINGS

Axelsson P, Lindhe J: Effect of fluoride on gingivitis and dental caries in a preventive program based on plaque control. Commun Dent Oral Epidemiol 3: 156–160, 1975

Bhussry BR, Bibby BG: Surface changes in enamel. J Dent Res 36: 409–16, 1957

Darling AI, Mortimer KV, Poole DFG, Ollis WD: Molecular sieve behaviour of normal and carious human dental enamel. Arch Oral Biol 5: 251–273, 1961

Dirks OB: Posteruptive changes in dental enamel. J Dent Res 45: 503–511, 1966

Ericsson Y, Hellström I, Jared B, Stjernström L: Investigations into the relationship between saliva and dental caries. Acta Odontol Scand 10–11: 179–194, 1952–54

Feagin F, Koulourides T, Pigman W: The characterization of enamel surface demineralization, remineralization, and associated hardness changes in human and bovine material. Arch Oral Biol 14: 1407–1417, 1969

Francis MD, Briner WW: The development and regression of hypomineralized areas of rat molars. Arch Oral Biol 11: 349–354, 1966

Groeneveld A, Purdell-Lewis DJ, Arends J: Remineralization of artificial caries lesions by stannous fluoride. Caries Res 10: 189–200, 1976

Gron P: Remineralization of enamel lesions in vivo. Oral Sc Rev 3: 84–99, 1973

Gustafson G: The histopathology of caries of human dental enamel. With special reference to the division of the carious lesion into zones. Acta Odontol Scand 15: 13–55, 1957

Head J: A study of saliva and its action on tooth enamel in reference to its hardening and softening. JAMA 59: 2118–2122, 1912

Kohelehmainen L, Rytömaa I: Increment of dental caries among Finnish dental students during a period of 2 years. Commun Dent Oral Epidemiol 5: 140–144, 1977

Koulourides T: Experimental changes of mineral density. In Harris RS (ed): Art and Science of Dental Caries Research. New York, Academic Press, 1968, pp 355–378

Koulourides T, Axelsson P: Experimental and clinical studies of caries arrestment (ORCA abstr). Caries Res 11(2): 130, 1977

Koulourides T, Cueto H, Pigman W: Rehardening of softened enamel surfaces of human teeth by solutions of calcium phosphates. Nature 189: 226–227, 1961

Koulourides T, Feagin F, Pigman W: Remineralization of dental enamel by saliva in vitro. Ann NY Acad Sci 131: 751–757, 1965

Koulourides T, Phantumvanit P, Munksgaard EC, Housch T: An intraoral model used for studies of fluoride incorporation in enamel. J Oral Pathol 3 (4): 185–195, 1974

Little MF, Posen J, Singer L: Chemical and physical properties of altered and sound enamel. 3. Fluoride and sodium content. J Dent Res 41: 784–789, 1962

Mannerberg F: The incipient lesion as observed in shadowed replicas ('en face pictures') and ground sections ('profile pictures') on the same teeth. Acta Odontol Scand 22 (3): 343–363, 1964

Meckel AH: The formation and properties of organic films on teeth. Arch Oral Biol 10: 585–597, 1965

Muhler JC: Stannous fluoride enamel pigmentation—Evidence of caries arrestment. J Dent Child 27: 157–161, 1960

Muhler JC, Spear LB, Bixler D, Stookey GK: The arrestment of incipient dental caries in adults after the use of three different forms of SnF_2 therapy: results after 30 months. J Am Dent Assoc 75: 1402–1406, 1967

Selye H: Calciphylaxis. Chicago, University of Chicago Press, 1962

Silverstone LM: Remineralization phenomena. Caries Res 11: 59–84, 1977

Silverstone LM, Poole DFG: Histologic and ultrastructural features of "remineralized" carious enamel. J Dent Res 48: 766–770, 1969

Stephan RM: Intra-oral hydrogen-ion concentration associated with dental caries activity, J Dent Res 23: 257–266, 1944

Ten Cate JM, Arends J: Remineralization of artificial enamel-lesions in vitro. Caries Res 11: 277–286, 1977

von der Fehr FR, Loe H, Theilade E: Experimental caries in man. Caries Res 4: 131–148, 1970

von der Fehr FR: A study of carious lesions produced in vivo in unabraded, abraded, exposed, and F-treated human enamel surfaces, with emphasis on the x-ray dense outer layer. Arch Oral Biol 12: 797–814, 1967

Weatherell JA, Deutsch D, Robinson C, Hallsworth AS: Assimilation of fluoride by enamel throughout the life of the tooth. Caries Res [Suppl] 11 (1): 85–115, 1977

20 Fluorides in Dentistry

CARL A. OSTROM

Introduction
Basic Biologic Properties of Fluorides
  Metabolic Fate of Ingested Fluoride
  Anticaries Mechanisms of Fluorides
    Fluorapatite
    Remineralization
    Antimicrobial Activity
  Toxicosis
    Chronic
    Acute
    Treatment for Acute Fluoride Toxicosis
Fluoridated Water Supplies
  Epidemiology
  The Fluorosis Index
  Optimal Fluoride Level
  Controlled Water Fluoridation
    Major Clinical Trials
    World-wide Implementation
    Adjustment of Water Fluoride Levels
    Economics of Water Fluoridation
    Substitute Methods for Systemic Fluoridation
Topical Fluorides
  Mechanisms of Action

    The Fluoride Ion
    Acid Etching
    Phosphate Ion
    Cariogenic Priming
    Stannous Ion
  Frequency of Application
  Concentrated Solutions for Clinical Application
  Topical Application Methods
    Fluoride Solutions
    Fluoride Gels and Trays
    Fluoride Mouth Wash
    Fluoridated Dentifrices
    Fluoridated Prophylactic Pastes
    Multiple Fluoride Treatment
    Special Methods of Flouride Therapy
      The Orthodontic Patient
      Rampant Caries
      Selected Carious Lesions
      Xerostomia
Summary
Glossary
Suggested Readings

INTRODUCTION

No other factor in preventive dentistry has been as thoroughly documented as the cariostatic benefits of the fluoride ion. In 1956, the Surgeon General of the United States officially stated that dental caries prevention and safety factors of controlled water fluoridation place it among the most conclusively proven public health benefits known. All major health organizations and five consecutive presidents of the U.S. have officially endorsed this statement. On this premise alone, it becomes a responsibility of every member of the dental profession to understand the mechanisms by which the fluoride ion acts, its safety, and its uses as they apply to dental health maintenance.

In addition to the major benefit of systemic fluorides that are consumed by children during the ages of tooth development, we also need to understand the numerous other mechanisms by which the fluoride ion may act to prevent or arrest dental caries. These additional mechanisms extend from the post-eruptive enamel maturation effect through the arrestment of existant carious lesions to the maintenance of an optimal dentition. The end result will be a sharp improvement in the quality of practice for those dentists who provide all of the benefits of the fluoride ion to their patients.

BASIC BIOLOGIC PROPERTIES OF FLUORIDES

Fluorine is a highly volatile halogen gas that, for practical purposes, is never found free in nature because it forms such a reactive ion. However, fluoride is present almost everywhere, either as bound fluoride or in ionic form in solution. The earth's minerals are its natural source, principally volcanic ash, deep lying rock strata and certain ores such as bauxite. Over the ages, water that has passed through or over fluoride rich minerals has dissolved fluoride, so that some is present in most waters, most soils, and virtually all foods. Thus fluoride is a naturally occurring constituent of our food and drinking water. In the body tissues it ranges from a high concentration in the skeleton and teeth, to a low level in the blood stream. In fact, recent research has shown that mice bred through four generations on a fluoride-free diet and water supply developed anemia and a reduction in reproductive capacity. On this basis, both the cariostatic values and the systemic effects justify the position that fluoride is an essential micronutrient.

Metabolic Fate of Ingested Fluoride

When flouride is ingested, that which is bound to organic material is almost entirely retained and then ultimately excreted in the feces. Only minute amounts are considered to be metabolized to ionic form and carried to the blood stream. Ingested fluoride ion appears in the blood plasma in minutes. From an ingested dose of 1.0 mg., the blood level will rise from its normal level of about 0.15 to about 0.25 ppm within one hour. Within the second hour this concentration will be cleared and the blood returned to its normal level of fluoride. From such an ingested 1.0 mg dose almost all appears in the urine within two hours, where the concentration may rise from a normal of 0.5–1.0 ppm to a peak of 2.5 ppm about 120 minutes after ingestion. With normal urine voiding the concentration usually returns to normal within 12 hours. While in the blood stream, fluoride ion may be incorporated into mineralizing tissues in the form of fluorapatite. Thus systemic deposition of fluoride in enamel is completed when enamel mineralization has been completed. Dentinal fluid circulation permits continuing deposition in that tissue to about 50 to 60 years of age. Similarly, bone metabolism supports changing skeletal fluoride concentration throughout life. The salivary glands secrete fluoride ion at such extremely low levels that this is considered to have a negligible effect on incorporation into hard tissues. It is known that fluoride ion in the blood plasma is responsible for conversion of hydroxyapatite to fluorapatite in the developing teeth, and that this is a continuing process during tooth mineralization. Since ingested fluoride is cleared from the blood stream within two hours, it would seem likely that daily ingestion of a single dose of 1.0 mg. should be considerably less effective for caries prevention than daily ingestion of the same total dose in numerous increments, such as a child obtains from drinking optimally fluoridated water.

Anticaries Mechanisms of Fluorides

The fluoride ion inhibits the progress of caries by at least three known mechanisms: (1) reduction of apatite solubility through conversion of hydroxyapatite to fluorapatite, (2) remineralization of the carious lesion with deposition of a mixture of fluoride salts, and (3) antimicrobial activity. Although the details vary, each action occurs in both dentin and enamel. Therefore, for simplicity, the following discussion will be in terms of enamel caries.

Fluorapatite

The mineral phase of dental enamel is a form of apatite that is commonly spoken of as hydroxyapatite $[(Ca_{10})(PO_4)_6(OH)_2]$. However, hydroxyapatite is usually impure to some degree. If for any reason one of the hydroxyl ions is absent or has been replaced by some other ion, the physical presence of fluoride ion in the local environment may be followed by uptake of fluoride at that position in the crystal to form fluorapatite (see Chap. 7). This deposition may occur during any stage of mineralization. Therefore, apatite-bound fluoride ions may be found at all levels of both dentin and enamel if a child's blood stream contained appropriate levels of fluoride during the period when those tissues were in the process of mineralization. It has been calculated that, during the original mineralization, up to a maximum of five percent of enamel apatite in the form of fluorapatite may be tolerated without clinical fluorosis resulting in a cariostatic level approaching optimum. After the tooth has erupted into the mouth, additional surface fluorapatite formation can occur. Electrical assymetry on the hydroxyapatite crystal's surface apparently sets up an electrical field that pulls in both water molecules and charged ions. Fluoride ion diffusion into the hydration shell permits the fluoride to exchange with hydroxyl ions at the crystal surface. Subsequently such a fluoride ion may migrate into the body of the crystal and be incorporated into the interior lattice. Because this ionic migration through the densely mineralized enamel is limited, the fluoride concentration is usually higher at the enamel surface than it is in the deeper areas. This process of surface deposition is a form of enamel maturation whose rate appears to vary with the subject's exposure to fluoride. People who reside in an area with less than 1.0 ppm fluoride in the drinking water require up to 20 years after tooth eruption to acquire the enamel surface fluoride concentration that is considered optimum for reduction of caries susceptibility. However, those who are exposed to drinking water that contains 1.0 ppm fluoride ion throughout the period of tooth mineralization have an enamel surface fluoride level that confers high caries resistance at the time of tooth eruption. In the normal oral environment, fluorapatite is relatively insoluble. Therefore, its benefit is of long duration but not necessarily permanent.

Remineralization

Whereas the facts concerning fluorapatite are well established, more recent research strongly indicates that the accumulation of a mixture of fluoride salts in the microspaces of the subsurface enamel carious lesion is a highly effective mechanism of fluoride anticaries activity. Described in the chapter on the dynamics of mineralized tissues as well as later in this chapter, the demineralization-remineralization equilibrium, together with fluoride incorporation within the earliest carious lesion, appears to be a fundamental mechanism of fluoride cariostasis.

Antimicrobial Activity

A growing number of reports indicate that, in addition to its mineralization activities, the fluoride ion contributes cariostatic effects because it influences the plaque microbial ecology. It is well established that microbial glycolytic enzymes are inhibited by the fluoride ion. Two cariostatic mechanisms may follow. Inhibition of sugar metabolism reduces acidogenesis with a resultant reduction of enamel demineralization and simultaneous interference with plaque polysaccharide formation resulting in a reduction of microbial adhesion to the tooth surface (see Chap. 14). After a topical fluoride application, the rate of plaque acidogenesis may be suppressed for as much as three or four days, and the *Streptococcus mutans* proportion of the total plaque flora that can be recovered from a tooth surface is known to be reduced for as long as a week. The duration of these effects is unlikely to relate to the free fluoride ions from the topical application because such ions are rapidly precipitated either on the enamel surface as calcium fluoride or in the plaque as bound fluoride. It is more likely that the transitory effects of topical fluoride applications on plaque microbial ecology follow reionization of the fluoride ion from those two sources. It is also unlikely that this mechanism results from systemic fluoride secreted in the saliva because that concentration is usually less than 0.15 ppm, whereas the minimum concentration that has a detectable inhibitory influence on microbial glycolysis is considerably greater than that. More pertinent is the ability of plaque to accumulate bound fluoride to concentrations up to 180 ppm. With the shifting equilibria of the oral environment, it is logical that some of the fluoride ion will be dissociated from plaque-bound fluoride and, in fact, concentrations sufficient to inhibit microbial glycolysis have been detected. Therefore, in the academic sense, it is possible that the fluoride ion contributes an antimicrobial activity that is of transitory benefit in addition to its predominant mineralization effects.

Toxicosis

Chronic

Fear of the unknown is a tremendously potent deterrent. Those in opposition to fluouridation play on this fear. Therefore, it is important that every dentist understand the safety of the fluoride ion as it is used for caries prevention, as well as the nature of its toxicity. The safety of 1 ppm fluoride in drinking water has been extremely well established. In 1955, the American Dental Association submitted a complete bibliography on the safety of public water fluoridation that has been entered in the Congressional Record where it occupies 70 pages. Virtually all health profession organizations have gone on record in support of water fluoridation as a safe, conclusively proven beneficial public health measure. Physical limitations of fluoridating equipment make it impossible to overdose city water supplies to an unacceptable level for conventional city water usage. Exception might be claimed in the 1979 Maryland case in which accidentally overdosed fluoridated city water (approximately 35 ppm for 2–4 days) was used at one dialysis clinic. Eight patients treated with hemodialysis on those days became ill, complaining of chest pains, vomiting, nausea, and violent diarrhea. One of those patients died. This must be weighed relative to the clinic's failure to use the standard procedure calling for deionized water in preparation of its dialysis solution. A nearby hospital that did (correctly) use deionized water performed dialysis for several patients on the same days and experienced no difficulties. In the city population no other toxic or untoward effects occurred. Thus, this extremely unfortunate accident must be attributed to inadequate preparation of dialysis solutions. Time and again the validity of claimed health hazards associated with fluoridation of water supplies

have been rebutted by overwhelming scientific evidence.

In communities with controlled water fluoridation, and in those that have naturally fluoridated water in concentrations of 1.2 ppm or less, the chronic dental effects that can occur are nonexistant or negligible. Ingestion of higher concentrations is associated with enamel fluorosis, which will be discussed later in this chapter.

Except for academic interest, higher levels resulting in chronic toxicosis hardly concern the dentist. Historically, men who had worked in a cryolite factory for upwards of 20 years, and who had inhaled 20 to 80 mg of fluoride daily, have shown a significant incidence of chronic crippling skeletal fluorosis. Such industrial problems no longer exist because industry has learned to control fluoride dust. American Indians who lived in areas with more than 20 ppm fluoride in their drinking water have shown significant skeletal fluorosis, but no known case of crippling fluorosis from drinking water has ever been reported. A high incidence of chronic fluorosis has been observed only in experimental animals. Rats drinking water with a concentration of 50 ppm show thyroid changes. Levels of 100 ppm yield retarded growth and 125 ppm fluoride results in kidney changes.

Acute

Little direct information is available on acute toxicity after ingestion of ionized fluoride in humans. From studies in rodents, extrapolated by standard pharmacologic procedures to a 150 lb adult human, it has been calculated that the minimum lethal dose is about 2 grams and the dose that may be lethal to 50 per cent of challenged humans might be about 5 grams. However, such calculations are more theoretical than real because ionized fluoride is a powerful emetic. In humans, ingestion of 250 mg will induce vomiting, nausea, and retching, with return to normal in 48 hours. From such a 250 mg dose, 20 to 25 per cent of the fluoride not expelled by vomiting will be excreted in the urine during the first 3 to 5 hours and another 20 to 25 per cent in the following 5 to 12 hours. The remainder will be deposited in the skeleton, from whence it will be lost over a period of years. This 250 mg dose has clinical application because it is approximately the amount contained in 15 ml of a solution used for topical application. However, since a topical application requires no more than 5 ml the wise dentist will not dispense more than that amount to the bracket table.

As will be discussed later in this chapter, fluorides may be prescribed for home use, both for the systemic effect and for the topical benefit. To avoid the possibility of accidental ingestion of an excessive quantity of fluoride, the ADA Council on Dental Therapeutics has recommended that fluoride preparations intended for home use be dispensed or prescribed in quantities containing no more than 264 mg of sodium fluoride, or 120 mg of fluoride ion. Based on a calculated maximum ingestion of one fourth of the lethal dose for a 20 lb child, this translates to 120 tablets each containing one mg fluoride. It also limits prescription of fluoride mouth washes so that one liter of 0.02 percent sodium fluoride contains approximately 90 mg of fluoride. An additional safety feature would be to use a "child-proof" container. In all cases, the label should contain a clear warning that the container should be stored in a place not accessible to children.

Treatment for Acute Fluoride Toxicosis

In clinical practice, the possibility of anyone inadvertently ingesting a toxic dose is remote. The dentist keeps fluoride supplies in clearly recognizable opaque plastic containers, stores them in a manner such that they are not easily accessible to other people, and dispenses amounts that are too small for a patient to obtain a toxic dose. Nevertheless, all dental personnel need to know how to treat a case of acute fluoride toxicosis. Immediate administration of intravenous glucose should be provided to maintain an adequate blood sugar level and to prevent shock. Gastric lavage with dilute lime water should also be initiated as soon as possible because fluoride is escharotic to mucosa. Third, one should wash away vomitus and excreta to prevent external burns. In subsequent hours, the patient should be induced to drink large volumes of dilute lime water or milk and a calcium solution should be available for intravenous administration if symptoms of shock occur. In the following days, continuing treatment should include parenteral fluids as necessary to maintain a high urine volume. In addition, the patient should be encouraged to drink large volumes of dilute lime water or milk.

FLUORIDATED WATER SUPPLIES

The accumulation of knowledge on the application of systemic fluorides for reduction of dental caries in a population has a long history that dates back almost 200 years. The key portions of this evidence can be enjoyed in a few hours of most interesting reading (See Suggested Readings, McClure, 1970).

In the earliest known report of interest, Morozza, in 1802, detected fluoride in the teeth of a fossilized mastodon. In 1823, Berzelius detected trace levels of fluoride that varied from zero to 3 ppm in the waters that he analyzed. In 1866, Magitot, a great man in the history of dentistry, observed that certain teeth decalcified more readily than others, and he related this finding to their fluoride content. The respect accorded to Dr. Magitot was so great that, with no further documentation, fluoride losenges ("pastilles") were widely used throughout Europe for about 30 years.

Then the pendulum swung the wrong way. In the early 1900's, observations on mottled enamel in southwestern United States, related to earlier reports of more severe cases, led Dr. McKay to travel to Italy, a site of extreme dental fluorosis, so that he might personally investigate this phenomenon. He found that the characteristic "black teeth" no longer occurred in children who resided in certain municipalities after installation of a new water system that drew from surface impoundments. However, children living in immediately adjacent rural areas where the ancient wells were still used continued to develop black teeth. Of course it was the high level of fluoride leached from the lava beds of Vesuvius that was present in the well waters. Speculations on the disfiguring effects of fluoridated water were resolved after 1925 when the city of Oakley, Idaho, with a high frequency of dental fluorosis and a high fluoride content in its artesian well water, switched to a shallow water source that had a low fluoride content. The result was that no new cases of fluorosis in that community were recognized thereafter.

Epidemiology

During those same years, the low incidence of dental caries in high fluoride areas was also recognized. In the early 1930's the United

TABLE 20-1. INVERSE RELATION BETWEEN CARIES EXPERIENCE AND COMMUNITY'S NATURAL WATER FLUORIDE LEVELS

ppm F in Water	No. Cities Examined	No. Children Examined	Average DMFT
<0.5	11	3687	7.5
0.5–0.9	3	1140	4.2
1.0–1.4	4	1430	3.2
>1.4	3	847	2.5

(Dean HT, Arnold FA, Elvove E: US Pub Hlth Rep 57: 1155–1179, 1942)

States Public Health Service, led principally by Dr. Trendly Dean, started significant studies that ultimately established the effectiveness and safety of systemic fluorides, and the pendulum slowly swung back again to acceptance of controlled water fluoridation as a dental public health measure. The series of epidemiologic surveys summarized in Table 20-1 shows the inverse relation between caries experience and water fluoride levels. These data are from overwhelming numbers of subjects and the interpretation can lead to only one conclusion.

The Fluorosis Index

The fluorosis index was developed as a clinical classification to permit correlation of the degree of enamel disfigurement with the water fluoride levels. A fluorosis index of 0.5 is so minimal that it might well be idiopathic. An index of 1.0 is assigned when very small white spots cover less than 25 per cent of the enamel surfaces. This degree of fluorosis might actually be considered attractive because the subject's teeth on casual viewing appear whiter than average. A fluorosis index of 2.0 is disfiguring; the teeth have larger white spots covering 25 to 50 per cent of the enamel surfaces. An index of 3.0 is assigned when distinct brown stain is seen, while 4.0 is scored when hypoplasia is present.

Optimal Fluoride Level

Continuing surveys of the caries incidence and degrees of fluorosis in communities with natural water fluoride levels varying from zero to high concentrations led to the realization that, in parallel with the inverse relation between caries prevalence and water fluoride

level, there was a direct relation between the water fluoride level and fluorosis. Figure 20-1 demonstrates a key feature. At a level of 1.0 to 1.2 ppm, the caries inhibition effect of the fluoride ion approaches its maximum. Fortunately, this is achieved with minimal risk of fluorosis as seen by a fluorosis index approaching zero. At concentrations lower than 1.0 ppm negligible reduction in fluorosis is obtained but significantly less protection from caries results. On this basis, the level of 1.0 to 1.2 ppm was accepted as optimum. This standard has been adopted world wide.

Controlled Water Fluoridation

Major Clinical Trials

From the preceding studies which were conducted in areas with water supplies that were naturally fluoridated, two key factors were established: optimum caries prevention occurred with 1.0 to 1.2 ppm fluoride in the water; and insignificant or no enamel fluorosis occurred at those same levels. These basic facts formed the basis for a series of studies that were designed to determine whether artificial fluoridation of city water supplies would reduce the caries prevalence in children who lived in those cities during the period of tooth formation. The results of four major independent studies are summarized in Table 20-2. The trials in Grand Rapids, Michigan, and in Evanston, Illinois compared the caries prevalence before and after 15 years of city water fluoridation. The other two trials, Sar-

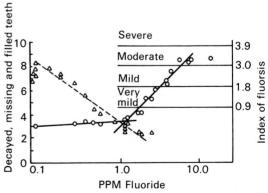

Fig. 20-1. Simultaneous graph of DMF teeth (dotted line at left) and average index of fluorosis (two solid lines) plotted against the water content of fluoride (logarithmic scale). (Hodge, HC: J Am Dent Assoc 40: 436–454, 1950)

TABLE 20-2. SUMMARY OF FOUR MAJOR TRIALS ON THE DENTAL BENEFITS OF ARTIFICIALLY FLUORIDATED CITY WATER SUPPLIES

City	Fluoride Status	Year Exam'd	Age, Years	DMF Teeth	Percent Reduction	Missing Teeth	Percent Reduction
Grand Rapids	−F	1945	12–14	9.5	56	0.84	66
	+F	1959		4.26		0.29	
Evanston	−F	1946	12–14	9.03	49	0.19	68
	+F	1959		4.66		0.06	
Sarnia	−F	1959	12–14	7.46	57	0.75	71
Brantford	+F			3.23		0.22	
Kingston	−F	1960	13–14	12.46	70	0.92	89
Newburgh	+F			3.73		0.10	

(Modified from Ast DB, Fitzgerald B: J Am Dent Assoc 65: 581–587, 1968)

nia/Brantford and Kingston/Newburgh, used paired cities. Sarnia and Kingston were control cities without fluoridated water, for comparison with Brantford and Newburgh after they had fluoridated water for 15 years. Statistically, the latter two trials are more significant than the studies done in Grand Rapids and Evanston. Detailed medical examinations that were conducted in conjunction with the Grand Rapids and the Kingston/Newburgh studies found no differences in growth, health, or development from the therapeutic level of city water fluoridation.

World-wide Implementation

The impressive success of those four major trials that were conducted in the United States and in Canada was followed by artificial fluoridation of water systems in many parts of the world. Due to lack of standardization, it is not feasible to summarize the benefits in various parts of the world, but the consistent high rates of benefit have been impressive. For example, the city of Tiel, The Netherlands, reported a 90 per cent reduction in the numbers of teeth extracted from 16 year-old children who had lived in that city since fluoridation of its water was started. This tremendous benefit parallels the results of the Kingston/Newburgh study, as shown in Table 20-2.

In the United States the number of people who are served with optimally fluoridated water has grown consistently over the years. At the present time, approximately 59 per cent of the people in the United States receive optimally fluoridated water. This provision varies widely from 100 per cent in the District of Columbia, through 85 per cent in Illinois, 46 per cent in Alabama, to three per cent in Nevada. Geographic and engineering features make it difficult to provide fluoridated water in areas

that are predominantly rural or have large ranch areas. In recent years, a growing number of states has legislated state wide fluoridation of piped water supplies. Connecticut was first and Minnesota, Illinois, Delaware, Michigan, South Dakota, and Ohio followed. Georgia and Nebraska joined those ranks recently.

Adjustment of Water Fluoride Levels

Since the amount of water consumed varies with thirst, and thirst varies with temperature, it has been recognized that the optimum water fluoride concentration should be adjusted to the prevailing temperature of the community. "Drinking Water Standards," published by the United States Public Health Service, provides a recommended range of water fluoride levels relative to a community's annual average maximum daily temperature. Some communities that have large seasonal variations in temperature also adjust their water fluoride level for each season. There are no published data suggesting a need for such seasonal control.

Economics of Water Fluoridation

Current data indicate that the cost of fluoridating a city's water supply is no more than 15 cents a year per capita. In contrast, the savings for unneeded childhood dental treatment as a result of 60 per cent reduction in caries increment would be on the order of $75.00 for the average seven year old child. Extended into adulthood, the savings would be infinitely greater, particularly for those persons who might otherwise require extensive dental reconstruction as a result of early loss of some teeth because of caries. Far more important than dollar savings are the dental health maintenance values. Fluoridated water contributes to enamel maturation. Caries prevention minimizes the loss of normal dental anatomy, contacts, and balanced occlusion. These factors favor minimization of periodontal disease. In fact, it is logical to expect that people who live in a fluoridated community may look forward to 50 to 60 per cent less dental treatment needs throughout their lifetime. Fluoridation of communal water has its greatest impact on the lower income portions of the population. Therefore, controlled water fluoridation would reduce the backlog of unmet dental treatment needs in future years, a period during which it is logical to expect that demand will be rising. Furthermore, studies have shown that dentists in a fluoridated community enjoy a finer level of dental practice. With a sharp reduction in the number of hours spent in restoration of extensive carious lesions, the average dentist has time to practice at a much more ideal level. Since patients will have a lower incidence of the sequelae of recurrent caries and periodontal disease, the dentist will be able to justify, and patients will desire, the finer levels of dental care. Smaller restorations and fewer endodontic problems will become the rule. Thus the finest in dental care would become more widely sought and practiced.

Substitute Methods for Systemic Fluoridation

Fluoridating equipment installed in schools has been moderately successful, but it fails to provide fluoride during school vacations, weekends, and non-school hours as well as during the post school years of enamel maturation. Substitute vehicles, (e.g., table salt or milk containing added fluoride) have shown a degree of effectiveness, but significantly less than fluoridated water. The primary disadvantage is that all children do not consume predictable quantities of these products. The marketing problem is a second disadvantage since it is not economical to vary milk or table salt's fluoride content to balance the amount of fluoride naturally present in each community's water supply. Vitamin capsules containing added fluoride or fluoride tablets may be prescribed, but these also have disadvantages. The prescribing dentist will need to know the natural water fluoride level in the community to calculate the supplementation required in the prescriptions to ensure

that a child will not receive a dosage sufficient to cause fluorosis. Perhaps more important is the fact that a single daily dose contained in a tablet or capsule will be cleared from the blood stream within two hours. However, optimally fluoridated water consumed eight or ten times daily to satisfy thirst, or in foods that were prepared with that water, will maintain an effective blood fluoride level eight or ten times longer each day and thereby permit much longer periods for fluorapatite formation in the developing teeth.

In general a great number of clinical trials have indicated that 50 to 80 per cent caries reduction in deciduous teeth may be anticipated if daily fluoride supplementation in the form of a single dose is started by two years of age, but only marginal to 40 per cent reduction in the permanent teeth may be expected among children started on tablets at about 5 years of age. On the contrary, the opposite effects have been observed with fluoridated drinking water, in that the permanent teeth obtain more protection than the deciduous teeth. Although numerous compounding factors may play partial roles in this disparity, a widely held interpretation is that parents monitor the fluoride supplementation more closely for infants and younger children than they do for older children.

Although the subject here is systemic fluoridation, it is important also to remember that fluoridated drinking water also has a topical effect on erupted teeth. As pointed out previously, people who live in an area served with water containing less than 1 ppm fluoride may require up to 20 years after tooth eruption to reach the enamel surface fluoride level that is considered optimum for caries prevention. Experimental rats that were tube fed fluoride received only half of the caries prevention that was observed in rats that drank the same fluoride dosage. Recognition of this post eruptive effect has led to the suggestion that prescriptions of fluoride tablets include the instruction that each tablet be chewed, dissolved in the saliva, and swished about the teeth before being swallowed. Similarly, fluoride solutions may be used. Appropriate prescriptions adaptable for children of various ages and for communities with suboptimal water fluoride concentration are described in *Accepted Dental Therapeutics*, which is published by the American Dental Association and is updated biannually. The natural water fluoride level for most communities is available from State Health Departments. To prescribe fluoride supplementation for patients who consume private well waters, the dentist usually can obtain a free analysis of a sample from the State Health Department.

TOPICAL FLUORIDES

The dental profession's interest in topical fluoride application developed in the early 1940's after demonstration that exposure of extracted teeth for a few seconds to dilute solutions of fluoride ion produced completely bound fluoride on the enamel surface which subsequently was less soluble than the original enamel surface. This was recognized as a new phenomenon, completely unrelated to deposition of systemic fluoride in the teeth during their original mineralization. Clinical trials of this concept showed that sodium fluoride in topical application produced a significant reduction in future carious lesions in the order of 30 to 50 per cent, depending on the methods used.

Discovery of the topical effect also suggested that a fluoride-containing dentifrice should be effective, but the avid nature of the fluoride ion appeared to be a problem. Fluoride ion combines so rapidly and completely with other agents in the dentifrice that few vehicles other than water are available to carry it to the tooth surface. Solution of this problem and clinical trials that conclusively demonstrated their effectiveness led the Council on Dental Therapeutics of the American Dental Association to establish fluoride-containing dentifrices in a new class, designated as therapeutic dentifrices.

A wide variety of other fluoride compounds has been tested, (e.g., potassium, lead, silicon, tin and zirconium). All yielded some cariostatic benefit, but less than stannous fluoride, which in the early 1950's was recognized as most effective. Next in development was acidulated sodium fluoride containing excess phosphate ions, which was as cariostatic as stannous fluoride and offered other advantages. Still more recently, stannous hexafluorzirconate was shown to be extremely effective in that it produced about 90 per cent caries reduction. Unfortunately, it was too caustic to the oral mucosa and is therefore not acceptable for clinical use. At the present time there is general agreement on the values of three

basic fluoride compounds for topical application—sodium fluoride, stannous fluoride and acidulated phosphate fluoride.

Mechanisms of Action

The mechanisms of action of topical fluoride solutions include the action of the fluoride ion alone, the effect of prior acid etching of the enamel surface, the effect of the phosphate ion in the fluoride solution, the effect of cariogenic priming and the action of the stannous ion in a stannous fluoride solution.

The Fluoride Ion

Immature enamel usually has on its surface a relatively small number of imperfect hydroxyapatite crystals. When ionized fluoride is applied to such a surface, those imperfect crystals may take up fluoride ions to form essentially insoluble fluorapatite. At the same time, and in direct relation to the fluoride concentration in the topical solution, calcium fluoride will be adsorbed on the enamel surface. This calcium fluoride will provide temporary resistance to acid attack, but most of it will be lost by dissolution back into the plaque and saliva within days. If during those days an acid attack makes available a free apatite bond, a fluoride ion from the calcium fluoride might be taken up into the crystal to form fluorapatite. Although this latter mechanism has not been clearly demonstrated in research, it is entirely logical in theoretical chemistry.

Acid Etching

Deliberate acid etching of the enamel surface prior to or simultaneous with topical application of ionized fluoride will free some bonds from the hydroxyapatite, making deficient crystals available for fluorapatite formation. Thus acid etching of the enamel surface will cause an increased number of fluorapatite crystals to be formed at the enamel surface and greater resistance to subsequent cariogenic attack will result. Again, of course, calcium fluoride will be deposited on the surface, at least for a few days.

Phosphate Ion

Addition of phosphate ion to acidulated sodium fluoride carried the concept of topical application one step further. This approach was based on the logic that an excess of phosphate ions would drive the mineral equilibrium of the enamel surface toward remineralization with maximum fluorapatite formation. Clinical trials have shown up to 70 per cent reduction in caries increment in children after topical application of acidulated phosphate fluoride.

Cariogenic Priming

To the extent that fluorapatite is formed by any of the preceding methods, the cariostatic benefit is essentially permanent. However, the protection is only partial and caries does still occur. Less widely understood, but highly effective, is the ability of the fluoride ion to arrest existing carious lesions. When this occurs at an early stage of caries, one can say that cariogenic priming of the subsurface carious lesion for fluoride deposition has occurred. Caries can be considered the end result of a number of cycles that consist of demineralization and remineralization phases (See Chap. 19). The demineralization phases produce a subsurface microscopic lesion that contains microspaces from which calcium and phosphate ions have been leached. Each time that the equilibrium is reversed and remineralization occurs, if fluoride ions are available, a mixture of calcium-fluoride-phosphate salts will be precipitated in the microspaces. Such minimally soluble fluoride-containing salts make the microscopic lesion more resistant to future demineralization attacks. Since each cariogenic attack is likely to remove the most soluble mineral that is present, subsequent remineralization phases with fluoride present will deposit increasing concentrations of fluoride salts that are less soluble than the apatite of the original enamel. Thus, with fluoride ion present, enamel becomes progressively more resistant after each cycle of a demineralization attack and remineralization phase. These observations support the demineralization-remineralization concept as potentially the most important mechanism in fluoride cariostasis.

Stannous Ion

Like the fluoride ion during remineralization phases, the stannous ion contributes to the formation of complex, relatively insoluble salts of tin. Thus the stannous ion from topical application makes a significant contribution to the arrestment of existing carious lesions, including those that have involved the dentin.

Frequency of Application

The dental profession has long sought a fluoride "magic bullet" that, in a single topical application, would confer a permanent state of high caries resistance to tooth surfaces. In so far as the first topical application of the fluoride ion will convert the available imperfect hydroxyapatite crystals on the surface of immature teeth to fluorapatite, any form of topical fluoride including fluoridated drinking water will serve the purpose, and topically applied acidulated phosphate fluoride is probably the most effective. However, it is also clear that enamel surface fluorapatite formation is but one of the mechanisms by which topical fluorides render teeth more resistant to cariogenic challenge. Therefore it becomes not only a question of what form of fluoride to use but, more importantly, one of frequency or constancy with which fluoride ion can be made available to the sites at which the cariogenic challenge occurs. Over a period of years, subclinical caries will occur at some sites, but frequent topical fluoride applications will contribute to increasing caries resistance at those specific enamel surface sites at which the demineralization-remineralization cycles occur. To repeat, it is the frequency, or even the constancy of fluoride ion availability that is the primary determinant of topical fluoride effectiveness.

Concentrated Solutions for Clinical Application

Only two forms of fluoride used for topical application have consistently been followed by highly significant reduction in new carious lesions. These are acidulated phosphate fluoride applied in the manner of Wellock and Brudevold (See Suggested Readings) and stannous fluoride applied in the manner of Bixler and Muhler (See Suggested Readings). Important factors in their effectiveness are, unlike home use of a fluoride mouthwash, their application is controlled by the dentist, and semiannual application coincides with an effective recall program.

Acidulated phosphate fluoride usually contains 1.23 per cent fluoride made available from 2.0 per cent sodium fluoride and 0.34 per cent hydrofluoric acid. To this is added ortho-phosphoric acid to a concentration of 0.98 per cent. A *p*H of about 3.0 results. When stored in an opaque plastic bottle this is a stable solution with a long shelf life. It is noninjurious to the mucosa. Although almost tasteless, it is commerically available with flavoring agent added. Acidulated phosphate fluoride currently is widely used for topical application in the dental operatory.

Stannous fluoride is usually used in a concentration of 8 per cent for children and 10 per cent for adults. These solutions have a *p*H close to 3.0 and fluoride concentrations of 1.10 and 1.37 percent respectively. Its disadvantages are that stannous fluoride has a bitter metallic taste, the solution has a short shelf life that makes it necessary to prepare a fresh solution for each half-day and, used in excess, it may cause a chemical burn of mucosa. With skill, each of those disadvantages can be managed. Often repeated is the misleading statement that stannous fluoride stains teeth. It does not stain sound enamel. Tin absorbed into a carious lesion forms tin phosphates that are brown, and the arrested lesion becomes brown. As the tin is leached out of the lesion over a period of months the color disappears. In the sense of arrestment, this may be considered an indicator that it is time to reapply topical stannous fluoride to continue the caries arrestment effect. In plaque, tin reacts with oxygen and sulfur to form sulfates which are also brown. This occurrence indicates that the patient's plaque control is inadequate. Plaque retained in porous surfaces and in defective margins of existing restorations will also be stained and, idealistically, such stains indicate the need to replace the defective restoration. Thus the dentist may justifiably use the stain as a disclosant. A feature unique to stannous fluoride is that it has been shown to arrest the frank carious lesion that has invaded the dentin. This may justify topical application of stannous fluoride in selected circumstances.

Topical Application Methods

Fluoride Solutions

Certain factors in topical fluoride methodology are empirical in origin. Since those empiricisms were employed in clinical trials that yielded high effectiveness, it seems logical to continue to use them until their contribution to cariostasis is disproven. Other empiricisms and substitutes are promoted periodically. Until such are proven at least as effective as the original methods, their adoption is not warranted. The following methodology is based on that logic. A thorough prophylaxis including pumice drawn by dental floss or tape across each interproximal surface is considered essential to provide a maximum exposure of reactive enamel to fluoride. The patient is allowed to rinse thoroughly. Either a quadrant or a half-mouth is isolated with cotton rolls and the teeth are dried with compressed air. To control fluoride application most effectively cotton pellets in forceps are more efficient than a cotton applicator stick. The fluoride solution is applied repeatedly and continuously to keep the teeth wet for four minutes. During this period, floss is drawn through each interproximal embrasure to ensure wetting of those surfaces. The cotton rolls and holder are removed and the patient is permitted to expectorate but not to rinse. Then the procedure is repeated for the remaining quadrants. Throughout these procedures, the operator is vigilant to avoid saliva contamination of the surfaces being treated, and if this does occur, the process must be started all over again. Before dismissal, the patient is advised to avoid eating, drinking, or rinsing for thirty minutes, to prolong the availability of fluoride ion to react with the tooth surfaces. These same procedures are used with either acidulated phosphate fluoride or stannous fluoride, with the exception that the operator uses greater skill and care with the latter due to its taste and its potential to burn the gingivae if used in excess.

Fluoride Gels and Trays

These preparations were developed on the premise that a gel form should hold the fluoride preparation in more intimate and prolonged contact with the reactive tooth surfaces. They are commonly used with acidulated phosphate fluoride or with sodium fluoride, but not with stannous fluoride. Gels may be applied in the same manner as topical solutions. More commonly, they are applied in a tray. After a thorough prophylaxis, a ribbon of gel is placed in the area of the tray that will approximate the teeth. The arch that is to be treated is dried with compressed air (as well as possible), and the tray is quickly seated in position, where it is held for four minutes. The patient may be advised to hold the tray in position with his opposing teeth and to keep it in motion by simulated light chewing to foster movement of the fluoride gel to all parts of the dentition. The procedure is then repeated on the opposing arch. The patient is permitted to expectorate but not to rinse, and is advised to avoid eating, drinking, or rinsing for 30 minutes. A variety of trays is available. The simplest consists of a set of reusable trays in various sizes together with a supply of sponge-like tray liners that are wetted with the fluoride gel or solution. Trays of heat-moldable material may be more closely adapted to the arch. Custom trays for each patient may be fabricated in the manner used to make an athlete's mouthguard. Numerous clinical trials have indicated that gels and the tray method are not more effective and often less effective in caries prevention than topical application of a fluoride solution. The usually low effectiveness of the tray method may be ascribed to two factors. First, it is difficult, if not impossible, to have all tooth surfaces of a given arch free from saliva as the tray is inserted. Second, and perhaps more important, a gel under pressure moves in the path of least resistance, which is toward the tray margins, rather than the paths of sharply greater resistance, into the caries susceptible pits, fissures, and interproximal surfaces of contacting teeth. The latter serious deficiency of the tray method can be minimized by fabrication of a closely fitting custom tray for each individual patient. However, the cost of custom trays and the failure of a stock tray to provide appreciable caries prevention when used to transport the fluoride gel agent make the use of topically applied solutions significantly more cost effective.

Fluoride Mouth Wash

Several clinical trials have shown that supervised daily use of a mouth wash containing fluoride may yield as high a degree of caries prevention as that obtained from semiannual topical application. However, numerous other trials have shown that unsupervised home use of a fluoride mouth wash conferred far less–to negligible protection. These experiences make it clear that most people cannot be depended upon to follow such a regimen. Therefore, routine prescription of a fluori-

dated mouthwash as the sole source of topical fluoride is likely to be relatively ineffective for most subjects, but may be quite effective for the most highly motivated patients. It may be especially appropriate for patients with fixed orthodontic appliances.

Many published reports of clinical trials support the conclusion that no other compound is more effective in mouth wash than neutral sodium fluoride for protection from caries. A number of trials indicate that a concentration of 0.05 per cent sodium fluoride may be optimum for daily use. Fortnightly use of 0.2 per cent has been shown to provide significant protection, albeit less than the protection afforded by daily use of a 0.05 per cent concentration. A recent study indicated highly significant benefits from daily use of 0.025 per cent neutral sodium fluoride mouth wash. This finding suggests the importance of two known factors. First, a heavier deposition of calcium fluoride is deposited on the surface by the higher fluoride concentration. Second, the effectiveness of such a low concentration used daily supports the interpretation that frequency of fluoride availability is more significant than the concentration that is applied.

It has also been shown that there is a potential risk of chronic fluoride overdose in patients who inadvertently swallow during daily fluoride mouthwashing. People with nasal congestion find it difficult to hold a mouthwash without swallowing. Young children apparently have difficulty in learning to breathe while holding a mouthwash, and the average 4 to 5 year old subject who held 7 ml. of mouthwash for 30 seconds swallowed about half. On this basis it may be calculated that a child might ingest about 1.7 mg. of fluoride from 30 seconds mouthwashing with 0.05 per cent sodium fluoride. If the child lived in a community with optimally fluoridated water, about 1.0 mg. would be ingested from that source. That total daily ingestion of about 2.7 mg. risks development of a disfiguring level of fluorosis of the permanent teeth. Alternatively 0.025 per cent sodium fluoride mouth wash used daily might yield total daily ingestion of 0.85 mg. fluoride in a nonfluoridated community, or 1.85 mg. in an optimally fluoridated community. These findings strongly suggest that optimum caries protection together with acceptably low fluoride ingestion for four to five year old children may be obtained from daily 30 second use of seven ml. of 0.025 percent neutral sodium fluoride.

Higher concentrations are used principally in school programs under close supervision. The subject is advised to rinse the teeth for 30 seconds, either weekly or biweekly, and then to expectorate the fluoride solution. Commercial preparations are available by prescription. The dentist is advised to consult *Accepted Dental Therapeutics*, published by the American Dental Association's Council on Dental Therapeutics, for current features and precautions.

Fluoridated Dentifrices

Three currently available commercial products have been accepted as therapeutic dentifrices by the American Dental Association's Council on Dental Therapeutics. This acceptance was based on each having been proven effective in an adequate number of well controlled clinical trials. Colgate's MFP contains 0.76 per cent sodium monofluorphosphate, which is a relatively stable inorganic salt, and 41.85 per cent insoluble metaphosphate as a polishing agent. Macleans' Fluoride dentifrice contains 0.76 per cent sodium monofluorphosphate, 1.15 per cent sodium lauryl sulfate, and 38 per cent calcium carbonate as polishing agent. The action of Crest is based on its content of 0.4 per cent stannous fluoride, together with 1.0 per cent stannous pyrophosphate to extend the time availability of the stannous ion, and 39.0 per cent calcium pyrophosphate as a polishing agent. Use of these dentifrices has been followed by 15 to 40 per cent reduction in caries increment depending principally on the frequency of daily use.

Fluoridated Prophylactic Pastes

Pumice prophylaxis reduces the enamel surface fluoride concentration. Either or both of two mechanisms may be responsible for this loss. Abrasion may remove a few microns from the enamel surface, which normally has a higher fluoride concentration than the subsurface enamel. Independently, heat generated by friction may result in thermodynamic conversion of fluorapatite to calcium fluoride which may be washed away. Use of a polishing agent that contains fluoride tends to prevent the loss, presumably by the mass action effect. However, clinical trials have shown relatively little cariostatic benefit from the use of fluoridated prophylactic pastes as the sole source for topical fluoride application. It should be stressed that polishing with an agent which contains fluoride is not a substitute for a topical fluoride application.

Multiple Fluoride Treatment

Research has clearly indicated that maximum benefit is obtained by multiple application, or even constant availability of the fluoride ion. Among the early demonstrations of this factor was the effectiveness of stannous fluoride used in three agents, a fluoridated prophylactic paste followed by topical application of a liquid solution and prescription of the stannous fluoride dentifrice for daily home use. Clinical trials indicated that use of all three agents was more effective than use of any one or combination of two. In fluoridated mouthwash studies and in fluoridated dentifrice studies, it became clear that supervised, controlled daily use of the agent was considerably more effective than more casual use of the same agent at home. These clinical research experiences support the concept that cariogenic priming of caries susceptible sites for remineralization and accumulation of fluoride salts in the microscopic lesion may be the most important mechanism in fluoride cariostasis. In addition, since the fluoride action on plaque microbiology is of such short duration, it is logical to assume that this fluoride benefit should be most effective with daily or constant availability of fluoride ion. Currently, research efforts are devoted to mechanisms for slow release of low levels of fluoride ion in the mouth. Several recent reports indicate that plastic sealants or varnishes are capable of providing such prolonged release of fluoride ion. Other current studies suggest that simultaneous exposure of enamel surfaces to solutions that contain both sucrose and fluoride at several widely spaced intervals each day may be highly cariostatic. Until such mechanisms have been proven successful and safe in clinical trials, it would seem logical that currently available methods be used to the maximum extent. To this end a preventive dentistry program logically should include a semiannual recall system for prophylaxis with a fluoridated polishing paste, followed by topical application of a fluoride solution and prescription of a fluoridated dentifrice for daily home use. For selected patients, other topical forms used in addition, but not substitution, may be justified. Dietary control of sugar intake and a program ensuring plaque control should not be overlooked.

Special Methods of Flouride Therapy

The Orthodontic Patient

The inability of most subjects to maintain a good level of plaque control while wearing fixed orthodontic appliances suggests that such persons would merit special consideration in fluoride therapy. In addition to prophylaxis and topical application of a fluoride solution on each occasion that the bands are removed, such patients might be well served by prescription of fluoride mouthwash as well as a fluoridated dentifrice for daily home use.

Rampant Caries

Occasionally the dentist meets the problems of a patient who has rampant caries, with numerous teeth in which carious exposure of the pulp appears imminent but immediate operative treatment is unfeasible. Topical stannous fluoride's arrestment of dentin caries provides a useful expedient for arrestment of such lesions until operative treatment is feasible.

Selected Carious Lesions

Semiannual topical application of ten per cent stannous fluoride solution has been used effectively to arrest caries in broad-surfaced buccal or lingual lesions. This may be especially appropriate when the only alternative is reduction of an otherwise sound posterior tooth for placement of a full crown. In such cases, the disclosant feature of stannous fluoride may be especially useful.

Xerostomia

The increased rate of caries formation in persons with a moderate reduction of salivary flow usually can be controlled by routine fluoride treatment together with excellent plaque control and restriction of dietary sugars. Alternatively, true xerostomia cases almost always develop severe caries, the prevention of which requires special treatment. This is especially

true of head and neck cancer patients who have had radiation therapy that included exposure of the major salivary glands and/or extirpation of the salivary glands. The MD Anderson Hospital and Tumor Institute of Houston, Texas has developed an effective program. Radiation dosage over 2,000 rads justifies a strenuous caries prevention regime. For each patient, custom made fluoride carriers (trays) are fabricated. After thorough prophylaxis and instruction in personal plaque control, the patient uses the fluoride carriers to apply, for five minutes each day, a fluoride gel that contains 1.0 per cent sodium fluoride, 1.0 per cent tribasic sodium phosphate, 0.5 per cent citric acid, 0.1 per cent red dye #3 (disclosant), and flavoring agents. After the five minute self application, the patient is instructed to perform additional plaque removal as indicated by the disclosant. Those patients in whom this schedule fails and caries appears may have their schedule increased to 15 minute applications made three times each day. The latter schedule rarely fails to prevent further caries.

SUMMARY

The fluoride ion has multiple actions in the prevention and arrestment of dental caries. Ingestion of optimal concentrations during childhood imparts fluorapatite cariostasis throughout the mineralizing enamel and dentin. Continued ingestion of fluoridated water during the posteruptive years contributes to topical maturation of the enamel surfaces. The effectiveness and safety of controlled fluoridation of water supplies is among the most conclusively proven public health measures. Exposure of the erupted teeth to fluoride ion appears to contribute cariostatic effects by three mechanisms: fluorapatite formation at the enamel surface; remineralization of early carious lesions; and inhibition of plaque microbial sugar metabolism. While fluorapatite is relatively permanent in its effectiveness, the latter two actions are intermittent and of relatively short effectiveness. Therefore, in clinical dental practice, frequent application of topical fluorides is essential for maximum caries prevention. Supervised daily topical application of the fluoride ion, either in water solution as a mouthwash or in gel-tray application, has yielded the greatest fluoride cariostatic benefit known to date. However, the casual use of such preparations at home appears to be responsible for considerably less benefit. The present state of knowledge supports the logic that the majority of dental patients will receive maximum fluoride benefit from a preventive dentistry program that, in addition to dietary control of sugar intake and plaque control, also includes semiannual prophylaxis with a fluoride-containing polishing paste followed by topical application of a fluoride solution in the dental operatory, and prescription of one of the approved fluoridated dentifrices for daily use at home. Additional forms of fluoride treatment may be considered for special situations.

GLOSSARY

Apatite. A family of minerals in crystalline form, of the general formula $Ca_{10}(PO_4)_6X$, wherein the X might include hydroxyl, carbonate, fluoride, oxygen, or sulfate ions.

Enamel maturation. Nonspecific posteruptive changes in enamel which appear to result in increased concentrations of some mineral ions such as F, Pb, Zn, and reduction in CO_3 concentration, as well as progressive increase in caries resistance.

Essential micronutrient. A nutritional trace element that cannot be synthesized by the organism and must be provided from the diet to maintain health and well being.

Fluorapatite. A form of hydroxyapatite in which fluoride ions have replaced some of the hydroxyl ions.

Fluorosis. General term for chronic fluoride toxicity that results in malformation of the mineralized tissues - teeth and bone. *Skeletal fluorosis* is a term applied when the skeletal bone contains an abnormally high level of fluoride. *Crippling skeletal fluorosis* is seen in livestock fed rockphosphates as feed supplement, or fluoride contaminated forage, and is manifested in bones reduced to brittle, chalky structures.

Hydration shell. A layer of tightly bound water that envelops the apatite crystal and provides a medium for ionic exchange within the crystal. This term is also sometimes used in reference to the first layer of water molecules surrounding an ion that is in aqueous solution. In demineralization of hydroxyapatite, water forms a hydration shell surrounding each dissolved Ca and PO_4 ion. In remineralization, crystallization occurs when Ca and PO_4 precipitate, converting the waters of the hydration shells to free water.

Hydroxyapatite. A form of apatite of the general formula $Ca_{10}(PO_4)_6(OH)_2$. The principal mineral component of teeth, bones, and calculus.

Hypoplasia. Defective or incomplete development of any tissue.

Idiopathic. Of unknown cause.

Lattice. Internal structure of a crystal wherein the atoms or ions are in definite relation to each other.

Mottled enamel. Defective enamel caused by excessive tissue fluid concentrations of fluoride ion during original mineralization.

Xerostomia. Dry mouth that results from functional or organic disturbances of the salivary glands.

SUGGESTED READINGS

Ast DB, Fitzgerald B: Effectiveness of water fluoridation. J Am Dent Assoc 65: 581–587, 1962

Birkeland JM, Charlton G: Effect of pH on the fluoride ion activity of plaque. Caries Res 10: 72–80, 1976

Bixler D, Muhler JC: Effect on dental caries in children in a nonfluoride area of combined use of three agents containing stannous fluoride: a prophylactic paste, a solution and a dentifrice. J Am Dent Assoc 68: 792–800, 1964

Bowen WH, Hewitt MJ: Effect of fluoride on extracellular polysaccharide production by Streptococcus mutans. J Dent Res 53: 627–630, 1974

Brudevold F, McCann HG, Nilsson R, Richardson B, Coklica V: The chemistry of caries inhibition problems and challenges in topical treatments. J Dent Res [Suppl] 46 (1): 37–45, 1967

Charlton G, Blainey B, Schamschula RG: Associations between dental plaque and fluoride in human surface enamel. Arch Oral Biol 19: 139–143, 1974

Council on Dental Therapeutics: Accepted Dental Therapeutics, 36th ed. Chicago, American Dental Association, 1975

Daly TE: Dental care of head and neck cancer patients receiving radiation therapy. In Chalian VA, Drane JB, Standish SM: Maxillofacial Prosthetics. Baltimore, Williams & Wilkins, 1972

Dean HT, Arnold FA, Elvove E: Domestic water and dental caries. II. A study of 2832 white children, aged 12–14 years of eight suburban Chicago communities. US Pub Health Rep 56: 761–799, 1941

Dean HT, Arnold FA, Elvove E: Domestic water and dental caries. V. Additional studies of the relation of fluoride in domestic waters to dental caries experience in 4425 white children, aged 12–14 years, of 13 cities in four states. US Pub Health Rep 57: 1155–1179, 1942

Englander HR, Keyes PH, Gestwicki M, Sultz HA: Clinical anticaries effect of repeated topical sodium fluoride applications by mouthpieces. J Am Dent Assoc 75: 638–654, 1967

Ercisson Y: Report on the safety of drinkin water fluoridation. Caries Res [Suppl] 8: 16–27, 1974

Forrester DJ, Schulz EM: Proceedings of the International Workshop on Fluorides and Dental Caries Reduction. Baltimore, University of Maryland, 1974

Friedman M, vander Merwe EHM, Bischoff JI, Fatti LP, Retief DH: Effect of a sealant used in conjunction with topical fluoride application, on fluoride concentrations in human tooth enamel. Arch Oral Biol 21: 237–241, 1976

Hodge HC: The concentration of fluorides in drinking water to give the point of minimum caries with maximum safety. J Am Dent Assoc 40: 436–454, 1950

Isaac S, Brudevold F, Smith FA, Gardner DE: The relation of fluoride in the drinking water to the distribution of fluoride in enamel. J Dent Res 37: 318–325, 1958

Jackson D, Weidmann SM: Fluorine in human bone related to age and the water supply of different regions. J Pathol Bacteriol 76: 451–459, 1958

Koulourides T: Experimental changes of enamel mineral density. In Harris RS (ed): Art and Science of Dental Caries Research. New York, Academic Press, 1968

Koulourides T, Phantumvanit P, Munksgaard EC, Housch T: An intraoral model used for studies of fluoride incorporation in enamel. J Oral Pathol 3: 185–196, 1974

McClure FJ: Water Fluoridation. The Search and the Victory. Bethesda, US Department of HEW, 1970

Mercer VH, Muhler JC: The clinical demonstration of caries arrestment following topical stannous fluoride treatments. J Dent Child 32: 65–72, 1965

Muhler JC, Spear LB, Bixler D, Stookey GK: The arrestment of incipient dental caries in adults after the use of three different forms of SnF_2 therapy: results after 30 months. J Am Dent Assoc 75: 1402–1406, 1967

Newbrun E: The safety of water fluoridation. J Am Dent Assoc 94: 301–304, 1977

Tinanoff N, Brady JM, Gross A: The effect of NaF and SnF_2 mouth rinses on bacterial colonization of tooth enamel: TEM and SEM studies. Caries Res 10: 415–426, 1976

Volker JF: Effect of fluorine on solubility of enamel and dentin. Proc Soc Exp Biol Med 42: 725–727, 1939

Wellock WD, Brudevold F: A study of acidulated fluoride solutions. II. The caries inhibiting effect of single annual topical applications of an acidic fluoride and phosphate solution. Arch Oral Biol 8: 179–182, 1963

21 Pit and Fissure Sealants

RUSSELL N. KEMPER

Introduction
    Occlusal Caries—a Major Dental Problem
    Historical Methods of Resolving the Occlusal Caries Problem
Sealants as a Method of Resolving the Problem
    Historical Use of Sealants
    Problems with Adhesion to Tooth Enamel
    Sealants—Physical and Chemical Properties
        Molecular Structure of Sealants
        Relationship between Sealant Physical Properties and Bonding

Clinical Procedure for Sealant Application
    Sealant Application
    Sealant Application as an Adjunct to Topical Fluoride
    Incipient Caries
    Clinical Application Problems
Evaluation of Clinical Effectiveness of Sealants
Effect of Sealants on Enamel Maturation and Caries
Summary
Glossary
Suggested Readings

INTRODUCTION

Dental caries has long been recognized as a major health problem. Much effort has been expended on improving methods of treating the disease. In recent decades increasing attention has been directed toward understanding the causes of this disease and developing materials and methods for prevention of dental decay. The importance of diet (see Ch. 16 and 17), good oral hygiene, and trace elements, especially fluoride (see Ch. 20), in reducing the incidence of caries has been well established.

Oral and tooth morphology affect carious attack. Relative caries incidence is low on smooth, self-cleansing surfaces but increases significantly on interproximal and occlusal surfaces.

Occlusal Caries—a Major Dental Problem

Several investigations have shown that the occlusal surfaces are especially susceptible to dental decay, accounting for nearly 50 per cent of all caries. Even fluoridation, which significantly reduces smooth-surface caries, provides only a slight reduction in occlusal caries. This has been demonstrated in studies in which the fluoride has been provided in many forms, such as a dentifrice, in fluoridated table salt, or as a tablet, and applied as a topical gel or prophylactic paste. These studies have all shown that the occlusal surfaces receive the least cariostatic effect from topical and systemic fluoride procedures. In light of these and other findings, there is a need to

461

protect the occlusal surface against caries by some other method.

The susceptibility of the occlusal surface to carious attack results from the saclike morphology of the pits and fissures (Figs. 21-1, 21-2). Occlusal fissures consist of deep narrow faults extending into the enamel and provide ideal sites for the entrapment of bacteria, food debris, and nutrients. Since the fissure widths usually measure only a fraction of the diameter of a toothbrush bristle, cleansing by conventional methods becomes almost impossible. Therefore, decay can readily occur.

Although pits and fissures are found predominantly in the occlusal surfaces of molars and premolars, pits are occasionally found at the cingulum of anterior teeth, particularly in lateral incisors. These cingulum pits are less common than occlusal pits. When, however, the cingulum is pronounced, it is usually accompanied by a deep pit.

Analysis of fissure contents indicates that the fissures are filled with food debris and plaque, which is made up of a variety of microorganisms. Studies by Theilade and co-workers in which surgically removed impacted molar crowns were placed in the mouths of volunteers, show that microorganisms invade the fissure areas within 24 hours following exposure to the oral environment. The numbers and types of microorganisms vary with time and from patient to patient.

The carious process in occlusal surfaces begins with the accumulation of microorga-

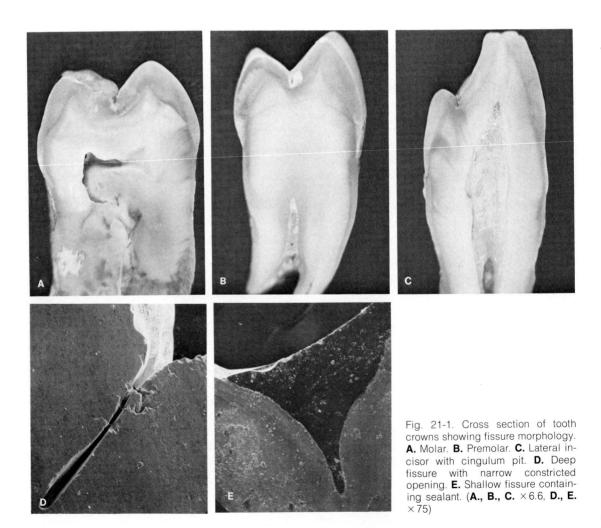

Fig. 21-1. Cross section of tooth crowns showing fissure morphology. **A.** Molar. **B.** Premolar. **C.** Lateral incisor with cingulum pit. **D.** Deep fissure with narrow constricted opening. **E.** Shallow fissure containing sealant. (**A., B., C.** ×6.6, **D., E.** ×75)

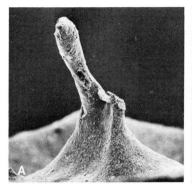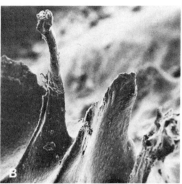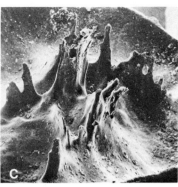

Fig. 21-2. Replicas of fissures. (Galil, K. A., Gwinnet, A. J.: Arch Oral Biol 20: 493, 1963) (×100)

nisms and nutrients within the pits and fissures. Fissures with steep walls and narrow openings are particularly susceptible. The thin enamel at the base of the fissure usually leads to early dentinal involvement.

Enamel rods fan out in a radial fashion at the base of a pit or fissure. Enamel decalcification during caries attack proceeds along the enamel rods. As a result fissure caries are characterized by a cone or triangular shaped lesion having the apex at the enamel surface and its base at the dentinoenamel junction (Fig. 21-3). This carious process spreads the area of attack across a large area of the dentin involving large numbers of dentinal tubules. This process can lead to considerable cavitation and undermining with little evidence of changes at the enamel surface.

Historical Methods of Resolving the Occlusal Caries Problem

Over the years various methods have been tried to solve the problem of occlusal caries. Hyatt made shallow cavity preparations along the occlusal fissures and filled them with amalgam (prophylactic odontotomy). Bodecher opened up the fissures with a round bur to make shallow, nonretentive grooves. Others have tried various chemical treatment methods such as silver nitrate, zinc chloride, potassium ferrocyanide, and copper cement with little success. More recently various adhesive materials that act as agents to seal the fissures from the oral environment have been investigated.

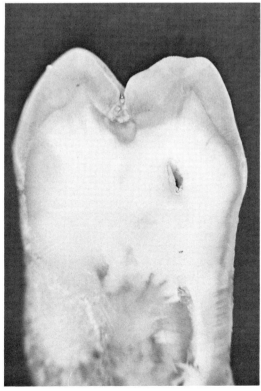

Fig. 21-3. Mode of caries attack in occlusal fissures. Note cone-shaped area of enamel demineralization and area of dentinal involvement.

SEALANTS AS A METHOD OF RESOLVING THE PROBLEM

Historical Use of Sealants

In the early 1960s a major breakthrough occurred in preventive dentistry: the development of acid etching of enamel and the use of adhesive dental techniques. Since that time a considerable effort has been directed toward perfecting sealants for the prevention of occlusal caries.

The use of acid-etching techniques to enhance the retention of adhesive dental materials grew out of earlier work by Buconocore and others. In 1955 Buconocore reported that acid etching tooth enamel significantly improved the bond between an acrylic restorative material and enamel. In 1965 Cueto and Buonocore published the results of studies on the use of adhesive techniques in sealing pits and fissures. The sealant consisted of a blend of methyl-α-cyanoacrylate and powdered methyl methacrylate.

Several other investigators have experimented with various cyanoacrylate formulations. However, as a class the cyanoacrylates have proved difficult to handle and provide only marginal retention to enamel. As a result they have not advanced much beyond the experimental stage.

Another class of materials studied by early investigators was the polyurethanes. One product containing fluoride in a polyurethane system was marketed briefly during the early 1970s as a long-term topical fluoride application under the trade name Epoxylite 9070.* Polyurethanes have, however, shown very poor retention and thus have not proved successful as sealants.

The only really successful class of sealants to date is the methacrylates, and in particular the higher molecular weight dimethacrylates. This class of materials includes Bis-GMA, the principal monomer in most dental composites and originally developed by Bowen.

Roydhouse was perhaps the first to employ Bis-GMA in a sealant formulation. His studies, reported in 1968, showed that a blend of Bis-GMA and methyl methacrylate significantly reduced the incidence of occlusal caries after 3 years.

Buonocore modified the Bis-GMA system so that the material cures by ultraviolet irradiation. This sealant, later marketed under the trade name Nuva–Seal,† proved to be an important advance at the time. Sealant retention and caries reduction were significantly improved.

In the latter part of the 1960s and early 1970s sealant research increased significantly. Several modifications and improvements were made in the methacrylate systems. As a result of this effort new sealants based on Bis-GMA or similar monomers have been developed and marketed under trade names such as EPOXYLITE 9075†, KERR‡ Pit and Fissure Sealant, CONCICE§ White Sealant and DELTON¶ Pit and Fissure Sealant. These materials all rely on the acid etching technique for bonding to tooth enamel.

Problems with Adhesion to Tooth Enamel

Successful adhesive bonding to enamel, whether chemical or mechanical, relies on tailoring the characteristics of the adhesive to those of the enamel surface. Bonding to enamel presents some difficult problems owing to surface contamination, the ever-present moist environment, and the nature of the enamel surface.

Tooth enamel has a rather complex structure consisting of about 95 per cent inorganic components, approximately 2 per cent to 5 per cent water, and less than 1 per cent organic material. The inorganic portion of enamel consists of five major elements: calcium, phosphorus, oxygen, hydrogen, and carbon, plus at least 16 trace elements in concentrations ranging from 1 to 5000 ppm. Included among the trace elements are magnesium, sodium, potassium, chlorine, and fluorine.

The organic component of enamel consists of proteinaceous material that seems to have low crystallinity and does not appear to consist of ordered fibers.

The principal crystalline structure in enamel is tricalcium phosphate, which exists in platelike apitite crystals of calcium hydroxyapitite, $Ca_{10}(PO_4)_6(OH)_2$ (see Ch. 7). These crystals form microscopic hexagonal rods or enamel prisms that are approximately $4\mu m$ in diameter and extend from the dentin to the free enamel surface. Between the enamel rods are minute interstices that contain small amounts of proteinaceous material. The enamel rods radiate from the dentin in a fanlike pattern that varies somewhat according to the location on the tooth, the tooth type, and individual characteristics (Fig. 21-4).

---

* Lee Pharmaceuticals.
† L. D. Caulk Company.

† Lee Pharmaceuticals.
‡ Sybron Corporation.
§ 3-M Company.
¶ Johnson & Johnson Dental Products Company.

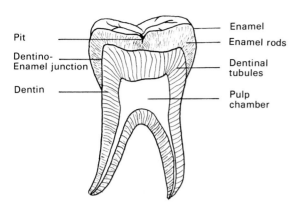

Fig. 21-4. Permanent molar showing typical enamel rod alignment.

A considerable effort has been expended during the last two decades in search of materials that will form durable bonds with the rather complex enamel surface. In general, effective adhesive bonding to a given surface can be achieved through a chemical and/or mechanical bonding. Chemical adhesion can occur by two mechanisms, primary chemical bonding (ionic, metallic, or covalent) and secondary chemical bonding (intermolecular forces such as hydrogen bonding or Van der Waal's forces).

Most adhesives do not rely on primary chemical bonding. In the case of pit and fissure sealants primary chemical bonding would require either direct covalent bonding between the tooth enamel and the sealant or incorporation of the sealant with the hydroxyapitite crystal lattice through ionic bonding.

Although isolated primary chemical bonds might be formed with certain adhesive materials, durable bonding by this mechanism would require widespread bonding, a condition not presently practical in the oral environment. Ionic bonding, for example, requires the deposition and incorporation of the appropriate ions into the crystal lattice. Such a precipitation would normally occur from solution or melt over an extended period of time. Secondary chemical bonding is, however, an important bonding mechanism in adhesives technology. Reagents are often used to cleanse and activate the substrate surface to set up a condition for electrostatic attraction between the adhesive and adherent.

Acid etching of tooth enamel, in addition to roughening the surface, also cleanses the surface and enhances the wetting or attraction between the sealant and enamel. Although the etching process does enhance bonding by providing sites for microscopic interlocking, it undoubtedly increases the electrostatic attraction or secondary chemical bondings. Because both micromechanical retention and secondary chemical bonding are undoubtedly involved in the sealant retention, it is difficult to isolate the contribution of each of the bonding mechanisms to the ultimate bond strength. Both are important.

In spite of many efforts at providing adhesion to enamel by various means, acid etching remains the only effective method of cleansing and conditioning enamel for bonding.

Much has been published in the dental literature concerning etching agents, ideal concentrations, and etching mechanisms. In 1971 Ohsawa of Japan published an extensive study on acid etching with various acids and acid concentrations. His results indicated that pyruvic and phosphoric acids give the greatest bond strengths under his test conditions. His work and the work of Silverstone and of others indicate that the ideal concentrations for effective etching with phosphoric acid lie between 30 per cent and 50 per cent. In fact Gwinnett and Buonocore have reported that higher concentrations produce less etching.

Chow and Brown have explained the concentration effects of phosphoric acid on etching by showing that monocalcium phosphate monohydrate $(Ca(H_2PO_4)2 \cdot H_2O)$ forms during etching. Using phase diagrams, they have shown that, at higher acid concentrations, early deposition of this salt onto the enamel seems to "protect" the surface from further dissolution. At concentrations of more than 60 per cent, this reduction in enamel solubility becomes significant. At lower concentrations, this precipitate is less readily formed, and etching proceeds to a greater extent. The $Ca(H_2PO_4)2 \cdot H_2O$ precipitate is readily dissolved by rinsing, leaving the enamel ideally prepared for adhesive bonding.

At concentrations less than about 27 per cent, a second but significantly less soluble precipitate $(CaHPO_4 \cdot 2H_2O)$ is formed. Formation of this precipitate also reduces the extent of enamel etching. Because of its low solubility this latter precipitate would not be readily removed during the rinsing procedure and could interfere with bonding.

Other etching agents have also been tested, and some have been offered commercially. Citric acid is used as an etching agent to some extent. Phosphoric acid is, however, the most studied and widely used. Preferred concentrations range from 30 per cent to 50 per cent. Phosphoric acid buffered with zinc oxide is also available. Evidence does not, however, indicate that the buffered acids offer any particular advantage over nonbuffered solutions.

Acid etching serves at least three interrelated purposes. It cleanses the surface of debris and oral fluids, roughens the surface for micromechanical retention, and conditions the surface, increasing its receptivity for the adhesive agent.

Figure 21-5 shows a photomicrographic comparison between unetched and etched enamel. The prism rod outlines are clearly discernible in the etched specimen. Here the rod cores were more soluble than the rod periphery, leaving tiny cells with thin shell walls.

The rod cores are not always more soluble. In Figure 21-6A an entirely different etching pattern is evident. In this case the rod cores are more resistant to acid etching. The rod peripheries have been dissolved, leaving tiny cone-shaped prism ends. Variations in etching patterns are seen between teeth from different patients, different types of teeth, and even with different sites on the same tooth (Fig. 21-6B).

Deciduous teeth show a somewhat different etching pattern from permanent enamel. Studies by Ripa and Cole and also by Buonocore indicate that sealant retention is lower on primary teeth than in the permanent dentition. Acid etching of primary surface enamel results in a roughened surface with randomly distributed micropores rather than in the characteristic ordered etching patterns of permanent enamel. Removal of this outer layer of primary enamel will give a surface that, when etched, will usually produce an etching pattern typical of permanent enamel. Microscopic studies have shown that resins do not penetrate adequately into etched primary enamel, and this perhaps explains the lower sealant retention reported for primary dentition. One explanation offered for the differences in etching and sealant retention between primary and permanent enamel is that the surface layer of primary enamel has no definite crystalline structure. This apparently amorphous structure has been called "prismless" enamel. Horsted's studies suggest, however, that prismless enamel is not commonly found on occlusal surfaces of primary or permanent enamel. Thus, the poorer etching and lower sealant retention reported for primary enamel may result from other factors.

Enamel solubility depends at least in part

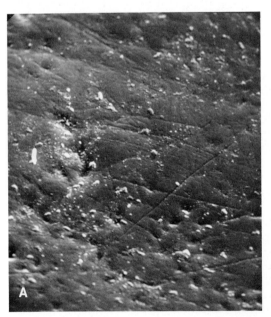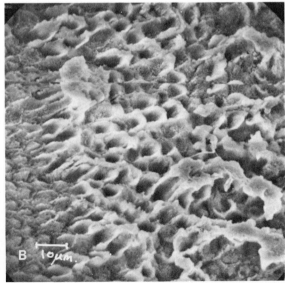

Fig. 21-5. Scanning electron photomicrographs of human enamel surfaces. **A.** Unetched enamel. **B.** Etched enamel (×1000)

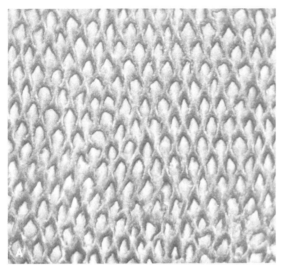 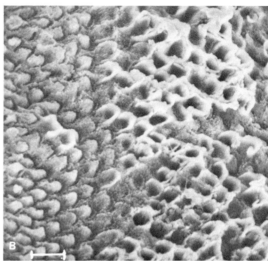

Fig. 21-6. Scanning electron photomicrographs. **A.** Etching pattern of enamel having rod cores with low solubility. **B.** Random etching pattern (×1000).

on the concentrations of various trace elements within the enamel structure. Inclusion of greater concentrations of fluoride, for example, leads to a reduction in enamel solubility. In the clinical situation this can lead to a condition in which the etching step must be repeated to achieve the proper etch.

Acid etching of tooth enamel effectively removes the surface layer of enamel. The depth of the etch depends on the acid and its concentration.

Silverstone, investigating the etching process, has measured the loss of surface contour and the depth of histologic change obtained with various phosphoric acid concentrations, including zinc oxide-buffered acid (Table 21-1). His results show that the greatest loss of contour and greatest histologic changes occur with acid concentrations in the 20 per cent– 30 per cent range.

With 30 per cent phosphoric acid there is a loss of contour some 10μm in depth. In addition the histologic change (micropores) reaches an additional 20μm. The resin flows into the micropores leading to the sealant "tags," which provide micromechanical retention.

Etched enamel not covered by sealant soon returns to a normal appearance. There seems to be general agreement among many investigators that this return to normal results from some degree of remineralization (see Ch. 19). It is, of course, possible that, rather than remineralization, rapid abrasion of the fragile

etched surface to a more durable virgin surface is what occurs. The prevailing view is, however, that at least some degree of remineralization does occur. The time reported for complete remineralization or return to a normal appearance varies among investigators.

Albert and Grenoble report remineralization within 96 hours (4 days); Retief reports remineralization within 1 week. Müehlmann found that complete remineralization took from 2 to 48 days. Arana reported different rates of remineralization in four patients of different ages. Although his study did not employ a statistically significant number of subjects, the indication is that remineralization

TABLE 21-1. DEPTH OF ETCH AND HISTOLOGIC CHANGE IN ENAMEL (TO NEAREST μm) AFTER A 1-MIN EXPOSURE TO VARIOUS CONCENTRATIONS OF PHOSPHORIC ACID

	Concentration of phosphoric acid (%)						
	20	30	40	50	50	60	70
					ZnO		
Depth of etch	14	10	9	7	6	2	2
Depth of histologic change	20	20	15	12	10	4	2
Total depth of enamel affected	34	30	24	19	16	6	4

(Silverstone LM: Caries Reg 8:2, 1974, Basel, S. Karger A6).

occurs faster in younger patients. In two patients under 25 years of age the enamel regained a completely normal appearance within four days, whereas the enamel showed only "almost complete" remineralization within the same time period in the two patients over 55 years of age. In the latter case the enamel returned to its normal appearance within 16 days.

Little information is available on the nature or quality of enamel that has remineralized *in vivo*. Several investigators have, however, analyzed enamel after *in vitro* remineralization. Wei, using an electron microprobe, showed that etching lowered the calcium and phosphorus (Ca/P) concentrations in enamel. After *in vitro* remineralization both the calcium and phosphorus concentrations, as well as the Ca/P ratio of the surface enamel, returned essentially to their normal values.

Krutchoff and Rowe showed by infrared spectroscopy that interatomic bond types changed after etching but returned to normal after remineralization. Thus, it appears that an etched enamel surface is returned to its normal condition by remineralization. If etching is restricted to the surface layer, no permanent damage should occur. Lost surface contour is not, however, replaced, and repeated etching or extended etching times could reduce the surface contour of the tooth, reducing the thickness of the enamel at the etched site.

Sealants—Physical and Chemical Properties

MOLECULAR STRUCTURE OF SEALANTS

Three principal classes of materials have been or are currently used as sealants: methacrylates, cyanoacrylates, and ionomer cements.

Methacrylates are, by far, the most important class of sealants. They include self-curing and light-activated sealants that may be either unfilled or filled. The reactive unit of the resin is the methacrylate end group of esters derived from methacrylic acid and an alcohol. The typical monomers used in sealants have two principal differences from their cousin methyl methacrylate, which is used in standard acrylic systems. Sealant monomers, generally, have higher molecular weights and are **difunctional**; *i.e.*, they have reactive groups at each end of the monomer. The higher molecular weight reduces their volatility, and the difunctionality leads to cross linking of the polymer chains to make a stronger and insoluble sealant.

Most sealants are based on bis-GMA or similar high molecular weight methacrylate. Bis-GMA by itself has the viscosity of cold honey and thus would not flow into the fissures and etched enamel well enough to produce a good seal. To reduce the viscosity of the bis-GMA and to improve the sealant's flow and surface-wetting characteristics, other, more fluid diluent monomers are added. Typical fluid monomers include glycol derivatives such as triethyleneglycol dimethacrylate and the more basic material methyl methacrylate.

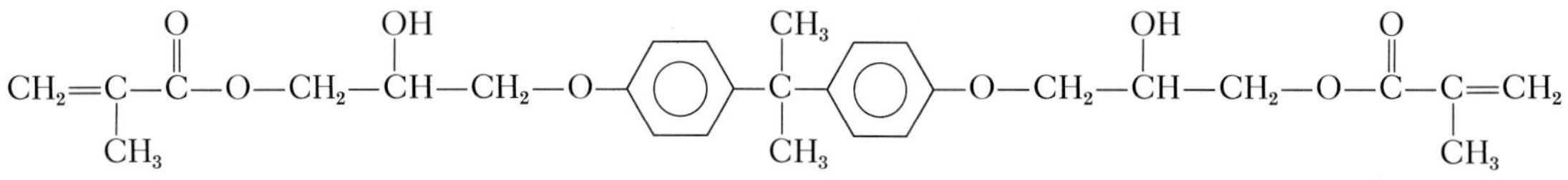

Bis-GMA

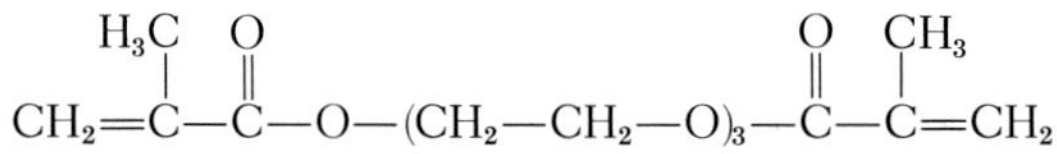

Triethyleneglycol dimethacrylate

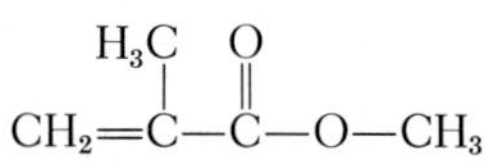

Methyl methacrylate

Most pit and fissure sealants are unfilled resins. Sealants are available containing filler that is added to reduce wear. The inclusion of filler necessitates, however, an extra step in the placement procedure to adjust occlusion after sealant placement. Further, is is not established that a more wear-resistant filled sealant has any advantage over unfilled sealants, since the sealant is acting as a barrier within the neck of the fissure, where abrasion is low.

Methacrylate sealants are applied to the tooth as fluid monomers and cured (hardened) by free radical mechanisms. This polymerization reaction may be initiated either chemically or by light irradiation. The type of curing mechanism employed determines the type of reactive additives included in a given formulation.

Chemically cured sealants are usually supplied as two liquids commonly called a catalyst and a universal or base. The catalyst contains sealant monomers and a peroxide, usually benzoyl peroxide, which is capable of producing polymerization–inducing free radicals.

The universal contains an aromatic tertiary amine accelerator in sealant monomers. When the catalyst and universal liquids are mixed, the peroxide (B) and amine (A) react chemically (Fig. 21-7), causing the peroxide to decompose to form free radicals ($R\cdot$). These radicals, in turn, react with the methacrylate monomers (M) to give methacrylate radicals ($M\cdot$). Progressive attack of methacrylate radi-

$$A + B \longrightarrow R\cdot$$
$$R\cdot + M \longrightarrow M\cdot$$
$$M\cdot + M \longrightarrow M\text{-}M\cdot$$
$$M\text{-}M\cdot \xrightarrow{M} [M]\cdot^n \longrightarrow [M]^n$$

A = Initiator (universal solution)

B = Peroxide (catalyst solution)

R · = Radical

M = Monomer

M · = Monomer radical

[M] n = Polymer

Fig. 21-7. Generalized reaction mechanism for chemically initiated free radical polymerization.

$$R \longrightarrow R\cdot$$
$$R + M \longrightarrow M\cdot$$
$$M + M\cdot \longrightarrow M\text{-}M\cdot$$
$$M\text{-}M\cdot \xrightarrow{M} [M]\cdot^n \longrightarrow [M]^n$$

R = Photoinitiator

R = Radical

M = Monomer

M = Monomer radical

[M]n = Polymer

Fig. 21-8. Generalized reaction mechanism for light-induced polymerization.

cals on methacrylate monomer leads to the buildup of the polymer chains. Since the sealant monomers are difunctional (reactive groups at both ends) the polymerization reaction leads to a cross-linked polymer network.

Light-polymerized sealants are usually supplied as a single sealant liquid that is painted onto the tooth surface and cured by exposure to an intense light of the proper wavelength. To ensure adequate shelf life, the photoinitiator may be supplied as a separate component that is mixed with the sealant before use.

Light-induced polymerizations occur by the same free radical polymerization mechanisms as that of chemically cured systems. In this case, however, the free radicals are generated by light activation of an appropriate photoinitiator (R) (Fig. 21-8). This radical then attacks the methacrylate monomer, inducing polymerization.

A commonly used photoinitiator is benzoin methyl ether. Its absorption lies in the long-wave ultraviolet (uv) region. Thus, under irradiation with the appropriate uv light wavelength and intensity, is becomes an efficient polymerization initiator.

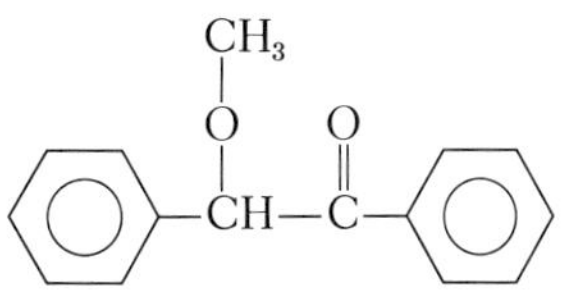

$$CH_3$$

Benzoin methyl ether

Both chemically cured and light-activated sealants contain trace quantities of phenolic stabilizers. These additives are included to control the rate of polymerization and to ensure an adequate shelf life for the methacrylate monomer system.

Cyanoacrylates are largely an experimental sealant in the United States but are commercially available in some countries. The three most commonly used cyanoacrylates are the methyl, ethyl, and isobutyl derivatives, which polymerize by a base-catalyzed anionic mechanism. The reaction is initiated by adding trace quantities of a weak base such as an amine. Cyanoacrylates are so reactive toward base catalysts that they will polymerize on contact with water, a property that was expected to be an asset in dentistry.

$$CH_2{=}\underset{\underset{CN}{|}}{C}{-}\underset{\underset{O}{\|}}{C}{-}O{-}CH_3$$

Methyl cyanoacrylate

$$CH_2{=}\underset{\underset{CN}{|}}{C}{-}\underset{\underset{O}{\|}}{C}{-}O{-}CH_2{-}\underset{\underset{CH_3}{|}}{CH}{-}CH_3$$

Isobutyl cyanoacrylate

Cyanoacrylates have, however, low tensile strength and do not form the strong bond to tooth enamel that can be achieved with methacrylates. In addition the cyanoacrylate bond appears to degrade over a period of months under moist conditions. This is made evident with clinical trials, which show that the experimental sealant retention rate is lower for cyanoacrylate sealants than for methacrylates. To weaken further the position of cyanoacrylates, questions have been raised about their chemical stability and about the toxicity of their possible degradation products. Thus, until there is adequate clinical and biologic proof to the contrary, cyanoacrylates should not be used for dental applications.

Glass ionomer cements have been advertised as pit and fissure sealants under the trade name ASPA.* These cements are powder/liquid systems in which the liquid is a polyacrylic acid solution and the powder is an aluminosilicate glass. The mixed cement forms a putty-like paste that hardens in 2 to 10 minutes. Hardening occurs by an acid–base reaction between the polyacrylic acid and leachable glass powder with the formation of a cementing hydrated salt.

* Amalgmated Dental Products.

Bond strengths are lower with glass ionomer cements than with methacrylate sealants. There is, however, evidence that the cements achieve some degree of chemical bonding with the enamel surface. Because these cements have a pastelike consistency, they must be packed into the fissure area and then contoured to adjust occlusion. For this reason they lend themselves more toward filling deep, open fissures or fissures that have been mechanically widened. In this sense, glass ionomer cements are in a different class from conventional sealants. Although ionomer cements are suggested for use as sealants, clinical studies are somewhat limited. Additional studies are needed to demonstrate long-term retention and efficacy.

RELATIONSHIP BETWEEN SEALANT PHYSICAL PROPERTIES AND BONDING

As discussed earlier, effective sealant bonding depends on microscopic mechanical interlocking and electrostatic attraction between the sealant and the etched enamel. Factors contributing to good bond strengths include the tensile strength of the sealant and the ability of the sealant to wet the enamel and to penetrate into the rough etched surface. Sealants that exhibit the greatest penetration into tooth enamel have low contact angles and low viscosities.

Contact angle is a measure of the ability of a liquid to wet a given surface. Specifically, contact angle is that angle formed between the surface of a liquid and a given surface at that point where the liquid contacts the surface. Differences in contact angle can be visualized by comparing water droplets on a waxed and an unwaxed surface (Fig. 21-9). In a sealant, a low contact angle with etched enamel indicates that the sealant will wet the surface, flowing into the etchings and providing intimate contact for good bonding.

Viscosity of the sealant also plays a role in bonding. A sealant with low viscosity will obviously flow more readily across the etched surface and into the fissures and etched enamel surface. A combination of low viscosity and low contact angle gives a sealant the wetting characteristics necessary to cause the sealant to spread across the surface and into the depths of the etched enamel, forming long sealant tags for strong bonding (Fig. 21-10).

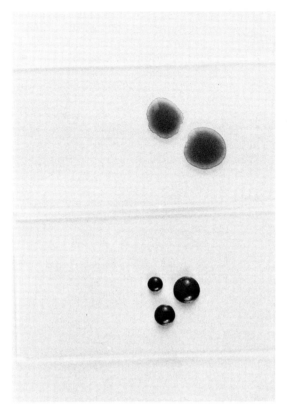

Fig. 21-9. Liquids showing high and low contact angles on surfaces. *Top,* water drops on clean glass surface. *Bottom,* water drops on silicone-treated glass surface. (Dye was added to improve visibility)

Fig. 21-10. Cross section of a sealed molar showing sealant tags reaching into etched enamel (×200).

strengths are calculated by dividing the breaking force by the unit area of the sample.

Tensile Strength = Force/Area

Results are usually reported in pounds per square inch (psi) or in Megapascals (MPa) or its equivalent kilonewtons per square meter (kN/m^2).

Another important factor in sealant retention is the tensile strength of the sealant material. A sealant with low tensile strength will not be retained adequately, even though it may have the wetting characteristics (low viscosity and low contact angle) necessary for good penetration and bonding. If the tensile strength of the sealant is low enough, the sealant tags can fracture, leading to loss of retention and apparent bond failure.

Various methods have been developed for measuring the bond strength of sealant materials. Although the apparatus and techniques for measurement may differ, most are similar in principle. Figure 21-11 shows one tensile bond strength measurement device that uses an alignment block to hold the sample in proper alignment for tensile bond strength measurement. A tooth section and sealant are placed in cups and held in alignment during bonding. The samples are then transferred to another alignment block and loaded until failure under tensile stress. Bond

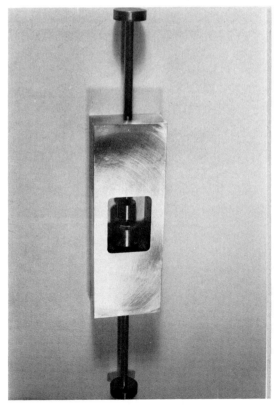

Fig. 21-11. Apparatus for measuring tensile bond strength of sealants. (Kemper, R. N. and Kilian, R. J.)

In Table 21-2 the tensile bond strengths of a commercial chemically cured sealant and an experimental isobutyl cyanoacrylate sealant are compared. Note that the bond strength of the methacrylate sealant is significantly greater than that of the cyanoacrylate sealant.

TABLE 21-2. COMPARISON OF TENSILE BOND STRENGTH OF A CYANOACRYLATE SEALANT AND A METHACRYLATE SEALANT

Sealant type	Enamel type	Bond strength*		
		(MPa)	(S.D.)	(PSI)
Isobutyl cyanoacrylate	Bovine	4.22	2.96	(592)
Commercial methacrylate†	Bovine	8.19	3.99	(1188)
Commercial methacrylate†	Human	16.45	6.64	(2386)

* Samples stored in water at 37°C for 24 hr before testing.
† DELTON™ Pit and Fissure Sealant, Johnson and Johnson Dental Products Company.
(Kemper RN, unpublished data)

Microleakage or its prevention in sealants is directly related to the bonding of the sealant. With good sealant penetration into etched enamel and strong durable bonding, microleakage will be virtually nonexistent. As long as the sealant bond remains intact, any leakage would have to proceed through a tortuous path of the hills and valleys of the interface between the sealant and enamel surface. With good sealant adaptation and bonding, microleakage cannot occur to any measurable degree. If, on the other hand, sealant retention is poor, owing to any number of factors, including poor sealant wetting characteristics, improper tooth etching, moisture contamination of the etched enamel surface, or sealant fracture, some leakage may be observed.

Microleakage has been evaluated *in vitro* for several commercial sealants. The usual method is to immerse sealed, extracted teeth in solutions containing a radioactive element, usually ^{45}Ca. After a specified immersion

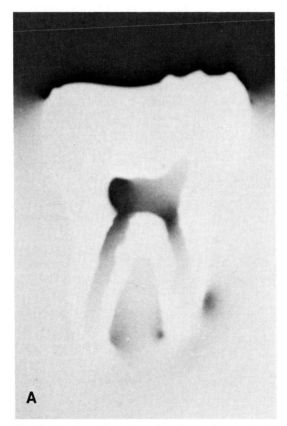 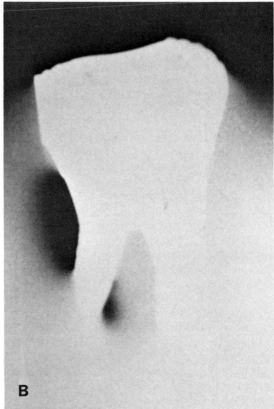

Fig. 21-12. Autoradiographs of tooth specimens showing no leakage (Phillips, RW and Swartz, ML unpublished data) Note: Specimen **A.** was stored at 37° for one week. Specimen **B.** was thermocycled 2500 times at a temperature differential of 40°C. That there is no microleakage is indicated by the absence of a thin black radiation exposure line at the fissure/sealant margins.

time, with or without thermocycling, the teeth are sectioned and placed on x-ray film, and autoradiographs are prepared (Fig. 21-12).

Microleakage shows up as thin, black lines between the sealant and enamel. Again, microleakage is not a problem with sealants that have good bonding characteristics and that have been properly placed.

CLINICAL PROCEDURE FOR SEALANT APPLICATION

Sealant Application

Selection of teeth for sealant treatment depends on the patient's oral health and the dental examination and treatment schedule. Ideally, teeth would be treated as soon after eruption as possible as part of a comprehensive caries prevention program. Large numbers of children do not, however, receive regular dental care. Under such circumstances sealants can play an important role in public health prevention programs. In such a program, candidate teeth are usually selected and sealed in a mass treatment operation. This is usually accomplished through a caries prevention program in public schools or local public health systems. The greatest success can be achieved by beginning a caries prevention program in the early school grades with children in the 6- to 7- year-old age bracket. At this age the first permanent molars have erupted. All fully erupted, sound molars and premolars should be treated. If possible, children should be examined annually. This ensures that newly erupted teeth can be sealed in a timely fashion. In addition, teeth sealed in previous visits can be reexamined. Sealant can be reapplied to any areas in which sealant may have been lost and thus continued protection is ensured.

In private practice the dentist can exercise a greater degree of flexibility. Visits can be scheduled to ensure that the teeth are treated as soon after eruption as possible. Sealant application can be carried out at 6- or 12- month intervals as a part of the dentist's regular prevention program.

Whether is a public health situation or in private practice, the selection of teeth for sealing is vitally important. Teeth should be free from caries and have the occlusal surface fully erupted. Often in newly erupting teeth, a gingival flap partially covers the distal pit. This flap interferes with acid etching of the area and prevents sealant from flowing into the fissure. It can also retain moisture, which can seep out onto the etched and dried enamel. At the present time sealing over small carious lesions is not recommended. Only fissures without soft spots or explorer catches should be sealed. The question of sealing over incipient caries is discussed in greater detail later in this chapter.

Although different sealant brands vary considerably in their physical form and curing mechanism, all use the acid etch technique. The various steps in this procedure must be followed closely to ensure success. Sealant application can be divided into five basic steps: 1) cleansing of the tooth, 2) acid etching, 3) isolation and drying, 4) sealant application, and 5) postapplication inspection.

Most clinical trials have been conducted using cotton rolls for isolation. With this isolation technique great care must be exercised to prevent moisture contamination, which reduces sealant adhesion. In the application technique shown in Figure 21-13 and discussed later, isolation is accomplished with cotton rolls. If rubber dam isolation is used, the dam should be placed prior to etching and left in place until after all sealant has been placed.

Prior to acid etching, candidate teeth should be cleaned by toothbrushing or pumicing lightly to remove any debris. Depending on office routine, this can be done before the initial examination.

After the selecting and cleansing, the candidate teeth should be isolated with cotton rolls or rubber dam and etched. Usually two quadrants can be etched and sealed simultaneously. Because of the difficulties encountered in keeping etched teeth clean and dry until sealant application, great care must be exercised during this period.

The etching procedure is performed by dabbing the etching liquid lightly onto the occlusal surface by using a cotton pledget. Although manufacturers' directions and etching liquids vary somewhat, usually a 60-second etch with 30 per cent– 50 per cent phosphoric acid is sufficient. Once etching is complete, the tooth should be rinsed and dried. A properly etched tooth will have a frosty white appearance. Occasionally a tooth will be more resistant to the etching process. If a tooth does not take on a frosty white appearance after

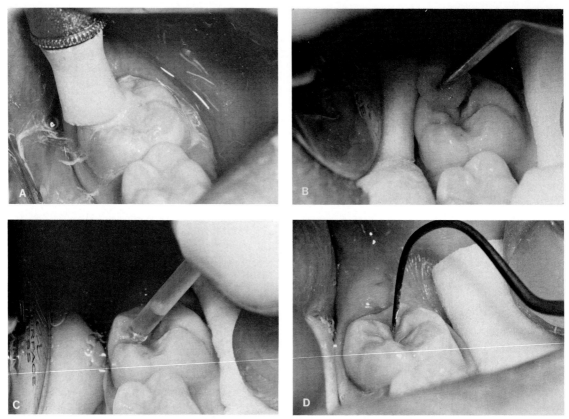

Fig. 21-13. Sealant application procedure. **A.** Cleansing; **B.** acid etching; **C.** sealant application to *dried* occlusal surface; **D.** post application inspection.

etching, it should be reetched one time. Resistance to etching does not mean that the tooth will necessarily be resistant to occlusal caries, since the fissures can still trap debris and harbor decay-causing bacteria.

The etching liquid should be removed from the tooth by flushing with water while evacuating the area. The patient should not expectorate, since this allows saliva to contact the etched surface. Such contamination reduces sealant adhesion. If saliva contamination should occur, a brief (30-second) reetch should be performed.

After the acid has been thoroughly flushed from the tooth, the area should be reisolated with dry cotton rolls. The teeth should be dried thoroughly by blowing for about 30 seconds each with dry, oil-free air from an air syringe. The teeth should be kept thoroughly dry until after the sealant has been placed and has cured. Various drying agents can also be used with air drying, but there is no clinical evidence that the use of a drying agent has any particular benefit. The importance of this drying step cannot be overemphasized. Be-

cause of the strong affinity of water for the etched tooth surface, any moisture contamination will be drawn into the etchings and will prevent the sealant from forming the tags that are critical to durable bonding.

Sealant should be applied as quickly as possible after drying the etched surface, to reduce the possibility of accidental surface contamination. Again the etched surface should be thoroughly dry; otherwise bond strength is reduced. Sealant application techniques vary from one manufacturer to another. Light-cured sealants are painted onto the etched surface and cured by exposure to a high-energy light source. The chemically activated sealants cure by mixing two or more components. The freshly mixed sealant is painted onto the etched enamel and allowed to harden. Although the polymerization activation methods may differ greatly, the polymerization mechanism and the finished sealant are essentially the same.

To the practitioner the important differences between brands of sealants lie not so much in the method of sealant activation, but rather in the handling characteristics of the sealant. Sealant retention is a direct result of how well the sealant can wet and adapt to the etched enamel surface. More viscous sealants must be pushed across the enamel surface in such a manner that air bubbles are not trapped in the sealant or in the rugged valleys of the etched surface. More fluid sealants tend to flow across the surface more readily and appear to be drawn into the etchings more quickly.

Sealant applicators vary considerably. The most common applicator is the brush. With proper care, brush application works well. The dentist must, however, recognize the problems that can arise with improper brush techniques. Rapid flicking of the brush can create air bubbles in the sealant. There is also a tendency to paint a very thin film with the brush. Because of the effects of air on methacrylate polymerization, the surface layer of a sealant will not cure. If the sealant is painted on in a very thin layer, no cured sealant will remain on the tooth. This can lead to spotty sealant coverage. The brush should be used as a sealant carrier to deliver sufficient quantities of sealant to give good surface coverage.

One manufacturer has designed a convenient dropper-type sealant carrier. With this device the sealant is easily carried to the tooth surface and is slowly expelled onto the surface with a fingertip lever as the applicator tip is moved across the tooth surface. This applicator appears to work equally well on both the maxillary and mandibular teeth.

After the sealant has fully cured, the surface should be wiped with a cotton roll to remove any unpolymerized surface liquid so that the surface may be inspected. The examination should be done by using a sharp explorer. The explorer tip should be drawn lightly across the tooth surface. The presence or absence of sealant in a given area can be detected tactilely. Sealant has a softer and smoother feel than enamel (filled sealants are rougher than enamel). Air bubbles in the surface show up as catches and can be detected visually. A properly applied sealant should be free of air bubbles, should fill the occlusal pits and fissures, and should extend up the more shallow channels toward the periphery of the occlusal surface. If fissure coverage is not complete or if air bubbles are present, the affected area should be reetched and retreated with sealant. Recently, dyes or pigments have been added to some sealants to aid in the inspection process.

The occlusion should also be examined, particularly if a filled sealant is used. With filled sealants any occlusal interference must be eliminated by conventional composite finishing techniques. Except in cases of gross occlusal interference, the unfilled sealants do not require mechanical adjustment. Unfilled sealants will wear in or facet under abrasion from an opposing cusp. It is possible, however, to fracture sealants if the occlusal interference is severe. Such interference can be corrected mechanically. However, gross interference represents poor sealant placement technique and should be avoided.

Although pit and fissure sealants have been available for several years, few long-term clinical data are available. No data exist on caries experience for young adults who received sealant as children. Various suggestions have been proposed for how long sealants should be reapplied during the lifetime of the patient. Some have argued that, once sealants have been applied, the sealant protection must be maintained. Further, if the sealant does come off, carious activity will begin. Others speculate that, once an individual has reached adulthood, carious activity decreases owing to changes in diet and in body chemistry. They suggest that sealant protection should be maintained only through the caries-prone adolescent years. Definitive answers to the questions of how long sealant maintenance should be continued will require long-term studies. Patients' histories will have to be followed from childhood through early adulthood, a process that will take many years to complete.

In the meantime one must rely on sound clinical judgment in a sealant maintenance program. Rather than forgo sealant placement until the sealant reapplication question is answered, it certainly seems more desirable to provide sealant protection through the caries-prone adolescent years. A sound caries prevention program will ensure that many young patients will reach adulthood with sound teeth. At that time additional data will be available and the patient can be counseled further about what preventive measures should be continued.

Sealant Application as an Adjunct to Topical Fluoride

Pit and fissure sealants should be considered as an adjunct to, and not a replacement for, fluorides. Fluorides offer their greatest protection on smooth surfaces of teeth, on the buccal, lingual, and aproximal surfaces. Sealants are designed to seal and protect defects, pits, and fissures within the enamel surface, sites in which debris can be trapped and support carious activity. Fluorides offer little protection in these areas.

Sealants and topical fluorides, then, are complementary. Sealant application and fluoride treatments can be combined in one visit as part of a comprehensive prevention program. Some attention should be paid to the sequence of sealant and fluoride treatments when combined in a single visit.

If topical fluoride treatment is done before the sealant application procedure, fluoride will be removed from any areas contacted by the etching liquid used with the sealant. Some investigators have suggested that fluoride treatment prior to sealant application may actually be beneficial since tiny amounts of fluoride may remain entrapped within the fissure. While this fluoride entrapment may be possible, if fluoride can reach this area, the etching liquid will also. Thus, it would seem doubtful that any appreciable amounts of fluoride could remain within the fissure areas. With prior fluoride application, fluoride ions would also be removed from any smooth surfaces contacted by the etching liquid. Thus valuable fluoride protection could be lost in the aproximal and gingival areas if the etching liquid is not judiciously maintained only on the occlusal surface.

The preferred sequence for fluoride and sealant treatments in one visit is to place the sealant first and then carry out the fluoride treatment. This sequence ensures that all areas not covered by sealant will receive fluoride protection. Since fluoride treatment materials have no apparent detrimental effects on sealants, routine fluoride application procedures may be employed. Further, any etched areas not covered by sealant will have enhanced fluoride uptake.

Incipient Caries

One of the principal concerns among clinicians is the possibility of inadvertently sealing over incipient caries. Some have speculated that bacteria remaining within a fissure will continue to multiply and destroy underlying tooth structure while, on the surface, the tooth appears sound. Because of the nature of the carious process in fissure caries, it is often difficult to detect incipient caries. This has led some clinicians to reject sealants as a sound preventive measure. Available clinical evidence does not, however, support the fears that carious activity will continue in sealed small carious lesions. On the contrary, clinical studies on bacteria viability in such sealed lesions indicate that the opposite is true. In one study by Handleman and coworkers, cultivatable microorganisms in infected dentin showed a 2,000-fold decrease over two years. Most of this reduction occurred during the first two weeks after sealant placement. Clinical and radiographic examinations indicate that carious activity did not progress in these sealed carious lesions. It appears that inadvertent sealing of incipient carious lesions does not endanger the health of the tooth. Further studies are needed, particularly with respect to lesion size, before deliberate sealing of small carious lesions could be considered as a sound clinical procedure.

Clinical Application Problems

The vast majority of sealant placement problems and early sealant failure results from moisture contamination. The necessity of maintaining a dry field, free from saliva contamination, cannot be overemphasized. Because sealant retention is derived primarily through mechanical bonding, the sealant must make intimate contact with the etched enamel. Foreign contaminants will reduce this contact and weaken the bond. Although sealants have a strong attraction to dry etched enamel, water is highly polar and also has a strong attraction for this surface. Thus the sealant liquid cannot displace water from a contaminated surface. Rather, the sealant will flow across the surface, trapping the water within the etchings. This prevents the sealant from forming tags within the surface and thus seriously weakening the bond.

Saliva contamination creates additional problems owing to its proteinaceous content. Water contamination can be corrected by redrying the surface, but redrying an area contaminated with saliva will leave a thin deposit or organic material (see Ch. 5). Sealant cured against this surface will not have a solid surface on which to bond; as a result, the bond will be weak.

If saliva contamination occurs, the surface

should be flushed with water and redried. Often, the saliva resists flushing from the surface. Since it is difficult to determine visually if the surface is thoroughly cleansed, an alternate procedure is to repeat the etching process. A shortened 30-second etch should be sufficient.

Even with careful scheduling the dentist will be faced with teeth in various stages of eruption. Often a gingival flap will cover, at least partially, the distal pit of molars. If sealant is to be applied under such circumstances, this flap should be raised with an explorer tip. This flap must be held away from the tooth throughout the etching, drying, and sealant application steps. Tucking a cotton pledget between the flap and the distal marginal ridge has been found to be useful in controlling seepage. Even if this gingival flap has receded to the point that it does not cover the distal pit, it provides a site for retaining moisture. If the moisture is not thoroughly removed from between the flap and the tooth, moisture will continue to seep out of this area onto the dried occlusal surface. In fact this problem is not entirely confined to cases in which a distal flap is present. Moisture can also seep from the gingival tooth margin onto the dried occlusal surface on any tooth on which the gingivae approach the perimeter of the occlusal surface.

EVALUATION OF CLINICAL EFFECTIVENESS OF SEALANTS

Sealants have received, perhaps, as much attention in controlled clinical studies as any single class of dental materials. Those sealants receiving an "Acceptable" seal from the American Dental Association, Council on Dental Materials and Devices, have been demonstrated to be effective through clinical studies. In clinical investigations a variety of study designs have been employed. Most investigations have used the half-mouth study design in which treated and control pairs are set up on opposite sides of the same mouth. In some reported studies, candidate teeth were carefully handpicked, selected teeth having deep, narrow fissures, while in other studies, all noncarious posterior teeth were selected in mass screening approaches. In some studies both molars and premolars were treated,

whereas other studies used molars only. Because of the tooth selection differences, care must be taken in comparing results from various studies.

Clinical efficacy studies require collection and analysis of the data to give a measure of the effectiveness of a sealant in preventing occlusal caries. Although the results from various clinical studies have been presented in a number of ways, the method of Cvar provides a convenient procedure for statistical analysis of caries reduction. For a realistic assessment of sealant effectiveness, a test for significance is employed, along with calculations of per cent effectiveness and net gain of caries-free teeth over carious teeth.

In calculating Net Gain, study pairs (treated-control pairs) are classified as (1) Both Teeth Sound, (2) Both Decayed, (3) Treated Sound–Control Decayed, and (4) Treated Decayed–Control Sound. Net Gain is the estimated number of teeth saved from decay or the number of Treated Sound–Control Decayed minus the number of Treated Decayed–Control Sound. The absolute numerical value of Net Gain depends on the caries attack rate of the patients in the study and varies from one study population to another. This disadvantage can be overcome by calculating the per cent effectiveness, which is simply the Net Gain divided by the total number of carious control teeth, multiplied by 100. Per cent effectiveness does not distinguish between high and low caries attack rates. For example, a sealant may have a high per cent effectiveness but have saved few teeth from decay because of a low caries attack rate on the population.

Net Gain = (Treated Sound
  – Control Decayed)
  – (Treated Decayed–Control Sound)

Per cent Effectiveness =
  Net Gain/Total Control Decayed × 100

To ascertain whether or not there has indeed been a positive treatment effect rather than positive results by chance, a test for significance should be applied. Care must be taken in reviewing results of clinical studies and in comparing results from various studies to ensure that the data are interpreted correctly.

Regardless of the specific details of a given study design, the purpose of these clinical investigations is to demonstrate sealant retention and caries reduction. Sealant retention is usually presented as per cent retention, or per cent of occlusal surfaces remaining sealed over the given time period. Often the results are reported as per cent total retention, per cent partial retention, and per cent total sealant loss.

In comparing one sealant with another the most meaningful conclusion can be reached if the materials are evaluated in the same clinical study. Such comparisons eliminate the variables associated with different procedures and study populations. The results of one side-by-side comparison of two commercial sealant materials by Brooks and coworkers are presented in Table 21-3. In this study an ultraviolet-light-cured sealant was compared with a leading chemically cured sealant. A half-mouth study design was employed in which contralateral pairs of treated and untreated teeth were followed over a three-year time period.

The light-cured sealant had a complete retention of 58.3 per cent, a Net Gain of 31 teeth saved from occlusal caries, and had a 38.8 per cent effectiveness. The chemically cured sealant had an 84.2 per cent complete retention and showed a Net Gain of 59 teeth and a 68.6 per cent effectiveness. Thus, both sealant materials showed a positive treatment effect after three years with less occlusal caries on the treated teeth than on untreated teeth. As the investigators in this study have pointed out, the half-mouth study design using untreated teeth as controls is no longer considered ethical. Comparisons can now be made

using sealants of known clinical effectiveness as controls. In selecting a sealant for use in practice, all supporting clinical study data should be examined carefully. Considerable differences exist in the retention and effectiveness of various sealants. Efficacy should be a primary consideration in the selection of a sealant for caries prevention.

EFFECT OF SEALANTS ON ENAMEL MATURATION AND CARIES

Before the subject of pit and fissure sealants is completed, some consideration should be given to the question of enamel maturation. In the past some have expressed concern that sealants will interfere with the natural process of enamel maturation of newly erupted teeth. This process of ion exchange and mineral deposition from the saliva begins as a new tooth emerges into the oral environment and continues throughout the life of the tooth. In a healthy environment the process is generally believed to be beneficial since it can lead to a hardening of the enamel as more resistant ions are deposited within the enamel surface (see Ch. 19).

Sealants present a barrier to this ionic exchange. Some have argued that this interference might be detrimental to the health of the tooth. In defense of sealants, however, there appears to be no published research documenting that maturation of enamel affects the incidence of dental caries. Moreover, with all

TABLE 21-3. RESULTS FROM 3-YEAR COMPARATIVE STUDY OF A LIGHT-CURED SEALANT AND A CHEMICALLY CURED SEALANT[1]

	Light-cured sealant[2]			Chemically cured sealant[3]		
	1 yr	2 yrs	3 yrs	1 yr	2 yrs	3 yrs
Number of sealant–control pairs examined		258			233	
Retention (%) for teeth present at all annual examinations						
Complete	86.3	58.9	58.3	96.4	86.1	84.2
Partial	8.3	25.0	20.8	1.2	10.3	9.7
None	5.4	16.1	20.8	2.4	3.6	6.1
Caries status, treated–control pairs at 3 years						
Both teeth sound			108			111
Both teeth decayed			32			23
Treated sound–control decayed			48			63
Treated decayed–control sound			17			4
Net gain (no. of teeth saved from caries)			31			59
Effectiveness (%)			38.8			68.6

1. J. D. Brooks et al, JADA, 99, 42–46 (1979).
2. NUVA-SEAL™ Pit and Fissure Sealant, L. D. Caulk, Co.
3. DELTON™ Pit & Fissure Sealant, Johnson & Johnson Dental Products Co.

the attention given to controlled clinical evaluations of sealants, there have apparently been no cases in which the incidence of occlusal caries was higher on teeth receiving sealant than on those receiving no treatment. This is true even for those experimental formulations that were considered clinical failures. From the point of view of the clinician as well as the patient, it would seem much more beneficial to seal the fissure and allow the underlying enamel to remain "immature" than to expose the teeth to the dangers of occlusal caries and the subsequent removal of "mature" enamel during cavity preparation and restoration.

SUMMARY

Since their conception in the mid 1960s, pit and fissure sealants have received considerable attention in academic circles. Several classes of sealants have been proposed and tested. One class of sealants, methacrylates, has proved to be superior to date. Methacrylate sealants are based on high-strength monomer systems such as bis-GMA and/or dimethacrylates of the ethyleneglycol series.

Several commercial sealants have been made available to the profession. These materials vary considerably in their handling and placement characteristics. Chemically cured and light-cured systems are available. All sealants use acid-etching procedures for cleansing and roughening the enamel surface for durable bonding.

Controlled clinical studies have been published and adequately demonstrate the safety and efficacy of pit and fissure sealants. Thus, with proper sealant selection, sound placement techniques, and adequate patient checkups, the clinician can be confident that pit and fissure sealants will protect the occlusal surfaces against occlusal decay as long as the sealant remains intact.

GLOSSARY

Acid etching. Process of using diluted acid, usually 30 per cent to 50 per cent phosphoric acid, to roughen the surface of tooth enamel by dissolution in order to enhance retention of adhesive dental materials.

Adhesion. The attachment or union of one object to another through intermolecular attraction or bonding.

Adhesive. A material or substance which is used to bond one substance to another. A dental adhesive material is a material which bonds to tooth structure or is used to bond a restorative material or device to tooth structure.

Chemical bonding. A mechanism of adhesion whereby two substrates are held together by forces which result from the formation of primary or secondary chemical bonds between the materials.

Cingulum. A small, sometimes pronounced developmental lobe occurring on the gingival one-third of the lingual surface of the crown of incisors and cuspids. A pronounced cingulum is sometimes accompanied by a pit within the enamel.

Contact angle. The angle formed between the surface of a liquid on a substrate and the surface of the substrate. A low contact angle indicates good attraction between the liquid and the substrate (wetting).

Cyanoacrylate. A class of adhesive materials which was used experimentally as a pit and fissure sealant in some early sealant investigations.

Enamel rods or prisms. Microscopic rod-like structures of hydroxyapatite which make up tooth enamel.

Fissure. A linear groove or fault in the occlusal surfaces of molars and premolars formed during tooth development and resulting from incomplete fusion of the enamel of the lobes of the cusps.

Glass ionomer cement. A class of dental materials consisting of a polyacrylic acid and a reactive glass filler which harden by an ionic interaction of the glass and the polyacrylic acid. They are sometimes used as a sealant as well as for other restorative purposes.

Hydroxyapatite. The principal mineral component of teeth having the general chemical formula, $Ca_{10}(PO_4)_6(OH)_2$.

Maturation of enamel. A continuing process of enamel surface change whereby a dynamic ionic exchange occurs between enamel and mineral-containing solutions in contact with the tooth resulting in the deposition of less soluble ions onto the enamel surface.

Mechanical bonding. Retention of a material on substrate by interlocking into cracks and microscopic pores. With acid etching, mechanical bonding plays a significant role in retention through the interlocking of sealant tags within the roughened enamel surface.

Methacrylate. The principal class of polymeric materials used in dental sealants and restorative materials. Methacrylates are derived from an alcohol and methacrylic acid and include the higher molecular weight compounds used in conventional sealants.

Microleakage. Process by which oral fluids and bacteria penetrate into microscopic cracks and margins of a dental material or at the interface of two materials such as with a sealant and the tooth.

Pit. A deep hole or shaft in the enamel usually found

where two or more enamel lobes meet. Pits occur within the fissures or at the cingulum.

Remineralization. A process by which the remaining enamel previously etched or decalcified returns to a normal appearance by apparent redeposition of minerals.

Sticky fissures. Fissures allowing a detectable catch with a sharp explorer tip which may be due to early stages of caries.

Viscosity. A measure of the resistance of a liquid to flow.

SUGGESTED READINGS

Albert M, Grenoble DE: An in vivo study of enamel remineralization after acid–etching. J S Calif Dent Assoc 39: 747, 1971

Arana EM: Clinical observations of enamel after acid-etch procedure. J Am Dent Assoc 89: 1102, 1974

Ast DB, Bushel A, Chase HC: Clinical study of caries prophylaxis with zinc chloride and potassium ferrocyanide. J Am Dent Assoc 41: 437, 1950

Ast DB, Smith DJ, Wachs B, Kantwell KT: Newburgh-Kingston caries fluorine study. XIV. Combined clinical and roentgenographic dental findings after 10 years of fluoride experience. J Am Dent Assoc 52: 314, 1956

Backer-Dirks O: Longitudinal dental caries. Study in children 9–15 years of age. Arch Oral Biol 6: 94, 1961.

Backer-Dirks O: The distribution of caries resistance in relation to tooth surfaces. In Wolztenholome GEW, O'Connor M (eds): Ciba Foundation Symposium. Boston, Little, Brown, 1965, p 66

Backer-Dirks O: The relation between the fluoridation of water and dental caries experience. Int Dent J 17: 583, 1967

Backer-Dirks O, Houwink B, Kwant GW: The results of 6 ½ years of artificial fluoridation of drinking water in the Netherlands. The Tielculembory experiment. Arch Oral Biol 5: 284, 1961

Besic FC, Bayard M, Wiemann MR Jr, Burrell KH: Composition and structure of dental enamel: elemental composition and crystalline structure of dental enamel as they relate to its solubility. J Am Dent Assoc 91: 594, 1975

Bodecker CF: Dental caries immunization without filling. NY State Dent J 30: 337, 1964

Bodecker CF: Enamel fissure eradication. NY State Dent J 30: 149, 1964

Brooks JE, Mertz-Fairhurst EF, Della-Giustina VE, et al.: A comparative study of two pit and fissure sealants: three-year results in Augusta, Ga, J Am Dent Assoc 99: 42, 1979

Brown WE, König KG (eds): Cariostatic Mechanisms of Fluorides. Proceedings of a Workshop Organized by the ADA Health Foundation and NIDR, Naples, FLA, 1976. Caries Res [Suppl] 11 (1): 1–327 1977

Brudevold F, Amdur BH, Messer A: Factors involved in remineralization of carious lesions. Arch Oral Biol 6: 304, 1961

Buonocore MG: A simple method of increasing the adhesion of acrylic filling materials to enamel surfaces. J Dent Res 34: 849, 1955

Buonocore MG: Adhesive sealing of pits and fissures for caries prevention with use of an ultraviolet light. J Am Dent Assoc 80: 324, 1970

Buonocore MG: Caries prevention in pits and fissures sealed with an adhesive polymerized by ultraviolet light: a two year study of a single adhesive application. J Am Dent Assoc 82: 1090, 1971

Buonocore MG, Matsui A, Gwinnett AJ: Penetration of resin dental materials into enamel surfaces with reference to bonding. Arch Oral Biol 13: 61, 1968

Buonocore MG, Wileman W, Brudevold F: A report on a resin composition capable of bonding to human dentin surfaces. J Dent Res 35: 846, 1956

Chow LC, Brown WE: Phosphoric acid conditioning of teeth for pit and fissure sealants. J Dent Res 52: 1158, 1973

Cueto E, Buonocore MG: Adhesive sealing of pits and fissures for caries prevention (abstr #400). International Association of Dental Research, 43rd General Mectg, July, 1965

Cueto E, Buonocore MG: Sealing of pits and fissures with an adhesive resin: its use in caries prevention. J Am Dent Assoc 75: 121, 1967

Cvar JF: Statistical analysis of half-mouth sealant studies. In Wachtel LW (ed): Proceedings, Symposium on Dental Biomaterials—Research Priorities, August 7–8, 1973, Des Plaines, Ill. DHEW Publ No. (NIH) 74-548, 1974, pp 111–114

Dennison JB, and Powers JM: Physical properties of pit and fissure sealants. J Dent Res 58: 1430, 1979

Englander HR, Carlos JP, Senning RS, Mellberg JR: Residual anti-caries effect of repeated topical sodium fluoride applications by mouthpieces. J Am Dent Assoc 78: 783, 1969

Fan PL, Seluk LW, O'Brien WJ: Penetrativity of sealants. J Dent Res 54: 262, 1975

Galil KA, Gwinnett AJ: Three-dimentional replicas of pits and fissures in human teeth: scanning electron microscopic study. Arch Oral Biol 20: 493, 1975

Gwinnett AJ: Morphology of the interface between adhesive resins and treated enamel surfaces as seen by scanning electron microscopy. Arch Oral Biol 16: 237, 1971

Gwinnett AJ, Buonocore MG: Adhesives and caries prevention: a preliminary report. Br Dent J 119: 77, 1965

Gwinnett AJ, Matsui A: A study of enamel adhesives. The physical relationship between enamel and adhesive. Arch Oral Biol 12: 1615, 1967

Handelman SL, Washburn F, Wopperer P: Two-year report of sealant effect on bacteria in dental caries. J Am Dent Assoc 93: 976, 1976

Hennon DK, Stookey GK, Muhler JC: Prevalence and distribution of dental caries in pre-school children. J Am Dent Assoc 79: 1406, 1969

Horowitz, HS, Heifetz SB, Poulsen S: Adhesive sealant clinical trial: an overview of results after four years in Kalispell, Montana. J Prev Dent 3: 38, 1976

Hørsted M, Fejerskov O, Joost Larson M, Thylstrup A: The structure of surface enamel with special reference to occlusal surfaces of primary and permanent teeth. Caries Res 10: 287, 1976

Hyatt P: Prophylactic odontotomy: the cutting into the tooth for the prevention of the disease. D Cosmos 65: 234, 1923

Johansson B: Remineralization of slightly etched enamel. J Dent Res 44: 64, 1965

Kemper RN, Kilian RJ: New test system for tensile bond strength testing (abstr No 308). J Dent Res 55B: 138, 1976

Klein H, Knutson JW: Studies on dental caries. XIII. Effect of ammoniacal silver nitrate on caries in first permanent molars. J Am Dent Assoc 29: 1420, 1942

Koulourides T: Remineralization of enamel and dentin. Dent Clin North Am July: 485–487, 1962

Krutchoff DJ, Rowe NH: The chemical nature of remineralized flattened enamel surface (abstr No. 776). International Association of Dental Research, 49th General Meeting, March, 1971

Lee HL, Ocumpaugh D: Sealing of developmental pits and fissures. V. Comparison of adhesive topical fluoride coating vs fluoride gels. Biomater Med Devices Artif Organs 1 (1): 163, 1973

Lee HL, Swartz ML: Sealing of developmental pits and fissures. I. In vitro study. J Dent Res 50: 133, 1971

Ludwig TG, Pearce EIF: The Hastings fluoridation project. IV. Dental effects between 1954 and 1963. N Ze Dent J 59: 298, 1963

Marthaler TM: The value in caries prevention of other methods of increasing fluorine ingestion, apart from fluoridated water. Int Dent J 17: 606, 1967

Marthaler TM: Caries-inhibiting effect of fluoride tablets. Helv Odontal Acta 13: 1, 1969

Marthaler TM, Schenardi C: Inhibition of caries in children after 5 1/2 years of fluoridated table salt. Helv Odontol Acta 6: 1, 1962

McCune RJ: Clinical applications of pit and fissure sealants. In Wachtel LW (ed): Proceedings, Symposium on Dental Biomaterials—Research Priorities, August 7–8, 1973, Des Plaines, IL. DHEW Publ No. (NIH) 74–548, 1974, pp 117–128

McCune RJ, Cvar JF: Pit and fissure sealants, preliminary results (abstr No. 745). International Association of Dental Research, 49th General Meeting, March, 1971

McLean JW, Wilson AW: Fissure sealing and filling with an adhesive glass ionomer sealant. Br Dent J 136: 269, 1974

Mitchum JC, Turner LR: The retentive strengths of acid-etched retained resins. J Am Dent Assoc 89: 1107, 1974

Monus A, Grenoble DE: An in-vivo study of enamel remineralization after acid etching. J S Cal Dent Assoc 39 (9): 747, 1971

Moskowitz DH, Ward GT, Woolridge ED (eds): Proceedings, Dental Adhesives Materials, Symposium. New York, New York Division of Dental Health, DHEW, Nov. 8–9, 1973

Muhlemann HR, Lenz H, Rossinsky K: Electron microscopic appearance of rehardened enamel. Helv Odontol Acta 8: 108, 1964

Muhler JC, Radike WW, Nebergall HW, Day HG: The effect of a stannous fluoride containing dentifrice on caries reduction in children. J Dent Res 33: 606, 1954

Ohsawa T: Studies on the solubility and grip of enamel in pretreatment for caries—preventive sealing. Jpn J Dent Health 21: (1): 53, 1971

Parkhouse RC, Winter GB: A fissure sealant containing methyl 2–cyanoacrylate as a caries preventive agent. Br Dent J 130: 16, 1971

Pigman WH, Cueto H, Baugh D: Conditions affecting the rehardening of softened enamel. J Dent Res 43: 1187, 1964

Ripa LW: Occlusal sealing: rationale of the technique and historical review. J Am Soc Prev Dent 3: 32–39, 1973

Ripa LW, Buonocore M, Cueto E: Adhesive sealing of pits and fissures for caries prevention: a report of two year study (abstr No. 247). International Association of Dental Research, 44th General Meeting, March, 1966

Ripa LW, Cole WW: Evaluation of an occlusal sealer in a mentally handicapped child population: results one year following initial application (abstr No. 320). International Association of Dental Research, 47th General Meeting, March, 1969

Ripa LW, Cole WW: Occlusal sealing and caries prevention: results 12 months after a single application of adhesive resins. J Dent Res 49: 171, 1970

Rock WP: Fissure sealants. Results obtained with two different sealants after one year. Br Dent J 133: 146, 1972

Roydhouse RH: Prevention of occlusal fissure caries by use of a sealant: a pilot study. J Dent Child 35: 253, 1968

Shafer WG, Hine MK, Levy BM: A Textbook of Oral Pathology, 3rd ed. Philadelphia, WB Saunders, 1974

Sharp EC, Grenoble DE: Dental resin penetration into acid etched subsurface enamel. J S Cal Dent Assoc 39: 741, 1971

Silverstone LM: Fissure sealants, laboratory studies. Caries Res 8: 2, 1974

Takeuchi M: Sealing of the pit and fissure with resin adhesive. III. Outlines of its progress at the present time. Jpn Dent J 4: 33, 1967

Takeuchi M, Shimizu, T, Kizu T, Eto M, Nakagawa M, Ohsawa T, Oishi T: Sealing of the pit and fissure with resin adhesive. IV. Results of five years field work and a method of evaluation of field work for caries prevention. Bull Tokyo Dent Coll 12: 295, 1971

Theilade E, Fejerskov, O, Prachyabrued W, Kilian M: Microbiologic study on developing plaque in human fissures. Scand J Dent Res 82: 420, 1974

Wei SHY: Remineralization of enamel and dentine, a review. J Dent Child 34: 444, 1967

Woody RD, Moffa JP, McCune RJ: Assessment of leakage of four pit and fissure sealant materials by Ca^{45} (abstr No. 717). International Association of Dental Research, 50th General Meeting, March, 1972

22 Toothbrushes and Toothbrushing

JOSEPH F. ALEXANDER

Introduction
Historic Background
Physical Properties of Toothbrush Filaments
  Natural Bristle
  Nylon
Biologic Effects of Brushing
Toothbrush Design and Function
Toothbrushing Techniques
  Bass Technique

Charters and Stillman Techniques
Other Techniques
Automatic Toothbrushes
Patient Factors
  Frequency of Brushing
  Wear
Summary
Glossary
Suggested Readings

INTRODUCTION

The mechanical removal of dental plaque from tooth surfaces has conclusively been demonstrated to be an effective method of controlling dental caries. No tool or device intended for the removal of dental plaque ranks higher in the armamentarium of preventive dentistry than the toothbrush, yet it is afforded little attention by patient and practitioner alike. The apparent simplicity of the toothbrush is deceptive, but if we can judge by the volume of literature that has been produced on the subject over the past 40 years, a great deal needs to be learned before the full potential of the toothbrush is realized. The search for the ideal toothbrush has been elusive due to the number of variables that must

be considered in any clinical evaluation of toothbrush performance. As is true in any scientific field of investigation, the measurement of complex interrelated variables encountered in evaluating toothbrush performance has frequently led to confusion and the development of a cynical attitude that one brush is as good as another. This is particularly true in studies in which subjective measurement criteria were used to evaluate toothbrush performance. All this has served to generate a skeptical attitude about toothbrushes and studies related to the use of particular types of toothbrushes. While intuition tells us that some toothbrushes may perform better than others, the results of various laboratory and clinical investigations have seemingly failed to provide convincing proof that measured differences between various toothbrushes are meaningful. This apparent dilemma can only be resolved through a comprehensive examination of the current dental literature and how this relates to the design and functionality of toothbrushes. The purpose of this chapter is to provide a comprehensive review of factors that may ultimately reflect on the ability of toothbrushes to effectively control the progress of dental caries. It has been written to provide answers, where they exist, to those questions most frequently asked by practitioners and patients alike, concerning the use of a toothbrush. Aside from providing an appreciation of the depth and scope of the work carried out in this area, it is hoped that this material will dispel some of the toothbrush myths that have sprung up over the years and lend direction to future work in the area.

HISTORIC BACKGROUND

Historically, the use of various mechanical devices to cleanse the teeth dates back to antiquity. While brushes similar in design to those used today first appeared in China as early as 1600 A.D., their introduction to Western Civilization occurred considerably later. In the United States, the first toothbrush patent was filed in 1857, but it was not until the early 1900's that toothbrushes became available in quantity to the public. A survey taken in 1924 showed that 37 different kinds of toothbrushes of all conceivable sizes and shapes were available on the market.

Little substantial change in basic design or fabrication of toothbrushes was noticed until 1938 when the first brushes made with nylon rather than animal bristle were produced. This change was based more on economic necessity than a conscious effort to improve an existing product. War both reduced the supply of high quality hog bristle from China and made the cost prohibitive. Nylon brushes were less expensive to produce and resulted in a durable brush of uniform and predictable texture. However, many dentists advised against their use because the brushes were too stiff. The first nylon brushes were, in fact, copies of the popular natural bristle brushes and, since the stiffness of nylon is little influenced by contact with water compared to natural bristle, nylon brushes were extremely harsh. The sensation of stiffness was further heightened by the presence of sharp, pointed cut ends which lacerated oral soft tissues and caused bleeding.

As the popularity and use of nylon brushes spread, it became important to the dental profession that the merits and disadvantages of both types of brushes be studied further. This resulted in a renewed interest in not only toothbrush materials, but in design, safety, and ultimately, performance. Prior to this, the toothbrush had been allowed to evolve into an incredible variety of forms, many of which were not adaptable to use in the human mouth. During this period of development, there was a general awareness that the formation of soft deposits on the teeth was in some way related to dental disease (see Chap. 5), and that regular cleansing of the teeth was efficacious in controlling the process. Mechanical removal of soft plaque deposits by toothbrushes became an area of increasing interest attracting many competent dental investigators. Heightened interest subsequently led to the development of a "second generation" of toothbrush designs, for the most part based on valid laboratory measurements and occasionally supported by adequate clinical testing.

PHYSICAL PROPERTIES OF TOOTHBRUSH FILAMENTS

Natural Bristle

The quality of natural bristle used in the fabrication of toothbrushes can vary. The best hog bristle is found in China, but India currently provides the most reliable source of supply for brushes made in the United States. Many factors influence the quality of available bristle material. Bristles taken from hogs in winter or from cold climates are thicker; bristles are also thicker near the root than at the free end. In addition, the color of the bristle is variable depending on the breed of the hog used. Since the diameter of natural bristle can vary from .0035 inches to .0190 inches, it is difficult to manufacture a brush of uniform quality and texture. However, texture variations, as found in natural bristle brushes, are largely smoothed out by blending and the effects of moisture on the modulus (stiffness) of the fiber. The water absorption rate is very rapid for dry bristle, which can absorb over 25 per cent moisture when soaked in warm water. The result is a drastic 40 per cent reduction in

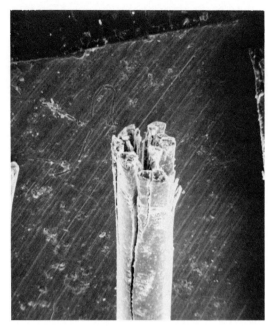

Fig. 22-1. Scanning electron micrograph of a natural bristle (×100)

fiber modulus. Natural bristle is also subject to more rapid wear due to its lower abrasion resistance. Since natural bristles contain a hollow central core, there is a tendency for the ends to break open and possibly encourage the entrapment of bacteria and other debris (Fig. 22-1). However, some observers are of the opinion that splitting of the bristle tips is desirable and can result in more effective cleaning at the gingival margin.

Nylon

Nylon is a totally synthetic material formed from long chains of polymer molecules linked together by selective chemical bonding. The many different types of nylon available are the result of the introduction of various side groups onto the polymer chains. Polymer strength is largely determined by the cold drawing process used to produce the filament. During extrusion, the polymer molecules are orientated in respect to the filament axis; this produces a material of high structural strength. Of the many types of nylon available, most brushes manufactured in the United States today are made from Nylon 66 or Nylon 612. One of the major differences between the two is the nature of their response to water. At 100 per cent relative hu-

midity, 66 nylon will absorb 9.0 per cent water, while 612 nylon will absorb only 3.0 per cent water. This differential response to moisture affects both the stiffness and bend recovery of the fiber. A higher percent water uptake results in a greater loss in wet stiffness, similar to the effects observed with hog bristle. With a slower rate of water uptake, however, the result is a brush of more uniform texture. These differences are by no means trivial. Natural bristle loses 40 per cent of its stiffness when immersed in water for ten *minutes*, while Nylon 612 loses only 23 per cent of its stiffness when immersed for 10 *hours* (Fig. 22-2). Moisture also affects the bend recovery of Nylon 66 more than Nylon 612. Bend recovery determines the ability of a material to return to its original shape after deformation, which will in turn ultimately affect the durability of the brush.

Humidity has little effect on the bend recovery of type 612 Nylon, while it does reduce the recovery of type 66 Nylon from 90 per cent to 82 per cent at 100 per cent relative humidity (Table 22-1). While hog bristle has good dry bend recovery, its fatigue resistance is very low; this results in breaking, splitting, or complete fracture after many cycles of flexing. While studying the effects of wear on bristle

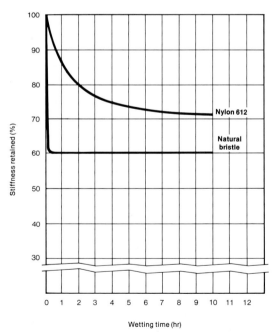

Fig. 22-2. Stiffness retained vs. wetting time for 10 m filaments and fibers submerged in water at 74°F

TABLE 22-1. BEND RECOVERY OF NYLON 612
AND NYLON 66 VS. RELATIVE
HUMIDITY

Relative Humidity at 73°F. (%)	Bend Recovery (%)	
	612	66
100	91	82
50	92	90
10	92	91

stiffness, it was shown that natural bristle brushes wore much more rapidly than nylon brushes. This conclusion was in agreement with clinical studies by others who determined that nylon brushes were more durable.

Excluding the variables of tuft density and total number of filaments in the brush head, the stiffness of any toothbrush (nylon or natural) is determined by the diameter and trim height of the filament used in the brush. Since filament stiffness is a function of the second power of the filament diameter, even a small deviation will have a large effect on stiffness. Additionally, the stiffness of a filament is inversely proportonal to the third power of the length of the fiber. Combining these relationships, a formula can be derived which relates filament diameter and trim height of one brush to another brush for equal stiffness:

$$\frac{h^3}{d^2} = \frac{H^3}{D^2}$$

h = Trim height of existing brush
d = Filament diameter of existing brush
H = Trim height of desired brush
D = Filament diameter of desired brush

By substituting the known values in this equation and assuming either a new trim height (h) or diameter (d), the texture of an unknown brush can be computed, assuming tuft arrangement or density has not changed. In effect, brushes of even radically different design can exhibit similar textural properties based on a calculation of the relationships between trim height and filament diameter.

In practical terms, this means that the texture of nylon brushes is highly controllable and predictable. Since a deviation as small as $1/16$ inch in trim height would result in a 49 per cent change in stiffness, demanding standards of quality control for nylon brushes must be maintained to produce a brush of uniform texture. Unfortunately, these benefits are frequently erased by the lack of uniform standards regulating the labelling of toothbrushes. Labelling brushes as soft, medium, hard, extra hard, etc., is thus often meaningless since this is left to the caprice of the brush manufacturer. In 1953, Hine examined the textures of 48 popular toothbrushes and compared his measurements against the package label grade of stiffness. He found, for example, that some brushes labelled "hard" were actually stiffer than brushes marked "extra hard", or some brushes labelled as "medium" were stiffer than brushes labelled as "hard." The grading of toothbrushes in the United States is quite arbitrary because of the lack of texture standards. This is not true in Great Britain where standards for toothbrush labelling are regulated by a precise grading system developed by Dr. Kenneth Wright, working for the National Engineering Laboratory. This grading system is unique, since texture is determined directly through the use of a sensitive, electronic pressure detector rather than by computation using trim height and filament diameter measurements. Brush labelling is, therefore, exact and takes into account the variables of tuft geometry and overall brush density.

BIOLOGIC EFFECTS OF BRUSHING

"The brush must not injure or irritate the tissues. It is irrational to brush unhealed or diseased gums, but, when healed, they can be strengthened by the judicious application of friction, just as the hands can be toughened and strengthened by labor. It's the amount of friction, and not its hardness, which strengthens the tissues." This statement made by T. Sidney Smith in 1940 probably describes as well as any other the prevailing opinion at the time regarding the selection of a good toothbrush. The view that the principal function of toothbrushing is to provide massage, which increases the resistance of gingival tissues by increasing keratinization, was expounded in the early 1920s. It was reasoned that a civilized diet failed to provide the mechanical stimulus necessary for gingival health. The development of a thicker gingival stratum corneum resulting from the frictional stimulation of toothbrushing was thought to result in a greater resistance to bacterial invasion. Studies on the effects of toothbrushing on gingival keratinization have shown that brushing can result in a significant amount of keratinization, but it has never been shown that these effects can alter gingival structure and enhance the resistance of these tissues to inflammatory changes. As pointed out by MacKenzie, it is difficult to determine the true keratinized state of healthy, non-mechanically stimulated gingiva since unbrushed gingiva tends to become inflamed because of the effects of plaque on this tissue. It appears that changes in gingival keratinization occurring after toothbrushing may not be a direct result of friction on the gingival epithelium but rather the result of the removal of plaque followed by a concomitant reduction in tissue inflammation.

While the rationale behind the use of hard brushes to promote gingival health remains somewhat suspect, the longer term effects of using hard brushes have been amply demonstrated by numerous clinical studies. Bass was one of the first to describe the harmful effects of the improper use of hard toothbrushes. "Frequent traumatizing and injuring the border of the thin gingiva upon the enamel-covered crown gradually wears it off from the enamel and forces it to recede beyond the cementoenamel junction. This occurs especially on the labial and buccal surfaces and on those teeth which are most exposed to the usual long-stroke harmful type of brushing." Once recession of the gingival tissues occurs beyond the cementoenamel junction, grooves may be cut in the exposed cementum and underlying dentin by the abrasive action of a dentifrice. Studies have demonstrated that brushing extracted teeth with a dentifrice produces abrasion to enamel and dentin. Other studies have shown that these abrasive effects were dependent almost entirely on the properties of the dentifrice abrasive and not the toothbrush. The type of bristle used in a toothbrush has little if any effect on abrasion to dentin or enamel. Hard tissues brushed experimentally with nylon or natural bristle brushes in conjunction with an abrasive dentifrice produce equal levels of abrasion. However, more recent studies have demonstrated the abrasive interactions with brushes of different hardness are related to brushing force and the concentration of dentifrice used.

An abrasivity index for dentifrices was developed in 1970 by the Council on Dental Therapeutics of the American Dental Association and has provided some basis of standardization for comparing the abrasiveness of various dentifrices. Since the act of toothbrushing is extremely complex and dependent upon many contributing variables, abrasiveness alone may only be a minor factor in assessing the potential of a dentifrice to damage the teeth. The amount of time spent brushing, force of brushing, frequency of brushing, bristle size and diameter, brushing motion, and speed of brushing have all been shown to affect the level of abrasion to hard dental tissues.

The mechanical removal of acquired dental deposits with the use of an abrasive dentifrice will inevitably be accompanied by some loss of hard tooth structure. Since individual brushing habits are known to vary widely, it is important that the abrasive effects of the dentifrice be minimized while still maintaining good cleaning and polishing action. The development of acceptable limits of overall abrasiveness is certainly desirable but does not take into account the actual cleansing requirements that will vary widely from one individual to another. From an examination of the literature in this area it appears certain that the use of hard abrasives in addition to a poor brushing technique can lead to early signs of gingival recession and hard tissue notching. Of course, the effect of toothbrushing is not the only causative factor related to gingival recession. Middle aged people usually show signs of gingival recession that may be considered the normal effects of physiologic aging or the result of either local or systemic disease. Another view is that recession could be related to thinning supportive bone due to tooth position or angulation. Where bone structure is reduced, the gingival margin becomes unsupported and could be further worn away by pressures related to toothbrushing.

While attempts to correlate gingival recession with specific, clinical etiologic factors has not been possible, the most common effects appear to be related to the regular use of a toothbrush. This has been most strikingly demonstrated by several clinical studies in which oral hygiene practices and the level of gingival recession were compared. Somewhat paradoxically, these studies have shown that patients with good oral hygiene have a greater degree of gingival recession than patients with poor oral hygiene. Frequent exposure of soft supportive gingival tissue to the abrasive action of toothbrushes, particularly hard brushes, may be responsible for the higher degree of gingival recession seen in patients with good oral hygiene. Older patients with a longer history of toothbrush use or misuse, would be expected to demonstrate a greater degree of cervical exposure. The strong positive correlation observed between age and the degree of gingival recession has been largely accepted by dental clinicians. While some form of gingival recession can be seen in almost all patients, the most pronounced cases are found in adults, and this has been shown to increase both in frequency and linear dimension with age. Again these effects correlate closely with the use of toothbrushes. In comparing the degree of cervical exposure and associated abrasion conditions existing in a good hygiene group with the same conditions in a poor hygiene group, Kitchin showed in his work that true abrasion had not been confused with loss of cervical tooth structure through some other mechanism, such as chemical erosion. The degree of segregation of abrasion in certain areas of the dentition also correlated well with patient dexteral preferences. Again, this further indicated that abrasion was closely related to brushing habits rather than other organic factors. In another study, subjects with greater recession were shown to have significantly lower mean gingival and mean plaque scores than subjects without recession. Presumably, patients with better oral hygiene habits, reflected by lower plaque scores, run a greater risk of developing gingival recession.

Once recession has progressed beyond the bounds of normal gingival contour, cementum and dentin become exposed. Also, the enamel coating itself is very thin at the gum margin so that abrasive attack on this tissue can lead to further exposure of the soft underlying dentin. Once exposed, these tissues are subject to abrasive attack which is likely to be accelerated by the use of incorrect brushing techniques. Therefore, it is not surprising that a strong correlation has been shown between gingival recession and cervical dentin abrasion. This further suggests that both gingival recession and cervical abrasion are related in some way to one or more variables associated with toothbrushing. It should be made clear, however, that while both may parallel each other as a clinical parameter, their etiologies are quite distinct. Recession is primarily a toothbrush factor, while cervical abrasion is more related to the abrasivity of the denti-

frice. Limiting the rate of soft tissue retraction will, in effect, act to reduce the level of cervical abrasion. While long term clinical studies measuring the effects of different types of toothbrushes on gingival recession are lacking, it appears safe to conclude from available evidence that hard toothbrushes are more likely to promote these effects than any other type of toothbrush. Excessive brushing pressure, improper brushing motion, and prolonged brushing are all factors that can accelerate the rate of gingival erosion, ultimately affecting cementum and dentin.

The use of toothbrushes with end-rounded bristle tips may also be one way to minimize soft tissue abrasion that results from brushing. The first nylon brushes, aside from being stiff, caused an unpleasant scratching sensation when used due to the presence of sharp, chisel shaped projections on the ends of the bristles formed during the trimming process (Fig. 22-3A). It was soon learned that these could be removed during the manufacture of the brush using a simple sanding technique. As a result, the bristle tips appear smooth and free from sharp, pointed barbs (Fig. 22-3B). The clinical value of end-rounding toothbrush fibers has long been a matter of well deserved skepticism. Early experiments gave credibility to the concept of end-rounding but failed to provide conclusive proof that such bristles acted to reduce trauma to soft, supportive tissues. It was not until recently that laboratory studies have shown that the level of abrasion to sensitive tissues can be significantly reduced using end-rounded toothbrushes. These results were also confirmed clinically in humans by using a dye visualization technique.

While many of the design features seen in today's professional quality toothbrushes were developed on a purely empirical basis, research has provided a considerable amount of clinical data which, by and large, supports the concept that some brushes perform better than others. Applied to a loosely defined category of brushes called "professional", it appears certain that brushes of this type better satisfy the functional requirements of brushing compared to brushes of poor design. As long as brushing remains necessary to maintain a healthy oral environment, some level of abrasion, either to the teeth themselves or the gingiva, will be inevitable. The goal of professional guidance, in regards to the mechanical removal of plaque deposits, is to achieve this

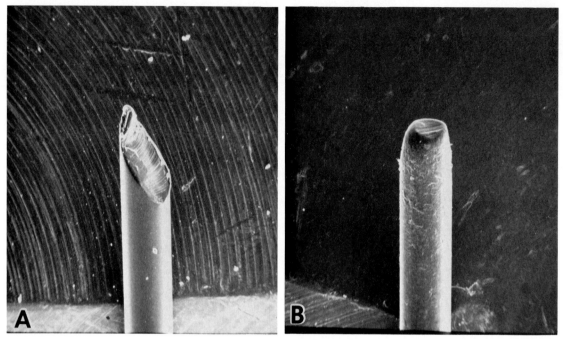

Fig. 22-3. **A.** S.E.M. of a trimmed, non-end rounded nylon bristle (×50) **B.** S. E. M. of a trimmed, end rounded nylon bristle (×50)

TOOTHBRUSH DESIGN AND FUNCTION

By the time synthetic bristle brushes became widely accepted by the dental profession, they were represented by an incredible variety of designs ranging from one extreme to the other. Some appeared to be the result of a conscious effort to satisfy the optimal functional requirements of an effective toothbrush, but many designs were considered arbitrary and oftentimes silly. As the importance of good plaque removal in controlling caries became obvious, more attention was given to the clinical effectiveness of toothbrush designs. In the process of attempting to answer which brush designs are superior, a large volume of clinical data was generated. Much of this proved of little value and somewhat contradictory, largely because quantitative and reproducible methods for measuring plaque were slow to be developed and/or accepted. As a result, the data from one study

could not be directly compared to another. Also, some studies were sponsored by brush manufacturers with the hope of establishing a measure of professional recognition for their unique design. While many studies were carried out with impartial scientific objectivity, the impact of the data they provided in understanding the physical functionality of the toothbrush often proved to be trivial. As a reminder of this, the dental literature today is bulging with reports showing how a newly invented toothbrush, featuring a precise range of various diameter filaments, placed at critically strategic angles and expertly trimmed to conform to every conceivable anatomical feature of the mouth, was clinically superior to all the other brushes tested.

At the time Bass embarked on a study of toothbrushes, the serrated head brush was one type of brush in vogue. It was reasoned that, cut in this fashion, the bristles in the center of the tuft, being longer than those around the periphery, were better able to enter into depressions and narrow spaces between the teeth. Bass observed the opposite effect. The longer bristles actually worked to hold off and prevent effective application of the shorter bristles. After experimentation and study he concluded that a flat trim head was best. With this type of brush, the bristles, when placed against the teeth, are deflected in such a way as to fan out and enter the interproximal areas between the teeth. This observation was one factor which led Bass to develop a method of brushing that has gained almost universal acceptance for its relative simplicity and effectiveness. The technique requires the use of a soft, flat-trimmed brush. The bristles are placed against the teeth at a 45° angle and gently worked down to the gingival margin using a vibratory motion.

Little else has been shown concerning the effectiveness or superiority of other types of trim design. Considering the diverse anatomic spacial relationships possible in the human mouth, it is not likely that any specific trim configuration will be found to meet all these requirements. The American Dental Association, in recognizing that toothbrush design is somewhat arbitrary, but should meet the requirements of efficiency and cleanliness, currently recommends a straight-trimmed brush for general adult use.

In addition to trim design, the number and arrangement of bristle tufts appears to have some measurable effect on the physical functionality of the toothbrush. In clinically testing these concepts, it has been shown that a positive correlation exists between plaque removal and the total number of filaments in a brush. In a similar comparison, it was found that soft multi-tufted brushes reached more areas of plaque than did harder brushes. While other studies have failed to provide additional, statistically valid evidence that tuft density is a positive factor in plaque removal, there is little doubt that the two are closely related. The overall density of a toothbrush is controlled by two factors: filament diameter and the number of tufts in the brush head. Filament diameter not only plays a passive physical role in determining the overall density of a toothbrush, but also may have an important effect on overall plaque removal.

Soft nylon toothbrushes were available prior to 1948, but they received little professional recognition until Dr. Charles Bass provided evidence that brushes constructed with narrow diameter filaments had important advantages over conventional hard brushes. He considered a 0.007 inch diameter nylon filament to be optimal, but did concede that a slight deviation in size was permissible. Bass reasoned that the bristles of these brushes were not only less abrasive to soft gingival tissue, but due to their narrow bristle diameter were better able to penetrate into the gingival sulcus. The key to successful plaque removal with these brushes was the use of a specific brushing technique. The necessity to use a particular brushing motion with soft brushes has never been clearly proven. The Bass technique and the Roll method appear equally effective with this type of brush. On the other hand, alterations in filament diameter appear to affect the ability of a brush to remove plaque particularly in regards to the type of motion used. A recent study showed that a soft brush used with the Bass technique failed to function as effectively as did a harder brush using the Roll technique. Other studies similarly highlight the fact that filament diameter is a critical factor in determining the effectiveness of a toothbrush in removing plaque, but much of this has been shown to depend on the method of brushing employed. This much appears certain, the use of well designed soft toothbrushes in conjunction with most conscientiously applied brushing techniques will result in effective plaque removal. How effective this technique will be in quantitative terms largely depends on the level of patient instruction, motivation, and dedication to a regular home hygiene program. Conversely, a good brush will produce disappointing results in the hands of uninstructed patients. Well controlled studies have shown that weekly supervised toothbrushing at school and regular cleaning by hygienists can greatly reduce caries incidence in children. In one study comparing the effectiveness of supervision and nonsupervision on gingival health, results showed that merely carrying out a prophylaxis on a child and giving the child a toothbrush without ensuring that the child knows how to use the brush effectively produced no improvement in oral hygiene.

The second factor that determines brush density is the number of tufts present in the head of the brush. The original brush described by Bass was a space-tufted brush, having only three rows of evenly spaced bristles, six tufts to the row. While several clinical studies have shown a positive correlation between plaque scores and the total number of filaments present in the brush, the effects of the number of tufts has not been considered equally as a separate parameter. In those studies where the effectiveness of a multi-tufted brush was compared to a conventional brush, interpretation of the clinical results rested on the quantity of filaments found in the brushes rather than the arrangement or number of tufts present. From the limited information available, it appears that the total number of filaments and the number of tufts in a brush show parallel correlations in terms of plaque removal. For example, it has been shown that a multi-tufted brush tested was equally effective when the head was reduced to half its original size. In a more meaningful study, the effectiveness of four identical brush heads differing only in the total number of tufts present was tested. It was shown that fully multi-tufted brushes were more effective than brushes of identical design with lower numbers of tufts.

The acceptance of soft, multi-tufted brushes by patients and dental professionals alike has been considerable. In a recent study among periodontists, 55 per cent recommended multi-tufted brushes and 76 per cent indicated a preference for soft brushes. While good plaque control can probably be achieved with almost any reasonably good toothbrush, provided motivation and instruction are adequate, certain brushes do appear to perform better in the hands of the average patient.

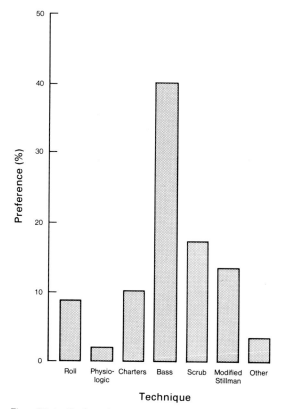

Fig. 22-4. Preferred toothbrushing techniques. (Reprinted with permission from: Thaller J., Reiser M., Ward H.: N.Y. State D.J. 38: 305–308, 1972)

TOOTHBRUSHING TECHNIQUES

Numerous techniques have been described to brush the teeth, but their sheer multiplicity merely highlights the fact that no one method has been shown to be the best for all individuals. Over the years, several methods have achieved a measure of popularity which does not necessarily correlate with any recognized level of professional acceptance. The popularity of one method over another is probably related more to patient factors, such as ease of instruction or simplicity of execution, rather than proven effectiveness. In 1972 Thaller surveyed the relative popularity of the major techniques of brushing among periodontists and showed that the Bass method was by far the most popular (Fig. 22-4).

Central to the success of any of these techniques is the action of the brush in the gingival crevice. If this cannot be accomplished effectively in relation to all anatomic situations, the prime objective of brushing will be de-

feated. We have already seen how brush design plays a role in achieving this requirement. The method of use is no less important.

While the horizontal scrub technique is probably the most popular method used by uninstructed patients, it fails to clean the cervicoproximal tooth areas, and may cause abrasion at the cementoenamel junction on the buccal and lingual surfaces of the teeth. Of the more orthodox techniques, none are able to satisfy every anatomic requirement expected from brushing. It is important, therefore, to understand the deficiencies inherent in each technique as well as the benefits.

Bass Technique

In the technique developed by Bass, the brush is placed in such a manner that the bristles are at a 45 degree angle to the tooth surfaces. The brush is moved back and forth with a vibratory motion until the brush reaches the gingival sulcus. This method has been shown clinically to clean equally as well the lingual and facial aspects of the proximal surfaces. In spite of its apparent popularity, particularly among periodontists, the Bass technique is one which is somewhat difficult to learn. In one study it was shown that only 24 per cent of those taught the technique practiced it in a satisfactory manner 14 to 21 days after instruction. In contrast, the Roll technique is considered the easiest to learn, requires the least correction during follow up visits, and is most appropriate when there is minimal change in the normal cementogingival relationship. In this technique the bristles are placed well up on the attached gingiva at a 45 degree angle. The sides of the bristles are pressed against the tissue and simultaneously moved incisally or occlusally against the gingiva and teeth in a rolling motion. This action is repeated 8 to 12 times in each area in a definite order so as not to neglect any buccal or lingual surfaces. The occlusal surfaces are brushed with a conventional, reciprocal motion. Despite its popularity, some investigators have stated that it can cause gingival recession and does not adequately clean the gingival crevice or the interproximal surfaces of the teeth.

Charters and Stillman Techniques

The Charters technique was developed primarily for interproximal cleaning, although it should be stated here that no brush, regardless of design, can adequately clean this area. For this, floss must be used. With the Charters technique, the bristles are placed into the interproximal areas, and with a gentle vibratory motion, the ends are forced between the teeth. For lingual brushing, the same procedure is used, except that only the tip of the brush is used. When cleaning the maxillary posterior teeth, the brush head is placed against the palate, and the bristles are worked between the teeth. Besides being difficult to learn, the Charters technique performs poorly on the proximal surfaces and cannot be used effectively where the teeth are poorly aligned. The Stillman technique is equally difficult to learn and execute. It was designed primarily to provide a good massaging action to the gums and promote gingival keratinization. Recognizing these drawbacks, the method has

been modified to promote better cleaning and reduce tissue trauma. The bristles are placed apically at a 45 degree angle on the gingiva, just coronal to the mucogingival junction. With the brush in this position, a slight mesiodistal vibratory motion is performed in conjunction with a movement of the brush to the occlusal plane. For obvious reasons, this technique has failed to gain a high level of acceptance.

Other Techniques

The Physiologic technique is recommended only for use with a soft toothbrush and has the advantage of being rather simple to learn. It is based on the premise that food is deflected apically during chewing and, therefore, brushing should be carried out in the same direction. Using a soft brush, the ends of the bristles are moved from the occlusal portion of the teeth toward the gingiva in a gentle, sweeping motion. While easy to learn, the Physiologic technique fails to achieve good interproximal cleaning.

The Fones technique of brushing is probably the simplest of all and has been shown to be effective for young children who cannot master a complex brushing motion. It is not recommended for patients with periodontitis, since it does not adequately clean the interproximal areas and can produce laceration of the gingival tissue if applied too vigorously. In the Fones technique, the brush is pressed vigorously against the teeth while applying a circular motion with as large a diameter as possible. Because this method employs essentially a circular scrubbing motion, it should only be used with a soft brush.

It is obvious from all this that there is no one, universally accepted technique used by all dentists for all patients. In fact, divergence of opinion is more the rule than the exception. In many cases, the most effective method for a patient is an adaptation or combination of one or more techniques (i.e., a combination of the Bass and Roll methods). In acute periodontitis, a combination of the Charters technique and Roll technique has been shown to be effective.

All the methods described here are undoubtedly effective if applied correctly. It should be remembered that regardless of which particular technique is recommended, the same general principles apply. The purpose of brushing is to remove dental plaque from all tooth surfaces, as well as the gingival margin, with the minimum amount of damage to the teeth and surrounding structures. If the patient is found to be achieving an acceptable level of oral hygiene with the method being used, no attempt should be made to change it unless signs of tissue trauma and gingival recession are evident. It also follows that when a clinician prescribes a particular toothbrushing method for an individual there should also be an evaluation of the patient's dexterity, the oral health status, and individual ability and interest in learning and adhering to the method prescribed.

Automatic Toothbrushes

The rationale behind the development and use of the automatic toothbrush is unambiguous. It should function in a way making it easier to remove plaque deposits. Several studies have shown significant improvements in oral health when automatic toothbrushes were used. The current professional consensus is that both automatic and manual toothbrushes are equally effective. In a review of mechanical methods of plaque removal it was reported that ". . . electric toothbrushes are no more effective than manual toothbrushes over a protracted period of time."

When automatic toothbrushes were first introduced, many dental practitioners had serious reservations about putting them in the hands of their patients, fearing that compulsive brushers would use them to excess causing damage to supportive soft tissues. From the clinical studies available, there is no evidence to show that automatic toothbrushes are any more abrasive to soft tissues than manual toothbrushes. Some studies have shown that automatic toothbrushes are highly beneficial in certain situations. It was pointed out in a 1971 evaluation of 40 clinical studies comparing power vs. manual brushing, that while the automatic toothbrush and the manual brush can be used with equal effectiveness in removing plaque, the automatic toothbrush may be especially useful in the hands of physically or mentally handicapped persons. Also, patients with extensive fixed bridge work or orthodontic appliances find automatic toothbrushes quite useful.

PATIENT FACTORS

Ultimately, the therapeutic benefits realized from good plaque control rests in the hands of the patient. Throughout this chapter, the role of patient motivation and learning in making the best possible use of a well designed toothbrush has been stressed. While it is possible to speak objectively about the potential benefits that can be realized from the use of specific types of toothbrushes shown to be clinically effective, subjective factors related to improper use could cancel these out. The full potential of a toothbrush can only be realized when the patient understands the importance and mechanics of total plaque control.

Frequency of Brushing

While numerous epidermiologic studies have shown that less plaque occurs as the frequency of oral hygiene procedures increases, there is ample confusion as to how regularly plaque must be removed. It has been demonstrated that as oral hygiene procedures are suspended, clinically evident gingivitis develops in 4 days. Based on these and other studies, the onset of gingivitis is more related to the age of the plaque rather than the amount. The brushing habits of individuals vary widely, particularly in regards to the amount of time spent brushing, total number of strokes, and brushing pressure. Another important factor is the manual dexterity of the patient. Because of all these factors, it is difficult to be dogmatic in suggesting a brushing regimen. One study showed that patients with the greatest number of plaque free teeth and the lowest gingival inflammation scores spent about 25 minutes a day in oral hygiene procedures. While it is true that brushing two or three times daily results in improved gingival health, frequency of brushing does not correlate well with reduction in caries. The quality of brushing is obviously a more important factor than frequency.

Studies have shown that the benefits of toothbrushing are primarily confined to the facial tooth surfaces while the posterior buccal surfaces are largely ignored. Areas missed during the first brushing are likely to be overlooked on the second and third session because most people develop a characteristic pattern of brushing. Therefore, it is more likely that the same areas would be neglected regardless of the frequency of brushing. If we assume that the patient is using an effective brushing technique, the question remains how frequently this needs to be carried out in order to maintain a clinically healthy mouth. Since it appears that the age of the plaque is more important than the amount, the longer the plaque remains undisturbed, the greater will be the severity of the insult to hard and soft tissue structures in the mouth. What this critical time period is probably depends on numerous variables related to diet, (see Chap. 16) microflora, (see Chap. 11) saliva flow (see Chap. 2), anatomy and others. It has been shown that removing plaque effectively every second day is sufficient to maintain a clinically healthy gingiva. It appears then, that complete removal of plaque to a zero level every day or possibly every other day is more efficacious than several inefficient brushings each day.

Wear

Toothbrushes that are worn cannot work effectively to remove plaque. As simple as this statement sounds, it is largely overlooked by patients. One study has shown that 45 per cent of toothbrushes in use are in reality already worn out. While the consequences of this fact largely benefit brush manufacturers, very little investigation has been carried out along these lines, although the American Dental Association has been vocal in urging patients to examine the condition of their toothbrushes.

Actually, very little is known about how long a toothbrush should last, since use is regulated by so many variables. From the meager amount of information available, it appears that the physical properties of the fiber used in the brush, combined with the type of mechanical force applied during use largely define the wear characteristics of a toothbrush. Of the physical fiber qualities affecting brush wear, bend recovery is probably the most important. The ability of a filament to return to its original vertical plane following a period of stress in another direction defines this property. The ultimate durability of the toothbrush using a particular fiber is determined by the resistance of the fiber to permanent deflection from its original vertical axis. Differ-ences in bend recovery between various types or grades of nylon probably explain why seemingly identical toothbrushes wear out at appreciably different rates. Brush texture, trim height, tuft design, and density also play a significant role in brush durability.

The second most important factor regulating brush wear is use by the patient. Here the variables are almost infinite in number and highlight the fact that time is probably the worst criterion for predicting the useful life of a toothbrush. In a controlled clinical study spanning two years, the relationship between brush wear, age of the brush, and gingival health were investigated. It was found that the method of brushing is more important than the length of time the brush was in use. The more worn a toothbrush appeared to be when discarded, the newer it tended to be.

Other studies have shown that progressive deterioration of the bristles and tufts results in the ineffectual use of the brush due to a loss of adaptability to oral structures, particularly at the gingival margin. Disorientation and splaying result in a loss of texture which reduces the ability of the brush to reach anatomic structures known to harbor plaque. One study, using mechanically deformed brushes showed that even a slightly worn brush removed 23 per cent less plaque than a new brush, and the use of a well worn brush resulted in an even greater reduction in plaque removal. Dental practitioners and hygienists alike should be prepared to provide realistic guidelines to patients in this area.

SUMMARY

Until the time that chemical or biologic agents are successfully developed to prevent or cure dental disease, the toothbrush will remain, in addition to dental floss, the primary physical agent used to control plaque. While the use of various forms of flouride, antibacterial agents, and professional treatment are effective in controlling dental disease, these do not obviate the need for thorough plaque removal on a regular basis. To carry this even further, there is good evidence to show that the effective use of preventive tools such as diet, therapy, and fluorides is largely negated when plaque is allowed to grow unchecked.

The limits of design and functionality, as related to toothbrushing, appear to be loosely defined only because much more needs to be learned about the effects of brushing on the progression of dental disease. The variation and spectrum of responses one can expect from dental professionals on any discussion of toothbrush selection highlights our basic ignorance of the quality of performance we should generally expect from toothbrushes. Some say the type of brush used doesn't matter, others maintain that a specific design is critical for good plaque control. Obviously, the answer lies between these two extremes. Again, this highlights the need for more basic research in this area.

In all this discussion, patients should not be forgotten because the toothbrush may be all they have to maintain a healthy oral environment. Skeptical attitudes expressed or implied about toothbrushes to a patient can undermine their confidence in a home plaque control program. Basic ignorance about how a toothbrush should work and how it should be designed to work effectively may be at the heart of this attitude. The thrust of this chapter has been to lend direction and provide information on the physical functionality of toothbrushes. Dental professionals should know something about toothbrushes because it is one of the most important preventive appliances available to the profession. The research described in this chapter has hopefully provided a base of information about toothbrushes to assist the professional in making an intelligent choice in the best interests of the patient. Proper instruction and follow up will help develop the proper motivational climate required for a good plaque control and the maintenance of a caries free state.

GLOSSARY

Abrasivity index. An index of abrasion employed by the A.D.A. to provide a means of standardization in comparing the abrasiveness of various dentifrices.

Bass technique. The brush is positioned at a 45° degree angle to the tooth/gum surface. A rocking motion is applied back and forth until the bristles move into the sulcus, over the gingival margin, and into the interproximal areas.

Bend recovery. The ability of a material to return to its original shape after deformation.

Charter technique. A brushing motion designed to achieve good cleaning of the interproximal areas. The bristles are moved interproximally with a gentle vibrating motion, forcing the filament tips between the teeth.

Filament stiffness. A major factor in the measurement of brush texture; derived as a function of filament diameter and length.

Fones technique. A brushing technique where the buccal surfaces are covered with a rotary motion. Lingual surfaces are cleaned with a back and forth movement.

Gingival recession. Loss of gingival contour due to mechanical traumatization of epithelial attachments at the cemento-enamel junction.

Modulus. A coefficient of bristle stiffness measured as a ratio of change in stress to a change in strain.

Natural bristle. Selected hog bristle blended and trimmed for use in toothbrushes; generally imported from India or China.

Nylon. A superpolymeric amide with a repetitive linear structure, used as a fiber or molding compound.

Physiological technique. A brushing method in which the teeth are cleaned by moving the brush apically from crown to root, simulating the direction of food movement during chewing.

Roll technique. A brushing method in which the bristles are slowly brought down on the teeth with a rolling motion towards the crown until a 180° degree arc has been made.

Trim. Characteristic arrangement of bristle tips at the brushing surface, e.g., flat, concave, scalloped, etc.

SUGGESTED READINGS

Alexander JF, Saffir AJ, Gold W: The measurement of the effect of toothbrushes on soft tissue abrasion. J Dent Res 56:722–727, 1977

Anneroth G, Poppelman A: Historical evaluation of gingival damage by toothbrushing. Acta Odont Scand 33: 119–127, 1975

Ariaudo A: How frequently must patients carry out effective oral hygiene procedures in order to maintain gingival health? J Periodont 42: 309–313, 1971

Ashmore H, Van Ablie NJ, Wilson SJ: The measurement in vitro of dentin abrasion by toothpaste: Brit Dent J 133: 60–66, 1972

Bass CC: The optimum characteristics of toothbrushes for personal oral hygiene. Dent Items of Interest 70: 697–718, 1948

Bay I: Quantitative evaluation of the roque-removing ability of different types of toothbrushes. J Periodont 38: 526–533, 1967

Berdon JK, Hornbrook RH, Hayduk SE: An evaluation of six manual toothbrushes by comparing their effectiveness in plaque removal. J Periodont 45: 496–499, 1974

Bergenholtz A, Hugoson A, Lundgren D, Ostgren A:

The toothbrush as an aid in oral hygiene. J Periodont Res 2: 247–248, 1967

Bjorn H, Lindhe J: Abrasion of dentin by toothbrush and dentifrice. Odont Revy 17: 17–27, 1966

Burgett FG, Ash MM: Comparative study of the pressure of brushing with three types of toothbrushes. J Periodont 45: 410–413, 1974

Carter HG, Barnes GP, Woolridge EW, Ward GT: Effect of various toothbrushing techniques on gingival bleeding and dental plaque. Vir Dent J 51: 18–29, 1974

Craig TT, Montaque JL: The 1974 oral health survey. JADA 92: 326–332, 1976

Dobbs HE, Abbott DJ: Sensitive method for measuring the relative abrasiveness of dentifrices. J Dent Res 47: 1072–1079, 1968

Downer MC: Evaluation of an unsupervised oral hygiene program. Brit Dent J 131: 152–156, 1971

Dunkin RT: Abrasiveness of automatic versus manual toothbrushes. Dent Survey 51: 36, 39–40, 44, 1975

Elliott JR, Bowers GM, Clemmer BA, Rovelstad GH: A comparison of selected oral hygiene devices in dental plaque removal. J Periodont 43: 217–220, 1972

Fanning FA, Henning FR: Toothbrush design and its relation to oral health. Australian Dent J 12: 464–467, 1967

Gibson JA, Wade AB: Plaque removal by the Bass and Roll techniques. J Periodont 48: 456–459, 1977

Gilson CM, Charbencau GT, Hill HC: A comparison of physical properties of several soft toothbrushes. J Mich Dent Assoc 51: 347–361, 1969

Glickman I, Petralis R, Marke RM: The effect of powered toothbrushing and interdental stimulation upon microscopic inflammation and surface keratinization of the interdental gingiva. J Periodont 36: 108–111, 1965

Gorman WJ: Prevalence and etiology of gingival recession. J Periodont 38: 50–56, 1967

Granath L, Holger R, Liliegren E, Holst K: Variation in caries prevalence related to combination of dietary and oral hygiene habits in 6-year-old children. Caries Res 10: 302–317, 1976

Hansen F, Gjermo P: The plaque removing effect of four toothbrushing methods. Scand J Dent 79: 502–506, 1971

Harte DB, Manly RS: Four variables affecting magnitude of dentifrice abrasiveness. J Dent Res 55: 322–327, 1976

Heath JR, Wilson HJ: Classification of toothbrush stiffness by a dynamic method. Brit Dent J 130: 59–66, 1971

Hine M: Variation in toothbrush textures. JADA 46: 536–539, 1953

Hiniker J, Forscher B: The effect of toothbrush type on gingival health. Periodont 25: 40–46, 1954

Huff GC, Taylor PP: Clinical evaluation of toothbrushes used in periodontics. Texas Dent J 83: 6–11, 1965

Kiplinger M, Wachti C, Fosdick LS: Some observations on the cleansing effect of nylon and bristle toothbrushes. J Periodont 25: 183–188, 1954

Kitchin PC: The prevalance of tooth root exposure and the relation to the extent of such exposure to the degree of abrasion in different age classes. J Dent Res 20: 565–581, 1941

Kitchin PC, Robinson HBG: The abrasiveness of dentifrices as measured on the cervical areas of extracted teeth. J Dent Res 27: 195–200, 1948

Kopczyk RA, Lenox JA, Saxe SR: Potential for keratinization of the sulcus epithelium in the dog. J Dent Res 53: 137, 1974

Lang NP, Cumming BR, Loe H: Toothbrushing frequency as it relates to plaque development and gingival health. J Periodont 44: 396–405, 1973

MacFarlane D: The dynamic stiffness of toothbrushes. J. Periodont Res 6: 218–226, 1971

MacKenzie I: Does toothbrushing affect gingival keratinization? Royal Soc of Med 65: 1127–1131, 1972

MacKenzie IC, Miles AEU: The effect of chronic frictional stimulation on hamster cheek pouch epithelium. Archs Oral Biol 18: 1341–1349, 1973

McAllen LH, Murray JJ, Brook AH, Crawford AN: Oral Hygiene instruction in children using manual and electric toothbrushes. Brit Dent J 140: 51–56, 1976

McCauley H: Toothbrushes, toothbrush materials and design. JADA 33: 283–322, 1946

McConnell D, Conroy CW: Comparison of abrasion produced by a simulated manual versus a mechanical toothbrush. J Dent Res 46: 1022–1027, 1967

McKendrick AJW, McHugh WD, Barbenel LM: Toothbrush age and wear. Brit Dent J 130: 66–68, 1971

Manly RS, Brudevold F: Relative abrasiveness of material and synthetic toothbrush bristles on cementum and dentin. JADA 55: 779–780, 1957

Manly RS, Wiren J, Manly PJ, Keene RC: A method for measurement of abrasion on dentin by toothbrush and dentifrice. J Dent Res 44: 532–540, 1965

Manly RS, Wiren J, Harte DB, Aheren JM: Influence of method of testing on dentifrice abrasiveness. J Dent Res 53: 835–839, 1974

Maurice CF, Wallace DA: Toothbrush effectiveness. Relative cleansing ability of four toothbrushes of different design. Ill Dent J 26: 286–292, 1957

Mehta F, Sanjana M, Shroff B, Ratan H: The effects of toothbrush type of gingival keratinization. All India Dent Assoc 36: 115–136, 1964

Merzel J, Viegas AR, Munhoz C: Contribution to the study of keratinization in human gingiva. J Periodont 34: 127–133, 1963

O'Leary TJ, Drake RB, Jiuiden GJ: The incidence of recession in young males: relationship to gingival and plaque scores. J Periodont 6: 109–111, 1968

Owen TL: A clinical evaluation of electric and manual toothbrushing by children with primary dentitions. J Dent Chil 39: 15–21, 1972

Padbury AD, Ash M: Abrasion caused by three methods of toothbrushing. J Periodont 45: 434–438, 1974

Phillips R, Swartz M: Effects of diameter of nylon bristles on enamel surface. JADA 47: 20–26, 1953

Radentz WH, Barnes GP, Cutright DE: A survey of factors possibly associated with cervical abrasion of tooth surfaces. J Periodont 47: 148–154, 1976

Robertson N, Wade A: Effect on filament diameter and density in toothbrushes. J Periodont Res 7: 346–350, 1971

Robinson H: Toothbrushing habits of 405 persons. JADA 33: 1112–1117, 1946

Robinson H, Kitchin P: The effect of massage with the toothbrush on keratinization of the gingivae. Oral Surgery 1: 1042–1046, 1948

Sangness G, Zachrissan B, Gjermo P: Effectiveness of vertical and horizontal brushing techniques in plaque removal. J Dent Chil 39: 94–97, 1972

Sangness G, Gjermo P: Prevalence of oral soft and hard tissue lesions related to mechanical tooth-cleansing procedures. Comm Dent Oral Epidemiol 4: 77–83, 1976

Schmid MO, Balmelli OP, Saxer UP: Plaque-removing effect of a toothbrush, dental floss and toothpick. J Clin Periodont 3: 157–165, 1976

Shkurkin GR, Almquist AJ, Peelhofer AA, Stoddard EL: Scanning electron microscopy of dentition: methodology and ultrastructural morphology of tooth wear. J Dent Res 54: 402–406, 1975

Skinner EW, Takata G: Abrasions on tooth structure by nylon and natural bristles (abstr). J Dent Res 30: 522, 1951

Stahl S, Wachtel N, Decastro C, Pelletier G: The effect of toothbrushing on the keratinization of the gingiva. Periodont 24: 20–21, 1953

Stookey GK, Muhler JC: Laboratory studies concerning the enamel and dentin abrasion of common dentifrice polishing agents. J Dent Res 47: 524–532, 1968

Swartz M, Phillips R, Hine M: Effect of certain factors upon toothbrush bristle stiffness. Periodont 27: 96–101, 1956

Swartz ML, Phillips RW: Cleansing, polishing and abrasion techniques (in vito). Ann NY Acad Sci 153: 120–136, 1968

Thaller J, Reiser M, Ward HL: A study to ascertain the oral hygiene practices by the members of the periodontal community. NY State Dent J 38: 305–308, 1972

Tucker G, Andlaw RJ, Burchell CK: The relationship between oral hygiene and dental caries incidence in 11-year-old children. Brit Dent J 141: 75–79, 1976

Van Huysen G, Boyd T: Cleaning effectiveness of dentifrices. J Dent Res 31: 575–581, 1952

Vogel RI, Sullivan AJ, Pascuzzi JN, Deasey MJ: Evaluation of cleansing devices in the maintenance of interproximal gingival health. J Periodont 40: 745–747, 1975

Volpe AR, Mooney R, Zumbrunnen C, Stahl D, Goldman HM: A long-term clinical study evaluating the effect of two dentifrices on oral tissues. J Periodont 46: 113–118, 1975

Vowles AD, Wade AB: Importance of filament diameter when using Bass brushing technique. J Periodont 48: 460–463, 1977

Wade AB: A clinical assessment of the relative properties of nylon and bristle brushes. Brit Dent J 114: 260–264, 1953

Warren WC, Rustogi KN, Hansen KR, et al: A plaque assessment index for measuring toothbrush efficiency. J NJ Dent Assn Winter: 38–45, 1977

Wolfram K, Egelberg C, et al: Effect of the tooth cleansing procedures on gingival sulcus depth. J Periodont Res 9: 44–49, 1974

Wright KHR, Swenson JI: The measurement and interpretation of dentifrice abrasiveness. Soc Cosmetic Chem 18: 387–411, 1967

PART FIVE

Caries Research

23 Caries Experimentation

LEWIS MENAKER

Introduction
Human Studies
   Epidemiologic Survey Methods
   Intraoral Caries Methods
   Legal and Ethical Requirements for the
      Protection of Human Research Subjects
   Laboratory Animal Models
   Rodent Models
   Other Animal Models
   Pathogen-Free and Germ-Free Models

   Diets
   Caries Scoring
In Vitro Studies
   The Artificial Mouth
   Laboratory Procedures
      Nondestructive Biophysical Methods
      Destructive Biophysical Methods
Glossary
Suggested Readings

INTRODUCTION

Much of the material presented throughout the body of this text is the direct result of the data gathered from experimentation in the broad field of cariology. Advances in pellicle and tooth biochemistry, apatite structure, demineralization–remineralization kinetics, microbiology and immunology, chemotherapy, and fluoride chemistry have given us an ever-expanding understanding of dental caries. It is only through further increases in our knowledge that the ultimate goal can be reached: the prevention and elimination of the disease itself.

The fruits of caries experimentation are already with us. While major control over dental caries is already a possibility through fluoride therapy, occlusal sealants, plaque control, and diet manipulation, it is a certainty that the future holds many other advances. It is now possible to speculate that experimentation will yield a caries vaccine, more efficacious fluoride compounds, sucrose substitutes, and inroads into behavioral modification to ensure patient compliance.

In this chapter the general objective will be to uncover the methodology used for investigations into dental caries, with the specific objectives designed to elaborate on the use of human, laboratory animal and *in vitro* models for studying the disease itself. Each approach has its advantages and disadvantages, the final selection dictated by the goals of the study and the host (Chaps. 1–7), agent (Chaps. 11–15), and environmental (Chaps. 16–22) variables under investigation. It is hoped that, through an exposure to research from a "behind-the-scenes" vantage point, three goals will be accomplished: first, that an appreciation for the thought processes involved in caries research will be developed; second, that an ability to evaluate the scientific literature critically will

499

evolve; and third, that, for those receptive individuals, a stimulus to participate in research will be evoked.

HUMAN STUDIES

As with any disease undergoing investigation, it is a logical choice of scientists to turn first to those patients demonstrating evidence of the condition as a source of material from which they can gain information and insights into the disease process. Any step away from use of the human model to animal and *in vitro* studies carries with it the inherent possibility that the entity under study is only an approximation of the true disease. This acquiescence to less than the ideal requires the acceptance of the various givens, assumptions, and compromises that demand caution in interpretation and application of the data generated.

Unfortunately the case for the use of human beings as experimental subjects in caries research also has its drawbacks. It soon becomes obvious that, relative to laboratory animal and *in vitro* experiments, human studies are limited by the inability to sequester people so as to allow for ideal control over all experimental variables. The number of subjects and the expense involved in many studies also dictate the use of animals. Added to the list of restrictions are the extended time factor for caries development in man, the complexities of overriding human living patterns, the inability to isolate or impose single experimental variables, and the limited manipulations and invasive techniques allowed under moral, ethical, and legal considerations. It is these constraints that have prescribed the conditions for caries studies involving human subjects.

Epidemiologic Survey Methods

Perhaps the most common methodology employed in human studies involving caries is the survey. The major objective of this approach is to determine the prevalence of the disease or the comparison of prevalences in two or more populations. This approach can be modified for the clinical trial of one or several levels of a therapeutic agent. In this case base line prevalence levels would be determined and an effort made to obtain study populations with similar backgrounds. Examples of such studies are dentifrice trials and the now classic Newburgh-versus-Kingston public water fluoridation study. The goal of the clinical trial is to measure differences in the caries increment between test groups during the test period. While this may seem straightforward and simple, the truth is that many pitfalls exist. These include compliance with the experimental protocol by the test subjects and the biases introduced by 1) prior knowledge of the experimental procedures, 2) a placebo effect, and 3) the individual's knowing that he or she is participating in an experiment (Hawthorne Effect). As with any investigation special care must be taken prior to the start of the trial to ensure proper experimental design and acceptable data presentation. Juggling of data by statistical manipulation to show "statistically significant" differences is meaningless if biological significance is obviously lacking. In these studies caries is determined by using parameters such as the the number of people with caries, the number of teeth with caries, the number of tooth surfaces with caries, or the size of the lesions in a given study population. Evaluation using the latter two categories is obviously complicated by the masking effect of restorative procedures and by the ravages due to neglect. In these instances a lesion only on the proximal surface would count as one unit. If restored, however, both the occlusal and proximal surfaces, because of the demands of the cavity design, would be included in the count. Further misleading data could result from the uncontrolled extension of a lesion left unrestored. Occlussal decay could progress into buccal and lingual developmental grooves so that use or nonuse of professional care rather than true caries prevalence would be measured. Another drawback to the use of the total number of lesions as the measure of prevalence is the contradiction that, as the caries lesions increase, their total number may actually be recorded as having decreased owing to enlargement and coalescence.

Employment of an index wherein a "yes" or "no" designation is recorded for the presence or absence of decay is also of limited use. A number generated using this system would be of little value for discriminating subtle differences in caries experience, especially in industrialized societies harboring many individuals with high levels of decay.

For these reasons the most widely used method for recording caries prevalence is the summation of the decayed, missing, and filled teeth (DMF-T). This index, in reality, measures the first attack of caries on the tooth and is relatively independent of the complicating factor of dental care. Furthermore, because of the much higher agreement between two examiners (or on reexamination by the same examiner) using the DMF-T, most of the increased sensitivity gained from the DMF-S (decayed, missing, and filled *surfaces*) is negated by the increased examiner error inherent in obtaining this index.

Use of any of these indices gives us a picture that is still far from the ideal. For instance, detection of the decay (D) component will vary from examiner to examiner, as well as within the same examiner at subsequent examinations. Furthermore, the quality of the examining conditions, including the amount and type of light, the sharpness of explorers, and the use or absence of radiographs will also determine the amount of decay reported. Errors in the missing (M) category can result from the inclusion of teeth lost for reasons other than caries. This could result from losses due to congenital defects, accidental trauma, orthodontic treatment, and periodontal disease. In primitive societies teeth are sometimes altered or removed as part of tribal rites. The detection of filled (F) teeth is also subject to errors that alter the precision of the data. Surveys done among populations with varying cultural attitudes toward dental care, or indeed the complete absence of such care, will obviously limit the validity of using the DMF scale as a comparative index.

While the DMF score is used for the permanent dentition, the *def* (decayed, indicated for extraction because of caries, filled) index is employed for deciduous teeth. In evaluating the primary dentition no "*m*" factor is included, owing to the normal shedding process. This index is useful up to the age of 6, after which shedding becomes the dominant factor. The weakness of this index can be seen in the individual with less caries attack whose score could show up as high simply because more teeth have survived and remain at risk and subject to counting. Various adaptations of the *def* have been used in children after the age of 6. A modified *dmf* index limited to the primary canines and molars has some usefulness up to the ages of 11–12. Whatever system the investigator chooses, it is generally accepted as not a good idea to combine caries scores in the primary and secondary teeth. If

the scores are combined, the experimenter runs the risk of obscuring the data for both sets of teeth.

The DMF approach to estimating caries is nonetheless a practical method for gathering comparative data, especially when combined with a "large number" statistical design. The comparison of a "norm" or control group to a "test" population is accomplished through establishing relative and not absolute prevalences. The relativity of the data is due to the built-in limitations of the DMF survey methodology. Clinical detection of caries is based on the investigator's ability to recognize the lesion at some point after it appears. Since caries is seen histologically well before it is detectible by the clinical examination (see Chap. 9), even the best clinical scoring will always be an underestimate of the "true" count. Unfortunately, the closer the examiner attempts to come to detecting the incipient lesion, the greater the increase in both examiner and interexaminer error.

The goal of the typical epidemiologic study is to identify a target population and evaluate the existence of a differential risk to caries. Factors commonly studied include differences in nutrient intake, genetic makeup, and trace element or fluoride content of water supplies. The ideal study group is a population ranging in age from 20 to 29 years. Such an age spread overcomes the contribution of varying eruption patterns among the individuals in the study and selects an age period in which relatively few teeth would be expected to have been lost by periodontal disease. Before the start of the survey a paired set of examiners should be selected. They should work closely to set up standards for the scoring procedure, both for procedures done in the mouth itself, as well as for the viewing of radiographs. Even if only one examiner is to be used, a standardization procedure should be employed to reduce to a minimum the estimated 10 per cent variability seen within the same individual clinician.

In the field the examination should be conducted with the aid of a second individual who serves as the recorder. The examining area should be screened against noise to allow the recorder to hear, and if at all possible, the examination should be taped and the records rechecked against the tape back in the office. The use of adequate light is essential. This should be in the form of an artificial light source so as to avoid the changing intensity of natural light, which will vary both with the time of day and with weather conditions. A portable examination chair will facilitate the examination and do much to avoid examiner fatigue. Dental explorers should be sharp; they must be resharpened after a fixed number of examinations or else discarded. The use of radiographs greatly enhances the ability to detect proximal lesions, and for this reason a portable x-ray machine is worth bringing along on field studies.

The data should be immediately transferred to a standard form (Fig. 23-1) and transcribed to punch cards for computer analysis. From there the data can be tabulated, the results analyzed, and conclusions drawn.

Whereas several other caries-scoring systems have been developed, including the Relative Index of Decay, the modified caries index of Bodecker, and a Scandinavian Moulage system, none has been shown to be superior to the DMF in terms of increasing the accuracy, precision, or efficiency of the survey. Perhaps in the future a weighted index

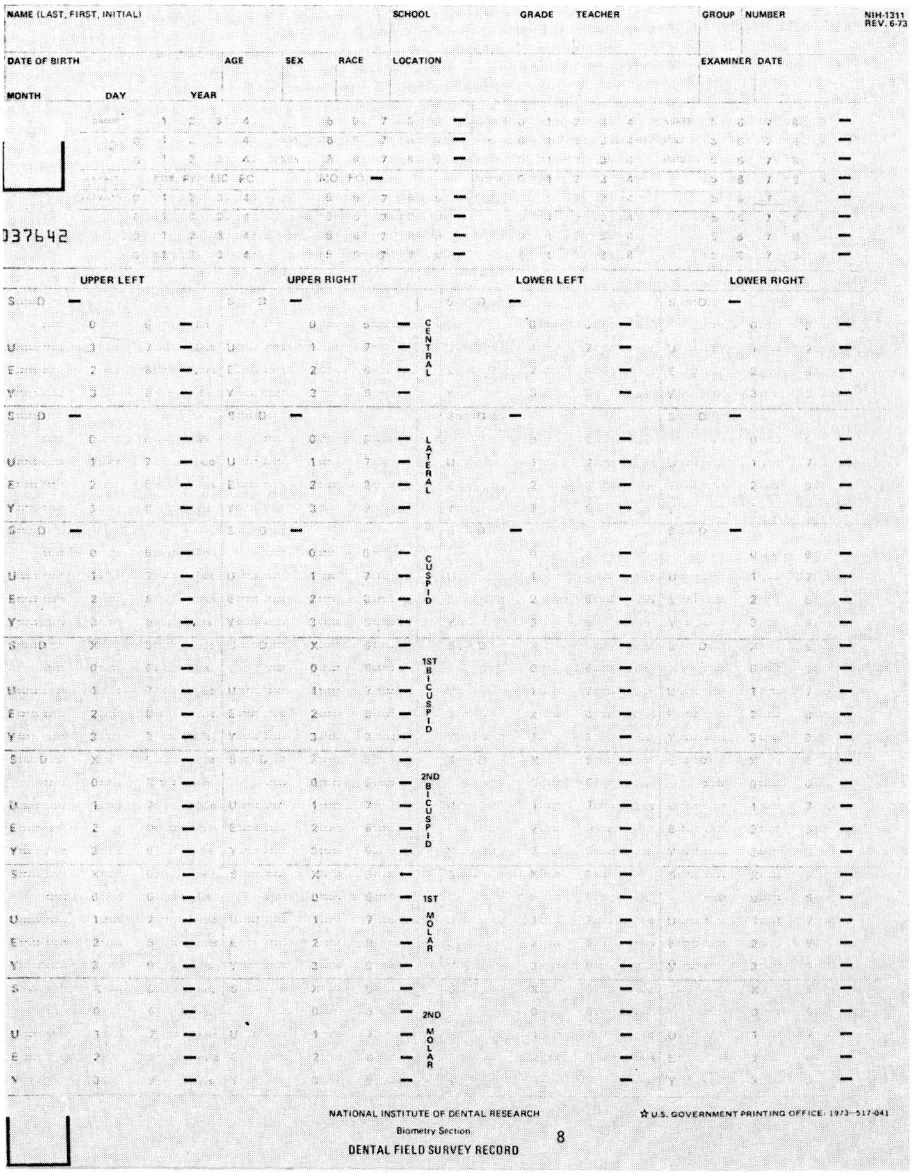

NAME (LAST, FIRST, INITIAL) | SCHOOL | GRADE | TEACHER | GROUP NUMBER | NIH-1311 REV. 6-73

DATE OF BIRTH: MONTH DAY YEAR | AGE | SEX | RACE | LOCATION | EXAMINER DATE

337642

UPPER LEFT | UPPER RIGHT | LOWER LEFT | LOWER RIGHT

CENTRAL · LATERAL · CUSPID · 1ST BICUSPID · 2ND BICUSPID · 1ST MOLAR · 2ND MOLAR

NATIONAL INSTITUTE OF DENTAL RESEARCH
Biometry Section
DENTAL FIELD SURVEY RECORD
8

☆ U.S. GOVERNMENT PRINTING OFFICE: 1973—517-041

Fig. 23-1. A sample of a standard dental field survey record developed by the Biometry Section of the National Institute of Dental Research.

designed in terms of susceptibility of each tooth surface to decay will be developed. Through the use of a computer a simple program could be constructed whereby the complex interrelationship resulting in the pattern of caries seen in each mouth could be used to take into account a "surface-at-risk" factor. This concept might more adequately be used to evaluate data gathered with the DMF index and give better interpretation of the efficacy of caries preventive agents.

Another epidemiologic method of interest in caries research is the diet survey. Through this approach the pattern and amount of food consumed can be assessed. The technique can be as complex and exact as a chemical analysis of duplicate servings of the food eaten by the individual. More often the survey will be in the form of a diet history. This can range from a 24-hour recall of foods eaten, obtained by interview, to the keeping of a diet diary for a fixed period of time, usually 5 days. Several drawbacks to this method include the difficulty in obtaining a complete as well as truthful listing; standarization of serving size is also a difficulty. Often the data from these diet surveys are subjected to computer analysis. These computer programs are usually generated from tables of nutrient content of foods published by various government agencies. Although these data are accurate, it must be realized that like-named foods can vary in nutrient content. For example, a potato grown in Maine is different from one grown in Idaho. Handling, storage, and preparation also alter nutrient values. With these facts in mind it can be seen that the "noise" in the diet survey approach is extremely high. For this reason one should not expect that a computer analysis of such data, with its set of inherent errors, will make the numbers generated any more scientifically meaningful. Computer experts often use the term *GIGO* (garbage in–garbage out) to describe such a situation, and the reader must view studies using this approach with extreme caution.

A final epidemiologic procedure to be discussed is microbiologic sampling. As with diet the microbial flora represents one of the major factors in the etiology of dental caries. Taking samples from the oral cavity demands great care. An appreciation for the concept of ecologic niches (see Chap. 12) is mandatory in any sampling technique. The flora of the gingival crevice will differ from that of the occlusal surface of a molar, which will in turn pre-

sent a different picture from that of a sample obtained from the interproximal area. Culture techniques, including growth media and atmospheric conditions, will greatly affect the survivability and growth of the isolated bacteria. And finally, procedures for identification of the microorganisms must be well documented. For a more in-depth coverage of this topic, see Chapters 11, 12, 13.

Intraoral Caries Methods

The epidemiologic approach to research has yielded a wealth of information on dental caries. The method has, however, various drawbacks and limitations, as stated previously. For this reason several other approaches using the human model have been developed. One such general approach involves the use of teeth destined to be extracted. Sources of such teeth include premolars to be removed for othodontic reasons and third molars. While these are still in the mouth they can be subjected to various local experimental manipulations and after extraction analyzed by a multiplicity of techniques including histologic, chemical, and other degradative procedures. Examples of studies that have used this approach include the testing of pulp capping materials, the evaluation of fluoride uptake into tooth structure after exposure to topical agents, observation of the effect of high-speed rotary instruments on pulp pathology, and analysis of microleakage around restorative materials.

A partial alternative to tooth extraction has been the development of an enamel biopsy procedure. Basically, this method involves the polishing off of approximately 0.2 mg of enamel from any accessible tooth surface. A small felt cone impregnated with an abrasive material such as silicon carbide is coated with glycerine, which acts as a trap for the ground enamel particles. The felt cone and tooth material can then be analyzed for such things as trace element and mineral content. This procedure removes an enamel layer of less than 5μ and is similar to a pumice prophylaxis.

Another interesting approach to caries research involving human subjects is the intraoral cariogenicity test (ICT). Briefly, sterilized slabs of either human or bovine enamel are placed in an appliance resembling a removable partial denture. The enamel is set into a slot in the plastic flange area and covered with a Dacron mesh to encourage the retention of dental plaque (Fig. 23-2). Experiments that expose the enamel to the intraoral environment in combination with extraoral exposure to cariogenic conditions, such as frequent submersion in sucrose solutions, allow for a unique, as well as ingenious, experimental model.

While the epidemiologic approach to caries research generally depends on expression of the data as a total DMF score or in terms of an increased increment above a base level over a finite time period, the ICT allows for chemical analyses and observation of physical parameters of decay such as changes in enamel microhardness. A more in-depth discussion of the ICT is given in Chapter 19. In the future several other procedures for detecting caries will most certainly be developed. One such method showing promise involves measuring differences in electrical resistance between carious and sound teeth. Such advances will greatly aid the cariologist involved in studies employing human subjects.

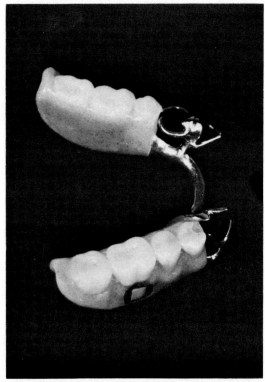

Fig. 23-2. A removable appliance used in the intraoral cariogenicity test (ICT). Note enamel slab in flange area. (Courtesy of Dr. Koulourides)

Legal and Ethical Requirements for the Protection of Human Research Subjects

Research involving human beings as experimental subjects is strictly regulated in most countries. In the United States the legal authority for these directives is described in Part 46 of Title 45, as amended, of the Department of Health, Education, and Welfare (DHEW) *Regulations on Protection of Human Subjects.* These guidelines, published in the March 13, 1975 edition of the *Federal Register,* establish the ground rules for the setting up of Institutional Review Boards at research facilities to approve, monitor, and review projects involving human beings. The composition of these boards is spelled out and includes provisions for representation of lay as well as professional membership. It is the function of these boards to determine if human beings are involved as research subjects, and if so, if they are at risk or not. Characterization of research as involving "human beings at risk" is not a disqualification. The ratio of risks to benefits is the major determining factor. In "at risk" studies the DHEW regulations require the use of informed consent. Even in studies deemed "not at risk" it is often a matter of courtesy, respect, and wisdom to acquire a signed and witnessed informed consent from each individual in the study.

The contents of an appropriate informed consent form are also discussed in the *Regulations of Protection of Human Subjects.* The form should be written in the second person and use language that the subject can understand. This requires the avoidance or defining of technical terminology and provision for translations into other languages when a portion of the anticipated subject population does not understand English. The document should cover the following items:

1. A statement of the general purpose of the study and an invitation to participate.
2. A description of the procedures to be followed and any risks involved.
3. A statement of expected benefits, if any. The suggestion of a benefit can be a strong inducement and therefore should be limited to substantial and likely benefits.
4. If any standard and accepted treatment is being withheld, it should be discussed.

In addition any appropriate alternative procedures that might be advantageous should be described.

5. The rights to withdraw from the study at any time and to receive an answer to all questions must also be stated.

6. A statement discussing whether or not monetary compensation will be provided in the event of physical injury resulting from the research procedures.

A sample of the format and material to be contained in the consent form is shown in Figure 23-3.

An obligatory consideration in human studies where new procedures or therapeutic agents are being tested is the definition of an end point. This is a preestablished level of success above which the control population (subjected to either no treatment or the standard treatment) is allowed to receive the benefits of the study. Another necessary preexperimental condition is the definition of an end point due to the harmful effects of the agent being tested. With these precautions in mind the quality of the clinical investigation will be greatly improved.

Laboratory Animal Models

The use of laboratory animals as models for experimentation is a well-accepted and widespread practice. Laboratory animal breeding farms have developed species and strains that are susceptible to and/or develop diseases and syndromes that parallel those naturally occur-

---

Institution: _____

Project: _____

Investigator: _____

Subject: _____

Legally authorized representative
 of subject: _____

The undersigned investigator has presented orally to me,
_____(subject) (legally authorized representative of subject),
the following information with respect to me giving information consent for participation
of _____ in the above project:

(1) A fair explanation of the procedures to be followed, and their purposes, including identification of any procedures which are experimental;

(2) A description of any attendant discomforts and risks reasonably to be expected;

(3) A description of any benefits reasonably to be expected:

(4) A disclosure of any appropriate alternative procedures that might be advantageous for the subject:

(5) An offer to answer any inquiries concerning the procedures; and

(6) An instruction that (I) (subject for whom I am legally authorized representative) am free to withdraw consent and and to discontinue participation in the project or activity at any time without prejudice to (me) (subject for whom I am legally authorized representative).

(7) A statement relative to compensation for physical injury during the experiment.

Based on the foregoing information, I give consent to (my participation) (participation by the subject for whom I am the legally authorized representative) in the above project.

The information presented to me did not include any language through which (I) (the subject for whom I am legally authorized representative) was required to waive, or to appear to waive any legal rights including any release of the institution or its agents from liability or negligence.

Date and time	Auditor witness to oral presentation & signature of subject or legal representative	Date	Subject
			or
		Date	Legally Authorized Representative of Subject
		Date	Investigator

Fig. 23-3. Sample of the format and material to be contained in an informed-consent form as used at the University of Alabama in Birmingham.

ring in man. The selection of an animal model for dental caries depends greatly on the animal's susceptibility to the condition, which in turn is greatly dependent on factors such as tooth form, occlusion, relationship of contiguous soft tissues, and eating patterns. Basically, there are three types of caries lesions, those occurring in the crevices of pits and fissures, which result from retention of food and bacteria by impaction; those occurring on smooth surfaces; and those seen on root surfaces of the teeth. The latter two categories are more dependent on the adhesiveness of bacteria than the pit and fissure lesions are. Animal models such as the rat and nonhuman primates demonstrate well-developed retentive areas, while dogs, gerbils, and hamsters have fewer retentive areas in their dentitions.

The general question involved in determining the appropriateness of using an animal model in caries research is identical to that asked in any experimental field: "Are the results obtained from the animal model study applicable to the condition as it occurs in man?" To help answer that question in the affirmative, researchers into the problem of dental caries have put tremendous efforts into imposing strict controls over conditions for their studies. Among these are the use of highly inbred strains of animals to approach genetic uniformity; the use of chemically defined, or at least purified, diets; and the use of a defined oral flora as with gnotobiotes.

The selection of an optimal species for caries research depends on many factors. These include animal availability, genetic uniformity, availability of background data and sources of information, housing and care requirements, disease problems, cost, and adaptability of the animal to experimental manipulations. From the outset attention must be given to all aspects of animal care. During shipment of animals care must be taken to prevent exposure to extremes of temperature. Long waits at air terminals or on trucks during summer or winter months can prove extremely hazardous. Improper packaging and rough handling, including excessive noise exposure, can cause irreversible trauma, especially to pregnant animals and newborn. Delayed delivery can result in food and water deprivation. This can be avoided by careful flight scheduling to avoid weekends. In addition, exposure to infectious agents both en route and upon arrival should be avoided by the use of air vents and filters.

Once the animals arrive at a housing facility, they are exposed to multiple environmental variables. Room variables include temperature, humidity, light (duration, intensity, and quality), air flow, barometric pressure, odor, noise, exposure to chemicals, and the relationship to man and other animals. Cage variables, such as bedding, area, venting, foods, and litter mates, must also be considered. For information on housing requirements and recommended environmental conditions for animals, see Guide for the Care and Use of Laboratory Animals (1970), DHEW Publication No. NIH-74-23, U.S. Government Printing Office, Washington, D.C. 20402.

Rodent Models

The major species of rodents used in dental caries research are the albino rat, the cotton rat, and hamsters. These are all rodents of the suborder *Simplicidentata*. These animals are all monophyodents with the dental formula I 1/1 (one upper and one lower incisor), M 3/3 (three upper and three lower molars). On inspection it can be seen that a large distema, or gap, exists between the incisors and first molars in each of these animals (Figure 23-4). Another characteristic of the dentition of these animals is the continuously growing incisor. This tooth is kept at a constant eruption level by the combined processes of eruption and incisal abrasion. This tooth is covered by enamel on the labial and cementum and dentin on the lingual.

While the incisors are an inappropriate model for studying dental caries, they have proved of value as a model for tooth development. The molars of these animals present certain important species differences. In the hamster the cusps are conical in shape with wide sulci separating them (Figure 23-5). For the rat the tips are flat with areas of exposed dentin, and the cusps are separated by deep, V-shaped sulci. It is these characteristics that make the hamster a good model for smooth surface caries, while the rat, because of the presence of deep sulci on the occlusal surface, better serves as a model for pit and fissure decay.

All three rat molars weigh a total of approximately 40 mg. One advantage of the hamster over the rat is the ability to open its mouth 180°. This accessibility allows for visual inspection of the dentition throughout the ex-

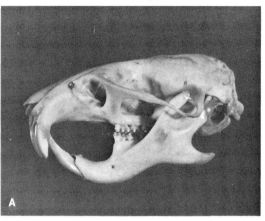
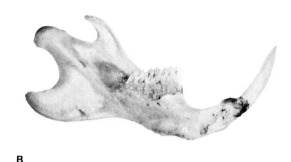

Fig. 23-4. **A.** Skull from an albino rat. **B.** Dentition of the albino rat. Note sagittally sectioned teeth.

periment, as well as for the ability to more easily incorporate the topical application of various agents into the research protocol.

Other rodents such as the gerbil and mouse have been used to a lesser extent in caries studies. The guinea pig and rabbit are seldom used as caries models. These animals have continuously erupting molars that further compromises their usefulness.

Other Animal Models

Whereas the majority of animal experimentation in the field of cariology has involved rodents, other animals have been used. These include the miniature pig and nonhuman primates. Although studies using the miniature pig have been reported, it should be recognized that these animals, although called "miniature," still grow to be 100–200 lb. For

obvious reasons, including housing, feeding, and handling, these animals have had limited use.

Several nonhuman primates have been adapted for caries studies. The South American marmaset, *Macaca mulatta* (rhesus monkey), *M. fascicularis* from the Philippines and Malaya, and the baboon are some of the more common of these. The dental characteristics of these animals are very similar to those of human beings. The nonhuman primates have both a deciduous and permanent dentition, an identical formula to man [2(I 2/2 + C 1/1 + P 2/2 + M 3/3 = 32], as well as a striking similarity in tooth morphology. Eruption patterns are also analagous to man, the permanent teeth erupting over the ages of 18 months to 7 years in *M. fascicularis*.

Domesticated animals such as the cat and dog are never used in caries studies. The teeth of these animals are conical in shape without the presence of deep sulci. This, plus diet habits, precludes their susceptibility to dental caries and eliminates them as appropriate animal models.

Pathogen-Free and Germ-Free Models

Since dental caries is a disease dependent on a microbial flora for its initiation and progression, investigations into the composition, biochemistry, and growth kinetics of cariogenic organisms have been seen as worthwhile endeavors. To accomplish these studies using an animal model, several approaches are available to the researcher. One such approach involves the use of conven-

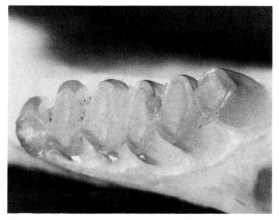

Fig. 23-5. Hamster molars.

tionally housed animals. The oral flora can be sampled both during the study and at the time of sacrifice. Obviously, the data gathered by this method will be greatly influenced by the flora already present at the start of the experimental period.

A second approach to microbiologic studies is the use of conventionally housed animals who are dosed with multiple antibiotics to suppress the oral flora. These animals are then infected orally with strains of bacteria resistant to the antibiotic regimen. Through this technique the effect of single organisms on the caries process can be tested without the use of complex housing equipment.

Another method commonly used in caries research involves the employment of sterile isolators (see Fig. 23-6). Just before birth the pregnant rat is anesthetized and taped to the outer wall of the isolator. The rat pups are obtained by Caesarian delivery directly into the isolator. Germ-free offspring are now commercially available, and there is no need to start a new colony by Caesarian delivery. Animals obtained in this manner are referred to as "germ free," but this is not exactly true or is at least hard to prove. A more appropriate term is *gnotobiotic*, which designates the fact that the resident microbial flora is known within the limits of detection. The gnotobiotic rat has been a tremendously valuable tool since the first studies in the early 1950s. Oral monoinfection of gnotobiotes with pure

strains of bacteria has resulted in a wealth of information on the role of specific bacteria in the etiology of dental caries. However, use of the monoinfection technique also has certain limitations. The investigator must first ensure implantation and infection with the microorganism, and this is often dependent on the type diet supplied to the animals. In addition the use of pure strains of virulent bacteria can often overwhelm the effect of other experimental variables such as diet or preventive agents. Again, care and preparation must be a major consideration in planning experiments using this technique.

Diets

The role of the diet in caries research is twofold. First, the diet must supply the 50-plus essential nutrients that the animal cannot biochemically synthesize by itself, as well as provide for ample energy sources. Secondly, in caries studies the diet must contain a cariogenic insult in the form of fermentable, and available, carbohydrate (sugar). It is this carbohydrate that helps in the selection, implantation, growth, and metabolism of the bacterial population.

For rodents a diet should contain 20%–25% protein of a good quality during the periods of growth, gestation, and lactation. A level of 15% protein is adequate for normal mainte-

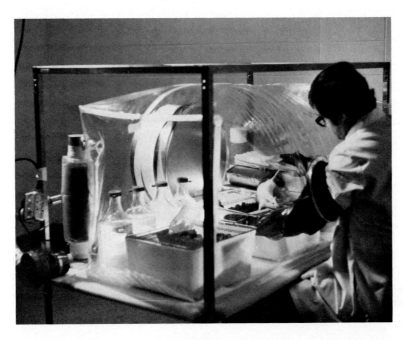

Fig. 23-6. Germ-free isolator. (Courtesy of Dr. Navia)

nance. A supply of essential fatty acids should be contained in the 5%–10% fat component. Vitamin requirements for rodents are the same as for man with the exception of vitamin C. Only the guinea pig requires this nutrient. Minerals (3%–5%) in the form of salt mixes are also needed. Bulk in the form of 4%–6% cellulose should also be supplied.

For nonhuman primates most is known about the nutritional requirements for the rhesus monkey. However, the question of minimal requirements versus optimal levels of nutrients for these animals remains obscure at this time.

Historically, attemps to formulate caries-promoting diets were first reported in the early 1930s. These diets were combinations of natural foodstuffs such as rice, whole milk powder, alfalfa leaf meal, and sodium chloride. Some decay in the sulci resulted from this type of diet, but the major result was fracturing of cusps because of the coarse texture of the meal. In addition, no smooth surface lesions could be induced with this diet. An advancement came in the 1940s with a change to a finely powdered diet consisting mostly of corn meal and whole milk powder. This diet and one composed of natural foods and 17% sucrose were the first to give rise to smooth surface lesions in rodents. The next improvement in diets came in the 1950s with the development of purified diets. While natural diets are made from natural foods such as corn, rice, alfalfa, and milk solids, purified diets are constructed from pure ingredients such as sucrose, casein, salts, vitamin mixtures, and vegetable oils. A further sophistication in diet preparation is the chemically defined diet. In this approach, pure amino acids are substituted for proteins, and specific fatty acids (linolenic, for example) would replace the oil. These diets are, however, extremely expensive and are only a slight improvement over purified diets for caries research. The purified diet still allows for changes in single ingredients, an impossibility when natural diets are employed.

For caries studies the ability of the diet to promote decay is obviously of great importance. In addition to the contents of the diet, especially the amount of fermentable carbohydrate, other factors such as particle size, palatability, eating and drinking patterns, retention and clearance of the diet, bedding material, and age of the animal also play an important role.

While this material refers to diets consumed by the weaned animal, there are times when the investigator desires to impose the nutritional intervention while the animal is still in the suckling stage. To accomplish this, several approaches are available. Some workers have surgically connected a tube directly to the stomach through the skin and fed the animals in this manner. Another approach used with a great deal of success is intubation (see Fig. 23-7). By this method an artificial milk made to simulate rat milk can be used alone or to supplement the mother's milk during the entire suckling period. By varying the content of the artificial milk, various nutrients can be tested while the teeth are going through their developmental stages.

In addition to presenting the food in a cup in a conventional cage several other methods of diet delivery exist for the postsuckling animal. One apparatus integrates the diet and water holders with an electrobalance (see Fig. 23-8). Through the use of a printout attachment the amount, frequency, and pattern of intake can be monitored. A second approach to controlling diet intake uses a pro-

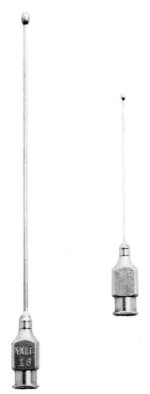

Fig. 23-7. Ball-tipped needle used for intubating baby rats.

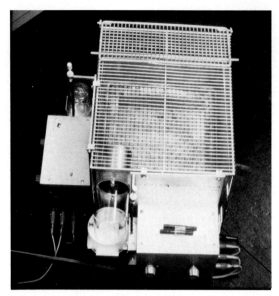

Fig. 23-8. Electrobalance feeding cage. These cages allow for food and water consumption to be monitored on a printout sheet.

grammed feeding machine (see Fig. 23-9). This device includes a rotary tray similar to a lazy-Susan controlled by a timer. In this manner food and liquid can be fed in "meals" and "snacks" to approximate human eating patterns more closely.

Whatever the approach to caries research, it must be understood that the diet is an extremely important experimental variable. Control of the contents, as well as frequency, amount, consistency, and pattern of dietary intake, is basic to the study if meaningful data are to be generated.

Caries Scoring

For almost all human and animal research in the field of cariology it is important to be able to make some estimate of the caries status in the experimental model. To accomplish this, several methods of caries scoring have evolved. For human studies (discussed earlier in this chapter) an evaluation based on decayed, missing, and filled teeth seems to be an adequate method of developing meaningful estimates of caries prevalence. Most often the caries increment over a finite period is used to compare two or more groups exposed to different experimental regimes.

In using an animal model, a similar goal to assess caries status exists. The factors that de-

termine the caries score include the species used, the age of the animal at the start of the experiment, the length of the experimental period, the site in the dentition to be examined, the progression of the caries attack, the diet used, and the method, if any, of flora inoculation. In rodents and nonhuman primates it is common to score caries on proximal, buccal, lingual, sulcal (fissures), morsal (cusp area), and root or cervical surfaces.

The jaws and teeth are usually prepared by dissection of the soft tissue from the jaws of decapitated animals. This step can be facilitated by boiling in a soap solution or autoclaving the severed heads. Depending on the scoring system used, a fixation and preservation step may or may not be required. Another method sometimes used to remove the soft tissue employs a dermestid beetle colony. These carnivorous insects can completely strip a jaw in a few days.

Some caries-scoring techniques call for the application of a stain. Commonly used stains include Kernechtrot B salt, silver nitrate, Alizarin blue S, Alizarin red S, and ammonium purpurate. These stains usually depend on the presence of free calcium or other reactive groups in the demineralized lesion.

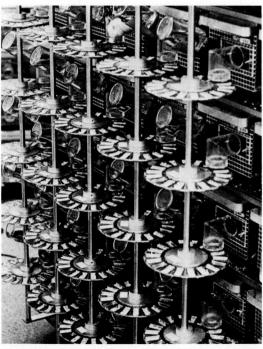

Fig. 23-9. König feeder. A programmable feeding machine.

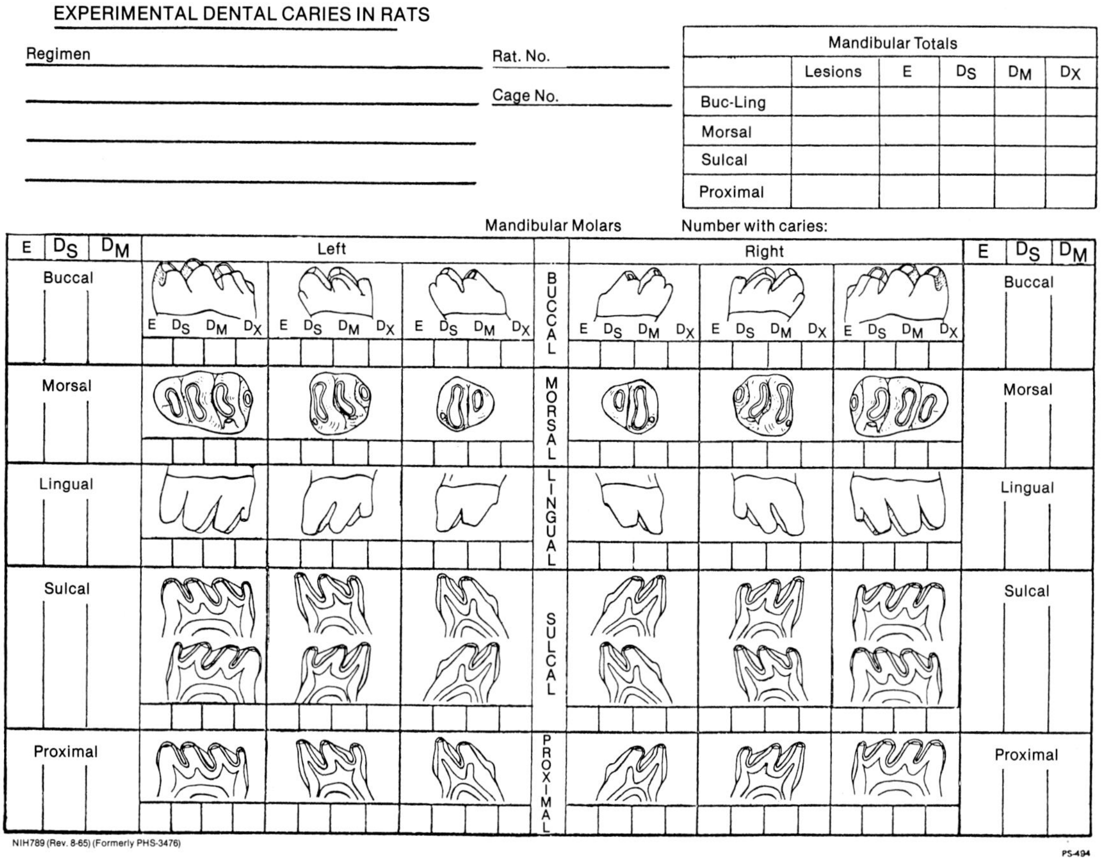

EXPERIMENTAL DENTAL CARIES IN RATS

Regimen _____

Rat. No. _____

Cage No. _____

	Mandibular Totals				
	Lesions	E	D_S	D_M	D_X
Buc-Ling					
Morsal					
Sulcal					
Proximal					

Mandibular Molars   Number with caries:

E	D_S	D_M	Left			Right			E	D_S	D_M
Buccal						B U C C A L			Buccal		
			E D_S D_M D_X	E D_S D_M D_X	E D_S D_M D_X	E D_S D_M D_X	E D_S D_M D_X	E D_S D_M D_X			
Morsal						M O R S A L			Morsal		
Lingual						L I N G U A L			Lingual		
Sulcal						S U L C A L			Sulcal		
Proximal						P R O X I M A L			Proximal		

NIH789 (Rev. 8-65) (Formerly PHS-3476)   PS-494

Fig. 23-10. Caries-scoring sheet for rat teeth (NIDR). E = enamel; D_s = slight dentin involvement; D_m = moderate dentin involvement; D_x = extensive dentin involvement; P = proximal.

The actual scoring procedure is done under magnification of approximately 15×. The various scoring systems have certain common points. Usually a set number of sites on specific teeth are assigned a value related to the area and depth of penetration of the lesion. Both tooth area and tooth depth affected by caries can then be estimated. Some techniques involve planimetric analysis of standardized photographs.

To assess the penetration of the lesion into the tooth, methods have been developed in which the teeth are ground away to known depths, scored, and ground again for further scoring. An improved approach has come with the advent of hard-tissue slicers that allow four or more sagittal sections to be made through each tooth. These sections are then placed on microscope slides and scored for caries progression.

The selection of the appropriate caries-scoring technique depends on the goals of the investigator. Does the experiment call for as-sessing the number of carious teeth, the total number of lesions, the volume of decay (area × depth) or the progression of the decay? Only after the researcher answers these questions can the proper scoring procedure for that study be determined. The final step is to transfer the data to a standardized scoring form. Shown in Figure 23-10 is a scoring sheet developed at the National Institute of Dental Research for studies involving rat teeth. Note that the system allows for scoring caries on all surfaces, as well as for scoring depth of penetration of the lesion.

In Vitro STUDIES

The Artificial Mouth

Dental caries is a disease initiated by the attack of acid products from bacterial metabolism on the external surfaces of the tooth.

This unifying concept of the disease makes dental caries a prime candidate for investigation using *in vitro* techniques. The origin of the concept of the artificial mouth is generally traced back to Magitot, who in the 1870s placed extracted teeth in sugar solutions for up to 2 years. In the group where the solution was sterilized, no caries resulted; in the group where creosote was added, no caries resulted. However, in the group of solutions inoculated with bacteria the teeth got caries. Magitot did a second classic experiment by using, not the bacteria, but their acid products to show the underlying cause of destruction in the carious tooth. These experiments were followed by the equally dramatic studies of W. D. Miller. To a vial containing extracted teeth Miller added sugar, bread, and other foods and human saliva. During the several months of incubation Miller was able to observe the pattern of carious attack on whole and sectioned teeth.

In the 1940s Dietz advanced the artificial mouth as a tool for caries research by sectioning teeth and placing them between two glass slides. The slides were then put into a chamber containing a nutrient medium, and the progression of the disease was followed. Another approach to an artificial mouth is to indent teeth into agar, remove the tooth, add saliva, and then replace the tooth for incubation. A more elaborate artificial mouth has been designed by Pigman that takes into account the pH, cleansing factors, saliva composition, and temperature. The progress of the disease can then be monitored through periodic photographs and radiographs.

The main drawback to the artificial mouth approach is that the lesion produced is usually a generalized decalcification rather than the penetrating lesion seen *in vivo*. A combination of *in vivo–in vitro* approaches was suggested as long ago as the 1860s. Mantagezza took sound extracted teeth and used them as replacements in dentures as well as for crowns, which he placed into the remaining roots of his patient's teeth. He observed that these prosthetic replacements were susceptible to decay and was the first to point out that tooth vitality was not a prerequisite for caries. This *in vivo–in vitro* technique has been greatly improved upon (see Chap. 19). The ICT developed by Koulourides (see Fig. 23-2) has allowed for great control over experimental conditions, a minimization of the risk of caries to the experimental subject, the ability to do many repetitions in a short time, extreme simplicity of approach, and low costs. However, the ultimate question of the applicability of the *in vitro* results to the *in vivo* condition still awaits a final answer.

Laboratory Procedures

In addition to the production of caries using the artificial mouth several laboratory procedures are available for the biophysical assessment of the lesion. These techniques can be classified as either destructive or nondestructive. The more commonly used methods are discussed here.

NONDESTRUCTIVE BIOPHYSICAL METHODS

Dental caries involves the production of microspaces in tooth structure. These spaces can be detected by a technique known as microradiography. Thin sections of the teeth are imbedded in methylmethacrylate and bombarded with x-rays. The penetration onto the photographic emulsion is a quantitative measure of the state of mineralization of the tooth area.

In autoradiography a radioactive isotope is injected into the living animal. Such tooth and bone seekers as calcium, strontium, fluorine, and phosphate are commonly used. The teeth are sectioned and placed on glass slides in contact with a photographic emulsion. The appearance of black silver grains on the developed film indicates the presence of the isotope in the tissue.

Various spectographic techniques are also available to the dental researcher. Basically they all depend on the interaction of nuclei, atoms, or molecules with a radiant energy source, resulting in the absorption or emission of a characteristic energy. For example, in infrared spectroscopy the external energy source has a wavelength of approximately 1–300μ. Another technique available is x-ray diffraction. With this procedure, when x-rays strike a crystal, such as hydroxyapatite, electrons scatter part of the energy, forming waves that enhance or interfere with each other. The patterns formed are characteristic for the crystal and are captured on films. These, and such other approaches as polarizing and electron microscopy, scanning electron microscopy, and the electron microprobe are in daily use in research laboratories.

DESTRUCTIVE BIOPHYSICAL METHODS

Whereas all these methods leave the tissue intact, it is sometimes essential to use destructive techniques in data collection. To get samples of tooth material for the analyses, it may be necessary to pulverize the teeth. A modified dental amalgamator has been found to be useful for this. Grinding with rotary instruments to get samples at varying depths may also be appropriate, as are punched biopsies from tooth sections. Acid etching with perchloric acid to calibrated depths has also proved valuable in tooth analysis. A biopsy technique on live patients has also been developed (see Intraoral Caries Methods.)

The separation of enamel and dentin from ground teeth is also possible. A differential flotation method in a bromoform:acetone mixture is available based on the different densities of enamel and dentin. Other commonly used analytic techniques include dry and wet ashing. Acid dissolution of enamel and microhardness testing (see Ch. 19) have also proved to be of value to dental researchers.

In general there is a limitless catalog of techniques available to the investigator, depending on the goals of the specific experiment. The listing here is simply intended to acquaint the reader with the more commonly used procedures. With this material as background the reader will hopefully be more capable of understanding the research literature in cariology and perhaps be stimulated to partake in the excitement of investigation.

GLOSSARY

Artificial mouth. An experimental *in vitro* approximation of the conditions in the oral cavity. The apparatus can vary in complexity from a test tube containing nutrients, a tooth, and bacteria to a machine designed to recreate the temperature, pH, salivary flow, clearance rates, etc., of an actual human mouth.

Caries increment. The increase/decrease in the number of caries lesions over a finite time period.

Chemically defined diet. A diet made up of ingredients based on their chemical constituents. For example, the individual amino acids rather than a protein would be used.

def. The decayed, indicated for extraction, and filled deciduous teeth. Used as an indication of caries prevalence in the primary dentition.

Dermestid beetle. A carnivorous insect used to clean the soft tissue from animal jaws in preparation for caries scoring.

Diastema. A space between two adjacent teeth in the same arch.

dmf. Decayed, missing, and filled deciduous teeth. Usually the "m" factor is limited to canines and molars in the primary dentition.

DMF-T. Decayed, missing, and filled teeth. The most commonly used index of caries prevalence in human populations.

DMF-S. Decayed, missing, and filled surfaces.

Enamel biopsy. A technique by which minute samples of tooth material from patients are obtained for analysis. The method utilizes a felt cone imbedded with a mild abrasive.

Epidemiology. The science of assessing the incidence and prevalence of diseases in human populations.

Gnotobiote. An animal in which all detectable bacteria, viruses, fungi, etc. are known to be absent or in which the organisms present are known to the investigator.

Hawthorne effect. The concept that bias is introduced into a study simply because research subjects react in an unnatural manner if they know that they are participating in an experiment.

ICT. Intraoral cariogenicity test. An intraoral method for assessing dental caries that combines the *in vivo* and *in vitro* approaches. Slabs of enamel are placed into removable prostheses which are worn by the test subject. These slabs are subjected to the experimental variables externally and are later removed from the appliance for analyses.

Incidence. The extent to which new cases of a disease occur in a given time period.

Increment. The increase in occurrence of an entity above a base line after a fixed time period.

In vitro. In a test tube. Refers to laboratory (nonanimal, nonhuman) studies.

In vivo. Studies done in the living body, either human or animal.

Monoinfection. Infection with a single variety of microorganism.

Monophyodont. Having only one set of teeth, therefore, no deciduous (primary) dentition.

Prevalence. The actual amount of a disease present in a population at a point in time.

Purified diet. A diet made from pure ingredients such as sucrose, casein, and vitamin mixtures, as opposed to using natural foods as the source of these nutrients.

SUGGESTED READINGS

Anbar M, St. John GA, Elward TE: Organic polymeric polyphosphonates as potential preventive agents of dental caries: *in vivo* experiments. J Dent Res 53: 1240–1244, 1974

Brown LR, Wheatcroft MG, Frome WJ, Rider LJ: Effects of a simulated skylab mission on the oral health of astronauts. J Dent Res 53: 1268–1275, 1974

Caldwell RC, Sandham HJ, Mann WV, Formicola AJ: The effect of a dextranase mouthwash on dental plaque in young adults and children. J Am Dent Assoc 82: 124–131, 1971

Cariostatic mechanisms of fluorides. Proceedings of a workshop organized by the American Dental Association Health Foundation and the National Institute of Dental Research, eds. WE Brown, KG Konig. Car Res 11: 1–327, 1976

Council on Dental Research, American Dental Association: Ethical guidelines for clinical investigation: ethical policy of the American Dental Association regarding the use of human subjects in clinical research. J Am Dent Assoc 86: 687–689, 1975

Donoghue HD: Composition of dental plaque obtained from eight sites in the mouth of a 10-year-old girl. J Dent Res 53: 1289–1293, 1974

Duany LF, Jablon JM, Zinner DD: Epidemiologic studies of caries-free and caries-active students: I Prevalence of potentially cariogenic streptococci. J Dent Res 51: 723–726, 1972

Fitzgerald RJ, Keyes PH: Demonstration of the etiologic role of streptococci in experimental caries in the hamster. J Amer Dent Assoc 61: 9–19, 1960

Green RM, Drucker DB, Blackmond DK: The reproducibility of experimental caries studies within and between two inbred strains of gnotobiotic rat. Arch Oral Biol 19: 1049–1054, 1974

Guide for the care and use of laboratory animals, DHEW Publication NIH 7423, U.S. Government Printing Office, Washington, D.C. 20402, 1975

Harris RS (ed): The art and science of dental caries research. Academic Press, New York 1968

Hunt CE, Navia JM: Pre-eruptive effects of Mo, B, Sr and F on Dental Caries in the Rat. Arch Oral Biol 20: 497–501, 1975

Ikeda T, Sandham HJ, Bradley EL Jr: Changes in *streptococcus mutans* and lactobacilli in plaque in relation to the initiation of dental caries in negro children. Arch Oral Biol 18: 555–566, 1973

Kelstrup J, Theilade J, Poulsen S, Moller IJ: Bacteriological, electron microscopical, and biochemical studies on dentogingival plaque of Moroccan children from an area with low caries prevalence. Caries Res 8: 61–83, 1974

Keyes PH: Dental caries in the molar teeth of rats. II A method for diagnosing and scoring several types of lesions simultaneously. J Dent Res 37: 1088–1099, 1958

Koulourides T: Remineralization methods. Ann New York Acad Sci 153: 84–101, 1968

Lehner T, Challacombe SJ, Cladwell J: An experimental model for immunological studies of dental caries in the rhesus monkey. Arch Oral Biol 20: 289–304, 1975

Menaker L, Navia JM: The effect of undernutrition during the perinatal period on caries development in the rat. II Caries susceptibility in underfed rats supplemented with protein or caloric additions during the suckling period. J Dent Res 52: 680–687, 1973

Navia JM: Animal models in dental research. Univ of Ala Press, Tuscaloosa, 1977

Navia JM: Evaluation of nutritional and dietary factors that modify animal caries. J Dent Res 49: 1213–1227, 1970

Research in Dentistry, Special Issue British Medical Bulletin 31:99–180, 1975

Takuma S, Ogiwara H, Suziki H: Electron-probe and electron microscope studies of carious dentinal lesions with a remineralized surface layer. Caries Res. 9: 278–285, 1975

Tanzer JM: Some important considerations with respect to food and water consumption in animal caries studies. J Dent Res 55: C215–C220, 1976

Taubman MA, Smith DJ: Effects of local immunization with *streptococcus mutans* on induction of salivary immunoglobulin A antibody and experimental dental caries in rats. Infect Immunity 9: 1079–1091, 1974

Van Reen R, Konig KG, Ostrom CA, McClure FJ: Evaluation of dental caries in the rat—a comparison of grinding and slicing techniques in two strains of rats fed a purified diet of high cariogenic capacity with orthophosphate supplements. Arch Oral Biol 7: 481–489, 1962

Wachtel LW, Brown LR: *In Vitro* Caries—factors influencing the shape of the developing lesion. Arch Oral Biol 8: 99–107, 1963

Index

Page numbers in *italics* indicate figures; "t" indicates tabular matter.

Acid(s). *See also Specific acids*
  conditions, survival of, by micro-
    organisms, 309
  demineralization of enamel, in
    caries, 248
  dissolution of enamel by, 202–
    203, 205–206, *203*
  in caries, 202, 214–215
  etching of enamel. *See* Enamel,
    acid etching of
  neutralization of, by saliva, 138
  organic, functional, 292
    production of, in amensalism,
    292
  plaque-mediated, penetration of
    enamel by, 253
  production, as prerequisite for
    cariogenic organism, 309
  plaque, carbohydrate metabo-
    lism in, 325–326
  volatile fatty, in plaque, 292–293
Acinus(i), of parotid gland, 19–20,
  23–28, *19, 21, 22, 26, 27, 28,*
  29
  of salivary glands, 8–13, *8, 9, 11,*
  12
    anatomic features of, 68, *68*
    autonomic effects on, 71–72
    during protein secretion, 76
    enzyme-mediated responses of,
      during eating reflex secretion,
      105
    submandibular, 40–41, *43*
Actinobolin, actions of, 400
  in caries control, 400–402
Actinomyces, on tooth surface(s),
  321
  cemental, 397
Actinomyces viscosus, in bacterial
  adherence, 284
  in plaque formation, second
    stage, 273
Activity coefficients, concept of,
  425–426
  definition of, 425
Adenosine monophosphate, cyclic.
  See cAMP
Adherence mechanisms, 280
Adrenergic receptors, salivary
  glands and, 70, 71
α-Adrenergic receptors, salivary secretion and, 70, 71
  stimulation of, parotid cellular
    changes in, *77, 78*
β-Adrenergic receptor(s), occupation to protein phosphoryla-

tion, sequence of events
  from, 79, *79*
  salivary secretion and, 70, *71*
  stimulation of, in protein secre-
    tion, 77–79
Age, as factor in saliva composition,
  141
  caries incidence related to, 218,
    218, 219
Agglutination, by saliva, 121
  direct, of bacteria, 125
Agglutinin(s), salivary, 120–122
Albumin, and digestive enzymes,
  115
  in salivary secretions, 115, 286
Albylamines, as antiplaque agents,
  411
Alcian blue stain, mucous secretions of salivary glands and,
  17–18, *17, 18*
  serous secretions of salivary
    glands and, 17
Aldosterone, in sodium extraction,
  138
Alexidine, 402, 404
Allysine, in cross linking of collagen, 176, *176*
Alveolus, of gland, definition on, 7, *8*
Ameloblasts, in formation of
  enamel, 187–188
Amelogenins, 187
Amensalism, of oral microorganisms, 292
Amino acid(s), analysis, of experimental pellicles, 158–159,
  161–163, *158, 163*
  of natural pellicle, 155–156,
    317, *156, 157*
  aromatic, salivary proteins rich
    in, 119–120
  in collagen, structures of, 170,
    171
  composition, of collagens and
    dentin phosphoprotein, 184t
  of enamel proteins, 188t
  metabolism, by plaque bacteria,
    326–327
  in plaque, 287, 318
  requirements, of oral microbiota,
    287
  in saliva, 287, 286t
β-Aminopropionitrile, in collagen
  studies, 177
Ammonia, and bacterial plaque, 142
  liberation of, plaque bacteria and,
    326–327

  salivary, 139
Ammonium compounds, quaternary, as antiplaque agents,
  411
cAMP, as intracellular mediator in
  secretory process, 79–80
  as second messenger, 79–80
  and calcium, in protein secretion,
    83
  concentration, rate of protein se-
    cretion and, 80
  dibutyryl, protein secretion and,
    80
  increase in, in β-adrenergic stim-
    ulation, 77–79
  influence of, on exocytosis, 80
  protein kinase and, 80, *79*
  ultrastructural changes in parotid
    gland caused by, *78*
Amphibians, salivary glands of, 4
Amylase, enzymes, isotypes of, 114,
  115
  salivary, 47, 54, 122
    functions of, 122
    isoelectric focusing of, on
      acrylamide gel, 122, *122*
    oral effects of, 323
Animals, laboratory, for caries research, recommended en-
  vironmental conditions for,
  506
    selection of, 505–506
    shipment of, 506
    species of, 507
    "germ free," 508
    gnotobiotic, 508
Antibiotics, broad spectrum, limitations of, in plaque control,
  398
  in caries, limitations of, 402
  description of, 397
  narrow spectrum, problems asso-
    ciated with, 399
  in plaque control and caries man-
    agement, 397–402
  systemic, long-term administra-
    tion of, caries incidence in,
    394
Antibody binding, to mucosal cells,
  125–126
Anticaries agents, fortification of
  food with, 328
Antimicrobial agents, in applicator
  trays, 392
  and bacterial equilibrium of oral
    cavity, 388

Antimicrobial agents (*continued*)
in caries management, 386–418
prospective applications of, 413–415
theoretical model for, 400, *401*
criteria for selecting, 390
delivery approaches for, 391–394
in dentifrices, 392
direct application of, 392–393
effectiveness of, errors in evaluation of, 387
ideal, properties of, 390–391
in mouthrinses, 391–392
for plaque control and caries management, 397–413
preventive strategies with, 389–390
selection and use of, 388–394
considerations in, 388–389
slow release delivery systems for, 393, *393*
systemically administered, 394
therapeutic strategies with, 389–390
topical applications of, 391–394
and vaccines, in combination therapy, 415
in varnishes, 393–394
Antiplaque agents, 388
Apatite(s), carbonate substitution in, 197, 202
chemical composition of, 196
crystallite, as aggregate of unit cells, 197, *200*
in enamel, dimensions of, 197, *196*
dissolution of, pH and, 138–139
and enamel, unit cell dimensions of, 198, 198t
of enamel, 188, 206
examples of, 197, 197t
fluoride-substituted, hydrogen bonds in, 201–202, *201*
mineral, 420
pure, and enamel, chemical composition of, compared, 198t
structure of, 196–197, 206
effects of ionic substitutions on, 199–202
pattern of, 199, *199*
synthetic and naturally occurring, formulae for, 197t
Apatitic precipitates, plaque pH and, 327
Apocrine glands, 5
Applicator trays, for antimicrobial agents, 392
Artificial mouth. *See* Mouth, artificial
Ascorbate deficiency, alterations in tooth development associated with, 346
ASPA, 470
Autoradiography, in caries research, 512

Bacteria. *See also* Microbiota, oral; Microflora, oral

acidogenic, in caries process, 214–215
aciduric, in caries process, 214–215
adhesion of, to plaque, 320–321
aggregation of, in whole saliva, 280
associated with caries, 395–397
attachment of, direct interspecies, 282–283, *283*
in interaction with dissimilar microbial species, 282–283, *283*
bypassing of surface crystallites by, in white spot enamel lesions, 237
in caries, 214
animal studies demonstrating, 300–301
colonizing pits and fissures of teeth, 321
direct agglutination of, 125
enzymes and, 323
filamentous, colonizing tooth surface, 321
interactions of, in plaque, 321
nutritional relationships between, 289
pellicles and, 159, 164, 314, *315*
physical entrapment of, in oral cavity, 284–285
plaque, adhesion, agglutination, and colonization by, 324–325
amino acid metabolism by, 326–327
biochemical activities of, 323–329
extracellular activities of, 323
intracellular activities of, 325–327
in plaque formation, 314, *315, 315*
four stages, 272–276, *272, 273, 274, 275, 276*
proliferation of, following tooth brushing, 118
reactions of salivary glycoproteins with, 121
site specific receptors of, 284
survival of, in carious dentin zone, following restoration, 256
on tooth, reduction of, in current research, 335
with peptidase or proteolytic activity, 288
Bacteriocins, bacterial interactions mediated by, 323
mode of action of, 293
and oral microflora, 293
selective activity of, 293
Staphlococcus epidermidis, S. mutans and, 293, 294
Streptococcus mutans and, 293, 294
Bass brushing technique, 489, 490–491
B-cells, 334–335
Benzoin methyl ether, 469
Bernard, Claude, investigations of salivary glands by, 66

Bicarbonate, changes in concentration of, and osmolality, in parotid secretion, 133, *134*
concentration, pH of saliva and, 138
secretory, and plasma, levels of, 135
Biopsy, enamel, in intraoral caries studies, 503
Birds, salivary glands of, 4
Bis biguanide(s), 402–405
mode of action of, 402
molecular configuration of, 402, *402*
and sodium fluoride, in combination therapy, 406–407
Bis-GMA, 464
and methyl methacrylate, 464
molecular structure of, 468
viscosity of, reduction of, 468
Blood, acquired covering of teeth and, 149
flow, blockage, selective, phenomenon of, in fluid secretion, 87, 88
increase, in fluid secretion, 87, 88
in salivary glands, changes in, evidence for, 96–97
salivary gland, and secretion, 66
and saliva, selected constituents of, compared, 140t
supply, as source of fluid, 84
Blood vessels, cholinergic-mediated changes in, in fluid secretion, 87
of salivary glands, 69
sympathetic effects on, 70
Bone(s), crystals, ionic pools around, 429, *429*
and mature enamel, physical properties of, compared, 192–193, 195t
mineral components of, 197
minerals, lability of, 428–430
support, as concern in dentistry, 421
Brushing, biologic effects of, 485–488
formation of new dental pellicle following, 117–118
frequency of, and quality of, as factors in oral health, 492–493
function of, view of, in 1920s, 485–486
gingival recession related to, 486–487
plaque formation following, 118
purpose of, 492
technique(s), 490–492
Bass, 489, 490–491
Charters, 491
Fones, 491
Physiologic, 491
relative popularity of, 490, *490*
Roll, 489, 491
Stillman, 491
Brushite, plaque pH and, 327

Calcification, abnormal 421
   induction of, 428, *428*
   activity coefficients and, 425–426
   chelation of calcium ions in, 423–425
   deficient, 421
   definition of, 420
   effect of pH on ionic product in, 421–423
   general problem of, 421–426
   ionic strength and, 425
   mechanism(s) of, alkaline phosphatase, 427
     booster, 427
     major factors in, 428
     template, 427–428
   studies of, historical background of, 420–421
Calcifying solutions, in remineralization of carious dentin, 256
Calciphylaxis, experimental, 428, *428*
Calcium, and cAMP, in protein secretion, 83
   as regulator of protein secretion, 83, 84
   citrate chelate, 424, *424*
   fluoride, on tooth surface, 453
   function of, in secretory process, 82–83
   hydroxyapatite, 227
   ion stabilization, surface, phosphoproteins and, 119
   ions, chelation of, in calcification, 423–425
   in parotid saliva, 139
   and phosphate, in plaque, 318–319
     saliva and, 142
     supersaturated, stabilization of, phosphoproteins in, 118–119
   -phosphorus ratio(s), of Alaskan Eskimo diets, 354–356, 356t
   of calcium phosphate salts, 426
   caries activity and, 350, *351*
   in enamel, 198, 346
   ideal, for caries resistance, 360
   in salivary aggregation of bacteria, 280
   in submandibular saliva, 139
   transport and deposition of, phosphoproteins in, 118
   triangles, of hydroxyapatite, 199–200, 201, *201*, 201t
Cancer, oral and gastric, relation of salivary components to, 144
Carbohydrate(s), caries and, 215–216, *216*
   dietary, in caries production, 352–353
     microbial activities mediated by, 352
     in oral disease, 352
     plaque metabolism and, 327–328
     reduction of intake of, for caries resistance, 359
   dissociation, from glycoproteins, in saliva, 286–287

exogenous, oral microorganisms and, 289–290
   of experimental pellicles, 159, 163, 316, *160*, *161*, *163*
   intake, relation of, to caries, 357–358, *357*
   metabolism, in plaque acid metabolism, 325–326
   of natural pellicle, 156, 316–317
   in plaque, 319–320
   restriction, during childhood, caries and, 358
   in saliva, 286t
   side chains of proteoglycans. *See* Glycosaminoglycan(s)
   soluble, composition of oral microbiota and, 290
   sources of, for oral microbiota, 286–287
Carbonate, in enamel, 198
   substitution, in apatites, 197, 202
Caries, acid dissolution of enamel in, 202
   crystallite core damaged by, 204, *204*, *205*
   rod regions damaged by, 202–203, *203*
   acute phase of, 227
   appearance of, variant picture of, 219–220
   arrest of, mechanisms in, 258
   arrested, 220, 227, 247–248, *221*
   as costly, 212
   as disfiguring disease, 212
   as ecologic consequence, 311
   as infectious disease, 337
   as multifactorial disease, 212, 214, 216, 433
     ecologic view of, 264
   bilateral occurrence of, 219
   cariogenic priming of, fluoride and, 454
   of cementum, 242–243
   cervical, clinical management of, 257
     fate of, 257, *257*
   chronic phase of, 227
   clinical course of, 223–224, *223*
   clinical management of, 256–258
   consolidation and regression of, studies of, 439
   correlations of, with civilization, 216–217
   crystallographic aspects of, 202–204
   deep, microflora of, 307
   definitions of, 212, 247
   in dentin. *See* Dentin, caries
   development of, age patterns of, 218, *218*, *219*
   factors involved in, 343, *344*
   familial patterns in, 217
   fluoride experience influencing, 223
   general comments on, 226–227
   geographical differences influencing, 217
   host factors influencing, 219–223
   national origins influencing, 217, *217*

salivary flow influencing, 222
   sexual patterns of, 217–218
   tooth composition influencing, 222–223
   tooth morphology influencing, 222
   and diet, epidemiologic relationships between, 353–356
   distribution of, in animal studies, 301–302, *302*, *303*
   in early man, 298
   and increase in, since Iron Age, 298–299, *299*
   present day, 297
   dysfunction in biologic mineralization in, 421
   ecologic concept of, importance of understanding, 297–298
     triad for, 297, 298
   ecologic triad for, 297, 298
   effect of sealants on, 478–479
   of enamel. *See* Enamel, caries
   epidemiologic considerations in, 216–219
   etiology of, acid dissolution in, 214–215
     bacteria in, 214
     carbohydrates in, 215–216, *216*
     chemoparasitic theory of, 213
     epidemiologic studies in, approaches in, 302–303
     areas of, 216–219
     major factors in, 214
     phosphoprotein phosphatase theory of, 213
     proteolysis-chelation theory of, 213
     proteolytic theory of, 213
     theory(ies) of, chelation causing mineral dissolution in, 424–425
     historical review of, 213–214, 299–300
   experimentation. *See* Experimentation, caries
   further exploration of, areas for, 247
   histopathology of, 226–246
   historical considerations of, 212–214
   immunity to, 222
     role of secretory IgA in, 337–338
   immunologic aspects of, 332–340
   immunology of, 335–338
   implications of, 211–212
     for dental profession, 223–224
     for society, 224
   incipient, as concern in sealant placement, 476
   increased prevalence of, statements explaining, 354
   index. *See* Index, caries
   in individuals aged twelve to seventeen, according to sex and age, *218*
   initiation of, bacterial specificity in, 300–307
     animal studies of, evidence

Caries (continued)
from, 300–301
microorganisms in, 301–
302, 301t, 302, 303
human studies of, evidence
from, 302–305
longitudinal studies in, 305–
307
interproximal, appearance of,
257–258
clinical management of, 257–
258
spontaneous arrestment of, 257,
258
management, antimicrobial
agents for, 397–413
microbial aspects of, 297–312
natural history of, 298–299, 299
neglect of, reasons for, 223–224
nutrition in. See Nutrition
nutritional modification of, prospects for, 359–362
occurrence of, intraoral patterns
of, 218–219, 219, 220
pain associated with, 212
pathogenesis of, stages in, 439
pit and fissure, 218, 219
clinical management of, 256–
257
plaque in initiation of, 214, 388
prevalence, recording of, in epidemiologic studies, 216, 500–
501
prevention, current methods in,
339
current research in, 335
factors for consideration in, 395
vaccine experiments in, 335–
337
rampant, 222, 222
fluoride therapy in, 458
onset of, microbial profile of,
305–307, 306
rate of tissue destruction in, factors influencing, 226–227
root surface, 219, 220
microbial agents of, 307
saliva composition and, 142–143
salivary endocrine theory of, fluid
movement through enamel
and, 137
salivary enzymes influencing, 143
scoring. See Index, caries
smooth surface, 218–219, 220
studies of. See Experimentation
caries
susceptibility to, and severity of,
factors influencing, 212
treatment of, emergency, 224
procedures in, 223
remineralization process in,
439–440
restorative measures in, 223
vaccine. See Vaccine
Cariogenesis, dentinal tubule fluid
movement and, 143–144
Cariogenicity test, intraoral, in caries studies, 433–438, 503–
504, 435, 436, 437, 438, 504

Cariology, clinical, 247–260
Cauque lesion, 346, 347
Cements, glass ionomer, 470
Cementum, 187
caries of, 242–243
Charters brushing technique, 491
Chelation, as term, origin of, 423
Chelator(s), characteristics of, 423
citrate anion as example of, 424
Chemoreceptors, in salivary secretion, 66
Chemotherapy, and caries, 400
in caries, prospects for, 387
combined, in caries, 406–407, 410
Children, nutritional counseling
for, 377–378, 379, 380
Chlorapatite, 197
Chlorhexidine, 388, 390, 394
absorption, 402
anticaries effectiveness of, 403–
404, 404t
as antiplaque agent, 402
bacterial resistance to, 403
characteristics of, 402–403
clinical trials with, 403–404
pellicle, and enamel surface, interaction between, 403, 403
retention halflife of, 403
side effects of, 403
and sodium fluoride, in combination therapy, 406–407
therapeutic uses of, 402
Chloride, concentration, changes
in, and osmolality, in parotid
secretion, 133, 134
range of, 135
secretion of, 135–136
Cholinergic receptors, salivary secretion and, 71
Chondroitin sulfates, 180, 180t, 180
Citrate, forms of, 424
Citric acid, carboxyl groups of, 424
Clinical examination, components
of, suggestive of nutritional
problems, 368t
in nutritional analysis, 367–368
Cocci, gram negative, of coronal
plaque, 268–269
on tongue, 268
gram positive, at gingival margin,
269
of coronal plaque, 268
on tongue, 267–268
Cocoa beans, factors from, as
cariostatic, 361
Collagen(s), amino acids in structure of, 170, 171
biosynthesis, 174, 173
catabolism of, 176–177
of cementum, 187
chains, cross linking of, 175–176,
176
in dentin, 184, 184t
extraction of, from tissues, for
study, 177
in fibril formation, 174–175, 173
in interstitial spaces, chain structure and distribution of, 171–
172, 172t

liberation of, from cells, 174
-like chains, 172–174
methods used to study, 177–179
molecules, extreme ends of, 170
native, proteases and, 170
organizational levels of, 169–170,
170
of periodontal ligament, 187
type I, 171, 172t
type I trimer, 172, 172t
type II, 171–172, 172t
type III, 172, 172t
types, 171–172, 172t
Collagenase, control of, 177
in destruction of collagen, 177
Complement system, activation of,
mucins in, 116
Compound glands, 6, 7, 6
Condensing vacuole(s), 74
and secretory granules, 74, 75
Connective tissues, collagen in. See
Collagen(s)
components of, necessity of understanding, 169
definition of, 168
protein constituents of, 169–179
proteoglycans of. See Proteoglycans
structural elements of, 168
Consent form, informed, contents
of, 504–505, 505
Copper, in saliva, plaque production and, 143
Corpuscles, salivary, 292
Crevicular fluid, as endogenous nutrient source, 286
Cuticle, 153, 153
Cvar method in evaluation of sealant effectiveness, 477
Cyanoacrylate(s), 464
as sealants, disadvantages of, 470
isobutyl, and methacrylates, bond
strengths of, compared, 472,
472t
molecular structure of, 470
methyl, molecular structure of,
470
polymerization by, 470
Cyanogen bromide, in collagen
studies, 177–179, 178

Defense mechanisms, mucosal, salivary proteins and, 124–127
Demilunes, of salivary glands, 14
Demineralization, cariogenic activity in terms of, 422–423, 423
Dental caries. See Caries
Dental plaque. See Plaque
Dental restorations, pellicle formation on, 164
Dentifrices, abrasive effects of, and
of toothbrushes, compared,
486
abrasivity index for, 486
effectiveness of, 392
fluoride, 453, 457
for patient application, 392
professionally applied, 392

penicillin-containing, studies of, 398
therapeutic, 453
Dentin, in acute cariogenic infection, 227
"blind tract," 255
canals of, foramina of, 239–240, *240*
caries, 253–256
active, indirect pulp capping in, 243
microscopic features of, 240–242, *241*
pathologic zones of, 240–242
spread of, 240
advancing front of, microflora of, 307, *308*
affected zone of, 254–255, 258
arrest of, factors enhancing, 248
arrested, microscopic features of, 242
pathologic zones of, 242
deep, microflora of, 307
hypermineralized zone of, 255, 258
infected zone of, 254, 258
microbial infection responsible for, fate of, 256
permanent restoration in, bacteria survival following, 256
zone(s), 254–255, 258
differentiation within lesion, 255
carious, therapeutic remineralization of, 255
cervical, abrasion of, gingival recession, and toothbrushing, 487
in chronic cariogenic infection, 227
collagen, 184
and skin collagen, compared, 184
and dentin phosphoprotein, amino acid composition of, 184t
composition of, 183
decalcification of, 184
development of, 239
and enamel, separation of, in caries research, 513
fluid flow in, 253–254
fluoride, 253
formation of, by odontoblasts, 185–187
radioautography in study of, 185–186
hydroxyapatite crystallites of, 253
intercanalicular, 239, *239*
intertubular, 239, *239*
matrix, dentinal tubules of, 253
mineral phase of, 253
organic phase of, 253
mature, structure of, 239
mineralization, external, 255–256, 258
internal, 255, 258
pericanalicular, 239, *239*
peritubular, 239, *239*

phosphoprotein of, 185
proteoglycans of, 184–185
and pulp, 238–239
reaction, 255
sclerotic, 255
sound, microanatomy of, 238–240
structural features of, 253
surface, and pulp, passage of molecules between, 254
transformation of predentin to, 185, 186
tubules of, in matrix, 253
Dentinogenesis, 185–187
radioautography in study of, 185–186
Dentist, in nutritional counseling, 365, 376, 278–379, 382
Dentition. *See* Tooth(Teeth)
Dermatan sulfate, 180, 180t, *180*
Detergents, definition of, 117
Dextran, in cell adhesion and agglutination, 324
in *S. mutans* aggregation, 283
Dextranase, in plaque disintegration, 411–412
Dialysis solutions, inadequate preparation of, fluoride toxicosis in, 448
Dicalcium phosphates, and fluoride, 410
Diet(s), analysis of, qualitative, in nutritional analysis, 368–369
semi-qualitative, in nutritional analysis, 369, *370–373*
as factor in saliva composition, 141
and caries, epidemiologic relationships between, 353–356
caries-promoting, formulation of, for diet survey, 509
composition of, modification of, 361–362
diary, computer-assisted dietary analysis of, 369, *370–373*
in nutritional analysis, 368–369
and ecology of oral microorganisms, 289
manipulation of, in caries control, 328
methods of delivery of, in diet surveys, 509–510, *509, 510*
and oral cavity, 343–344
patterns of, factors influencing, 376
plaque metabolism and, 327–328
physical consistency of, as influence on oral microflora and salivary gland function, 290
recommendations, for caries control, 328
for rodents, in diet survey, 508–509
role of, in caries, ignored by oral health professionals, 365
sugar in, influence of, on oral ecosystems, 289–290
supplementation, guidelines for, 383–384

in nutritional analysis, 374
survey(s), formulation of caries-promoting diets for, 509
methods of delivery of diet in, 509–510, *509, 510*
using animals, in caries research, 508–510
using humans, as epidemiologic study, 503
Dietary counseling. *See* Nutrition, counseling
Dietary trials, clinical, 356–359
Digestive enzymes, and salivary proteins, 115
Digitalis toxicity, salivary calcium-potassium ratios in, 145
Dihydrochalcones, 328
Dimethacrylates, 464
Disease, systemic, saliva composition and, 144–145
DMF scale, 216, 500–501, 502–503
for children, 501
factors limiting validity of, 501
and sucrose intake, in males and in females, compared, 356, *356*
Dumping syndrome, 138
Duraphat, 393, 394

Eccrine glands, 5
Ecosystem(s), definition of, 278
microbial, colonization of, 278–279
Electrolyte(s), content, of fluid, modification of, during secretion, 84
and fluid, secretion of, salivary secretion and, 65
major, concentrations of, in parotid gland, over range of flow rate, 133, *134*
and salivary gland secretory mechanisms, 136
salivary water and, and oral health, 132–147
secretion of. *See* Fluid and electrolyte secretion
Embedocles, and cause of disease, 429–430
Enamel, acid dissolution of, in caries, 202
crystallite core damage in, 204, 206, *204, 205*
rods in, 202–203, 205–206, *203*
acid etching of, action of topical fluorides and, 453
and adhesive dental techniques, historical use of, 463–464
agents for, 465–466
for bonding, importance of, 465, 466
depth of etch in, 467, 467t
etching patterns in, compared, 466, *467*
etching procedure for, 473–474
remineralization following, 467–468

Enamel (*continued*)
    unetched and etched specimens
        in, compared, 466, *466*
    adaptation, at sites of caried ini-
        tiation, enhancement of, 248
        to cariogenic challenge, condi-
            tions for, 430–431, *431*
        effects of local reactions in,
            431–432, *432*
        implications of, 432–433
    adhesion of sealant to, by chemi-
        cal bonding, primary, 465
        secondary, 465
        problems with, 464–468
    apatite, and caries, 191–207
    apatite crystals of, 188
    and apatites, unit cell dimensions
        of, 198, 198t
    as active chemical system, 191
    as three component system, 248–
        249
    bacterial flora of, 329
    biopsy procedure, in intraoral car-
        ies studies, 503
    brown spot lesions of, 257–258,
        433
    calcium-phosphorus molar ratio
        of, 198, 346
    carbonate content of, 198
    caries, biological mechanisms of,
        248–250
        clinical detection of, stage of le-
            sion for, 251
        development of, 250–253
        developmental stages and zones
            of, 250–253, *251*
        early, mineral content of, 253
        lesion in, definition of, 250
        microscopic examination of,
            250
        plaque pH and, 249
        Stage 3 lesion, micropores in,
            252, *252*
        Stage 4 lesion, white spots in,
            252, *252*
        subsurface demineralization in,
            251, *252*
        surface layer retention in, 252–
            253
    composition, during maturation,
        249
        following tooth eruption, 249
    coverings of, acquired after erup-
        tion of teeth, 149–165
        acquired pellicle, 152–165
        classification of, 149–165
        disagreement concerning, 148
        of embryologic origin, 149, *149,*
            150
        food debris, 150
        materia alba, 150–151
        nonmineralized, 148–166
        plaque, 151–152
    crystallites, 192–193
        arrangement of, 195–196, 228,
            195, 196, 230, 231
        core, acid dissolution of, 204,
            206, *204, 205*
        mature, 192, *194*
        precursors, 192, 205, *193*

    structural patterns of, 196, 205
    cuticle, primary, 149
    demineralization of, cariogenic
        activity in terms of, 422–423,
        454, *423*
    dental, water permeation of, 137
        "weeping phenomenon," 137
    and dentin, separation of, in car-
        ies research, 513
    diffusion pathways of, 228–237,
        238, *238*
    epithelium, reduced, 149, *149,*
        150
    fluid, 351
    fluoride, 249
        caries susceptibility and, 203–
            204, 310–311
        distribution of, in young adult
            from area of low water fluo-
            ride level, 249–250, *250*
        formation of, ameloblasts in, 187–
            188
        proteins in, 187, 188
    ground, microscopic examination
        of, in caries studies, 250
    hydroxyapatite in, 249
    intercrystallite matrix of, 228
    ionic substitution in, 201–202,
        249, *201*
    lamellae, 230–231, 232
        as inroads for caries producing
            bacteria, 231, 233
        and prism sheaths, 231, 233
    major inorganic component of,
        227
    maturation, 222–223, 228–230,
        249
        effect of sealants on, 478–479
        effects of nutrition on, 350
        posteruptive, 230
    mature, and bone, physical prop-
        erties of, compared, 192–193,
        195t
    undulating topography of, 227–
        228, *229*
    mineral, chemical composition
        of, 197–198
        and composition of apatites,
            compared, 198t
        variations in, factors causing,
            198
        structural composition of, 196–
            197, 198
    mineral phase of, 248, 249
    octacalcium phosphate in, 249
    pathological alterations in, zones
        of, 237
    penetration of, by plaque-me-
        diated acid, 253
    perikymata of, 227–228, *228*
    perikymata-Retzius diffusion
        pathways of, 233, *235*
    primary and secondary, etching
        and sealant retention of, dif-
        ferences in, 466
    "prismless," 466
    prisms of, 228, *231*
        sheaths of, 228, *230*
        and lamellae, 231, 233
    proteins, fetal, 187, 188

    mixture of, amino acid compo-
        sition of, 188t
    remineralization, 253, 419, 441
        concept of, 419–420
        experimental evidence support-
            ing, 433–439
        factors promoting, 350
        fluoride in, 430, 447
        following acid etching, 467–468
        impact of, on oral health pro-
            grams, 440–441
        Intraoral Cariogenicity Test in
            study of, 433–438, *435, 436,*
            437, 438
        lesions during, subsurface min-
            eral dissolution in, 433, *434*
        in treatment of caries, 439–440
        on removable appliance, in in-
            traoral cariogenicity test,
            503–504, *504*
    rod(s), 192
        acid dissolution of, 202–203,
            205–206, *203*
        arrangement of, in enamel,
            193–195, 464, *195, 465*
        crystallite orientation in, 195–
            196, *195, 196*
        structure of, 195–196, *195, 196*
    sieve concept, 250
    solubility, factors influencing,
        466–467
    solubility product of, 426
    sound, elements in, 249
        microanatomy of, 227–237
    spindles, 232, *234*
    Striae of Retzius of, 232, 233–
        237, *234, 236*
    structure of, crystalline, 464, *465*
        inorganic components of, 464
        levels of, 192–202
        organic component of, 464
        studies of, results of, 191–192
        subsurface structures of, 228–237
    surface of, sieve-like structure of,
        238, *238*
    surface topography of, 227–228,
        244, *228, 229*
    trace elements in, 249
    water phase of, 248–249
    white spot lesions of, 232, 237,
        250, *234*
        bypassing of surface crystallites
            by bacterial toxins in, 237
        fluorides in surface crystallites
            or intercrystallite matrix areas
            in, 237
        in interproximal caries, 257–258
        noncavitated, enigma of intact
            surface zone in, 237–238
        transport of internal minerals
            during dissolution and, 237
Endocrine glands, description of, 5
Enolase, fluoride and, 329
    inhibition of, by fluoride, 405, *405*
Environmental factors, changes in,
    effects of, on plaque flora,
    294–295
    influencing oral microbiota, 279
Enzyme(s), homopolysaccharide
    synthesizing, 323–324

-mediated reactions, sequential, in exocytosis, 81–82
oral bacteria and, 323
preparations, in plaque control, 411–412
protein carboxyl-methylase, in exocytosis, 81
proteolytic, proteoglycans and, 183
salivary, 122–123
caries and, 143
effects of, 323
Epidemiologic studies, approaches in, 302–303
design of, 500
diet survey in, 503
examples of, 500
facilities and equipment for, 501–502
factors studied in, 216–219, 501
microbiologic sampling in, 503
objective of, 500, 501
personnel for, 501
pitfalls of, 500
recording caries prevalence in, 500–501
recording of data from, 502, 502
relating diet to caries, exceptions to, 354–356
problems associated with, 354
Epidemiology, definition of, 216
Epithelium(a), cell surface of, half-life of, 127
enamel, reduced, 149, 149, 150
"leaky," junctional resistance in, 97–98
oral, cells of, bacterial adherence to, 282
"tight" and "leaky," classification of, 97
freeze-fracture studies of, 102
transepithelial channels of, 97–98
"very tight," 102
Epoxylite 9070, 464
Excretory ducts, of parotid gland, 21–22, 32, 24, 25, 41, 42
of salivary glands, palatine, 51, 53
submandibular, 42–44, 46
Exocrine glands, classification of, 6, 6
description of, 5
Exocytosis, 74, 75–77
influence of cAMP on, 80
possible sequential enzymatic events in, 81–82
role of transmethylation in, 81
Experimentation, caries, 499–514
biophysical methods in, destructive, 513
nondestructive, 512–513
caries scoring in, 510–511, 511
diet surveys in, 503, 508–510
epidemiologic survey methods in. See Epidemiologic studies
human studies in, 500–505
in vitro studies in, 511–513
intraoral caries methods in, 503–504
laboratory animal models in, 505–506

legal and ethical requirements for protection of subjects in, 504–505, 505
pathogen-free and germ-free models in, 507–508
rodent models for, 506–507, 507
Extralobular ducts, of salivary glands, 16

Family differences, caries incidence related to, 217
Fats, anti-caries effect of, 353
exogenous, oral microorganisms and, 290
Feeding cage, electrobalance, for diet survey, 509, 510
Feeding machine, programmed, for diet survey, 509–510, 510
Fish, mucous secretion by, 4
salivary glands in, 4
Flora, oral, acquisition of, 271–272
composition and ecology of, 263–277
microbial succession of, 270–276
Fluid(s), blood supply as source of, 84
crevicular, as endogenous nutrient source, 286
and electrolyte secretion, cellular site of, evidence for, 99–100
definition of, 84
energy for, 67
primary site for, 67
salivary, micropuncture studies of, 86–87
modern view of, 85
salivary secretion and, 65
flow, in dentin, 253–254
gingival, mixed saliva, and aqueous phase of plaque, compared, 317, 318t
gingival crevice, whole saliva, and plaque components, compared, 318t
hypotonic, bathing oral tissues, advantages of, 136
direct generation of, through gap junctions, evidence for, 101–102
movement, dentinal tubule, 143–144
oral, effects of nutrition on, 351
foods, and plaque, interrelationships of, 316
resorption, sodium transport and, 101
secretion, by salivary glands, potassium concentration and, 136
energetics of, 85
hypotonic, functional significance of, 136–138
mechanisms of, during eating reflex stimulated secretion, 90
recent hypothesis of, energetics of secretion in, 95, 95
experimental evidence rela-

tive to, 94–95
fluid transfer channels in, 87–92
hypotonic saliva as result of transepithelial countercurrent mechanism in, 92–94
observations related to, 100–101
vascular events in, 87, 88
secretory, functions of, 136
transfer channels, evidence for, 97–99
paracellular, 87–88, 90
transcellular, 87–88, 90
Fluor Protector, 393
Fluorapatite, 197, 447
cariostatic benefit of, 454
formation of, acid etching and, 453
fluoride ions in, 453
and hydroxyapatite, calcium triangles of, compared, 200–201, 201t
Fluoridation, systemic, methods for, 452–453
of water supply, 335, 445
benefits of, major studies of, 450–451, 451t
controlled 450–453
early studies influencing, 449
economics of, 451–452
epidemiologic surveys in, 449–450, 450t
fluoride levels for, adjustment of, 451
optimal, 450, 450
fluorosis index for, 450
safety of, 448
substitutes for, 452–543
world-wide implementation of, 451
Fluoride(s), acidulated phosphate, 454–455
acidulated sodium, 453
and phosphate ion, for topical application, 453–454
antibacterial properties of, 405, 405
anticaries mechanisms of, 446–448
antimicrobial activity of, 447–448
biologic properties of, 446–449
and bis biguanide, in combination therapy, 406–407
cariogenic priming for, 454
cariogenicity of S. mutans and, 307, 306
cariostatic effects of, 328–329, 353, 405–406, 432, 438, 406
clinical and laboratory investigations of, 405–406
in dentifrices, 453, 457
effectiveness of, 392
dentin, 253
in dentistry, 445–460
dietary, and caries, 346
effects of, as factors influencing anticaries effect, 407
early studies of, 449
on pellicle formation, 329

Fluoride(s) (*continued*)
  enamel, 249
    caries susceptibility and, 203–204, 310–311
  in enamel remineralization, 447
  and enolase, 329
  gel(s), acidulated phosphate, topical, effect of, on *S. mutans*, 394, *406*
    in trays, application of, 455–456
      problems associated with, 456
      for radiation therapy patients, 458
  for home use, prescriptions for, 449
  ingested, metabolic fate of, 446
  intake and exposure, as factors in caries process, 223
  ion, action of, in topical fluoride, 453
    remineralization of enamel and, 253
  in ionic pools, 430
  laminates, 393, *393*
  microencapsulation of, 393, *393*
  mouthrinses, 440
  mouthwashes, chronic fluoride overdose associated with, 456
    effectiveness of, 456
    prescriptions for, 449
    in school programs, 457
  natural sources of, 446
  near enamel surface, white spot enamel lesions and, 237
  pellicle and, questions concerning, 164–165
  and phosphates, in combination therapy, 410
  in plaque, 142, 319
    bacteria and, 329
    calcium and, 142
  in prophylactic pastes, 457
  and remineralization, 430
  salivary, 139–141
  solutions, application of, 455
  stannous, 453
    concentrated solutions of, 455
    disadvantages of, 455
    in remineralization of carious dentin, 256
    stannous ion in, 454
  Streptococcus mutans and, 406, *406*
  substitution, in hydroxy columns of hydroxyapatite, 200–202, 206, *201*
  tablets, disadvantages of, 452
    for patients from areas of suboptimal water fluoridation, 452–453
    prescriptions for, 449
  topical, 453–458, 459
    application of, concentrated solutions for, 454–455
    frequency of, 454
    methods of, 455–458
    effect of, discovery of, 453
    mechanisms of action of, 453–454

  sealant application as adjunct to, 475–476
  toxicosis, acute, 448–449
    treatment of, 449
    chronic, 448
  trays, types of, 456
  treatment, multiple, 457–458
    occlusal surfaces in, 461
    special methods of, 458
  in varnishes, 393–394
Fluorine, properties of, 446
Fluorosis, in high fluoride content of water, studies of, 449
  index, 450
  skeletal, 448
Fones brushing technique, 491
Food(s), additives, phosphates as, 409–410
  cariogenicity of, effects of food processing on, 361
  chemical composition of, enamel remineralization and, 350
  and ecology of oral microorganisms, 289
  exchange lists, 378
  fortification, processing and organoleptic properties of, 360–361
  with anticaries agents, 328
  four groups of, in dietary education, 368
    in nutritional counseling of children, 377–378
  intake, behavioral aspects of, 376–377
  intake patterns, modification of, 361–362
  local effects of, on oral cavity, 343, 350
  oral fluids, and plaque, interrelationships of, *316*
  residue time of, in oral cavity, 327
  selection, preference for sweet in, 360
Food debris, instruction of patients concerning, 150
  removal of, 150
Formic acid, in plaque, 325
Fructan, 319–320, 324, *320*
Fructosyl transferase, 324, 352–353

Gallbladder, junctional channel of, 98
Gap junctions, direct generation of hypotonic fluid through, evidence for, 101–102
  "fractured," freeze-fracture studies on, 102
Geography, United States, caries incidence related to, 217
Gingiva, keratinization of, brushing and, 485–486
  recession of, causes of, 486, 487
    dentin abrasion in, 487
    oral hygiene habits related to, 486–487
Gingival crevice, as ecosystem of oral microbiota, 269–270

  fluid, whole saliva, and plaque components, compared, 318t
Gingival flap, management of, in sealant procedure, 477
Gingival fluid, 351
  mixed saliva, and aqueous phase of plaque, compared, 317, 318t
Gingivitis, age of plaque and, 492, 493
  microflora in, 270
  plaque and, 263, 388
Gland(s). *See also Specific types of glands*
  anatomic classification of, 5–7
  classification of, according to ducts, 5
    according to mode of action, 5
    according to nature of secretion, 5–6
  salivary. *See Salivary glands*
Glass ionomer cements, 470
Glucan(s), as polymer in plaque, 324
  in cell adhesion and plaque formation, 324
  extracellular, formation of, by cariogenic organisms, 309, *310*
  plaque formation by *S. mutans* and, 283
  synthesis, from plaque streptococci, 319, *319*
Glucose, in experimental pellicles, 161
Glucosyl transferase(s), 323, 324, *319*
  caries vaccines against, 413
  characteristics of, 352–353
  and glucans, 324
Glycolysis, plaque bacteria and, 325–326
Glycoprotein(s), carbohydrates in, dissociation of, 286–287
  salivary, in bacterial adherence, between dissimilar species, 281
    between similar species, *281*
    to epithelial cell, 282
  reactions of, with bacteria, 121, 292
  in salivary aggregation of bacteria, 280
  structure of, 74
  synthesis, in salivary gland cells, 74–75
Glycosaminoglycan(s), of cartilage proteoglycans, 179
  -protein linkage, in proteoglycans, 181–182, *181*
  structure of, 179, *180*
  types of, 179–181, 180t
GMP, cyclic, protein secretion and, 82
Gnotobiotes, 508
Golgi apparatus, of serous acinar cells, 9
Gustin, function of, 114, 119–120
  levels, caries and, 142
  taste and, 141–142, 144
  zinc content of, 114–115

Hamster, in caries research, 506–507, *507*

Hemin, in oral cavity, 286

Heparan sulfate, 181, 180t, *180*

Heparin, distribution of, 181
  structure of, 181

Hexafluorzirconate, stannous, 453

Hibitane. *See Chlorhexidine*

Histidine, salivary proteins containing, 119–120

Holocrine glands, 5

Hopewell House study, 358

Host defense(s), and cariogenicity, 309–311
  malnutrition and, 349–350

Host factors, as influence on caries development, 219–223

Host resistance, optimal, maintenance of, 359–360

Humans; as experimental subjects, advantages of, 500
  drawbacks of, 500
  in epidemiologic studies, 500–503
  in intraoral caries studies, 503–504
  legal and ethical requirements for protection of, 504–505, *505*

Hunter, John, studies of calcification by, 420

Hyaluronic acid, 179, 180t, *180*

Hydrogen bonds, in fluoride-substituted apatites, 201–202, *201*

Hydrogen ion concentration. *See* pH

Hydroxyallysine, in cross linking of collagen, 176, *176*

Hydroxyapatite, activity product of, 425
  calcium triangles of, 199–200, 201, *201*, 201t
  calcium-phosphorus ratio of, 426
  composition of, 197
  crystal, dissolution of, effect of pH on, 422
  crystal structure of, 197, 206, *199*
  dissolution of, resistance to, ionic strength and, 425
  in enamel, 249
  equilibrium of two forces in, 421
  and fluorapatite, 447
  heteroionic exchange of, 430
  hydroxy groups of, columnar arrangement of, 199–200, *199*, *200*
  incorporation of fluoride into, 200–202, 206, *201*
  pellicle and, 164

Hydroxylysine, in cross linking of collagen, 176, *176*

Hypogeusia, zinc levels in, 144

IgA, secretory, 123–124, 333–334
  antibodies, Peyer's Patches and, 335
  binding to mucosal cells, 125–126
  biologic function of, 334
  booster response to microorganisms, 127
  in direct agglutination of bacteria, 125, 291
  in immunity to caries, 337–338, 412
  output of, in response to infection, 126
  in saliva, 291
  structure of, 334

IgG, salivary, 124

IgM, salivary, 124

Immune reactions, T- and B-cells in, 335

Immune response, secretory, 125–126

Immunity, cellular, caries and, 349
  gut-associated lymphoid tissues in, 335
  humoral, caries and, 349
  local vs. systemic, demonstration of, 333
  non-specific, caries and, 349

Immunization, active, against caries, animal studies of, 336–337
  human studies of, 337
  significance of, 335–336

Immunocompetence, nutrition and, 349–350

Immunoglobulins, and antibodies, in secretions, 333–334
  classes, 333. *See also Specific immunoglobulins*
  heterogeneity of, demonstration of, 333
  in pellicle, 314
  in plaque, 317, 318t
  salivary, 54, 123–124, 127
    in inhibition of oral microbiota, 291
  structure of, 333, 334

Index, caries, 216, 500–501, 502–503
  advantages of, 501
  for animal model, caries-scoring sheet for, 511, *511*
    technique for, 510–511
  for children, 501
  factors limiting validity of, 501
  and sucrose intake, in males and in females, compared, 356, *356*

Infection(s), as noxious stimulus to local tissues and nerves within mucosa, 126
  bacterial, management of, prior to discovery of sulfa drugs and penicillin, 397–398
  induction of antibodies of secretory system and systemic immune system in, 126
  microbial, responsible for dentin caries, fate of, 256
  neonatal, hypoplastic developmental defects in, 346, *347*

Informed consent form, contents of, 504–505, *505*

Intercalated ducts, of parotid gland, 20–21, 28–30, *22*, *23*, *31*, *32*

of salivary glands, 14, *8*, *9*
  anatomic features of, 68
  palatine, 51, 53
  submandibular, 41

Intralobular ducts, of salivary glands, 14–16, *8*, *9*, *16*

Intraoral caries methods, in caries experimentation, 433–438, 503–504, *435*, *436*, *437*, *438*, *504*

Intraoral Cariogenicity Test, 503–504, *504*
  in study of demineralization-remineralization reaction, 433–438, *435*, *436*, *437*, *438*

Invertebrates, salivary glands in, 4

Iodine, antimicrobial properties of, 408
  bactericidal effectiveness of, 407–408
  chemical characteristics of, 408
  clinical and laboratory investigations using, 408–409
  early uses of, 407
  intraoral usage of, 407
  salivary, 141
  Streptococcus mutans and, 408

Ionic strength, calculation of, 425

Iron, deficiency, in sucrose diet, caries and, 346–348
  levels, related to caries, 143
  in oral cavity, lactoferrin and, 123
  in saliva, 141

Isolator, germ-free, 508, *508*

Isoproterenol, effects of, on parotid gland, 81
  ultrastructural changes in parotid gland caused by, *78*

Kanamycin, effect of, on bacteria on precarious and sound enamel surfaces, 400, *401*
  mode of action of, 400
  molecular configuration of, *400*

Keratan sulfate, 179, 180–181, 180t, *180*

Kidney, and salivary glands, cytologic features of cells of, compared, 100

Koch, R., caries and, 300, 301

Laboratory procedures, in caries research. *See* Experimentation, caries

Laboratory tests, in nutritional analysis, 369–374, 376, 374t

Lactate dehydrogenase, defective strain, replacement of S. *mutans* with, 414

Lactic acid, caries and, 352, *352*
  in plaque, 325

Lactobacilli, adherence to tooth surfaces, 397
  characteristics of, 321
  locations of, 321
  on tooth surface, 321

Lactobacillus, in caries, 301, 305–307, 397, 301t, *306*
 deep dentin, 307, *308*
Lactoferrin, antimicrobial activity of, 126, 291
 description of, 120, 123, 291
 functions of, 120, 123
Lactoperoxidase, antimicrobial activity of, 126, 143
 functions of, 115, 120, 122–123
 hydrogen peroxide and thiocyanate, in anti-lactobacillus system, 291
Laminates, fluoride, 393, *393*
Lathyrism, production of, in collagen studies, 177
Lectins, in inhibition of bacterial salivary aggregation, 280
 salivary, 320
Leukocytes, salivary, 292
Levan, 319–320, 324, *320*
Ligament, periodontal, 187
Lipases, functions of, 123
Lipids, in plaque, 318
Lipoteichoic acid lattice, peptidoglycan and, 123
Lithium, cariostatic effect of, 410
Local immunity vs. systemic immunity, demonstration of, 333
Ludwig, Carl Von, studies of salivary secretion by, 66–67
Lymphocytes, T- and B-, and subclasses, demonstration of, 334–335
Lymphoid tissues, gut-associated, in immunity, 335
Lysine, in cross linking of collagen, 176, *176*
Lysosomes, membrane material for resynthesis and, 77, *73*
Lysozyme(s), antimicrobial activity of, 126, 127, 291
 distribution of, 291
 functions of, 115, 123, 291
 sources of, 123

Magitot, Emil, caries and, 213
Magnesium, salivary, 141
Malnutrition, developmental, immunocompetence and, 329–350
 in elderly, pathophysiological problems resulting from or contributing to, 383t
 host defense decrease in, 349–350
 hypoplastic developmental defects in, 346, *347*
Mammals, salivary glands of, 4, *5*
Materia alba, definition of, 150–151
 and plaque, compared, 151
Mechanoreceptors, in salivary secretion, 66
Medical history, factors in, suggestive of nutritional problems, 367t
 in nutritional analysis, 366
Medulla, salivary center of, 71–72
Merocrine glands, 5

Metabolism tests, in nutritional analysis, 376, 374t
Methacholine, in studies of secretion, 85
Methacrylate(s), application and curing of, 469
 and isobutyl cyanoacrylate, bond strengths of, compared, 472, 472t
 molecular structure of, 468
 types of, 468, *479*
Methyl methacrylate, and Bis-GMA, 464
 molecular structure of, *468*
 powdered, and methyl-α-cyano-acrylate, *464*
Microbial succession, allogenic, 270
 autogenic, 270
 during development of coronal plaque, 270, *271*
 definition of, 279
 of oral flora, 270–276
Microbiologic sampling, as epidemiologic study, 503
Microbiota, crevicular, 269–270
 oral, 263
 composition of, 264–270
 ecologic determinants of, 278–296
 adherence factors as, 280–285
 inhibitory factors in, 290–294
 nutritional factors as, 285–290
 physical factors as, 279–280
 sets of factors as, 279
 ecosystem(s) of, 264–265
 coronal plaque as, 268–269
 determination of composition of, isolation and culture procedures in, 266
 methods of expressing results following, 266–267
 preservation and dispersion methods for, 266
 problems in, 265–267
 sample collection in, 265–266
 development of, 272–276, *272, 273, 274, 275, 276*
 gingival crevice as, 269–270
 microbial, 264
 primary, 267–270
 types and distribution of cultivable bacteria in, 267, 268t
 saliva as, 270
 tongue as, 267–268
 effects of environmental changes on, 294–295
 major habitats of, 264–265
 distribution of bacterial types in, 265, *264*
 oxidation-reduction potentials of, 279–280
Microcapsules, polymer-coated, in caries treatment, 393, *393*
Microflora, oral, characteristics of, of ecological significance, 285t
 distribution of, availability of

nutrients influencing, 286
 elimination of, as goal in early caries management, 387
 nutrient requirements of, 285
 nutrition of, 285–290. *See also* Nutrient(s)
Microhardness test, in demineralization-remineralization studies, Kentron Microhardness Tester in, 434, 436
 technique of, 434, 436, 437
Microorganisms, oral, amensalism of, 292
 antagonistic interactions of, 292
 barriers to, host-associated, 291
 host-derived, 290–291
 cariogenic, acid-producing ability of, 309
 aciduric potential of, 309
 ecology of, 311
 formation of extracellular glucans from sucrose by, 309, *310*
 formation and utilization of polysaccharides by, 309
 types of, in animal studies, 301–302, 301t, *302*
 virulence of, 308–311
 in carious dentin, 307, *308*
 in dental caries, early claims of, 300
 habitat sites for, 314
Micropuncture studies, during pilocarpine-stimulated acinar secretion, 101
 of salivary glands, 85–87
Microradiography, in caries detection, 512
Milk, containing fluoride, 452
Miller, W. D., caries and, 213, 299–300, 332–333, 387
Mineral(s), apatites, 420
 bone-tooth, lability of, 428–430
 exchange, enamel in, 350
 in soft and hard tissues, differences between, 420
 trace, relationship of, to caries, 346, 346t
Mineralization, biologic. *See also* Calcification
 definition of, 420
 dynamics of, applied to caries, 419–444
 dysfunction in, in caries and periodontal disease, 421
Miraculin, 328
Mixed glands, 6
Morquio's disease, 180
Mouth, artificial, in caries research, drawback of, 512
 history of, 511–512
 in vivo–in vitro technique of, 512. *See also* Cariogenicity test, intraoral
Mouthrinses, convenience of, 391
 disadvantages of, 391–392
 fluoride, 440
Mouthwashes, fluoride, 456–457
 prescriptions for, 449

Mucin(s), definition of, 13
  reactions of, with bacteria, 121
  and salivary precipitates, 115–116
  secretion of, by salivary glands, 47, 115
Mucoproteins, high molecular weight viscous, 114
Mucous glands, 6
Mucous secretion, as defense mechanism against oral microbiota, 293
Mucous secretory cells, palatine, of salivary glands, 51, 52–54, 51, 52, 53, 55, 56, 57, 58, 59, 60
Mutan(s), 319 319
Myoepithelial cells, of parotid gland, 20, 28, 21, 22, 23, 30
  of salivary glands, 14, 8, 12, 15
  sympathetic effects on, 70–71

Nasmyth, Alexander, discovery of pellicle by, 152
Nationality, caries incidence related to, 217, 217
Nerve(s), in activation of fluid secretory cells, effects of, 100
  of salivary glands, 69–70
Nervous system, autonomic, effects of, on ancinar and ductal cells, 71–72
  in salivary secretion, 66
  and secretory cells of salivary glands, 70
  sympathetic, effects of, on myoepithelial cells, 70–71
    on vasculature of salivary glands, 70
Nitrite, salivary, cancers and, 144
Nitrogen, requirements, of oral microflora, 285
Nitrosamine, formation, in saliva, 144
NRRL 1768, in plaque control, 412
Nutrient(s), endogenous, amino acids as, 287
  carbohydrates as, 286–287
  peptides as, 287
  proteins as, 287–289
  sources of, 286
    essential, lacking ecological significance, 286
  exogenous, carbohydrates as, 289–290
  proteins and fats as, 290
  sources of, 289–290
  requirements, of oral microflora, 285–286
Nutrition, in caries, 343–365
  counseling, 376–382
    for adults, 378
      application of principles of behavioral modification in, 377
    behavioral aspects of food intake and, 376–377
    "caveats" associated with, 376
    for children, 377–378, 379, 380
    for elderly, 377, 382

    personalized approach in, 377–378
    in preventive dentistry program, 379–381, 381
    special problems in, 382, 382t
    team approach in, 378–379, 378
  developmental aspects of, and caries, 344–350
  education, need for, 362
  effects of, on disease, in extreme cases, 349, 349
    on enamel maturation, 350
    on oral fluids, 351
    and immunocompetence, 349–350
    in modification of caries, prospects for, 359–362
    of oral microflora, 285–290
    post-eruptive effects of, on caries process, 350–353
    problems of, alterations in salivary gland composition and function associated with, 348–349
    alterations in tooth alignment associated with, 348
    alterations in tooth development associated with, 346–348
  research, challange for, 362
Nutritional analysis, 366–376
  problems to confront in, 366
  triphasic, 366–376, 384
    clinical dietary trials in, 374
    clinical examination in, 367–368, 368t
    laboratory tests in, 369–374
    medical and social history in, 366–367, 367t
    metabolic function tests in, 375–376, 374t
    qualitative dietary analysis in, 368–369
    semi-quantitative dietary analysis in, 369, 370–373
    tabulation of data gathered during, 376, 375
Nuva-Seal, 464

Octacalcium phosphate, in enamel, 249
Odontoblast(s), formation of dentin by, 185–187, 239
  structure and location of, 185, 239, 186, 234
"Oral bioassay," 367–368
Oral flora, acquisition of, 271–272
  composition and ecology of, 263–277
  microbial succession of, 270–276
Oral fluids. See Fluid(s) and Specific sources of fluids
Oral health, programs, impact of remineralization on, 400–441
  salivary proteins and, 113–131
Oral mucosa, cells of, antibody binding to, 125–126

Oral tissues, differential growth patterns of, 344, 345
Organogenesis, "critical periods" during, 344–346, 345
Orthodontic patient, fluoride therapy for, 458
Osmolality, and four major osmolytes, 132–136
Osmolytes, four major, osmolality and, 132–136
Oxidation-reduction potentials, of oral microbiota, 279–280

Pain, dental caries and, 212
Pancreas, exocrine, morphologic characteristics of, 20t
  secretory processes in, gastrointestinal hormones in demonstration of, 72
Pancreozymin-CCK, pancreatic secretion and, 72
Parmly, L. S., caries and, 213
Parotid duct, 18–19
Parotid gland, acini of, 19–20, 23–28, 19, 21, 22, 26, 27, 28, 29
  apical zone of, 23, 24–27, 27, 28, 29
  basal region of, 23–24, 26, 27
  intercellular attachments of, 27–28, 27, 28, 29
  microfilaments and microtubules of, 27, 29
    in protein secretion, 76–77
  mitochondria of, 27, 26
  collagenous fibers of, 22
  concentrations of major electrolytes in, over range of flow rate, 133, 134
  excretory ducts of, 21–22, 32, 24, 25, 41, 42
  gross features of, 18–19
  innervation of, 19
  intercalated ducts of, 20–21, 28–30, 22, 23, 31, 32
  light microscopy of, 19–23, 19, 21, 22, 23, 24
  location of, 4, 7, 18
  in mammals, 5
  morphologic characteristics of, 20t
  myoepithelial cells of, 20, 28, 21, 22, 23, 30
  parenchymal elements of, 19–22, 8
    innervation of, 32–34
  secretory tubules of, anatomic features of, 69
  striated ducts of, 21, 30–32, 24, 33, 35, 36, 37
  stroma of, 22–23, 19, 23, 24
  ultrastructure of, 23–34
  veins and arteries of, 19
PAS reaction, mucous secretions of salivary glands and, 17–18, 17, 18
  serous secretions of salivary glands and, 16–17, 17
Pastes, prophylactic, fluoridated, 457

Pasteur, L., caries and, 213, 300
Pellicle(s), acquired, 152–165, 272, 314
    attachment of organisms to, in adherence situations 281
    and chlorhexidine, 403, 403
    composition and origin of, 316–317
    and overlying plaque, relationship of, 154
    amorphous, 154
    as lubricating medium, 164
    bacteria formation and, 159, 164, 314, 315
    definition of, 152
    experimental, amino acid composition of, compared, 158–159, 161–163, 158, 163
        bacteria and, 159
        carbohydrate composition of, compared, 159, 163, 160, 161, 163
        carbohydrates of, 159, 163, 316, 160, 161, 163
        composition of, and saliva of formation, compared, 159–161, 160, 161, 162
        model system(s) for, in situ, 161–164, 162
        in vitro, 157–158, 158
        in vivo, 157, 157
        morphologic and compositional studies of, 157
        pellicle formation in, 159, 161
        protein of, 161
    fluoride and, questions concerning, 164–165
    formation, 164
        fluoride and, 329
        following tooth brushing, 117–118
        water permeation and, 137
    function of, 164–165
    immunologically categorized proteins in, 314
    mineralization of, 165
    natural, 152–157
        carbohydrates of, 156
        chemical composition of, analysis of, amino acid, 155–156, 156, 157
            conclusions from, 156–157
            methods in, 155
        contributors to, 154
        protective function of, 164
        scalloped border, 154, 155
        stained, 152–153
        structureless character of, 152, 152
        subsurface, 153–154, 153, 154
        thin organic surface, 153, 153
Penicillin(s), and analogues, in plaque control, 398–399
    antibacterial action of, 398
    in caries prevention, 389, 390, 394
    systemically administered, 398–399
    topically applied, 398
Penicillium funiculosum, enzymes

produced by, in plaque control, 411, 412
Pepsin, in collagen studies, 177–178
Peptides, salivary, as growth substrates for oral microflora, 287
Peptidoglycan, and lipoteichoic acid lattice, 123
    and lysozymes, 123
Periodic acid Schiff reaction, mucous secretions of salivary glands and, 17–18, 17, 18
    serous secretions of salivary glands and, 16–17, 17
Periodontal disease, dysfunction in biologic mineralization in, 421
Periodontal ligament, 187
Periodontosis, gram negative organisms in, 270
Peyer's Patches, in immunity, 335
pH, critical, 139, 325
    effect of, on hydroxypapatite crystal dissolution, 422
    on ionic product, 421–423
    levels, at plaque-enamel interface, caries and, 215, 215
    oral, oral microbiota and, 279
    of plaque, factors influencing, 325, 326–327
    rise factor, 138, 327
    salivary, 138
Phenylephrine, ultrastructural changes in parotid gland caused by, 78
Phenylthiocarbamide, tasting of, 144
Phosphatase(s), acid, activity of, on enamel, 143
    secretory cycle and, 82
Phosphate(s), anions, three types of, 422
    as cariostatic agents, 328
    as food additives, 409–410
    as sugar substitutes, 361
    and calcium, in plaque, 318–319
        saliva and, 142
    cariostatic effects of, 409
    dental caries and, 213
    and fluoride, in combination therapy, 410
    ion, and acidulated sodium fluoride, for topical application, 453–454
    salivary, 138–139
    various types of, 409
        mechanism of action of, 409
        specific properties of, 409
Phosphoenol pyruvate, fluoride and, 405, 405
Phospholipids, in protein secretion, 81
Phosphoprotein(s), 114, 115, 117t
    as model for surface ion stabilization, 119
    charge-charge interactions of, 117–118
    dentin, 185
        dentin collagen, and skin collagen, amino acid composition of, 184t

detergent-like properties of, 117
    interaction of, with negative charges, 121
    phosphatase, caries process and, 213
    regulation of remineralization by, 118–119
Phosphoric acid, dissociation of, 421–422
    for enamel etching, 465–466
        depth of etch at various concentrations of, 467, 467t
Phosphorus, and calcium. See Calcium -phosphorus ratio
Physiologic brushing technique, 491
Pigs, miniature, in caries research, 507
Pits and fissures. See Tooth(Teeth), pits and fissures
Plaque(s), acid production, carbohydrate metabolism in, 325–326
    adhesion of bacteria to, 320–321
    age of, gingivitis and, 492, 493
    amino acids in, 287, 318
    aqueous phase of, 317
        mixed saliva, and gingival fluid, compared, 317, 318t
    bacteria, adhesion, agglutination, and colonization by, 324–325
        amino acid metabolism by, 326–327
        biochemical activities of, 323–329
        composition of, in health of oral tissues, 388
        control of, 388
        extracellular activities of, 323
        interactions of, 321
        intracellular activities of, 325–327
        polysaccharide formation by, 323–324
    bacterial, dietary substrates for, 352–353
    differences in composition of, 215, 321, 215
    biochemistry, 313–331
    calcium and phosphate in, 318–319
        saliva and, 142
    carbohydrates in, 319–320
    cariogenic potential of, ecologic factors influencing, 311
    collection, for studies of composition of oral microbial ecosystems, 265–266
    compartments of, 317
    components, whole saliva, and gingival crevice fluid, compared, 318t
    composition of, 151, 316, 329
        chemical, 317–323
        factors influencing, 321, 323
    control, antimicrobial agents for, 397–413
        for prevention of caries, 388
    coronal, as ecosystem of oral microbiota, 268–269
        development of, adherence sit-

uations in, 281, *281*
autogenic microbial succession during, 270, *271*
shifts in microbial composition during, over nine day period, 272, *272*
flora of, 268–269
limitation of, oral hygiene measures in, 293–294
structure of, extracellular polysaccharides in, 290
culture of, procedures in, for studies of composition of oral microbial ecosystems, 266
results of, methods of expressing, for studies of oral microbial ecosystems, 266–267
definitions of, 151, 214, 268
-dependent diseases, control of, 388
dispersion methods, for studies of composition of oral microbial ecosystems, 266
extracellular phase of, 317
flora, cultivable, variations of, on same tooth, 269, 269t
effects of environmental changes on, 294–295
fluid, 317
fluoride, 142, 319
bacteria and, 329
calcium and, 142
formation of, as natural process, 388
bacteria in, 272–276, 314, 315, *272, 273, 274, 275, 276, 315*
bacterial structures in, 314, *315*
and development of, important considerations in, 315–316
following tooth brushing, 118, 314
pellicle and, 314
salivary proteins and, 118
sites of, 314–315
stages in, 272–276
"free floating," 269
"gelatinous microbic," 263
and gingivitis, 263, 388
glycolysis and, 325–326
hypothesis, nonspecific, 395
specific, 394–395
identification of isolates of, for studies of composition of oral microbial ecosystems, 266
in initiation of caries, 214
inorganic components of, 318–319
interphases of, 314
interrelations of, with food and oral fluids, *316*
isolation of bacteria in, for studies of composition of oral microbial ecosystems, 266
lipids in, 318
and marginal gingivitis, 263
and materia alba, compared, 151
metabolism, copper and, 143
dietary carbohydrates and dietary patterns modifying, 327–328

factors modifying, 327–328
plaque thickness as factor in, 142
zinc and, 143
microbial components of, 320–323
morphogenesis, 314–316
one day, 273, *272, 274*
one-week, 275, *275*
microcolonies in, *151*
oral diseases influenced by, 313
organisms, turnover rate of, 395
pathogenic potential of, 151
and pellicle, amino acid composition of, compared, 156, *157*
pH of, factors influencing, 325, 326–327, 427
pit and fissure, flora of, 269
polysaccharides in, 319–320, 323–324
biologic significance of, 320
pooled, *S. mutans* in, 304
preservation, for studies of composition of oral microbial ecosystems, 266
proteins in, 287, 317–318, 318t
qualitative differences between, 394
quantity of, in oral disease, 394, 395
removal, frequency of brushing and, 492–493
toothbrush design and, 488–489
saliva and, 139, 317
saliva components influencing, 142
Streptococcus mutans in, 283, 301, 305–306, 311
structural features of, 315, 316, *315*
thickness, as factor in plaque metabolism, 142
three day, 275, *275*
three week, 275–276, *276*
trace elements in, 319
two day, 273, *273, 274*
and underlying pellicle, relationship of, 154
Plasma membranes, and secretory granules, fusion of, 75, 76, 81, 83
Polyglucan hydrolases, plaque formation and, 283
Polymers, synthesis of, bacterial adherence to plaque by, 283–284
Polysaccharide(s), bacterial, interaction of saliva with, 121
extracellular, adhesion due to, 283–284, *284*
formation of, by cariogenic organisms, 309, *310*
functions of, 325
in structure of coronal plaque, 290
formation, 323–324
and utilization of, by cariogenic organisms, 309
intracellular, in plaque, 320

plaque bacteria and, 326
in plaque, 319–320, 323–324
biologic significance of, 320
Polyurethanes, 464
Potassium, changes in concentration of, and osmolality, in parotid secretion, 133, *134*
channel, fluid transfer channel as, 98–99
concentration, at unstimulated flow rates, 135
and fluid secretion by salivary glands, 136
elevation of, at lowest flow rates, 135
during eating reflex secretion, 105, 106
permeability, fluid transfer and, 92
salivary, levels of, 145
secretion, rate of fluid production and, 135
and water secretion, sodium-potassium pump and, 100–101
Predentin, proteoglycans of, 185
transformation of, to dentin, 185, 186, 239
Preventive dentistry program, nutrition counseling in, 379–381, *381*
Primates, in caries research, 507
immunization of, against caries, 336–337
Procollagen, α-chains, posttranslational modifications of, 174, *175*
in collagen biosynthesis, 174, *173*
Proline, salivary proteins rich in, 116
Protease inhibitors, in mucosal secretions, 124
Protein(s), anti-caries effect of, 353
carboxyl-methylase, in exocytosis, 81
components, phosphorylation of, protein kinase catalyzing, 81
conjugated, 74
in connective tissues, 169–179
core, of proteoglycans, 182, *179, 182*
deficiency, alterations in salivary gland development associated with, 348
alterations in tooth development associated with, 348
neonatal, adult alteration of resistance to caries in, 349
of enamel, 187, 188
exogenous, oral microorganisms and, 290
-glycosaminoglycan linkage, in proteoglycans, 181–182, *181*
immunologically categorized, in pellicle, 314
link, in cartilage, 182
methyl acceptor, in parotid and in adrenal medulla, 81
packaging of. *See* Secretory granule(s)

Protein(s) (*continued*)
of pellicle, 161
phosphorylation, β-adrenergic receptor occupation to, se-
quence of events in, 79, 79
in plaque, 287, 317–318, 318t
salivary, 287, 117t, 286t
aggregation phenomenon of,
120–121
as mechanisms for defense,
124–127
attack on, by *S. mutans*, 288–
289
binding to microorganisms,
120–121
biochemical aspects of, 114–
115
biochemical considerations and
biologic significance of, 116–
124
classification of, 114–116
concentration of, measurement
of, 120
digestion of, 115
direct agglutination of bacteria
by, 125
histidine-rich, 120
immunological aspects of, 114–
115
modified, 124
and mucosal defense mechanisms, 124–127
nonenzymatic antimicrobial,
123–124
and oral health, 113–131
positively charged, 114
proline-rich, 116
acidic. *See* Phosphoproteins
quantitative analysis of, 120
rich in aromatic components,
119–120
separation of, 114, 115
total, altered levels of, in systemic disease, 144–145
tyrosine-rich, 119
well-studied, classification of,
125t
with antimicrobial activity, 126
secretion, in absence of secretory
granules, 77
cAMP as intracellular mediator
in, 79–80
cAMP concentration and, 80
background of, 72–74
by parotid acinar cell, after activation of protein kinase, 80,
81, 80
calcium and, 82–83, 84
conservation of secretory granules following, 77
dibutyryl cAMP and, 80
energy for, 67
events leading to, summary of,
83–84
important events in, 74, 75–77,
76
mechanisms of, in serous and
mucous salivary glands, 72–
74

microfilaments and microtubules in, 76–77
protein synthesis and, 74
role of β-adrenergic stimulation
in, 77–79
salivary glands in, 72–74
salivary secretion and, 65
secretory sympathetic activity
and, 70
secretory cycle, events in, 72–74
production of secretory granule
in, 74
protein synthesis in, 74
protein transport in, 74
secretory protein segregation
in, 74
terminal event in, 75–77
terminating of controlling of,
82
simple, 74
synthesis, and protein secretion,
74
secretory granule formation
and, 83
tooth, biochemistry of, 168–190
tyrosine-rich, 116
Protein kinase, and cAMP, 80, 79
calcium distribution and, 83
phosphorylation of protein catalyzed by, 80, 81, 80
phosphorylation of protein components catalyzed by, 81
protein inhibiting, 82
Proteoglycans, aggregation of, 182,
182
"bottle brush" model for, 179, 179
of connective tissues, 179–183
core protein of, 182, 179, 182
degradation of, in transformation
of predentin to dentin, 186
glycosaminoglycan-protein linkage
in, 181–182, 181
glycosaminoglycans in, disaccharide units of, 179–181,
180t
heterogenity of, 182
metabolism of, 183
microheterogeneity of, 182
molecular structure of, 179, 179
molecular weights of, 179
of predentin and dentin, 184–185
proteolytic enzymes and, 183
significance of, 183
Pseudomembrane, proline-rich proteins forming, 116
Pulp, and dentin, 238–239
passage of molecules between,
254
tissue fluid pressure in, 254
Pulp capping, indirect, controversy
concerning, 243
criteria to be met prior to, 243
philosophy of, 243
procedures in, 243
Pulpodentinal complex, 238–240,
244
Pyridoxine, anti-caries effect of, 353
Pyruvic acid, for enamel etching,
465

Radiation, effects of, on oral microflora, 295
Radioautography, in study of dentinogenesis, 185–186
Rat, albino, in caries research, 506,
507
Reflex(es), eating, and hemodynamic changes in glands, 96–
97
secretion stimulated by, mechanisms in, 103–106
mechanisms of fluid secretion
during, 90
and resting secretion, mechanisms in, compared, 104
oral, in salivary secretion, 66
Remineralization, of decayed tooth
surfaces, phosphoproteins in,
118–119
of enamel. *See* Enamel, remineralization
therapeutic, 440–441
Reptiles, salivary glands of, 4
Research, caries. *See* Experimentation, caries
Reticulum, rough endoplasmic, 74
in glycoprotein synthesis, 74–75
in protein synthesis, 74
Rodent(s), baby, intubation of, for
diet survey, 509, 509
bacteria-initiated caries in, types
of, 301–302, 301t, 302, 303
diet for, in diet survey, 508–509
experimental calciphylaxis of,
428, 428
gnotobiotic, 508
immunization of, against caries,
336
models, for caries research, 506–
507, 507
Rods, gram positive, at gingival
margin, 269
in coronal plaque, 268
Roll brushing technique, 489, 491

Salicylates, effects of, on parotid secretion, 97
Saliva. *See also* Fluid(s)
agglutination by, 121
agglutinins in, 120–122
and antibacterial agents, 391
antibacterial factors in, 291
as ecosystem of oral microbiota,
270
as host defense mechanism, 309–
310
as hypotonic fluid, 84–85
calcium and phosphate in, 138–
139
carbohydrate, amino acids and
protein in, 286t
components of, relation of, to
oral and gastric cancer, 144
composition, age as influence on,
141
as factor in caries process, 222
and caries, 142–143
and composition of experimen-

tal pellicle(s) formed in, compared, 159–161, *160, 161, 162*
diet as influence on, 141
micropuncture studies of, 86–87
sex as influence on, 141
and systemic disease, 144–145
and taste, 144
contamination, in sealant procedure, 476
and dental plaque, 139
diet-related factors influencing, 351
enzymes of. *See* Enzyme(s), salivary and *Specific enzymes*
flow, as defense mechanism against oral microbiota, 293
as factor in caries process, 222
reduction of, taste perception alterations in, 144
fluoride, urea, and ammonia in, 139–141
function(s) of, 54, 65, 114
nutrition and, 351
glandular, 115
human parotid, osmolarity of, 84
hypotonic, bathing oral mucosa, 136–137
physiologic purposes of, 145–146
result of transepithelial countercurrent mechanism, 92–94
hypotonicity of, and adjustment of osmolality of gastric contents after eating, 138
and low salt content of, taste and, 137–138
immunoglobulins in, 54, 291
interaction of, with bacterial polysaccharides, 121
lectins of, 320
lipolytic activity in, 123
magnesium, iodine, and thiocyanate in, 141
mixed, gingival fluid, and aqueous phase of plaque, compared, 317, 318t
neutralization of acid by, 138
osmolality, 145
osmolytes causing, 133
pH in, 138
and plaque concentrations of calcium and phosphate, 142
in plaque formation, 118
precipitates of, mucins and, 115–116
protease inhibitors in, 124
in remineralization of carious dentin, 255–256
resting, content of, 103
functions of, 103
secretion of, as eating reflex, 65, 145, 146
activation of, 103–105
events and responses in salivary glands during, 105
mechanisms in, 105–106
as product of metabolic activity of secretory cells, 67

as specific homeokinetic response of specialized organs, 65
biologic processes in, under neural control, 72
energetics of, 66–68
history of investigations of, 65
initial perspective on, 65–68
mechanisms of, 64–112
motor control of, 71–72
physiological, oral reflexes and nerve pathways in, 66
processes of, principal activities in, 67
resting, 65, 145
energy for, 103
mechanism of, 103
stimulation of, 103
and serum, selected constituents of, compared, 140t
tests of, for systemic monitoring in disease, 145
trace metals in, 141
type of, in parasympathetic stimulation of salivary glands, 72
in sympathetic stimulation of salivary glands, 72
urea in, 139, 351
studies of, in fluid secretion studies, 89–91
volume, minor salivary glands and, 47
whole, 115
aggregation bacteria in, 280–282
buffer capacity of, caries and, 142
cloudy appearance of, 116
plaque components, and gingival crevice fluid, compared, 318t
zinc in, 141–142
Salivary glands, acini of, 8–13, *8*
anatomic features of, 68, *68*
as site of fluid secretion transfer, 99–100
attachment mechanisms of, 13
autonomic effects on, 71–72
cellular composition of, 8–10, *9*
during protein secretion, 76
enzyme-mediated responses of, during eating reflex secretion, 105
intercellular tissue spaces between, 10–13, *12*
luminal surface of, 10, *11*
mucous, secretions of, 13, 17–18, *16, 17, 18*
structure of, 13
secretion by, pilocarpine-stimulated, 101
serous, secretions of, 13, 16–17, *16, 17*
structure of, 8–13, *8, 9, 11, 12*
surface morphology of, *9, 10, 11*
in animals, invertebrates and vertebrates, 4–5
as models for study, by biologists, 3

of glandular structure and function, 3–4, 54–60
blood flow of, and secretion, 66
buccal, 49
classification of, histochemical, 16–18
structural, 7
composition of, 5
concept of fluid transfer channels and, 91
definition of, 4
demilunes of, 14
development of, effects of nutrition on, 348–349
duct system of, importance of, 54
ductal cells of, autonomic effects on, 71–72
ducts of, transepithelial fluid transfer via gap junction in, 101–102
events and responses in, during eating reflex secretion, 105
extralobular ducts of, 16
functions of, 3, 5
consistency of diet and, 290
glossopalatine, 49–50
glycoprotein synthesis in, 74–75
hemodynamic changes in, during resting conditions and during reflex-stimulated secretion, 88
evidence for, 96–97
human, microanatomy of, 3–63
innervation of, 69–70
intercalated ducts of, anatomic features of, 68
intralobular ducts of, 14–16, *8, 9, 16*
and kidney, cytologic features of cells of, compared, 100
labial, 49, *49*
lingual, 50–51, *50*
major, 7, 18–47
morphologic characteristics of, 20t
microfilaments and microtubules of, in protein secretion, 76–77, 84
micropuncture studies of, 85–87
minor, 7, 47–54, *6*
distribution of, 47
function of, 47
structure of, 47–49
monostomatic, 7
mucous, protein secretory mechanisms in, 72
mucous secretions of, 13, 17–18, *16, 17, 18*
myoepithelial cells of, 14, *8, 12, 15*
sympathetic effects on, 70–71
palatine, intercalated ducts of, 51, 53
mucous secretory cells of, 51, 52–54, *51, 52, 53, 55, 56, 57, 58, 59, 60*
striated and excretory ducts of, 51, 53
stroma of, 51–52, 54
parenchymal cells of, neurotransmitter-mediated responses of,

Salivary glands, serous:
(*continued*)
    during eating reflex secretion, 105–106
    phylogenetic considerations in, 4–5
    polystomatic, 7–8
    position of, 4–5
    in protein secretion. *See* Protein, secretion
    secretion by, cAMP as intracellular mediator in, 79–80
    secretion of saliva by, 145
    mechanisms of, 65
    secretions of, osmolality of, 145
      osmotically active particles in, ions in, 145
    secretory cells of, patterns of innervation of, 69–70
      pharmacologic blocking of, 70
    secretory mechanisms of, electrolytes and, 136
    secretory parenchyma of, method of picturing, 67
    secretory tubules of, anatomic features of, 69
      as site of fluid secretion transfer, 100
    serous, protein secretory mechanisms in, 72
      of von Ebner, 50–51, *51*
    serous secretions of, 13, 16–17, *16, 17*
    slice systems, 79
    stimulation of, parasympathetic, secretion produced by, 72
      sympathetic, secretion produced by, 72
    striated ducts of, 14–16, 54, *9, 16*
      as secretory structures, 100
      cells of, during eating reflex secretion, 105–106
      during resting secretion, 103
    structural plan of, 7–16
    structure and innervation of, 68–72
    sublingual, gross and light microscopic features of, 44–47
      location of, 7
      minor, 49
      morphologic characteristics of, 20t
      ultrastructure of, 47
    submandibular, acini of, 40–41, 43
      excretory ducts of, 42–44, *46*
      gross and light microscopic features of, 34–38, *16, 17*
      intercalated ducts of, 41
      location of, 7
      morphologic characteristics of, 20t
      striated ducts of, 41–42, *44, 45*
      ultrastructure of, 38–44
    transepithelial resistance compared to junctional morphology in, need for studies of, 102
    tubules of, 13

vasculature of, elements of, 69
    sympathetic effects on, 70
Salivation. *See* Saliva, secretion of
Salt, table, containing fluoride, 452
Scleromyxederma, resembling experimental calciphylaxis, 428, 429
Sealant(s), adhesion of, to enamel, problems with, 464–468
    application, as adjunct to topical fluoride, 475–476
      basic steps in, 473
      clinical procedure for, 473–477, *474*
      drying procedure prior to, 474, 476
      etching procedure prior to, 473–474
      examination following, 475
      isolation for, 473
      problems associated with, 476–477
      selection of teeth for, 473
      techniques for, 474
    applicators, 475
    bond strength(s) of, compared, 472, 472t
      measurement of, 471
      device for, 471, *471*
    bonding, effective, factors influencing, 470
    chemically-cured, 469, 470, *469*
      and light-cured, effectiveness of, compared, 478, 478t
    clinical effectiveness of, evaluation of, 477–478, 478t
    contact angle of, 470, *471*
    effect of, on enamel maturation and caries, 478–479
    filled, 469
    historical use of, 463–464
    light-cured, 469, 470, *469*
      and chemically-cured, effectiveness of, compared, 478, 478t
    maintenance, continuance of, 475
    microleakage in, 472–473, *472*
    molecular structure of, 468–470
    physical and chemical properties of, 468–473
    physical properties and bonding, relationship between, 470–473
    pits and fissures, 461–481
    tensile strength of, 471
    viscosity, 470, *471*
      as factor in retention, 475
Sebaceous glands, 7, *6*
Secretin, pancreatic secretion and, 72
Secretory cycle, protein. *See* Protein, secretory cycle
Secretory granule(s), and condensing vacuoles, 74, 75
    conservation of, following secretion, 77
    formation of, protein synthesis and, 83
    timing of, 75
    in parotid gland, 73

    and plasma membranes, fusion of, 75, 76, 81, 83
    protein content of, 75
    resynthesis of, lysosomes in, 77, 73
    serous salivary glands and, 72
    size of, 75
    structure of, 75
Secretory pressures, high, experimental, source of, 96
Selenium, cariogenic effect of, 410
Seromucous glands, 6
Serous glands, 5–6
Sex, as factor in saliva composition, 141
    caries incidence related to, 217, *218*
Sialin, 138, 327
Sialography, 18–19
Simple glands, 6, 7, *6*
Simplicidentata, as models for caries research, 506, 507
Skeletal system, minerals and, 429
Smoking, iodine in saliva and, 141
    thiocyanate levels in, carcinogenesis and, 144
Social history, in nutritional analysis, 366–367
    in nutritional counseling, 377
Sodium, changes in concentration of, and osmolality, in parotid secretion, 133–134, *134*
    concentration, in parotid secretion, under resting conditions, 133
    extraction, aldosterone in, 138
    during eating reflex secretion, 106
    transport, in recent hypothesis of fluid secretion, 93
Sodium-potassium pump, potassium and water secretion associated with, 100–101
Sodium trimetaphosphate, as cariostatic agent, 328
Solubility product constant, of hydroxyapatite, 421
Sorbitol, in dietary regime, 328
    fermentation of, plaque acid and, 326
Spectographic techniques, in caries research, 512–513
Staphlococcus epidermidis, bacteriocins, S. mutans and, 293, 294
Starch(es), and plaque, 327
    in plaque metabolism, 323
Statherin, 116, 117, 119
    functions of, 119
    in maintenance of saliva supersaturated state and prevention of apatite dissolution, 139
    structure of, 119
Stillman brushing technique, 491
Streptococci, colonizing tooth surface, 321
    and extracellular polysaccharides, in development of plaque, 118
    in oral microbiota, 265, *264*
    on tongue, 267–268
Streptococcus, mitior, fuzzy surface coat of, 284

mutans, acid-producing ability of, 309

aciduric potential of, 309

adherence of, glucan-mediated, 283, *284*

adherence to tooth surfaces, 395

antigens in, and antigenic determinants of human heart muscle, 338

as "target" organism, 413

bacteriocins, 293, *294*

cariogenicity of, 303–304, *305*, 307

in animal studies, 301, 301t, *302*

characteristics as determinants of, 308–309

fluoride influencing, 307, *306*

colonization by, extraoral determinants of, 395–396

intraoral determinants of, 395

distinguishing characteristics of, 321

five biotypes of, 303, *304*

fluorides and, 406, *406*

formation of extracellular glucans from sucrose by, 309, *310*

formation and utilization of polysaccharides by, 309

iodine and, 408

long-term suppression of, 413

in mutan synthesis, 319, *319*

mutant effector strains of, replacement with, 414

in plaque, 283, 301, 305–306, 311

protein patterns of saliva supernatant and, 288–289, *288*

protein subfraction of, growth-promoting activity in, 288

recolonization by, aspects of organism limiting, 395

replacement of, with non-*S. mutans* antagonists, in caries control, 413–414

role and ecology of, in caries, 395–396

serotypes of, 321, 322t

adherence of, 321

growth of, 288, *288*

-*Streptococcus sanguis* ratio, 413–414

shift in, in caries control, 414

suppression of, vancomycin in, 399, 399t

transmission of, between adult humans, 396

vaccine against, rationale for directing, 336

salivarius, fuzzy surface coat of, *284*

sanguis, inhibitor interactions of, 321–323

in plaque formation, second stage, 273

-*Streptococcus mutans* ratio, 413–414

shift in, in caries control, 414

Striae of Retzius, of enamel, 232, 233–237, *234*, *236*

Striated ducts, of parotid gland, 21, 30–32, *24*, *33*, *35*, *36*, *37*

of salivary glands, 14–16, 54, *9*, *16*

anatomic features of, 69

as secretory structures, 100

cells of, during eating reflex secretion, 105–106

during resting secretion, 103

palatine, 51, 53

submandibular, 41–42, *44*, *45*

Strontium, cariostatic effect of, 410

Sublingual gland. *See* Salivary glands, sublingual

Submandibular gland. *See* Salivary glands, submandibular

Substrates, dietary, for bacterial plaque, 352–353

Sucrose, and cariogenicity, 309, 353, *310*

glucosyl transferase and, 352–353

metabolism, by-products of, in plaque, 304–305, *304*

plaque formation by *S. mutans* and, 283, 304–305

in plaque metabolism, 323–324

in smooth surface caries, 352

Sugar(s), alternatives to use of, 360, 361t

compounds tested as, 361

industrial research in, 360–361

contributions of, to organoleptic properties of foods, 360

conversion of, by enzyme systems of oral organisms, 290, 285t

in diet, influence of, on oral ecosystems, 289–290

effects of, on teeth, explained to child, 379

fermentable, and plaque, 327

in initiation of caries, 215–216, 299, *216*

and other substances, relative sweetness of, 361t

refined, estimated per capita consumption of, for selected periods, 355t

simple, cariogenesis by, 353

substitutes, fortification, processing and organoleptic properties of, 360–361

Sweeteners, noncaloric, under development, 328

Systemic immunity vs. local immunity, demonstration of, 333

Taste, hypotonicity and low salt content of saliva and, 137–138

impaired, conditions displaying, 144

saliva composition and, 144

T-cells, 334–335

Temperature, oral, oral microbiota and, 279

Template, in calcification, 427–428

Tetracyclines, in caries prevention, 389, 390, 394

Thiamin, caries-promoting effect of, 353

Thiocyanate, -mediated inhibitory systems, 291

salivary, 141

of smokers, 144

Thirst, during water deprivation, 138

Tin, absorption, by carious lesion, 455

in saliva, 141, 143

Tissue(s), calcification. *See* Calcification

connective. *See* Connective tissues

destruction, in caries, factors influencing, 226–227

mineralized, biological complexities of, 426–427

mineral phase of, variability of, 426

organic-mineral bonding in, 426

unattainable equilibrium of, 426–427

oral, differential growth patterns of, 344, *345*

soft and hard, minerals in, differences between, 420

of tooth, 183–188

Tongue, as ecosystem of oral microbiota, 267–268

Tooth(Teeth), accessibility of areas of, for chemotherapy, 391

albino rat, 506, *507*

alignment, effects of nutrition on, 348

poor, problems associated with, 348

anatomy of, as defensive factor, 310

brushing of. *See* Brushing

calcification of. *See* Calcification

cemental-dentinal lesions of, arrestment of, 440

cervical lesions of, clinical management of, 257

fate of, 257, *257*

cleaning, by food, 350

composition of, as factor in caries process, 222–223

crown, as ecosystem of oral microbiota, 268–269

crystals, ionic pools around, 429, *429*

decayed, missing, and filled. *See* DMF scale

defensive factors associated with, 310–311

development, alterations in, nutritional problems associated with, 346–348

interproximal lesions of, appearance of, 257–258

clinical management of, 257–258

consolidation of, 440

Tooth (Teeth) (*continued*)
  spontaneous arrestment of, 257, 258
  lingual lesions of, fluoride therapy in, 458
  minerals, lability of, 428–430
  morphology, as factor in caries process, 222
  occlusal surfaces of, caries of, as major dental problem, 461–463
    historical methods of resolving, 463
    method(s) of resolving, historical, 463
      sealants as. *See* Sealant(s)
  fissure morphology of, 462, *462*, *463*
  fissures of, carious attack in, *463*, *463*
  fluoride therapy and, 461
  pits and fissures, as caries susceptible areas, 218, *219*
    assessment of, for restoration, 440
    caries of, clinical management of, 256–257
    organisms colonizing, 321
    sealants, 461–481. *See also* Sealant(s)
  proteins, biochemistry of, 168–190
  pulverization of, in caries research, 513
  remineralization of, caries arrest in, 227
  root surfaces of, caries on, 219, *220*
  smooth surfaces of, caries on, 219, *220*
    assessment of, 440
  "soft," 349
  subsurface lesion of, development of, ionic diffusion as factor in, 422–423, *423*
  surface, decreasing of bacterial assault on, methods under evaluation of, 335
  tissues of, 183–188
  to be extracted, preextraction studies on, 503
Toothbrush(es), abrasive effects of, and of dentifrice, compared, 486
  automatic, 492
  design, effectiveness of, studies of, 488
    and function, 488–490
    interest in, 483
    "professional," 487
  durability, factors influencing, 493
  effectiveness of, patient factors influencing, 492–493
  evaluation of performance of, confusion in, 482–483
  filaments, density of, factors controlling, 489–490
    and plaque removal, 489

end-rounded, abrasion of tissues and, 487
  physical properties of, 483–485
  texture of, calculation of, 485
flat trim head, 488–489
hard, harmful effects of, 486
historic background of, 483
natural bristle, factors influencing quality of, 483
  properites of, 483–484
  splitting of tips of, 484, *484*
  wear of, 484–485
nylon, end-rounded, 487, *488*
  humidity and, 484, 485t
  introduction of, 483
  soft, 489
  texture of, control of, 485
  labelling of, 485
  types of, 484
  water uptake of, 484, *484*
  wear of, 485
serrated head, 488
straight-trimmed, 489
tufts in, number and spacing of, as factor in effectiveness, 489–490
wear characteristics of, 493
worn, plaque removal by, 493
Trace elements, in caries prevention, 410
  differences between studies of, 410–411
  in enamel, 249
  in plaque, 319
Trace metals, in saliva, 141
Trace minerals, relationship of, to caries, 346, 346t
Transferrin, 291
Transmethylation, role of, in exocytosis, 81
Tubule(s), of gland, definition of, 7
  of salivary glands, 13
Turku Sugar Studies, 358–359
Tyrosine, salivary proteins containing, 119–120

Urea, in gingival fluid, 351
  salivary, 139, 351
    plaque pH and, 326–327
    studies of, in fluid secretion studies, 89–91

Vaccine(s), and antimicrobial agents, in combination therapy, 415
  caries, against bacterial enzymes, 413
    development of, problems associated with, 412
    feasibility of, findings promoting, 338, 412
    possible side effects of, 338
  experiments, against *S. mutans*, rationale for, 336
    in animals, 336–337

immunologic principles of, 333–335
  significance of, in caries prevention, 335–336
  periodontal disease, chances for development of, 412–413
Vancomycin, in caries management and *S. mutans* suppression, 399, 399t
  characteristics of, 399
  prolonged use of, problems associated with, 399
Varnishes, antimicrobial agents in, 393–394
Veillonella, metabolic interaction of, 321
Vipeholm Dental Caries Study, 357–358, *357*
Virulence, definition of, 308
Vitamin(s), requirements, of oral microflora, 285
  of surgery patients, 383t
  supplementary, administration of, 383–384
Vitamin A deficiency, alterations in tooth development associated with, 346, *347*
Vitamin D deficiency, alterations in tooth development associated with, 346

Water. *See also* Fluid(s)
  deprivation, secretion during, 138
  extracellular, permeation of dental enamel by, 137
  fluoridation of. *See* Fluoridation, of water supply
  oral microbiota and, 279
  salivary, and electrolytes, and oral health, 132–147
  secretion, potassium link to, sodium-potassium pump and, 100–101

Xerostomia, and caries, 139, 222
  fluoride therapy in, 458
  radiation-induced, effects of, on oral microflora, 295, 305, *305*
X-ray diffraction, in caries research, 512
Xylitol, as cariostatic agent, 361
  benefits of, outlined in Turku Sugar Studies, 358
  future use of, 328
  plaque streptococci and, 326
  potential side effects of, 359

Zinc, antibacterial effects of, 410
  in oral tissues, variance in, 143
  in saliva, 141–142
    plaque production and, 143
  taste perception and, 144
Zymogen granules. *See* Secretory granules